CRITICAL CARE IMAGING

LAWRENCE R. GOODMAN, M.D.

Professor of Diagnostic Radiology and
Director of Pulmonary Radiology
Medical College of Wisconsin
Milwaukee County Medical Complex
Froedtert Memorial Lutheran Hospital
Veterans Administration Medical Center
Milwaukee, Wisconsin

CHARLES E. PUTMAN, M.D.

James B. Duke Professor of Radiology and
Professor of Medicine
Duke University School of Medicine
Executive Vice President for Administration
Duke University Medical Center
Durham, North Carolina

CRITICAL CARE IMAGING

THIRD EDITION

W.B. SAUNDERS COMPANY
Harcourt Brace Jovanovich, Inc.
Philadelphia   London   Toronto   Montreal   Sydney   Tokyo

W. B. SAUNDERS COMPANY
Harcourt Brace Jovanovich, Inc.

The Curtis Center
Independence Square West
Philadelphia, Pennsylvania 19106

Library of Congress Cataloging-in-Publication Data

Critical care imaging / edited by Lawrence R. Goodman,
Charles E. Putman.—3rd ed.
    p. cm.

Rev. ed. of: Intensive care radiology. 2nd ed. 1983.

Includes bibliographical references and index.

ISBN 0–7216–3449–4

1. Critical care medicine.   2. Diagnosis, Radioscopic.
3. Critically ill.   I. Goodman, Lawrence R.
(Lawrence Roger)   II. Putman, Charles E.
(Charles Edgar)   III. Title: Intensive care radiology.

[DNLM: 1. Critical Care.   2. Emergencies.
3. Intensive Care Units.   4. Radiography.
WX 218 C9338]

RC86.7.C72   1992

616.07′57—dc20

DNLM/DLC   91–16760

Editor: Lisette Bralow
Designer: Karen O'Keefe
Production Manager: Bill Preston
Manuscript Editors: Jody Murphy
Illustration Coordinator: Walt Verbitski
Indexer: Peter Pelogitis
Cover Designer: Megan Costello

CRITICAL CARE IMAGING   ISBN   0–7216–3449–4

Printed in the United States of America.

Last digit is the print number: 9   8   7   6   5   4   3   2   1

CONTRIBUTORS

Michael A. Bettmann, M.D.
Professor of Radiology, Boston University School of Medicine; Chief of Cardiovascular Imaging, University Hospital, Boston, Massachusetts.
Systemic Effects of Radiologic Procedures

Janice Bitetti, M.D.
Assistant Professor of Anesthesiology, George Washington University School of Medicine and Health Sciences; Co-director, Intensive Care Unit, George Washington University Hospital, Washington, D.C.
A Clinician's Perspective of Critical Care Imaging

Roger C. Bone, M.D.
Professor and Chairman of Internal Medicine, Rush Medical College of Rush University; Rush-Presbyterian-St. Luke's Medical Center, Chicago, Illinois.
Adult Respiratory Distress Syndrome: Clinical Perspective

Jeffrey C. Brandon, M.D.
Assistant Professor of Radiology, University of California, Irvine, College of Medicine; University of California, Irvine, Medical Center, Orange, California.
Acute Gastrointestinal Disorders

Frank Casty, M.D.
Fellow, Pulmonary Medicine and Critical Care, University of Vermont College of Medicine, Burlington, Vermont.
Adult Respiratory Distress Syndrome: Clinical Perspective

Caroline Chiles, M.D.
Associate Professor of Radiology, Virginia Commonwealth University Medical College of Virginia, School of Medicine, Richmond, Virginia.
Acute Thoracic Trauma

Dewey J. Conces, Jr., M.D.
Associate Professor of Radiology, Indiana University School of Medicine; Indiana University Hospital, Indianapolis, Indiana.
The Immunocompromised Patient

N. Reed Dunnick, M.D.
Professor of Radiology, Duke University School of Medicine; Director, Imaging Division, Duke University Hospital, Durham, North Carolina.
Acute Genitourinary Disease

Lawrence R. Goodman, M.D.
Professor of Diagnostic Radiology, and Director of Pulmonary Radiology, Medical College of Wisconsin; Milwaukee County Medical Complex, Froedtert Memorial Lutheran Hospital, Veterans Administration Medical Center, Milwaukee, Wisconsin.
A Radiologist's Perspective of Critical Care Imaging
Pulmonary Support and Monitoring Apparatus
Acute Inflammatory Disease
Imaging After Thoracotomy
Imaging After Cardiac Surgery

Virgil B. Graves, M.D.
Professor of Radiology and Neurosurgery, University of Wisconsin Medical School; University of Wisconsin Hospital and Clinical Science Center, Madison, Wisconsin.
Imaging Evaluation of Acute Neurologic Disease

Jud W. Gurney, M.D.
Assistant Professor of Radiology, University of Nebraska College of Medicine; University Hospital—University of Nebraska, Omaha, Nebraska.
Pulmonary Embolism

David L. Harshfield, M.D.
Assistant Professor, Department of Radiology, University of Arkansas for Medical Sciences; Chief of Radiology, John L. McClellan Memorial Veterans Hospital, Little Rock, Arkansas.
Acute Gastrointestinal Disorders

Roberta L. Itzkoff, M.D.
Assistant Professor, University of Arkansas for Medical Sciences; University Hospital of Arkansas and John L. McClellan Memorial Veterans Hospital, Little Rock, Arkansas.
Acute Gastrointestinal Disorders

R. Brooke Jeffrey, Jr., M.D.
Professor of Radiology, Stanford University School of Medicine; Chief of Abdominal Imaging, Stanford University Hospital, Stanford, California.
Acute Hepatobiliary and Pancreatic Disease

Elliot O. Lipchik, M.D.
Professor of Radiology, Medical College of Wisconsin; Chief of Angio-Interventional Section, Milwaukee County Medical Complex, Milwaukee, Wisconsin.
Acute Aortic Disease and Peripheral Venous Disease

Barbara L. McComb, M.D.
Assistant Professor of Radiology, Jefferson Medical College of Thomas Jefferson University, Philadelphia, Pennsylvania.
Pericardial Disease

Richard McKenzie, M.D.
Clinical Instructor, University of California, Irvine, College of Medicine; Fellow, Angio and Interventional Radiology, University of California, Irvine, Medical Center, Orange, California.
Acute Gastrointestinal Disorders

Gerald A. Mandell, M.D.
Professor of Radiology and Pediatrics, Jefferson Medical College of Thomas Jefferson University, Adjunct Associate Professor of Radiology, University of Pennsylvania School of Medicine, Philadelphia, Pennsylvania; Associate Director of Medical Imaging, Chief of Nuclear Medicine, and Director of Clinical Research, Alfred I. duPont Institute, Wilmington, Delaware.
Imaging Evaluation of the Neonate

Glenn E. Newman, M.D.
Assistant Professor, Departments of Radiology and Surgery, Duke University School of Medicine; Chief, Vascular Interventional Radiology, Duke University Hospital; Consultant, Veterans Administration Medical Center, Durham, North Carolina.
Acute Myocardial Infarction

Curtis R. Partington, M.D., Ph.D.
Assistant Professor of Radiology and Neurosurgery, University of Wisconsin Medical School; Staff Neuroradiologist, University of Wisconsin Hospital and Clinics, Madison, Wisconsin.
Imaging Evaluation of Acute Neurologic Disease

Charles E. Putman, M.D.
James B. Duke Professor of Radiology and Professor of Medicine, Duke University School of Medicine; Executive Vice President for Administration, Duke University Medical Center, Durham, North Carolina.
A Radiologist's Perspective of Critical Care Imaging
Cardiac and Noncardiac Edema: Radiologic Approach
Acute Thoracic Trauma

Carl E. Ravin, M.D.
Professor and Chairman, Department of Radiology, Duke University School of Medicine, Durham, North Carolina.
Cardiovascular Monitoring Devices

Hemendra R. Shah, M.D.
Associate Professor of Radiology, University of Arkansas for Medical Sciences; Staff Radiologist, John L. McClellan Hospital of Arkansas, Memorial Veterans Hospital; Courtesy Staff, Arkansas Children's Hospital, Little Rock, Arkansas.
Acute Gastrointestinal Disorders

Robert M. Steiner, M.D.
Professor of Radiology and Associate Professor of Medicine, Jefferson Medical College of Thomas Jefferson University, Philadelphia, Pennsylvania; Consulting Radiologist, Deborah Heart and Lung Center, Browns Mills, New Jersey.
Pericardial Disease

Steven K. Teplick, M.D.
Director, Radiology Residency Training Program, Professor, and Vice Chairman, University of Arkansas for Medical Sciences, Little Rock, Arkansas.
Acute Gastrointestinal Disorders

M. Kristin Thorsen, M.D.
Associate Professor of Radiology, Medical College of Wisconsin; Milwaukee County Medical Complex, Froedtert Memorial Lutheran Hospital, Veterans Administration Medical Center, Milwaukee, Wisconsin.
Acute Aortic Disease and Peripheral Venous Disease

Irena Tocino, M.D.
Clinical Associate Professor of Radiology, University of Utah School of Medicine; LDS Hospital, Salt Lake City, Utah.
Abnormal Air and Pleural Fluid Collections

Connie Mitchell Vail, M.D.
Staff Radiologist, Salt Lake Clinic, Salt Lake City, Utah.
Cardiovascular Monitoring Devices

Jack E. Zimmerman, M.D.
Professor of Anesthesiology and Medicine, George Washington University School of Medicine and Health Sciences; Director, Intensive Care Unit, George Washington University Hospital, Washington, D.C.
A Clinician's Perspective of Critical Care Imaging

PREFACE

Since publication of our first edition in 1978, critical care medicine has expanded dramatically. Critical care units, once unique facilities in tertiary referral centers, have become a necessary component of every general hospital. Major diagnostic and therapeutic advances have enlarged the scope of critical care medicine for acute medical illnesses and postoperative problems, and innovative procedures such as organ and bone marrow transplantation have expanded treatment to previously untreatable patients. Changing social patterns have added additional patients with acquired immunodeficiency syndrome (AIDS), drug-related diseases, and increasingly violent trauma. Intensive care medicine, once managed by a few interested physicians, is now a multidisciplinary specialty with board certification available in several disciplines.

The growth of critical care medicine has led to greatly expanded basic research and a better understanding of the pathophysiology of such acute injuries as blunt trauma, overwhelming sepsis, multiple-organ failure, and respiratory insufficiency. The development of new drugs, of new monitoring and life support technologies, and of modified or new surgical intervention has expanded the role of critical care medicine but has made health care delivery more complex and expensive.

The public, through personal experience and the mass media, has also become more aware and more accepting of the critical care unit as a part of modern medicine. Public expectations have also increased the demand for services. While one segment of the population demands more high-tech care, another segment grapples with the financial and ethical issues of life-sustaining treatments in terminally ill patients.

Against this background, diagnostic imaging has made tremendous strides in the last 14 years. Conventional bedside images have improved tremendously, and digital imaging is starting to make inroads in bedside radiography. The history, physical examination, and portable chest radiograph remain the mainstay in the initial assessment of patients with acute medical and surgical problems. It is hard to believe that many supplemental imaging techniques that we take for granted in the daily evaluation of acutely ill patients—such as computed tomography (CT), ultrasonography, and interventional radiography—were either not available or in their infancy when our first edition was written. In addition, many nuclear medicine procedures have become more sophisticated, and some are even available at the bedside. Magnetic resonance imaging (MRI) is now available to a limited number of critically ill patients. Interventional procedures (e.g., abscess drainage, inferior vena cava filters, and so forth) have added a new dimension to the nonsurgical care of the critically ill.

This third edition is intended for use by radiologists and clinicians concerned with care of the acutely ill or injured. We emphasize the importance of interpretation of all images within the clinical setting as well as a focus on the pathophysiologic events responsible for the radiographic changes. These acutely ill patients have extremely complex problems, and only with free and frequent communication between the radiologist and the clinician can maximum benefit be derived from the imaging studies. Good communication also leads to the more efficient choice of examinations and to quicker and more accurate diagnosis, which hopefully improves outcome while cutting costs.

The current edition has been enlarged from 13 to 22 chapters. New chapters have been added for discussion of acute neurologic and acute vascular disorders. The topic of acute cardiopulmonary disease has been greatly expanded to include individual chapters on pneumothorax, pulmonary embolism, and infection in the immunocompromised patient. The discussions of adult respiratory distress syndrome (ARDS) and acute cardiac disorders have been expanded greatly. The sections on acute abdominal diseases have been completely revised to include individual chapters on gastrointestinal, hepatobiliary, and genitourinary disorders. These topics include a comprehensive approach to diagnosis and interventional techniques. Neonatal imaging is also covered in greater detail.

We are very grateful to the many experts who contributed to this third edition. Some of our colleagues have been with us since the first edition, and others have been added because of their interest and expertise in acute care imaging. We hope that we have achieved our primary purpose of providing a text that is both practical and complete for the day-to-day imaging problems encountered by radiologists, intensive care clinicians, pediatricians, surgeons, and anesthesiologists in the management of the critically ill. We are particularly appreciative of the support shown by our departments and to past and current colleagues and residents.

One of us (L.G.) worked many hours on this text while on sabbatical at London's Royal Postgraduate Medical School (Hammersmith Hospital): Many thanks to Dr. David Allison and the entire radiology staff for their support.

Outstanding secretarial help was provided by Mrs. Sylvia L. Bartz and Mrs. Mary A. Cody.

LAWRENCE R. GOODMAN
CHARLES E. PUTMAN

CONTENTS

8
Abnormal Air and Pleural Fluid Collections 137
Irena Tocino

PULMONARY INTERSTITIAL EMPHYSEMA, 138 ■
PNEUMOMEDIASTINUM, 139 ■ SUBCUTANEOUS
EMPHYSEMA, 141 ■ PNEUMOTHORAX, 142 ■ Anteromedial
Pneumothorax, 144 ■ Subpulmonary Pneumothorax, 145 ■ Apicolateral
Pneumothorax, 147 ■ Posteromedial Pneumothorax, 149 ■ Air in the
Fissures, 149 ■ Tension Pneumothorax, 149 ■ Occult Pneumothorax, 151 ■
PNEUMOPERICARDIUM, 152 ■ PNEUMOPERITONEUM AND
PNEUMORETROPERITONEUM, 152 ■ PLEURAL FLUID, 152

9
Pulmonary Embolism 161
Jud W. Gurney

SCOPE OF THE PROBLEM, 161 ■ PATHOPHYSIOLOGY, 161 ■
Deep Vein Thrombosis, 161 ■ Pulmonary Embolus, 162 ■ CLINICAL
MANIFESTATIONS, 162 ■ DIAGNOSIS, 163 ■ IMAGING OF PULMONARY
EMBOLISM, 163 ■ Chest Radiography, 163 ■ Ventilation-Perfusion
Scanning, 167 ■ DEEP VEIN THROMBOSIS, 172 ■ PULMONARY
ANGIOGRAPHY, 173 ■ Indications, 174 ■ OTHER IMAGING
TECHNIQUES, 175 ■ Computed Tomography, 175 ■ TREATMENT, 175 ■
Anticoagulation and Fibrinolysis, 175 ■ Inferior Vena Cava Filter, 175 ■
RESOLUTION, 175 ■ Serial Lung Scintigraphy, 176 ■ CHRONIC
EMBOLISM, 177 ■ SUMMARY, 177

10
The Immunocompromised Patient 181
Dewey J. Conces, Jr.

HISTORICAL INFORMATION, 181 ■ Nature of Immune Defect, 181 ■
Temporal Relationship to Transplantation, 184 ■ Therapy, 186 ■ Epidemiologic
Risk Factors, 186 ■ Rate of Progression, 187 ■ Extrapulmonary Findings, 187 ■
LABORATORY STUDIES, 188 ■ CHEST RADIOGRAPHY, 188 ■
Consolidative Patterns, 189 ■ Nodular Patterns, 189 ■ Diffuse Patterns, 191 ■
Pleural Effusion, 192 ■ Lymphadenopathy, 193 ■ NONINFECTIOUS ETIOLOGIC
FACTORS, 193 ■ Pulmonary Edema, 193 ■ Neoplasm, 193 ■ Drug Reactions, 194
■ Radiation Pneumonitis, 194 ■ Interstitial Pneumonia, 195 ■ Other Noninfectious
Disease Processes, 195

11
Acute Thoracic Trauma 199
Caroline Chiles ■ *Charles E. Putman*

PULMONARY PARENCHYMAL INJURY, 199 ■ Pulmonary Contusion, 199 ■
Pulmonary Laceration, 201 ■ Fat Embolism, 201 ■ Pulmonary
Edema, 202 ■ Atelectasis, 203 ■ Aspiration, 203 ■ Lobar Torsion, 203 ■
ABNORMALITIES OF THE PLEURAL SPACE, 203 ■
CARDIOVASCULAR TRAUMA, 204 ■ Aortic Transection, 204 ■ Cardiac
Contusion, 205 ■ Pneumopericardium, 206 ■ Intravascular Missiles, 206 ■
TRACHEOBRONCHIAL FRACTURE, 207 ■ ESOPHAGEAL
RUPTURE, 208 ■ FRACTURES OF THE THORACIC SKELETON, 208 ■
DIAPHRAGMATIC RUPTURE, 208

12
Imaging After Thoracotomy 213
Lawrence R. Goodman

NORMAL RADIOGRAPHIC APPEARANCE FOLLOWING LUNG
SURGERY, 213 ■ Pneumonectomy, 213 ■ Lobectomy, 214 ■ Segmental or Lesser

CRITICAL CARE IMAGING

PART

I

1

A Radiologist's Perspective of Critical Care Imaging

■

Lawrence R. Goodman
Charles E. Putman

Over the last several decades, imaging of the critically ill has expanded beyond the bedside radiograph to include several other bedside examinations (e.g., ultrasonography and nuclear medicine techniques) and numerous other procedures that require the patient to be transported to the radiology department, such as computed tomography (CT), magnetic resonance imaging (MRI), and nuclear medicine techniques. Nonetheless, the portable chest or abdominal radiograph remains the initial diagnostic image and the imaging triage keystone. In many large hospitals, portable chest radiographs now account for one half of inpatient chest radiographs. Although the emphasis of this book is the conventional examination, each chapter emphasizes the role of supplemental imaging studies in arriving at a speedy and accurate diagnosis. As the number of intensive care unit (ICU) beds increases, as the complexity of patient problems increases, and as the number of imaging modes increases, an organized approach to the critically ill becomes more important for both quality medical care and a more efficient use of personnel and resources.

In this chapter, we present some of our thoughts about organizing a critical care imaging service, optimizing imaging and diagnosis, and improving communications. Some of the material presented is fact; much of it is opinion. The opinion is based on more than 30 years of our combined experience in running critical care radiology services in teaching hospitals. We hope that the facts are accepted and the opinions are evaluated in light of the reader's own hospital experience.

EFFICACY STUDIES

Bedside examinations are time-consuming, labor-intensive, and expensive. The surcharge for portable examination approximately doubles the technical charge for the radiograph. At best, portable radiographs produce adequate images. We perform the least sophisticated imaging procedure in our entire diagnostic armamentarium on the sickest patients in the hospital—those needing the most sophisticated diagnosis. Before delving into this textbook of critical care imaging, the reader may reasonably question how much information is actually gained from portable chest radiographs. Especially open to question is the "routine A.M. examination," given that routine screening studies for tuberculosis, lung cancer, and preoperative lung disease in the asymptomatic patient have proved to have a low yield.

In several recent studies, investigators have considered the diagnostic yield of portable radiographs based on the indication for examination and have tried to identify both high-yield and low-yield groups. A study involving more than 1300 radiographs on 167 respiratory ICU patients revealed 35% of radiographs showed new or progressive cardiopulmonary disease or tubes and catheters in unexpected positions (Bekemeyer et al., 1985). The radiographic finding led to a change in patient management in 30% and a change in tube or catheter position in 20%. Overall, 50% of *nonroutine* examinations resulted in a change in action. A surprising 39% of *routine* examinations resulted in a change in action. Table 1–1 summarizes changes in diagnosis and changes in therapy based on the indication for the radiograph. Strain and colleagues (1985) reviewed more than 500 routine morning portable radiographs and found 15% demonstrated unsuspected abnormalities, 93% of which required a change in management. Authors of similar studies involving medical and surgical units rather than respiratory units also document new or unsuspected findings in 37% to 65% of examinations (Greenbaum and Marschall, 1982; Henschke et al., 1983; Janower et al., 1984).

Table 1–1. EFFICACY OF PORTABLE CHEST RADIOGRAPHY IN THE ICU

Indication	New or Progressive Disease (%)	Changed Diagnosis or Therapy (%)	Adjusted Tubes or Catheter (%)
Admission radiograph	73	50	4
Routine examination	30	24	21
Routine follow-up	17	17	0
Post-procedure radiograph	8	25	27
Clinical change	50	43	19
Existing abnormality	17	43	13
All radiographs	27	30	20

Based on Bekemeyer, W. B., et al.: Efficacy of chest radiography in a respiratory intensive care unit: A prospective study. Chest 88:691, 1985.

Following the insertion of various tubes and catheters, Bekemeyer and associates (1985) found that 27% were improperly positioned and 6% resulted in radiographically visible complications of insertion (e.g., pneumothorax or pleural effusion). Improper tube location was most frequent after Swan-Ganz catheterization (24%), followed by endotracheal tube insertion (15%), central venous pressure (CVP) catheters (12%), and tube thoracostomy (7%). Many of the malpositioned vascular catheters could be suspected clinically (e.g., from abnormal wave forms) and many were not of immediate threat to the patient's well-being. Pneumothorax was uncommon (6 of 306 cases), but this complication is potentially lethal in a patient with marginal cardiopulmonary reserve or in a patient receiving mechanical ventilation. Endotracheal tube malposition, however, was a potential hazard needing rapid correction.

Strain and co-workers (1985) found that almost all patients with important radiographic changes showed clinical evidence of acute pulmonary disease or unstable cardiac disease or had indwelling tubes and catheters. The yield was low in patients with uncomplicated myocardial infarctions and in patients who were admitted for extrathoracic problems (e.g., diabetes or renal disease). All of these studies assume that an examination with negative results is not valuable (e.g., when no pneumothorax is present to account for a patient's respiratory difficulty). This assumption is not always valid, however.

Bedside examinations appear to be valuable in diagnosing and managing patients with acute cardiopulmonary disease or unstable cardiac disease, or those with support and monitoring devices, but such examinations are not required for other patients unless specific clinical indications arise. Common sense and a little advance planning can also reduce the number of radiographs required. If a catheter change or other intervention is planned, the routine daily film can often be delayed until after the procedure. Similarly, a chest or abdominal radiograph can often be eliminated on days that CT scans of those areas are planned.

Bedside studies are only of value when they are performed and viewed in a timely manner. A study by Greenbaum and Marschall (1982) emphasized the need for prompt and efficient handling of portable radiographs from the time of request to the interpretation of the final image. In a 1-month study in a medical ICU, approximately one third of radiographs were not of immediate use in patient management. Three major stumbling blocks were (1) failure to take the radiograph in a timely fashion (13%), (2) unavailability of the completed radiograph for morning rounds (14%), and (3) technically inadequate films (6%). An organized system, with good communication at all levels, should help eliminate many of these problems.

For chest disease, CT is the single most effective imaging mode after the bedside radiograph. It is particularly valuable for detecting pleural disease and mediastinal disease and for differentiating parenchymal from pleural disease. Two recent retrospective studies involving more than 100 CT scans on critically ill patients have shown that new, significant information affecting diagnosis, the understanding of the extent of disease, or the need for treatment was obtained in 70% to 75% of cases (Golding et al., 1988; Mirvis et al., 1987). The majority of diagnoses were related to mediastinal and pleural disease. Computed tomographic or ultrasonographic guidance for diagnostic aspirations of fluids results in a 95% success rate, and therapeutic drainage of effusions and empyema involves a 75% to 90% success rate with relatively few complications (O'Moore et al., 1987; Reinhold et al., 1989; Westcott, 1985). Thoracentesis under ultrasonic guidance decreases the post-procedure pneumothorax rate by a factor of six (Raptopoulos et al., 1991). The efficacy of CT in abdominal and pediatric work is discussed in later chapters.

TECHNICAL CONSIDERATIONS

Optimizing Techniques

Good radiographs require good technologists and good equipment. "Portable" radiography is not glamorous work and is often assigned to technologists with the least seniority or to a technologist who is "in the doghouse." The poor results are often predictable. We have found that some technologists enjoy the challenge and freedom of being out of the department and in a more clinical environment. By giving them encouragement and working with them, either through formal in-service conferences or day-to-day interaction, the radiologist can help them become valuable members of the intensive care team. Technologists are required to screen all radiographs for quality and frequently are the first to detect pneumothorax, a misplaced catheter, and so forth. At Duke University, experienced portable radiographers are considered "specialized technologists" and are treated accordingly.

An occasional in-service talk to the ICU nursing staff also helps improve cooperation between the ICU personnel, the technologist, and the radiologist. A team approach rather than an "us versus them" approach leads to better imaging, a more pleasant work environment, and less turnover among portable radiographic technologists.

Choosing a technique for portable radiographs requires a number of compromises to accommodate to the realities of bedside radiography. Kilovoltage is usually limited to the 80- to 85-kV range to minimize the deleterious effects of scattered radiation. Constant-potential, battery-operated, or capacitor-discharge mobile units are capable of a 100- to 400-mA output, and most chest exposures can be made between 2 and 4 mAs. Erect radiographs are usually obtained at 60 to 72 inches, and semi-erect radiographs are usually obtained at approximately 40 to 50 inches. For supine radiographs, the height of the tube stand usually limits the target film distance to approximately 40 inches.

Prager and associates (1984) have shown that a high-kilovoltage grid technique can be used successfully at the bedside. They compared 50 sets of *supine* bedside chest radiographs using standard kilovoltage (60 to 80 kV) with high-kilovolt radiographs (125 kV, 10:1 grid, 40 line pairs/cm). High kilovoltage was judged to produce superior results for all 11 anatomic areas assessed. The greater latitude of the high-kilovoltage technique provided a longer scale of contrast and reduced repeat examinations by a factor of six. The occasional repeat for "grid cutoff" was far outweighed by the improved film quality and consistency. Patient dose is reduced because of fewer repeat examinations, and the higher kilovoltage results in lower milliamperage. (All radiographs were done supine. It is likely that "grid cutoff" is more of a problem with erect positioning.) A fixed-distance arm for mobile x-ray units should help eliminate many artifacts from off-center or nonperpendicular tube alignment (MacMahon, 1988).

Attempts to improve radiographic consistency through the use of a phototimer or the use of 240-kV radiographs with grids have not gained widespread acceptance (Fisher et al., 1982; Tabrisky et al., 1980).

The choice of film screen combinations also involves compromises. Theoretically, the fastest film screen combination, which provides the shortest exposure, should decrease motion unsharpness and should provide the best images. Unfortunately, the fastest film screen combinations have decreased spatial resolution and increased noise due to quantum mottle, as fewer photons strike the screens. Noise varies with the square root of film speed: For every fourfold increase in speed, noise doubles. The increased noise is especially deleterious for detection of low-contrast lesions with ill-defined borders (Weaver and Goodenough, 1983). Vucich and colleagues (1979) and Weaver and Goodenough (1983) have emphasized the difficulty in choosing film screen combinations on the basis of physical data derived in the laboratory. Such data do not always translate into practical clinical use. The choice of appropriate film screen combinations must be based on matched comparisons of various film screen combinations in conjunction with the available mobile equipment. Such comparisons represent a practical approach to making these clinical determinations in lieu of a formal receiver operating characteristic (ROC) analysis.

Radiographic Consistency

"Is the patient getting better or getting worse?" is the clinician's greatest concern and not an unreasonable question to ask regarding an expensive diagnostic study. Day-to-day consistency of films removes much of the guesswork involved in trying to answer this fundamental question. Every effort must be made to ensure consistency, both in film quality and in patient positioning. This problem is multifocal, and the following steps may prove helpful:

1. Individual technique chart—A card at the bedside or logbook on the mobile unit where technologists can record successful techniques on a given patient eliminates guesswork. In addition, a generic "portable technique chart" should be available on each mobile unit.

2. Fixed kilovoltage—A constant kilovoltage should be used so that milliamperage is the only variable. This practice helps maintain constant subject contrast.

3. Kilovolt peak (kVp) greater than 100 kV—The use of high-kilovolt films with grids was discussed previously (Prager et al., 1984). Mirvis and colleagues (1988) have described a fixed overhead x-ray unit for intensive care work.

4. Altering the receptor—Wilkinson and Fraser (1975) recommend two pairs of screens with a film between each in the same cassette. The front film has twice the density of the back film because of absorption of the radiation by the front screens. The front film is optimal for the mediastinum and the back film is optimal for the lungs. Image phosphor plates have a dynamic range of 10,000 to 1 compared with 100 to 1 for conventional film. This range virtually assures consistent radiographs with ideal optical density (see later).

5. Minimum equipment requirements—Functioning collimators, collimator lights, positioning lights, and a tape measure on the collimator are needed to

ensure correct positioning, distance, and adjustment of technique selection. Good collimation also reduces scatter and patient dose.

6. Routine maintenance—A regular quality-control program for automatic processing machines and a scheduled maintenance and calibration program for portable equipment are essential.

7. Radiographic quality control—It should be departmental policy that suboptimal radiographs are not acceptable and that technologists are responsible for their own work. This places the initial quality control in the processor room, where it belongs.

Radiographic Projections

The ideal film is exposed at 6 feet with the patient sitting erect. This minimizes magnification. The erect radiograph also provides the best position for detecting and quantitating pneumothorax, evaluating the size of the pulmonary vessels, and detecting pleural effusion. If the patient is too ill or out of touch to assume the upright position, a semi-erect or supine radiograph that is well positioned and motion-free is preferable to an attempt at an upright radiograph of a struggling patient.

Although the vast majority of bedside radiographs are taken in the anteroposterior (AP) position, one should not hesitate to use other projections. If the first six AP radiographs do not yield the answer, the seventh is not likely to. In moderately ill patients, posteroanterior (PA) radiographs can be taken with the patient sitting at the bedside, hugging the cassette. When pneumothorax or pleural effusion is suspected and sitting erect is not possible, the patient can often be rolled onto his or her side for a lateral decubitus film. For pneumothorax, the technologist should center on the nondependent hemithorax, and for pleural effusion, on the dependent hemithorax. Tocino prefers horizontal beam lateral radiographs for the diagnosis of pneumothorax (see Chapter 7).

When performing decubitus radiographs for fluid, rolling the patient onto a cardiac arrest board prevents the dependent hemithorax from sinking into the mattress. The decubitus position shifts the blood, mediastinum, and abdominal viscera to the dependent side, which increases the functional residual volume of the nondependent lung by as much as 1 liter and maintains that lung in inspiratory apnea. This procedure is particularly helpful in visualizing the nondependent lung base in patients who cannot inspire deeply and in differentiating pleural effusion from underlying parenchymal consolidation (Lerner, 1978). Air trapping on the dependent side may also be visible.

Quality lateral films are difficult to obtain in the ICU and are seldom used other than to verify the position of tubes and catheters or large areas of opacification. Oblique radiographs are often helpful for evaluating the lung behind the heart, for determining tracheal narrowing, and for determining whether a lesion is anterior or posterior. Right posterior oblique (RPO) films are helpful in determining whether an endotracheal tube or nasogastric tube is in the esophagus or trachea (see Chapter 3). Supine, oblique films may also help in verifying pleural effusion. An erect and supine radiograph can help distinguish between a pleural effusion and lower lobe consolidation.

A radiograph centered on the diaphragm ("high KUB") provides superior visualization behind the heart and diaphragm. This view may facilitate the distinction between consolidation and effusion. With the central ray parallel to the diaphragm and lung base, this radiographic position also makes a subpulmonic pneumothorax easier to detect.

Self-adhesive labels should be affixed to every radiograph and should indicate the date, time, patient position, distance, and radiographic technique. An additional label that includes information on assisted ventilation, such as mode of ventilation, peak pressure, presence or absence of positive end-expiratory pressure (PEEP), and pulmonary capillary wedge pressure, is extremely helpful (Milne, 1986). This label is supplied and filled out by the nurse with the x-ray study request form or by the technologist, who can be taught where to obtain the information from the chart.

Upright or Supine? AP or PA?

Even under the best circumstances, one is occasionally faced with films that are not labeled to indicate the patient position and direction of beam.

The following clues help determine supine versus erect positioning:

1. The presence of air–fluid level indicates an erect-position film. The absence of air–fluid level does not exclude an erect-position film, because the x-ray beam may not be horizontal.

2. In a buxom female patient, the position of the breast may indicate upright or supine positioning.

3. An inclinometer, taped to the cassette, eliminates guesswork. A simple homemade example is presented in Figure 1–1 (Gallant et al., 1978). Of course, an erect cassette does not ensure an erect patient.

4. Magnification is considerably more pronounced on the supine radiograph.

Even the determination of whether a chest x-ray study was performed in the AP or PA projection is often difficult. Sometimes, the position of the flash plate on the film provides a clue. This parameter varies from hospital to hospital. Kattan and Wiot (1973) found that the appearance of the vertebral bodies of C6, C7, and T1 often provide the answer. On an AP radiograph, the vertebral body and joints

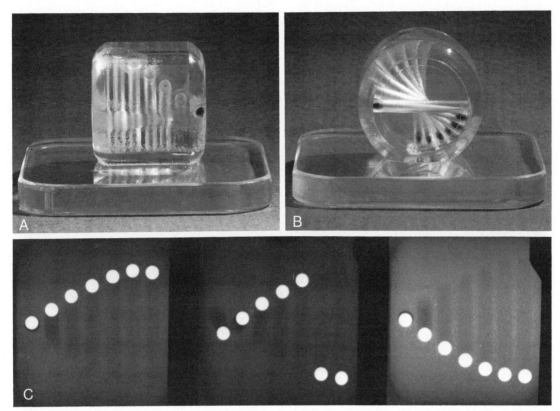

Figure 1–1. Inclinometer. The lucite cylinder has holes drilled, each at 15 degrees to the next. A BB is placed in each hole, and the ends are sealed. The cylinder is fixed to the rectangular plate so that when the plate is horizontal, one BB rolls down. *A,* Front view. *B,* Side view. When the plate is tilted forward, one BB rolls down for each 15 degrees. (Modified from Gallant, T.E., et al.: Technical notes: Simple device to measure patient position on portable chest radiographs. AJR 131:169–170, 1978, with permission, © by American Roentgen Ray Society.) *C,* Radiograph of Inclinometer. *Left,* Trendelenburg's position; all BB's are at the top when the plate tilts backward. *Center,* 15 degrees erect; two BB's have rolled down. *Right,* 90 degrees erect; all BB's have rolled down.

of Luschka should be visible. In this projection, the divergent x-ray beam travels tangentially to the endplates, as it does in the cervical spine view (with 20-degree angulation), which is designed to study the endplates and the joints of Luschka. On a PA radiograph, the neural arch, the articular processes, and the apophyseal joints are well visualized. The spinous processes are often pointed upward, because the divergent PA beam is parallel to the spinous processes and facet joints (Fig. 1–2). With 100 test films and six readers, Kattan and Wiot found that 78 films were correctly interpreted by all six readers, and that 15 were correctly interpreted by three or four readers. When mistakes were made, AP films were mistakenly considered PA films. The sign is least helpful in kyphotic patients, in AP radiographs exposed at 6 feet (because of less beam divergence), and when the central ray is high in the thorax. (As more and more portable radiographs are exposed at 6 feet, the value of this sign diminishes.)

Magnification may also help in determining which radiographs are AP and which are PA. Anterior structures such as the clavicle, the sternum, sternal wires, and anterior mediastinal clips are larger and less sharp on AP radiographs than on PA radiographs. On AP radiographs, the medial border of the scapula often projects several centimeters over the lateral lung.

Degree of Inspiration

Despite one's best efforts to obtain an inspiratory radiograph with the patient fully erect, this goal is often not achieved in the critical care unit. Harris (1980) studied 22 postoperative cardiac patients and found that the height of the diaphragm on "inspiratory" postoperative bedside radiographs was identical with that on preoperative expiratory radiographs (Table 1–2). In such cases, differentiation of significant basal atelectasis or lung edema from the effects of poor inspiration may be difficult. Expiration causes a decrease in thoracic blood volume; therefore, no vascular redistribution into the upper lobes should occur, and no vascular or peribronchial edema should be present (Milne, 1986). Crowded vessels should not be confused with enlarged vessels.

Magnification and Rotation

Accurate estimation of the degree of cardiac magnification on a given AP radiograph is difficult. One

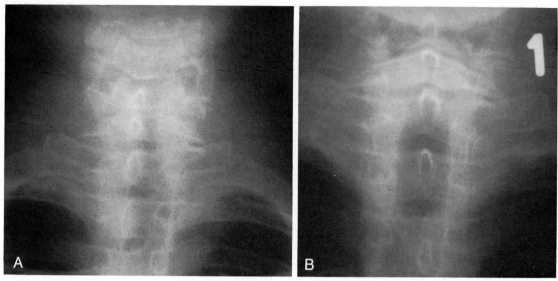

Figure 1–2. The direction of the x-ray beam (AP or PA) can often be determined by the appearance of the vertebral bodies of C6, C7, and T1 (see text). *A*, Anteroposterior radiograph. Vertebral bodies and joints of Luschka are visible. *B*, PA radiograph. The neural arch, articular processes, and apophyseal joints are visible. The spinous process may point cephalad (Kattan and Wiot, 1973).

would have to know the target-film distance and the patient's AP diameter to determine magnification. The degree of magnification also varies with the diameter of the patient's heart. With a large heart, the maximal transverse diameter is deeper in the chest and closer to the cassette. Less magnification occurs. Harris (1980), studying patients, and Milne (1986), studying phantoms, both concluded that on a 40-inch AP radiograph, a heart with a thoracic ratio of approximately 0.56 would have a cardiothoracic ratio of less than 0.5 on a 72-inch PA radiograph. On AP radiographs, as the target-film distance increases from 40 to 72 inches, Milne noted less than 5% reduction in the cardiothoracic ratio because both the heart and the thoracic width decreased proportionately. Harris found that the average mediastinum increased 15% in width between the 72-inch PA and 40-inch AP supine radiographs. It increased 49% on an expiratory AP radiograph (see Table 1–2). This

may explain the apparent radiographic change in mediastinal width after coronary artery surgery, when the patient's clinical condition is stable.

Rotation may change the relative density of the two lungs. If the patient is rotated to the left, the left pectoral muscle and breast are rotated off the left lung into the axilla, and the right muscles and breast are rotated over the right lung. Therefore, the density diminishes on the side to which the patient is rotated and increases on the contralateral side. The rotation to the left also causes an apparent elevation of the left hemidiaphragm in relation to the right (Milne, 1986). The illusion occurs because the anterior portion of the diaphragm, which is usually highest, is accentuated on the left, whereas the posterior portion of the diaphragm, which is usually lowest, is now more visible on the right. Rotation to the left also causes the left border of the heart to move laterally, causing apparent cardiac enlargement. Rotation to

Table 1–2. EFFECT OF PATIENT POSITION AND PHASE OF RESPIRATION ON PORTABLE RADIOGRAPHS

	Preoperative				Postoperative
	Standing (72-in. TFD)		*Supine (44-in. TFD)*		*Supine (44-in. TFD)*
	Insp.	*Expir.*	*Insp.*	*Expir.*	*Insp.*
Heart transverse diameter (cm) (n = 21)	14.6	15.6 (+7%)	16.3 (+11%)	16.7 (+14%)	16.3 (+11%)
Cardiothoracic ratio (n = 21)	0.47	0.55 (+17%)	0.51 (+9%)	0.59 (+25%)	0.57 (+25%)
Width of superior mediastinum (cm) (n = 20)	5.5	6.1 (+10%)	6.4 (15%)	8.2 (49%)	8.3 (51%)
Right lung height (cm) (n = 22)	22.5	19.3 (−14%)	23.2 (+3%)	18.6 (−17%)	19.1 (−15%)

(% = % change from posteroanterior inspiration)
TFD, Target film distance; Insp., inspiratory; Expir., expiratory.
Adapted from Harris, R. S.: The pre-operative chest film in relation to postoperative management—effects of different projection, posture, lung inflation. Br. J. Radiol. 53:196, 1980, with permission.

the right unfolds the aorta, which widens the mediastinum, and it moves the heart more to the midline, which decreases its apparent size.

RADIATION CONSIDERATIONS

The critically ill patient undergoes many diagnostic procedures during the course of a prolonged illness. Although a single portable chest x-ray study adds little to the patient's total radiation dose, the cumulative effects of multiple examinations can be considerable. Boles and colleagues (1987) found that the average portable radiograph exposed at 76 kV, 15 mA, and 40 inches provides a marrow dose of 49 millirads, a thyroid dose of 40 millirads, and a gonadal dose of less than 1 millirad. Careful collimation, relatively fast film screen combinations, the highest possible kilovoltage, greater target patient distance, and shielding of the lower abdomen all minimize this dose. The use of the optimal technique by experienced personnel decreases the number of repeat examinations. Likewise, photostimulable plates allow further dose reduction, as well as fewer repeat examinations. The greatest patient protection, however, remains the careful consideration of which radiographic studies are necessary and which are unlikely to yield helpful information. The marrow dose and gonadal dose from abdominal and spinal examinations and the lens dose from skull or sinus examinations are several orders of magnitude greater than the dose from chest examinations. These studies should be ordered only when absolutely necessary.

Radiation exposure of technologists and ICU personnel can be minimized with the use of basic precautions and common sense. The scattered radiation values for portable chest radiographs and lateral lumbar spine radiographs at 1 m are approximately 0.2 millirads and 1.3 millirads, respectively. Doubling the distance reduces the dose by a factor of 4 (0.05 and 0.35 millirads, respectively). Current equipment provides a 6-foot cord for the exposure controls. The technologist should fully extend the cord. Most scatter is backscatter directed *toward* the technologist. Most forward scatter is absorbed by the patient, the cassette, and the bed (North, 1985; Vogel and Löhr, 1976; Drafke, 1989). Placing the mobile machine between the technologist and the patient further reduces scatter. For closer work, use of a lead apron reduces exposure to scatter to less than 10% of the incident dose.

Nursing stations need not be abandoned every time the portable unit comes into view. Herman and associates (1980) found that a nursing station 11 to 17 feet from four ICU beds was exposed to 0.05 millirads per week for every 80 exposures. This value is approximately 1/200 of the maximal permissible whole body exposure for nonoccupational workers. The yearly exposure would be 2.6 millirads, which must be compared with an annual, naturally occurring background exposure of approximately 90 millirads.

In another study, Boles and co-workers (1987) placed four dosimeters at an ICU nursing station for 2 months and found no measurable radiation. If critical care personnel are required to hold a patient, lead aprons and gloves must be worn.

FILM INTERPRETATION AND COMMUNICATION

Organizing a Service

Critical care unit images must be available for review immediately after processing, they must be interpreted in a timely and knowledgeable fashion, and the results must be communicated rapidly. Staffing and hospital geography often dictate the arrangement, but an organized approach to displaying, interpreting, and storing images is needed. Mechanical alternators dedicated to ICU radiographs are the most practical, least expensive way of organizing such a service.

We prefer to have the mechanical viewer in the radiology department. It provides better quality control, less film loss, and more timely interpretation. Many hospitals have located the reading area adjacent to the ICU, which provides easier access for the clinicians. Each patient is assigned one or more panels on the alternator, and the most recent radiographs remain posted on the designated alternator 24 hours a day. The patient's jacket remains in a file cabinet adjacent to the viewer. This system markedly reduces file room requests for these high-demand radiographs and guarantees rapid availability of radiographs. In addition, the decreased film handling reduces the inadvertent filing of one patient's radiographs in another's jacket. More important, this practice assures radiologists and clinicians alike that images on their critically ill patients are always available. This system requires a mutual understanding between the radiologist and the clinician that the radiographs must not be taken off the alternator except for special circumstances, such as trips to the operating room, biopsy, and grand rounds.

All reviewing, reading, and conferences take place at the alternator. Because the patient's main jacket is housed there as well, all studies from throughout the department can be reviewed and integrated with other studies. A daily review conference, with open discussion between the radiologist and the clinician, maximizes information from the imaging studies and aids in planning future studies. Baker and Stein (1986) found that a daily meeting with the acute surgical ward staff helped direct the course of the imaging work-up by the choice of appropriate examinations, by the elimination of low-yield or redundant examinations, and by establishing the proper sequence of the studies. Such consultations decreased the use of five of six commonly ordered imaging procedures (Table 1–3) and decreased hospital stay by approxi-

Table 1–3. CHANGES IN DIAGNOSTIC
PROCEDURES DURING PERIOD OF
RADIOLOGIC CONSULTATION

Abdominal radiographs	+16%
Ultrasonography	−29%
Nuclear scans	−33%
Computed tomography	−39%
Barium enema	−42%
Upper gastrointestinal series	−73%
Colonoscopy	+6%
Gastroscopy	+8%

Adapted from Baker, S. R., and Stein, H. D.: Radiologic consultation: Its application to an acute care surgical ward. AJR 147:637–640, 1986, with permission, © by American Roentgen Ray Society.

mately 18% (approximately 2.8 days per patient). No increase occurred in mortality or morbidity due to misdiagnosis between the 8-month control group and the 8-month test group. Although this study was performed on a surgical ward, not in an ICU, similar, but perhaps less dramatic, results are likely to be achieved in the critical care unit.

Over the last decade, subspecialty critical care units have proliferated (e.g., cardiothoracic surgery, respiratory care, and neurosurgery), with a growing sophistication among the physicians operating them. This trend has culminated in board certification in critical care by several subspecialty groups. Radiologists must also increase their sophistication to provide a valuable service. They must understand the basic workings of the ICU, the unique problems of the ICU patient, the various drugs and interventions in daily use, and the strengths and limitations of the imaging procedures for the critically ill.

Radiology training must be strengthened in this area. Magnetic resonance imaging, color Doppler ultrasonography, and other newer imaging techniques are certainly more alluring to trainees of the 1990s, but specific training in the problems of the critically ill is needed as well. At large hospitals and teaching hospitals, the reading of the images should be assigned to members of the chest radiology section or the general radiology section. In smaller practices, these solutions are not practical. One or two members of the group should become expert and be accessible, even if they are not reading these radiographs on a daily basis. A major complaint from clinicians in smaller hospitals is a lack of continuity and an inconsistency of reading day to day. The potential solution is rotation of the assignment in 2-, 4-, or 8-week blocks, so that continuity in both interpretation and communication is provided. Consistent quality control by a given radiologist also leads to better portable radiographs.

The daily conferences, specialty conferences, and perhaps a text such as this one may also make the clinician a better reader of radiographs. Just as the radiologist must recognize the problems of the critical care unit, clinicians forced to look at images on a daily basis can better understand the strengths and weaknesses of a given study and some of the problems the radiologist faces.

Teleradiology and Picture Archiving Communication System (PACS)

We are currently witnessing a high-technology revolution that will fundamentally alter how radiographs are taken, displayed, transmitted, and stored. Teleradiology systems are limited-purpose units that allow the transmission of an image from one location to another with local image display and perhaps storage at the receiving station. The long-term goal is to have a larger, more comprehensive digital-based system that displays, stores, and transits all images and radiology data (reports, schedules, and so forth) throughout the department and, potentially, throughout the hospital. Picture archiving communication systems (PACS) will potentially link to information-management systems. Several currently available systems provide digital radiographs or electronic transmission of conventional radiographs to the critical care unit for viewing, either on a soft display (video monitor) or hard display (laser printer). The systems should become more versatile, more user-friendly, and perhaps less expensive in the next decade.

A basic teleradiology system involves digitization of conventional portable radiographs through the use of either a laser scanner or a video scanner (Aberle et al., 1990; Cho et al., 1988; Fraser et al., 1989; Goodman et al., 1988; Slasky et al., 1990). A more sophisticated system uses an image receptor that consists of a plate coated with photostimulable phosphor housed in a cassette. The cassette is exposed in a conventional manner but has a laser image reader that interrogates the latent image on the plate and produces a digital image that can be processed and displayed as a video image or hard copy (Sagel et al., 1990).

At the Medical College of Wisconsin, we have used a laser film digitizer with conventional portable radiographs to provide images for our new critical care unit, which is located two blocks from the main radiology department. This system provides the ICU with the current images within minutes of processing. Previously digitized images for comparison are stored in local memory and are presented on a second monitor. Approximately 8 to 10 images per patient are stored locally. The viewing physician has control of window, level, and magnification ($\times 2$, $\times 4$) at the receiving console. The original radiograph is displayed, interpreted, and stored in the x-ray department.

This system and a similar system at the University of Pennsylvania have met with rapid acceptance from radiologists, clinicians, and technologists. The system speeds interpretation because the images can now be in more than one place at one time, and the radiographs are less likely to become lost. Arenson and associates (1988) have shown that this system also shortens the time between production of the radiograph and changes in clinical management. The system provides acceptable video images with a maximum resolution of 2.5 line pairs per millimeter, which is approximately one-half the resolution of a standard radiograph. The final interpretation is made on the original radiograph. The disadvantages of the system include reduced spatial and contrast resolution, increased cost, and the need to produce conventional radiographs as the input images.

The phosphor plate technology offers several major benefits over the previously described system. The images are digitized directly without going through an intermediate film, and the dynamic range is approximately 1 to 10,000, as compared with 1 to 100 for conventional radiographs. The increased latitude essentially guarantees an acceptable optical density over a wide range of exposures and is especially valuable for viewing mediastinal disease and large opacities with indistinct margins (Schaefer et al., 1989). Tubes and catheters are detected equally well on digital and conventional radiographs, although the entire course of the device can be seen more confidently on digital images (Thompson et al., 1989). The disadvantages of such a system include high cost, limited processor throughput, complex technologic equipment, and decreased spatial resolution.

Teleradiology, if it is used simply to export images rapidly to other locations in the hospital, can potentially decrease communications with clinicians and decrease the input of radiologists in the diagnosis. Reading of the images must be timely, and the information must be conveyed rapidly to the critical care unit. Communications may be as basic as a phone call, handwritten wet reading, or "faxed" wet reading, or as sophisticated as voice recognition typing systems or phone access voice playback systems. These improved image and report management systems should allow better communications and should also decrease some of the stresses and strains between radiologist and clinician, such as those arising from the control and loss of radiographs or delayed reports. The long-term goal of the PACS is further improvement in efficiency; it will provide immediate access to all patient images at viewing stations throughout the radiology department and the rest of the hospital.

References

Aberle, D.R., Hansell, D., and Huang, H.K.: Current status of digital projectional radiography of the chest. J. Thorac. Imaging 5:10, 1990.

Arenson, R.L., Seshadri, S.B., Kundel, H.L., et al.: Clinical evaluation of a medical image management system for chest images. AJR 150:55, 1988.

Baker, S.R., and Stein, H.D.: Radiologic consultation: Its application to an acute care surgical ward. AJR 147:637, 1986.

Bekemeyer, W.B., Crapo, R.O., Calhoon, S., et al.: Efficacy of chest radiography in a respiratory intensive care unit: A prospective study. Chest 88:691, 1985.

Boles, J.M., Boussert, F., Manens, J.P., et al.: Measurement of irradiation doses secondary to bedside radiographs in a medical intensive care unit. Intensive Care Med. 13:60, 1987.

Cho, P.S., Huang H.K., Tillisch, J., and Kangarloo, H.: Clinical evaluation of a radiologic picture archiving and communication system for a coronary care unit. AJR 151:823, 1988.

Drafke, M.W.: Trauma and Mobile Radiography. Philadelphia, F.A. Davis, 1989.

Fisher, M.R., Mintzer, R.A., Rogers, L.F., et al.: Evaluation of a new mobile automatic exposure control device. AJR 139:1055, 1982.

Fraser, R.G., Sanders, C., Barnes, G.T., et al.: Digital imaging of the chest. Radiology 171:297, 1989.

Gallant, T.E., Dietrich, P.A., Shinozaki, T., et al.: Technical notes: Simple device to measure patient position on portable chest radiographs. AJR 131:169, 1978.

Golding, R.P., Knape, P., Strack van Schijndel, R.J., et al.: Computed tomography as an adjunct to chest x-rays of intensive care unit patients. Crit. Care Med. 16:211, 1988.

Goodman, C.R., Wilson, C.R., and Foley, W.D.: Digital radiography of the chest: Promises and problems. AJR 150:1241, 1988.

Greenbaum, D.M., and Marschall, K.E.: The value of routine daily chest x-rays in intubated patients in the medical intensive care unit. Crit. Care Med. 10:29, 1982.

Harris, R.S.: The pre-operative chest film in relation to postoperative management—some effects of different projection, posture, lung inflation. Br. J. Radiol. 53:196, 1980.

Henschke, C.I., Pasternack, G.S., Schroeder, S., et al.: Bedside chest radiography: Diagnostic efficacy. Radiology 149:23, 1983.

Herman, M.W., Patrick, J., and Tabrisky, J.: A comparative study of scattered radiation levels from 80-kVp and 240-kVp x-rays in the surgical intensive care unit. Radiology 137:552, 1980.

Janower, M.L., Jennas-Nocera, Z., and Mukai, J.: Utility and efficacy of portable chest radiographs. AJR 142:265, 1984.

Kattan, K.R., and Wiot, J.F.: How was this chest roentgenogram taken, AP or PA? Am. J. Roentgenol. Radium Ther. Nucl. Med. 117:843, 1973.

Lerner, M.A.: Inspiration chest radiography by lateral recumbency. Clin. Radiol. 29:155, 1978.

MacMahon, H.: A new approach to bedside chest radiography: Early clinical experience with a fixed geometry mobile system. *In* Peppler, W.W., and Alter, A.A. (eds.): Proceedings of the Chest Imaging Conference—1987. Madison, WI, Medical Physics Publishing Corporation, 1988, p. 371.

Milne, E.N.: A physiological approach to reading critical care unit films. J. Thorac. Imaging 1:60, 1986.

Mirvis, S.E., Fritz, S.L. Siegel, J.H., and Ramzy, A.: Radiographic system for use in emergency and intensive care units. AJR 150:691, 1988.

Mirvis, S.E., Tobin, K.D., Kostrubiak, I., and Belzberg, H.: Thoracic CT in detecting occult disease in critically ill patients. AJR 148:685, 1987.

North, D.: Pattern of scattered exposure from portable radiographs. (Published erratum appears in Health Phys. 50:317, 1986.) Health Phys. 49:92, 1985.

O'Moore, P.V., Mueller, P.R., Simeone, F.J., et al.: Sonographic guidance in diagnostic and therapeutic interventions in the pleural space. AJR 149:1, 1987.

Prager, P., Neumann, D., Geiger, K., et al.: Supine thoracic images with a mobile roentgen unit: Comparison between the soft-ray and hard-ray technics. Rontgenblatter 37:409, 1984.

Raptopoulos, V., Davis, L.M., Lee, G., et al.: Factors affecting the development of pneumothorax associated with thoracentesis. AJR 156:917, 1991.

Reinhold, C., Illescas, F.F., Atri, M., and Bret, P.M.: Treatment of pleural effusions and pneumothorax with catheters placed percutaneously under imaging guidance. AJR 152:1189, 1989.

Sagel, S.S., Jost, R.G., Glazer, H.S., et al.: Digital mobile radiography. J. Thorac. Imaging 5:36, 1990.

Schaefer, C.M., Greene, R.R., Oestmann, J.W., et al: Improved control of image optical density with low-dose digital and conventional radiography in bedside imaging. Radiology 173:713, 1989.

Slasky, B.S., Gur, D., Good, W.F., et al.: Receiver operating characteristic analysis of chest image interpretation with conventional, laser-printed, and high-resolution workstation images. Radiology 174:775, 1990.

Strain, D.S., Kinasewitz, G.T., Vereen, L.E., and George, R.B.: Value of routine daily chest x-rays in the medical intensive care unit. Crit. Care Med. 13:534, 1985.

Tabrisky, J., Herman, M.W., Torrance, D.J., and Hieshima, G.B.: Mobile 240-kVp phototimed chest radiography. AJR 135:295, 1980.

Thompson, M.J., Kubicka, R.A., and Smith, C.: Evaluation of cardiopulmonary devices on chest radiographs: Digital vs. analog radiographs. AJR 153:1165, 1989.

Vogel, H., and Löhr, H.: X-ray protection zones during x-ray exams in intensive care. [Author's translation.] Rontgenblatter 29:459, 1976.

Vucich, J.J., Goodenough, D.J., Lewicki, A.M., et al.: Use of Anatomical Criteria in Screen/Film Selection for Portable Chest Procedures. Proceedings from symposium on "Optimization of Chest Radiography." The University of Wisconsin, Madison, Wisconsin, 1979. HHS Publications (FDA) 80–8124. HE 20.4102:042.

Weaver, K.E. and Goodenough, D.J.: Physical aspects of the portable radiograph. *In* Goodman, L.R., and Putman, C.E. (eds.): Intensive Care Radiology: Imaging of the Critically Ill. Philadelphia, W.B. Saunders, 1983, p. 300.

Westcott, J.L.: Percutaneous catheter drainage of pleural effusion and empyema. AJR 144:1189, 1985.

Wilkinson, G.A., and Fraser, R.G.: Use of double screen-film combination in bedside chest roentgenography. Radiology 117:222, 1975.

2

A Clinician's Perspective of Critical Care Imaging

■

Janice Bitetti
Jack E. Zimmerman

Most readers of this chapter have probably worked in an intensive care unit (ICU). Nonetheless, we think it worthwhile to define intensive care and provide some perspective about today's units: the kinds of patients treated there, the services provided, and some of the challenges to be faced in the 1990s. We also want to share some information about life support techniques that might be helpful in interpreting ICU films and to discuss some common reasons for consultation in the ICU. Finally, we hope to convince readers that imaging for ICU patients is far too critical to be left to either radiologists or clinicians alone and that we must collaborate, communicate, and coordinate our efforts to promote optimal patient care.

THE MODERN ICU

Today's ICU is best defined as a technology consisting of people and machines whose main purpose is to detect and treat acute life-threatening physiologic abnormalities. Historically, ICUs evolved from postanesthesia recovery rooms and from experiences with the polio epidemics of the early 1950s. Developments such as arrhythmia monitoring, cardiopulmonary resuscitation, mechanical ventilators, and other devices and techniques provided further impetus for development of the ICU. These advances created problems in care delivery; concentration of the patients, caregivers, and machines in one location provided an expedient solution. In large hospitals, ICUs are typically organized according to department or specialty; in smaller hospitals, they are usually multidisciplinary (i.e., with mixed medical and surgical staff).

The ICU Patient

Patients in the ICU are best characterized through diagnosis, determination of prior health status, and most important, description of the severity of illness. Knowing that a patient is elderly, was in poor health previously, and has heart failure or pneumonia conveys a little information about the need for intensive care; the severity of physiologic abnormality is the factor that usually explains why the patient is in the ICU. To describe severity of illness, many clinicians use the Acute Physiology and Chronic Health Evaluation (APACHE) system (Knaus et al., 1985). The APACHE III system uses a point score based on the degree of derangement of 17 physiologic measurements plus points for age and prior health status to reflect increasing severity of disease.

A general description of today's ICU patient is provided by a recent survey of 40 medical-surgical ICUs in a nationally representative sample of hospitals with over 200 beds (Zimmerman, 1989). In teaching hospitals, the average age of an ICU patient is 57 years; 18% of ICU patients are in severely failing health, and 53% are admitted after surgery. In general, patients in nonteaching hospitals are older and less frequently admitted postoperatively. The proportion of patients with low severity of illness in nonteaching hospitals (41%) is much greater than in teaching hospitals (27%), but the proportion of severely ill patients is similar. Three diagnoses—peripheral vascular surgery, congestive heart failure, and upper gastrointestinal (GI) bleeding—account for about 19% of all ICU admissions in the United States. In large tertiary care centers, the most frequent diagnoses are cardiac surgery (13.5%), major vascular surgery (11%), trauma (7.6%), and craniotomy for neoplasm (6%).

ICU Services

Patients in the ICU can also be described by the services they receive. Approximately only 60% of ICU patients actually receive life-support therapy. The remaining 40% are admitted for monitoring or a perceived risk of developing instability (Wagner et al., 1987). The types of monitoring and treatment vary widely. Among large tertiary care hospitals, almost all patients undergo electrocardiography, and 64% undergo intra-arterial monitoring; 35% have central venous catheters and 18% have pulmonary artery catheters: Use of pulmonary artery catheters is approximately half as frequent in nonteaching hospitals. Surprisingly few patients receive life-support therapy; for example, only 38% receive mechanical ventilation, and 28% receive vasoactive drug infusion.

Challenges for the 1990s

Over the past three decades, advances in ICU technology have rarely been rigorously evaluated; in fact, no study has ever proved that ICUs save lives. Instead, philosophy, logic, and pragmatism have dictated that the technologic equipment and methods, the nurses, and the patients who might benefit from them be concentrated in ICUs. As a result of this lack of rigorous evaluation, many aspects of critical care practice—from the decision to insert a pulmonary artery catheter to the decisions of which patients to admit and how vigorously to treat them—are characterized by controversy and uncertainty. While physicians remain uncertain about the best way to treat critical illness, patients and society are increasingly concerned about the economic, social, and personal costs of current practices.

Cost, Allocation, and Ethical Challenges

Recent estimates suggest that during the 1980s, ICU costs in the United States grew to almost 1% of the gross national product (GNP) and 20% of total hospital costs, or $13 billion to $15 billion (Knaus and Ihibault, 1982). Medicare's diagnosis-related group (DRG) prospective payment system represents just one policy response to these rising costs. What is the impact of DRGs on ICUs? At one large teaching hospital, Medicare payments over 1 year were $4.7 million below the actual care cost (Butler et al., 1985); three California teaching hospitals reported a 31% reduction in ICU beds and a 14% decrease in length of stay (Mayer-Oakes et al., 1988). Rationing is *not* a challenge for the 1990s. Intensive care unit resources are already being rationed. The challenge is to develop a better understanding of the needs, benefits, and efficacy of ICU care, to develop just and rational allocation of resources, and to practice within an ethical framework (Kalb and Miller, 1989).

Diseases, Technology, and Other Challenges

Improvements in therapy have resulted in improved survival for patients with trauma, burns, and infection. For these patients, better therapy not only has reduced mortality, but has also changed the major cause of death to a relatively new entity, multi-organ system failure (MOSF) (DeCamp and Demling, 1988). This process is characterized by sequential failure of organ systems, primarily the lungs, followed by the liver, kidneys, and the GI tract. Although few in number, these patients generate enormous costs, owing to the use of ICU resources, blood products, and nursing staff. In the 1990s, continuing improvements in therapy are likely to increase the frequency of MOSF.

Advances in immunosuppressive and surgical techniques have dramatically increased transplantation procedures. Transplantation of livers, hearts, and lungs are complex, are costly, and may require extensive postoperative intensive care. Many ICUs have expanded dramatically to care for these patients; their numbers are likely to grow during the 1990s.

The increasing number of patients with acquired immunodeficiency syndrome (AIDS) represents another major challenge for the 1990s. Several analyses during the mid-1980s indicated an 87% to 100% mortality for AIDS patients requiring intubation and mechanical ventilation (Rosen et al., 1986). Recent reports, however, suggest improved ICU outcome results (50% to 64% mortality) for AIDS patients (Efferen et al., 1989; El-Sadar and Simberkoff, 1988). Selected patients with *Pneumocystis* pneumonia are now managed in ICUs with continuous positive airway pressure masks instead of mechanical ventilation (Gregg et al., 1990). The development of new therapeutic techniques, along with prognostic uncertainty and the projected increase in case load, promises future challenges for hospitals that have so far cared for only small numbers of AIDS patients (Wachter et al., 1989).

LIFE SUPPORT TECHNIQUES AND THE RADIOLOGIST

In this section, we discuss the common diseases requiring life support and aspects of monitoring that affect the radiograph. We also discuss some aspects of life support that have implications for the radiologist.

Respiratory Support

Indications

The reasons to support ventilation fall into three broad categories: airway obstruction, disorders of gas exchange, and failure of the airway's protective mechanisms. Although some patients' diseases overlap, we discuss the radiologic implications of each category separately.

AIRWAY OBSTRUCTION

Upper airway patency can be compromised when soft tissue alterations or foreign substances obstruct the free passage of air. In the postoperative patient, loss of muscle tone due to residual anesthesia often leads to upper airway obstruction. This problem is easily corrected by extension of the neck and elevation of the base of the tongue from the posterior pharyngeal wall. Space-occupying lesions of the airway such as edema, infection, tumor, hematoma, or scar tissue are more difficult to correct and may require bypass or stenting. Foreign substances can lead to partial or complete airway obstruction and may require bronchoscopic removal.

Chest radiographs are usually normal early in the course of airway obstruction. Neck films, however, may be helpful in identifying the location and extent of a space-occupying airway lesion. With epiglottitis and croup, for example, characteristic changes on neck radiographs can distinguish two clinically similar diseases (Mayo Smith et al., 1986; Shapiro et al., 1988). Later in the course of upper airway obstruction, the chest radiograph may become helpful by revealing pneumonitis, volume loss due to obstruction by aspirated particles, or pulmonary edema if obstruction involved extreme inspiratory effort. The last entity, known as postobstructive pulmonary edema, is noted almost immediately after relief of severe obstruction involving extremely negative pleural pressures.

DISORDERS OF GAS EXCHANGE

For the lungs to be effective, they must provide an arterial oxygen content adequate for metabolic needs and eliminate metabolically produced carbon dioxide. The components of lung function that determine how these goals are met include ventilation, perfusion, and ventilation-perfusion matching. Abnormalities of any one of these components can lead to respiratory failure manifested as hypoxemia, hypercarbia, or both.

Well-perfused but nonventilated alveoli create a "physiologic shunt" and predominately cause hypoxemia. Well-ventilated alveoli that are not perfused constitute wasted ventilation ("physiologic dead space") and result in both hypoxemia and hypercarbia. Shunt and dead-space ventilation represent the extremes of a spectrum of ventilation-perfusion mismatch. This mismatch can contribute to hypoxemia, hypercarbia, or both.

The chest radiograph is invaluable in distinguishing the cause of gas-exchange abnormalities. Infiltrates, poor inspiratory volumes, and collapse suggest shunt. Redistribution of vascular markings may reflect a low cardiac output state; increased interstitial markings may indicate that diffusion is compromised as well. Common processes that result in hypoxemia due to shunting include pneumonia, cardiac and noncardiac pulmonary edema, and lobar atelectasis.

The other major manifestation of disordered gas exchange is hypercarbia. By definition, hypercarbia is caused by an absolute reduction in alveolar ventilation, that is, hypoventilation. Alveolar hypoventilation can be associated with reduced air movement (e.g., drug overdose), normal air movement, or even elevated air movement (e.g., chronic obstructive pulmonary disease, COPD). With elevated air movement, hypoventilation is due to wasted ventilation, that is, ventilation-perfusion mismatch. Hypercarbia is usually accompanied by hypoxemia that is typically easy to correct with a relatively low (<40%) inspired oxygen concentration.

In the ICU, hypoventilation with carbon dioxide retention is often due to narcotic or sedative-induced suppression of respiratory drive. The chest radiograph in this situation is normal except for decreased inspiratory volumes. If hypoventilation due to inadequate muscle and chest wall movement occurs, then the chest radiograph may reveal fractured ribs or phrenic nerve palsy. Hypercarbia due to ventilation-perfusion mismatch is usually accompanied by parenchymal changes, as in COPD. Patients with acute changes in ventilation-perfusion matching, however, like patients with pulmonary embolism, may demonstrate no radiographic abnormality.

FAILURE OF AIRWAY PROTECTIVE MECHANISMS

The laryngeal and pharyngeal nerves and muscles constitute a finely tuned system with complex interactions that prevent secretions or solids from entering the airway. Drug overdose, stroke, and head trauma are some of the situations in which this protective system fails. If respiratory function is intact, then placement of a cuffed endotracheal tube (ETT) to prevent aspiration is adequate therapy. If central nervous system (CNS) function is compromised, then mechanical ventilation must be initiated. In either case, the chest radiograph is usually normal but may show evidence of aspiration pneumonitis.

Therapy

OXYGEN SUPPLEMENTATION

Support during respiratory failure ranges from simple oxygen supplementation to intubation and mechanical ventilation. Use of nasal cannulae, face masks, or 100% oxygen nonrebreathing masks has no significant effect on the radiograph. In contrast, continuous positive airway pressure (CPAP) delivered by a face mask (mask CPAP) or by an ETT does affect the radiograph. Therapy with CPAP is provided by delivering oxygen at high flow and under continuous pressure throughout inspiration and expiration for spontaneously breathing patients. The positive pressure during exhalation provides a positive end-expiratory pressure (PEEP) and improves oxygenation by increasing functional residual capacity (FRC) and opening alveoli. The same mechanism is responsible for the improved oxygenation that occurs when PEEP is added during mechanical ventilation. Therapy with CPAP is most often used to relieve hypoxemia in patients with pulmonary edema or pneumonia, or in patients undergoing ventilator weaning (Gregg et al., 1990).

We have repeatedly observed radiographic changes during mask CPAP therapy that are similar to those seen with PEEP during mechanical ventilation: lung volume is increased, vascular markings are attenuated, and pulmonary infiltrates seem improved in comparison with prior films. Complications of CPAP include mediastinal emphysema, pneumopericardium, and pneumothorax. Mask CPAP may also produce gastric distention.

TRACHEAL INTUBATION

The indications for tracheal intubation are few and simple: airway obstruction, mechanical ventilation, tracheobronchial toilet, and prevention of aspiration. The decision to intubate is primarily clinical and based on general appearance, physical findings, disease progression, laboratory aids, and radiographic appearance. Physiologic variables including respiratory rate greater than 35/min, arterial oxygen pressure (Pa_{O2}) less than 60 mm Hg, arterial carbon dioxide pressure (Pa_{CO2}) greater than 55 mm Hg, and vital capacity less than 15 cc/kg are also considered indications to support ventilation.

Intubation can be performed with an oral or a nasal ETT, cricothyroidotomy, or tracheotomy. Each method has important radiographic implications.

Oral intubation can be performed with the greatest speed and is the method of choice in emergencies. Another advantage of oral intubation is the ability to accommodate a large tube, which lowers resistance to breathing, facilitates suctioning, and allows passage of a fiberoptic bronchoscope. Radiographs following emergency oral intubation may reveal tube malposition and other complications, such as broken teeth and pneumothorax (Taryle et al., 1979). Oral ETTs are difficult to secure and thus have a greater likelihood of malposition than other tracheal tubes. Neck flexion can displace the tube caudad and cause main bronchus intubation; extension can cause displacement cephalad, which creates a risk of extubation. With any type of intubation, upward displacement of the diaphragm or Trendelenburg's position can move the carina upwards and cause main bronchus intuba-

tion (Heinonen et al., 1969). Therefore, the position of the ETT must be carefully assessed on a daily basis (Brunel et al., 1989) (see Chapter 3).

Nasotracheal intubation provides greater patient comfort, better oral hygiene, and less movement in the larynx than does oral intubation. Pulmonary toilet is more difficult, however, and plugging, collapse, or obstruction is more likely than with the use of oral ETTs. Nasal intubation increases the tendency of patients to swallow air, which results in gastric distention and small bowel dilatation (Cooper and Malt, 1977). Isolated cecal dilatation without any colonic obstruction occurs in some patients receiving mechanical ventilation and may be related to aerophagia (Golden and Chandler, 1975) (see Fig. 3–20). In addition, a significant but often overlooked complication of nasotracheal tubes is sinusitis (Kronberg and Goodwin, 1985). Simple removal of the tube can be adequate therapy, but antibiotics and surgical drainage are often necessary (Caplan and Hoyt, 1982) (see Chapter 3). Figure 2–1 demonstrates some low-pressure cuffed ETTs in common use.

Cricothyroidotomy is usually reserved for emergencies in which oral intubation is either impossible (e.g., extensive facial injuries) or inadvisable (e.g., cervical spine injuries) (Cole and Aguilar, 1988). Cricothyroidotomy is more readily performed and requires less skill than a tracheotomy, and in most centers, it has replaced the emergency tracheotomy. On the radiograph, a cricothyroidotomy is practically indistinguishable from a tracheotomy.

Current practice favors prolonged oral or nasal intubation rather than early tracheostomy because modern plastic ETTs cause less laryngeal damage than do older devices (Bishop, 1989; Colice, 1987; Heffner et al., 1986a). At present, the major indications for tracheostomy are upper airway obstruction, patient comfort, and avoidance of laryngeal injury when prolonged ventilatory support is anticipated. The major mechanisms causing laryngeal injury are necrosis from tube pressure and abrasion of the mucosa due to tube movement. Ulceration of the laryngeal mucosa and cord granulomas or web formation still cause concern, but long-term follow-up suggests that most complications resolve over several months (Colice et al., 1989). Minimization of tracheal cuff pressures and cuff distention (which is often detected on the chest radiograph) is important in preventing tracheal ulceration and eventual stenosis *regardless* of the route of intubation.

The risks of aspiration around a cuff and of nosocomial pneumonia from chronic instrumentation are not obviated by tracheotomy. Indeed, tracheotomy produces its own complications (Heffner et al., 1986b). Early ones include bleeding and dissection of air into mediastinal tissues; after removal, stenosis at the cuff or at stomal sites may occur. Although early tracheotomy may help avoid primary laryngeal injury, tracheotomy after several days of translaryngeal intubation can aggravate subglottic inflammation and allow synechiae formation at sites of previous vocal

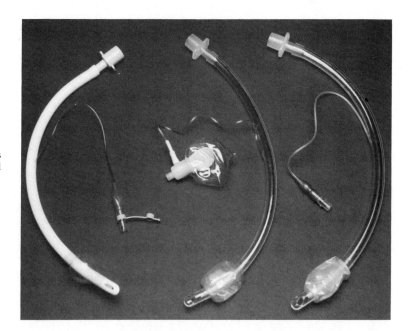

Figure 2–1. Low-pressure cuffed endotracheal tubes (ETTs). *Left,* Portex ETT. *Center and right,* National Catheter Corporation ETTs.

cord damage (see Chapter 3). Some commonly used tracheotomy tubes are shown in Figure 2–2.

MECHANICAL VENTILATION

Once mechanical ventilation is begun, a mode of ventilation must be chosen. The major alternatives are assist/control (AC) mode, intermittent mandatory ventilation (IMV), and pressure support (PS). Positive end-expiratory pressure may be added with any mode, but it carries the risk of barotrauma if lungs are stiff and airway pressures are high (McCloud et al., 1977).

The AC mode assures a minimum number of machine breaths as determined by the rate set on the ventilator. In addition, the patient's inspiratory effort can also initiate a machine breath. The AC mode minimizes patient workload and ensures a consistent tidal volume.

The IMV mode also assures a minimum number of machine breaths determined by the ventilator rate setting. Patient inspiratory effort, however, opens a "demand" valve, which permits any tidal volume that the patient can generate. The IMV setting (high rate) can totally control ventilation, or this mode (lower rate) can force the patient to do some or all of the work of breathing and can thus be used for weaning.

The PS mode was recently introduced as an alternative to the IMV mode for weaning. Although the demand valves in most modern ventilators respond rapidly to minimal inspiratory effort, they still require a certain amount of patient work. In the PS mode, a preset pressure is delivered following inspiration to help compensate for this added work. The PS stops once inspiratory flow drops below a preset level. The patient determines the inspiratory time, rate, and flow pattern, but lung compliance and pressure setting determine how much volume is delivered by machine

work. Stiffer lungs and lower PS cause less volume delivery and require more patient work.

Prior to initiation of mechanical ventilation, the radiograph may show low lung volumes, dense infiltrates, or areas of collapse. Once ventilatory support has commenced, the radiograph often reflects improved lung expansion. The degree of expansion is determined by tidal volume and PEEP (Zimmerman et al., 1979) (Fig. 2–3). In addition, the lung may appear less consolidated, and areas of collapse may resolve. Findings from the chest radiograph at high IMV rates are similar to those observed with the AC mode. At lower IMV rates, however, the radiograph may demonstrate poor inspiration or collapse if exposure occurred during a particularly weak inspiratory effort by the patient. At high PS levels, the chest radiograph is similar to that observed with the AC mode. At lower PS levels, hypoventilatory changes may occur; these changes may be more pronounced than those seen with IMV, in which a few machine breaths still provide intermittent expansion.

Weaning

The ability to be weaned from ventilator support is primarily influenced by the degree of resolution of the acute disease. Other determinants are ability to cough, secretion volume, nutritional status, hemodynamic stability, and fluid balance. These factors are assessed clinically, radiographically, and by physiologic measurements such as inspiratory and expiratory force, vital capacity, and tidal volume.

Weaning is accomplished by decreasing IMV rate, reducing PS, or alternating ventilator support with periods of either CPAP or T-piece breathing. Administering CPAP requires opening of a demand valve; T-piece breathing obviates this work, but its inability to stent alveoli may lead to more atelectasis. The

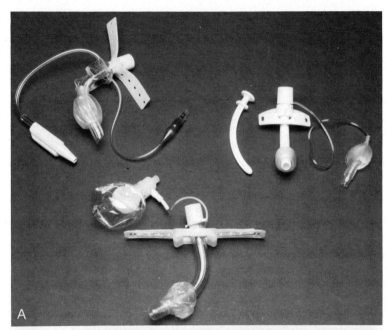

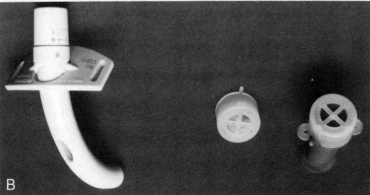

Figure 2–2. Tracheotomy tubes. *A,* Cuffed tracheotomy tubes. *Upper left,* Pitt Trach speaking tube. *Center,* Hi-Lo tracheotomy tube with large-volume, low-pressure cuff. *Right,* Shiley's cuffed/fenestrated tracheotomy tube with cannula. *B, Left,* Uncuffed Shiley's fenestrated tracheotomy tube. *Right,* Kistner's tracheal buttons.

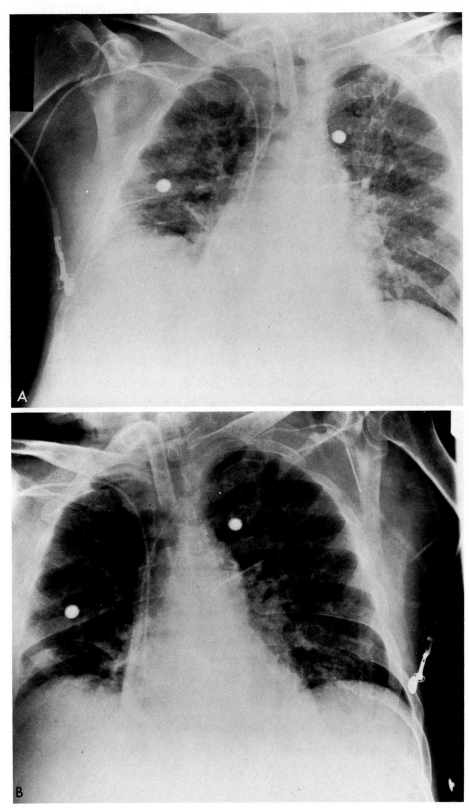

Figure 2–3. Effect of respiratory inflation volume and positive end-expiratory pressure (PEEP) on chest radiographs. All films were taken within 15 minutes by the same technician, who used the same equipment and technical factors. Note that the central venous pressure catheter is coiled in the superior vena cava. *A*, Pulmonary edema in a patient receiving an 800-ml tidal volume without PEEP. *B*, Repeat film with a 1200-ml sigh without PEEP.

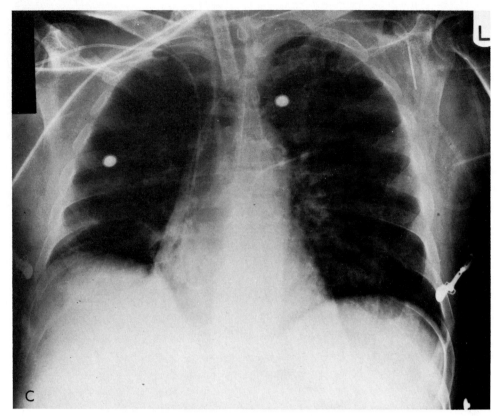

Figure 2–3 *Continued C*, Repeat film with an 800-ml tidal volume and 12-cm PEEP.

radiographs of patients being weaned from ventilatory support often appear worse than previous radiographs (Fig. 2–4). The paradox of a worsened radiograph together with a clinically improved patient suggests a change in ventilatory support. One should also consider, however, changes other than alterations in lung inflation as possibly resulting from changes in ventilatory support. A decrease in PEEP, a decrease in ventilator rate, or resumption of spontaneous breathing also causes increased venous return and increased central blood volume. These changes in ventilatory support can result in increased prominence of vascular markings on the radiograph. Thus, when the clinician substantially lowers PEEP or IMV rate, the increased blood return, a lower tidal volume, or both may cause the appearance of a fuller vasculature. Changes in lung volume as well as in blood return may contribute to the "wet" appearance that follows support changes. One must consider fluid balance, cardiac status, and lung volume before interpreting the film.

Complications

The radiographically detectable complications of ventilator therapy include barotrauma, nosocomial pneumonia, oxygen toxicity, gastric distention, increases in lung water, hyperexpansion, and atelectasis (see Chapter 3).

Frequently, patients who require ventilatory support have diseases that predispose them to pneumo-thorax (e.g., emphysema, asthma, or necrotizing pneumonia). High airway pressures developed in non-compliant lungs can also cause pneumothorax. Subcutaneous air and mediastinal emphysema are important warning signs that often precede pleural air and should be looked for in any ventilated patient (Altman and Johnson, 1979; Goodman and Putman, 1981) (see Chapters 3 and 8).

Patients receiving ventilatory support are particularly vulnerable to respiratory infections. Critical illness can suppress the immune system, and the ETT inhibits ciliary clearance and decreases ability to cough and clear secretions. An additional risk is aspiration of gastric or oral secretions around an ETT cuff (see Chapter 5).

High oxygen concentrations promote absorption atelectasis, and inspired fractions of 0.8 to 1.0 for more than 48 hours involve the risk of development of pulmonary toxicity. Dyspnea may occur within 12 hours, but the radiographic manifestations of interstitial edema and fibrosis do not appear for several days. Positive end-expiratory pressure is used to prevent a need for high inspired oxygen fractions. Gastric distention in ventilated patients is probably due to aerophagia. When severe, it can interfere with lung expansion and should be treated by suction through a nasogastric tube. The increase in lung water observed in ventilated patients may be caused by overhydration or left ventricular (LV) failure and is promoted by humidification of ventilator gases and

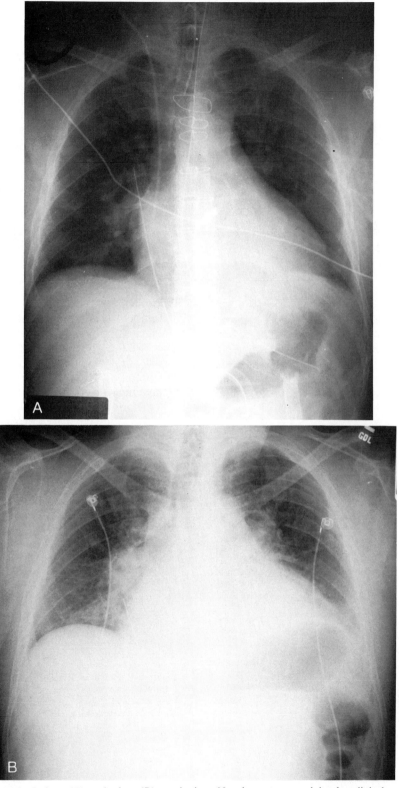

Figure 2–4. Chest radiographs before *(A)* and after *(B)* extubation. No change occurred in the clinical status between films. The postextubation film is underpenetrated; it shows smaller lung volumes and has a "wetter" appearance.

elevations in antidiuretic hormone and norepinephrine due to positive pressure ventilation. Hyperexpansion on the chest radiograph suggests excessive tidal volume, PEEP, or auto-PEEP (gas trapping caused by incomplete exhalation); it should prompt a review of the ventilator settings and airway pressures. In contrast, poor expansion or atelectasis on the chest radiograph can be due to film exposure at less than full inspiration.

Cardiovascular Support

Indications

Hypotension, with poor perfusion and oliguria, is the most common indication for cardiovascular support in the ICU. Although the causes are diverse, the underlying physiologic disturbance typically includes one or more of the following: insufficient preload, poor contractility, or abnormal afterload.

INSUFFICIENT PRELOAD

Preload refers to the ventricular end-diastolic volume. Hypovolemia, which is often due to bleeding or third spacing of intravascular fluid, leads to low blood pressure and decreased urinary flow. On Starling's curve, shown in Figure 2–5, Point A represents a reduced preload with low stroke volume; volume infusion increases ventricular end-diastolic volume and forward flow.

INADEQUATE CONTRACTILITY

Poor cardiac contractility, regardless of the etiology, causes inadequate stroke volume by shifting Starling's curve to the right (see Fig. 2–5, Point B to

C). For any level of preload, less forward flow results from reduced cardiac function. Clinically, signs and symptoms of congestive heart failure are present, and radiographically, pulmonary congestion and interstitial or alveolar edema are present.

An increase in LV end-diastolic pressure from poor cardiac function is transmitted to the pulmonary vasculature, causing pulmonary venous hypertension. On the radiograph, this "high-pressure" (hydrostatic) pulmonary edema may be difficult to distinguish from "low-pressure" pulmonary edema (otherwise known as adult respiratory distress syndrome, ARDS) because of increased capillary permeability (Sibbald et al., 1983; Sprung et al., 1981) (see Chapters 6 and 7).

Radiographic features typical of hydrostatic edema, which include widened vascular pedicle, pleural effusions, peribronchial cuffs, and septal lines, may also be observed in cases of increased permeability (Aberle et al., 1988; Milne et al., 1985; Smith et al., 1987). A Swan-Ganz catheter is often needed to distinguish the two entities (Matthay and Chatterjee, 1988). A pulmonary capillary wedge pressure (PCWP) in excess of 18 mm Hg indicates hydrostatic pulmonary edema. A reduction in PCWP to less than 18 mm Hg should be accompanied by clinical and roentgenographic improvement within 24 hours if the cause of the edema is cardiac failure. Edema that persists for a prolonged period (e.g., 24 hours) despite reductions in PCWP suggests increased capillary permeability (see Chapter 6).

The radiographic resolution of pulmonary edema may lag behind clinical improvement by several hours to several days (McHugh et al., 1972). Conversely, interstitial edema is often noted immediately after an increase in PCWP: Because it precedes alveolar edema, it occurs before rales can be detected by auscultation.

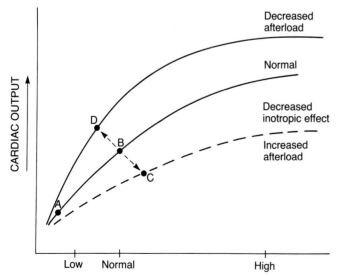

Figure 2–5. Modified Starling's curve. The middle curve reflects normal left ventricular function. Volume depletion in a hydrated, normal patient causes a move from Point A to Point B. Elevated afterload or worsening contractility shifts the curve rightward (Point B to Point C). Decreasing afterload improves function and shifts the curve upward (Point B to Point D).

ABNORMAL AFTERLOAD

Changes in impedance to ejection affect the heart's ability to pump. Elevation of afterload (e.g., in malignant hypertension) shifts Starling's curve (see Fig. 2–5) to the right (Point B to C) and decreases forward flow. Lowering of afterload (e.g., in the use of nitroprusside) improves flow by shifting the curve upward (Point B to D).

Monitoring

The most commonly used monitors in ICUs are central venous and pulmonary artery (PA) catheters. A central venous catheter (CVC) measures right-sided cardiac filling pressures; it is also used for hyperalimentation and venous access. The triple-lumen CVC has three separate ports and is useful for patients requiring multiple infusions. The PA catheter measures pressures of both the right and left sides of the heart as well as cardiac output through use of a thermodilution technique. It is employed in situations in which pressures of the right side of the heart do not reflect those of the left side; pulmonary disease and isolated LV failure are the most common examples.

Correct placement of all types of catheters is essential for accurate pressure recording and avoidance of complications (Wechsler et al., 1988). For measurement of central venous pressures, the tip of the CVC must be intrathoracic, that is, visualized beyond the first rib. For a triple-lumen CVC, the distal port is located 2 cm, and the proximal port 5 cm, from the tip. Ideal placement of the tip is 2 to 3 cm above the atrium with the proximal port inside the thorax at the junction of the superior vena cava and the internal jugular vein.

Complications related to PA catheter positioning include arrhythmias, pulmonary infarction, and arterial rupture (Goldenheim and Kazemi, 1984; Wiedemann et al., 1984). To avoid these complications, the tip of the PA catheter should be in the right or left pulmonary artery. Positioning the tip in the pulmonary outflow tract or right ventricle leads to arrhythmias, endothelial damage, or perforation; in intralobar arteries, it leads to persistent "wedging" and possible hemorrhage or infarction (see Chapter 4).

Complications related to insertion of PA and central venous catheters are pneumothorax, bleeding, and infusion of solutions into nonvascular spaces such as the pleural cavity. The route of insertion determines the likelihood of pneumothorax: The subclavian route carries a higher risk than the internal jugular route. A radiograph is needed immediately after insertion to assure correct positioning and to detect complications (Fig. 2–6).

Therapy

Pulmonary artery and central venous catheters provide useful information, but they do not save lives.

The data they provide are used to devise therapeutic strategies involving drugs and mechanical devices.

DRUGS

Vasoactive drugs affect preload, afterload, and contractility. α-Adrenergic agents increase afterload and preload. Dopamine agonists cause renal vascular dilatation at low doses and increase afterload and contractility at higher doses. β-Adrenergic drugs increase heart rate and contractility. Vasodilators lower afterload and preload, and many drugs have a combination of properties. Clinicians using potent vasoactive agents must be certain that infusion catheters are located centrally because backward leaking or subcutaneous infusion of vasoconstrictors causes serious ischemic sloughing.

MECHANICAL DEVICES

Intra-aortic balloon counterpulsation uses volume displacement to assist cardiac perfusion and function; deflation decreases afterload, and diastolic inflation enhances coronary flow. The intra-aortic balloon, in conjunction with vasoactive drugs, is used when LV function is impaired or when coronary flow is inadequate, as in cases of unstable angina. The tip of the device is ideally located just distal to the aortic arch. High positioning compromises subclavian flow or causes dissection; low positioning reduces therapeutic effectiveness.

Nutritional Support

Parenteral Nutrition

Parenteral nutrition consists of lipids, proteins, carbohydrates, and electrolytes delivered in high concentrations via a CVC. For long-term nutritional support, the catheter is tunneled subcutaneously before venous insertion. This practice reduces infection, the most common complication of parenteral nutrition. The distal catheter tip should be in a large vein to prevent sclerosis from hyperosmolar solutions. Considerations about positioning and complications of other CVCs also apply to parenteral nutrition lines. Despite the risk of pneumothorax, the subclavian route is preferred, because it improves access for catheter care.

Enteral Nutrition

Use of the enteral route, when feasible, is preferred to total parenteral nutrition (TPN) because it obviates the complications of line placement and infection. Because the gut receives a substantial portion of its nutrition via its lumen, enteral feeding is superior to TPN in maintaining the structural integrity of the gastrointestinal mucosa; thus, it has physiologic advantages. Enteral feeding, however, requires a func-

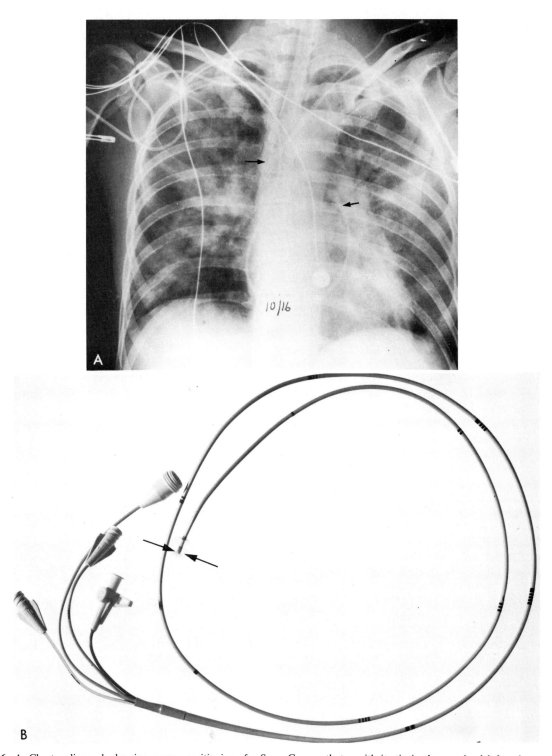

Figure 2–6. *A,* Chest radiograph showing proper positioning of a Swan-Ganz catheter with its tip in the proximal left pulmonary artery *(lower arrow).* The tip of the left central venous pressure catheter is in the superior vena cava *(upper arrow). B,* No. 7 French thermodilution catheter with the balloon inflated *(arrows).*

tioning gastrointestinal tract with intact motility and mucosal absorption. Postsurgical ileus and decreased intestinal motility from the use of narcotics are common and may prevent feeding via the enteral route.

Enteral feeding tubes are placed in the stomach and, in patients at increased risk for aspiration, beyond the pylorus. If long-term enteral feeding is anticipated in patients who lack airway protection, a gastrostomy or a jejunostomy may be created. Newer enteral feeding tubes are small-bore, soft, flexible, and less likely than standard nasogastric tubes to lead to sinusitis and esophagitis. They are radiopaque, and positioning should always be checked by radiography prior to feeding. These tubes can easily be slipped past an ETT cuff and into a peripheral bronchus. Some tubes, when placed with wire stylets, may even perforate the lung. Figure 2–7 shows some common parenteral and enteral feeding devices (see Chapter 17).

Renal Support

Sepsis, trauma, major surgery, hypovolemia, cardiogenic shock, and contrast agents are common causes of acute renal failure in ICU patients. Obstruction is a less common cause. When renal failure is severe, indications for dialysis include hyperkalemia, fluid overload, mental status abnormalities, acidosis, and pericarditis. In addition, dialysis may be performed to prevent uremic bleeding or when blood urea nitrogen (BUN) and creatinine levels are high. The three modes of dialysis are hemodialysis, peritoneal dialysis, and continuous arteriovenous hemofiltration. The major questions of radiographic interest during dialysis are, Does the chest radiograph show a reduction in volume overload? Does the heart shadow suggest a pericardial effusion? Has the instrument for vascular access been safely inserted and properly positioned?

Hemodialysis

Chronic hemodialysis is performed through a surgically created arteriovenous shunt, but in ICU patients, large catheters are inserted in the femoral or subclavian veins for immediate access. Hemodialysis rapidly removes toxic substances and fluid, but it requires anticoagulation because the patient's blood is passed through pumps and filters. The patient must be able to tolerate dialysis-induced fluid shifts, and well-trained personnel and expensive and complex equipment are necessary.

Peritoneal Dialysis

Percutaneous or surgical placement of a peritoneal catheter allows dialysis to be performed with the peritoneal surface serving as an exchange membrane. Because exchange is less efficient than hemodialysis, peritoneal dialysis is used infrequently for emergency dialysis. It may be used for patients with unstable blood pressure or for removal of large amounts of fluid, and it does not require a dialysis machine or highly trained personnel.

A complication of peritoneal dialysis is bowel perforation during catheter placement. Because air can be introduced through the catheter, however, the finding of free air on the abdominal examination must be clinically evaluated. Chest radiographs obtained during peritoneal dialysis may show elevated diaphragms, pleural effusions, or free air.

Continuous Arteriovenous Hemofiltration (CAVH)

Continuous arteriovenous hemofiltration (CAVH) was devised to manage hemodynamically unstable patients with acute renal failure. It is commonly used for continuous fluid removal in patients whose primary problem is volume overload. Toxin and electrolyte removal with CAVH is less efficient than with hemodialysis, but the hemodynamics are better preserved. In the CAVH technique, intravenous and arterial catheters are placed in position, and the patient's blood pressure is used as a driving force for continuous fluid removal across a membrane. The gradual nature of the process reduces the risk of hypotension (Horton and Godley, 1988). As with other vascular catheters, the internal jugular or subclavian approach can cause bleeding or pneumothorax, and the femoral approach can lead to retroperitoneal hemorrhage.

RADIOLOGIC CONSULTATION IN THE ICU

General Policies

The activity in an ICU is constant and in a continual state of flux. Despite the unpredictable nature of critical disease, a daily routine is attempted with scheduled rounds, changes in shift, and educational conferences. Communication with the radiology department is crucial in coordinating these activities. Clinicians and radiologists should jointly outline procedures for obtaining daily and "stat." films and policies for transport.

Timing Routine Films

In general, the earlier that films are available for review, the better. Members of the ICU team and most consultants formulate a care plan early in the day, and radiographic information may alter therapeutic decisions. In addition, plain films may suggest further diagnostic testing, and scheduling is best performed early. Timing should coordinate both departmental and ICU daily routines. In the ICU, some important considerations include surgical scheduling,

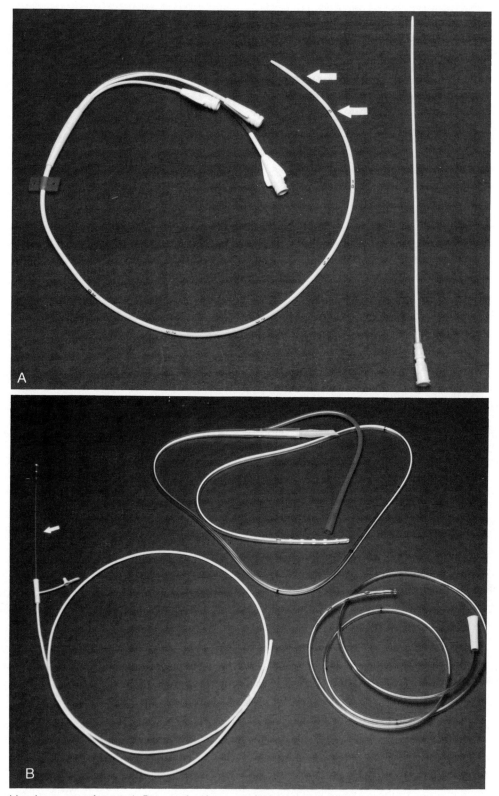

Figure 2–7. Nutritional support catheters. *A,* Parenteral catheters. *Left,* Triple-lumen catheter. *Arrows* indicate the two proximal ports. *Right,* Single-port catheter. *B,* Enteral feeding tubes. *Left,* Keofeed small-bore tube with stylet for insertion. *Right,* Levin tube. *Center,* Salem's sump tube.

timing of physician rounds, and nursing shift changes. These considerations must be coordinated with the capabilities of the radiology department.

We know of one ICU in which, like a "satellite" pharmacy, the radiology department moved closer to the patient. For ICU patients, all films and jackets were maintained at a multiviewer located adjacent to the unit. Each day, the radiologist would come to the ICU, conduct a joint conference, and after clinical correlation dictate interpretation via a telephone link. This step-saving, communication-enhancing mechanism was made possible by the collaboration of the radiology chairman and the ICU medical director.

Radiologic technologists and ICU nurses must also cooperate to ensure safe exposure. Technologists must understand how to work without causing decannulation, extubation, or disrupting other ICU functions. Conversely, nursing personnel should help position patients and ensure that support devices are not dislodged.

The "Stat." Film in the ICU

Stable ICU patients develop sudden crises with remarkable frequency. The "stat." call from the ICU for the radiology department's help frequently signals a respiratory disaster—for example, the oxygen saturation is dropping, the airway pressure is rising dangerously, or the blood pressure has plummeted. The major concerns are tension pneumothorax or a sudden change in the large airways, such as extubation, main bronchus intubation, mucous plugging, or collapse. Not only must the radiologist and radiologic technologist respond quickly, but also the ICU team must rapidly communicate the patient's history and clinical problem. The radiologist should call the results of stat. films to the ICU, and in some circumstances, the technologist should bring the film to the ICU. This plan allows direct communication between the radiologic and ICU teams and is helpful in determining a course of action. Stat. requests should be used judiciously to prevent lessening of their perceived urgency.

Transporting the ICU Patient

Most radiologists are familiar with the ICU patient who arrives in the radiology suite punctured by tubes, covered with intravenous (IV) lines, and connected to numerous pumps and monitors. We regularly send such patients to the radiology department. One hopes that despite the confusing and complex picture, nothing catastrophic will happen. Catastrophes do occur during transport, however, and just one cardiac or respiratory arrest in the radiology department is one too many.

The most common complications occurring during transport are respiratory and hemodynamic alterations (Indeck et al., 1988). Patients who require mechanical ventilation in the ICU are usually man-

ually ventilated during transport. Currently available manual devices can deliver 100% oxygen, and PEEP of up to 15 cm of H_2O, during transport. Several recent studies indicate that transport is safe if the levels of inspired oxygen, minute ventilation, and PEEP are similar to those supplied in the ICU (Braman et al., 1987; Weg and Haas, 1989). The patient's ventilator should be moved to the radiology suite for use throughout the procedure.

Pulse oximetry (which should be used during transport whenever possible) has allowed early recognition of hypoxemia. It is a simple, portable, and noninvasive method of determining the oxygen saturation of hemoglobin. The theoretic basis is the difference in visible red light absorption between saturated and unsaturated hemoglobin. Its use has revolutionized intraoperative monitoring and has expanded to intensive care, interventional radiology, and postoperative recovery as well. In addition, pulse oximetry can detect hypoxemia due to retained secretions, changes in patient position, worsening cardiac failure, altered tube position, and bronchospasm; all can appear during transport or imaging in the radiology suite.

Patients who are unstable hemodynamically should not be transported unless absolutely necessary. For some unstable patients (e.g., those with pelvic hemorrhage requiring embolization), radiologic diagnosis and therapy are both necessary and life-saving. For such patients, physicians and nurses must provide continuous monitoring and resuscitation throughout the procedure. Portable electrocardiogram (ECG) and intraarterial pressure monitors are helpful in these situations, but monitors must be watched closely. Massive volume infusion, vasopressors, or both may be required to maintain adequate blood pressure, particularly following sedation or paralysis. Care must be taken to avoid catheter displacement, disconnection, infusion of incompatible medication, or a sudden vasopressor bolus due to drug remaining in the line.

Changes in patient position can alter blood pressure, ventilation, or both. The lateral decubitus or head-up position, for example, can cause venous pooling and decreased preload. Many ICU patients are so sensitive to changes in cardiac preload that even small alterations can reduce cardiac output or blood pressure. Movement can also stop vasopressor infusion, owing to kinks in the lines. Another cause of hypotension is hypoxemia resulting from changes in ventilation or hypocarbia resulting from manual overventilation (Braman et al., 1987). Because hemodynamic and ventilatory changes are particularly likely to occur during positioning, careful monitoring for both are needed during any patient movement.

Sedation and paralysis are frequently needed for transporting and imaging ICU patients. Sedation should be administered with extreme caution to a spontaneously breathing patient. The dose required to calm a combative patient may be just adequate to suppress respiration several minutes later when the patient is lying unstimulated in a scanner. Radiology suites need to be equipped to handle emergencies, but prevention is preferable to resuscitation. Cautious administration of sedatives is warranted even in the intubated patient because of the hemodynamic side effects of virtually all available agents.

Our policy is to provide the same level of patient care during transport and imaging as the patient received in the ICU. Despite precautions, disaster strikes in the radiology department, just as it does in the ICU. All suites that handle such patients should be equipped with suction, oxygen, airway equipment, and resuscitation drugs. Radiology personnel must be attuned to the particular conditions of ICU patients and be prepared to provide outpost management.

Questions Clinicians Ask Radiologists

The radiologist can anticipate many of the questions clinicians will ask about ICU chest radiographs. The questions easiest to answer are related to tube and catheter placement; we recommend highlighting of each with a grease pencil. The more difficult questions involve complications and correlation of radiographic findings with clinical trends. A checklist summarizing some of these questions is presented in Table 2–1. Before attempting correlation, however, the radiologist should first ask the clinician several questions. These are listed in Table 2–2. Ideally, this information should be on the requisition, but it rarely is.

Position is a key factor in interpretation and should be clearly marked if it is not marked already by the technologist. The radiologist must obtain from the clinician information that is helpful in focusing the radiologic search. Physicians in the ICU often approach clinical problems on the basis of organ system, and if the radiologist's line of questioning follows this sequence, then a well-integrated response is more likely. The respiratory system in ventilated patients is often of paramount interest, and information regarding changes in lung function and mechanical support is essential to the radiologist. The state of the cardiovascular system naturally follows because cardiac function and the hemodynamic profile are

Table 2–1. QUESTIONS CLINICIANS ASK ABOUT ICU CHEST RADIOGRAPHS

Where is the tube or catheter? Is there a complication?

Devices	Check Location of	Optimal Location	Complications
Endotracheal tube	Tip	5–7 cm from carina	Cuff overinflation
	Cuff	≤ width of trachea	Gastric distention
Pulmonary artery catheter	Tip	Main PA trunks	PTX
			Pleural or mediastinal fluid
Central venous catheter	Proximal port	5 cm from tip	PTX
	Tip	Within thorax; outside atrium	Pleural or mediastinal fluid
Chest tubes	Tip	Within area to be drained	Persistent pleural fluid or PTX
	Side holes	Within pleural cavity	
Transvenous pacemaker	Tip	Apex of RV	PTX
			Pericardial effusion
			Pleural or mediastinal fluid
			Wire fracture or kink
Intra-aortic balloon pump	Tip	At aortic arch distal to origin of left subclavian artery	Evidence of aortic dissection
Nasogastric and enteral feeding tubes	Tip	In stomach or duodenum	Tracheobronchial placement
	Side holes	Beyond GE junction	PTX
			Pulmonary infiltrate

Why did the patient develop sudden respiratory distress?
Check for plugging with secretions, pneumothorax, atelectasis, and pulmonary edema. Consider thromboembolism.

Why did the P_{O_2} fall?
Check for increased fluid, new infiltrate, atelectasis, pneumothorax, hypoventilation, and pleural effusion.

Can you identify a source of the fever?
Check for infiltrates, collapse, atelectasis, and pleural effusions.

Why are pulmonary secretions increasing?
Check for infiltrates.

Has intubation caused any changes?
Check for lung expansion, barotrauma, aspiration, resolution of plugging, and collapse. Improvement in fluid overload or infiltrates is often more apparent than real.

Has extubation caused any changes?
Compare films for inspiratory effort. If they are comparable, look for increased fluid, aspiration, and atelectasis. Consider hypoventilatory changes before diagnosing pulmonary edema or new infiltrates.

Is there an explanation for a rise in airway pressures?
Check for barotrauma, plugging, collapse, increased fluid, and infiltrate.

GE, Gastroesophageal; PA, pulmonary artery; PTX, pneumothorax; RV, right ventricle.

Table 2–2. QUESTIONS RADIOLOGISTS SHOULD ASK CLINICIANS WHEN INTERPRETING
ICU CHEST RADIOGRAPHS

Has there been a change in ventilatory support?
(Including tidal volume, ventilatory mode, rate, level of pressure support, and PEEP)

Has there been a change in lung function?
(Including arterial blood gases and airway pressures)

What is the patient's fluid balance and cardiac status?
(Particularly if infiltrates have changed or appear to shift location)

Has there been clinical improvement or deterioration?
(Particularly when changes are marked or technique has changed)

Is the patient febrile, or is infection suspected?

Have any procedures been performed?
(Particularly suctioning, chest physiotherapy, bronchoscopy)

Are specific complications anticipated?

Does the patient have any unusual dressings or apparatus?
(Particularly in cases of unusual densities or linear shadows)

---

linked to any interpretation of pulmonary changes. Obviously, the systems of interest vary from patient to patient, but a systematic approach should be used.

THE RADIOLOGIST'S ROLE IN THE ICU

Daily Rounds

In our hospital, a radiologist is an integral part of the ICU team, both as an interpreter and as a consultant. Daily rounds are held in the radiologic suite with the ICU team, a radiologic resident, and an attending radiologist. A multiviewer, dedicated to ICU films, allows daily progress to be followed with ease. These rounds provide a trafficking of ideas, which benefits both radiologists and intensive care clinicians and improves patient care. Our radiologists, through familiarity with patient history and close clinical correlation, believe that rounds greatly enhance their experience and ability to interpret films. The clinicians obtain critical information, instruction in interpretation, and suggestions that could not be transmitted in formal reports. Discussions often proceed beyond the images of the day, with the radiologic team providing consultation for diagnostic and therapeutic planning.

Common Problems Requiring Consultation

As occurs in any specialty area, ICU patients often develop similar problems, and certain clinical situations arise repeatedly. A review of these circumstances and of their implications for the radiologist follows.

Sudden Respiratory Deterioration

Respiratory deterioration, characterized by a sudden drop in oxygen saturation or acute patient dis-

tress, often leads to a request for a stat. examination. The clinician responds immediately by manually ventilating the patient, excluding airway obstruction, examining the heart and lungs, and considering a circulatory disorder. An arterial blood gas study is obtained, and a radiograph is ordered. The differential diagnosis is great, and findings that are explanatory include new infiltrates suggesting aspiration pneumonia, pulmonary edema, lobar collapse, main bronchial intubation, and pneumothorax. Radiographic findings in each instance usually result in immediate changes in therapy.

If the chest radiograph does not provide an explanation, then the radiologist might suggest a number of potential problems that cause abrupt deterioration in oxygenation with little or no impact on the chest radiograph. Before suggesting pulmonary embolism, one should first consider plugging with secretions, bronchospasm, reversal of hypoxic pulmonary vasoconstriction by vasodilators, and microatelectasis. If pulmonary embolus is a reasonable possibility, then the radiologist and the clinician should jointly consider a diagnostic and therapeutic approach. Pulmonary hypertension, contraindications to anticoagulation or contrast load, and stability for transport are all considerations (see Chapter 9).

Change in Neurologic Status

Deterioration in mental status is another frequent problem in the ICU. Before imaging is requested, the level of consciousness, verbal and motor responses, cranial nerve function, and breathing pattern should be evaluated. This information, along with laboratory assessment, helps distinguish mass lesions from metabolic ones. If a mass lesion is suspected, then diagnostic studies are indicated. If elevated intracranial pressure is suspected, therapy should precede imaging. Computed tomography (CT) of the head can differentiate most of the treatable causes of neurologic deterioration: intracerebral, subarachnoid, and epidural and subdural hemorrhage; hydrocephalus; edema; and abscess. Although CT of the head does not help in diagnosing meningitis, it is often performed prior to a lumbar puncture to assure the absence of significant cerebral edema. The need for further studies such as angiography or magnetic resonance imaging (MRI) must be determined in a collaborative fashion by both radiologist and clinician (see Chapter 20).

The neurologic changes that most often lead to spinal imaging are peripheral sensory or motor findings suggesting spinal cord compression. Patients recovering from surgery for abdominal aneurysm, those with metastatic tumor, and those with subarachnoid or epidural catheters are at risk. Because urgent decompression is required, an expedient work-up is necessary.

Sepsis Without an Obvious Source

Some ICU patients are admitted with sepsis, but many develop infections during their stay. The usual scenario is a sudden increase in temperature or white blood count (WBC). These signs prompt clinical and laboratory evaluation including physical examination, Gram's stain, and cultures. Common sources of infection include urinary catheters, IV lines, and surgical or traumatic wounds. The radiologist is asked to assist in searching for the source. The chest radiograph may reveal pneumonia. Sinus films should be obtained if any nasal tube is present, and a technetium-labeled acetanilidoiminodiacetic acid (HIDA) scan may be warranted if cholecystitis is suspected. Chest or abdominal CT, when clinically appropriate, can be invaluable. Imaging may be combined with therapy because advances in interventional radiology have allowed nonsurgical drainage of the biliary tract, of the gallbladder, and of abdominal abscesses (see Chapters 17 through 19).

Upper and Lower Gastrointestinal Bleeding

Upper GI endoscopy is the most useful procedure for ascertaining the source of upper GI bleeding. With the advent of electrocoagulation, heat coagulation, and lasers, the therapeutic range of endoscopy has expanded as well. Sclerotherapy via the endoscope is now performed as first-line therapy for variceal bleeding. Ongoing bleeding that does not respond to endoscopic therapy, however, may require radiologic intervention. Examples of such situations are tears from Mallory-Weiss syndrome and hemorrhage in poor surgical candidates. In general, considerations for surgical or radiologic intervention include age, multiple coexisting diseases, amount of blood transfused, hemodynamic stability, and potential for recurrence of bleeding.

Colonoscopy is inferior to radiologic techniques for localizing the source of lower GI bleeding. After the site of bleeding has been pinpointed, usually via radionuclide scanning, considerations similar to those for upper GI bleeding determine whether surgery or interventional radiologic treatment is appropriate.

Hemodynamic Instability

Severe hypotension is a common problem in the ICU, but imaging is rarely required for diagnosis. When acute pericardial tamponade or valvular insufficiency is involved in the differential diagnosis, however, portable echocardiography is usually diagnostic. The presence of diastolic collapse indicates pericardial tamponade, which requires placement of a drainage needle under sonographic guidance or, in postsurgical patients, reoperation (see Chapter 14). Valvular insufficiency is suspected from the physical examination and can be confirmed by portable echocardiography. Retroperitoneal hemorrhage, another cause of hemodynamic instability, is best confirmed or refuted with CT.

Interpretation: Hedging vs. Helping

Patients in the ICU often present complex and confusing problems in clinical and radiologic diagnosis. The radiologist is frequently asked to help, but the clinician needs more than a list of all possible diagnoses that the radiograph suggests. In our experience, such a list represents hedging more than helping. Unquestionably, a differential diagnosis is useful. What is more useful, however, is a radiologist who is willing to make a commitment—to say, "I can't be sure, but in my experience, this probably represents . . ." In other words, we think that despite the uncertainty involved, a radiologist's best judgment is invaluable to a clinician who must also make a best judgment in the face of clinical deterioration.

Determination of the Appropriate Imaging Technique

Clinicians need, but too infrequently seek, advice about the choice of an imaging technique. The choices are overwhelming, and many clinicians simply do not have the expertise to make them. Again, communication between the ICU and radiologic teams is essential. The clinician needs to present background information and to frame the questions that the study should answer. A radiologist who understands the clinical problem can weigh the advantages and disadvantages of each study and recommend an approach. This interaction is essential if patients are to be prevented from being transported for studies that when reviewed by the radiologist could not possibly answer the clinical question.

Therapeutic Intervention

The last major category in which the radiologic and ICU teams interact is therapeutic intervention. Many ICU patients are poor surgical candidates, and embolization, ultrasonography- or CT-guided drainage, or angiographic placement of catheters and drugs may be preferable to operation. Details of these procedures are covered in later chapters.

As clinicians who care for critically ill patients, we need support from our radiologic colleagues. We need their interpretation and advice on the right study to order. Radiologists should visit the ICU in the hospital, look at the patients, and talk to the nurses and technologists. We need to understand each other's problems, and we need the experience and judgment of radiologists. Through communication, teamwork, and mutual respect, we can deliver the best patient care.

References

Aberle, D.R., Wiener-Kronish, J.P., Webb, W.R., and Matthay, M.A.: Hydrostatic versus increased permeability pulmonary edema: Diagnosis based on radiographic criteria in critically ill patients. Radiology 168:73, 1988.

Altman, A.R., and Johnson, T.H.: Rocntgcnographic findings in PEEP therapy. JAMA 242:727, 1979.

Bishop, M.J.: Mechanisms of laryngotracheal injury following prolonged tracheal intubation. Chest 96:185, 1989.

Braman, S.S., Dunn, S.M., Amico, C.A., and Millman, R.P.: Complications of intrahospital transport in critically ill patients. Ann. Intern. Med. 107:469, 1987.

Brunel, W., Coleman, D.L., Schwartz, D.E., et al.: Assessment of routine chest roentgenograms and the physical examination to confirm endotracheal tube position. Chest 96:1043, 1989.

Butler, P.W., Bone, R.C., and Field, T.: Technology under Medicare diagnosis-related groups prospective payment: Implications for medical intensive care. Chest 87:229, 1985.

Caplan, E.S., and Hoyt, N.J.: Nosocomial sinusitis. JAMA 247:639, 1982.

Cole, R.R., and Aguilar, E.A.: Cricothyroidotomy versus tracheotomy: An otolaryngologist's perspective. Laryngoscope 98:131, 1988.

Colice, G.L.: Prolonged intubation versus tracheotomy in the adult. Journal of Intensive Care Medicine 2:85, 1987.

Colice, G.L., Stukel, T.A., and Dain, D.: Laryngeal complications of prolonged intubation. Chest 96:877, 1989.

Cooper, J.D., and Malt, R.A.: Meteorism produced by nasotracheal intubation and ventilatory assistance. N. Engl. J. Med. 287:652, 1977.

DeCamp, M.M., and Demling, R.H.: Posttraumatic multisystem organ failure. JAMA 260:530, 1988.

Efferen, L.S., Nadarajah, D., and Palat, D.S.: Survival following mechanical ventilation for *Pneumocystis carinii* pneumonia in patients with acquired immunodeficiency syndrome: A different perspective. Am. J. Med. 87:401, 1989.

El-Sadar, W., and Simberkoff, M.S.: Survival and prognostic factors in severe *Pneumocystis carinii* pneumonia requiring mechanical ventilation. Am. Rev. Respir. Dis. 137:1264–67, 1988.

Golden, G.T., and Chandler, J.G.: Colemic ileus and cecal perforation in patients requiring mechanical ventilatory support. Chest 68:661, 1975.

Goldenheim, P.D., and Kazemi, H.: Cardiopulmonary monitoring of critically ill patients. N. Engl. J. Med. 311:776, 1984.

Goodman, L.R., and Putman, C.E.: Radiological evaluation of patients receiving assisted ventilation. JAMA 245:858, 1981.

Gregg, R.W., Friedman, B.C., Williams, J.F., et al.: Continuous positive airway pressure by face mask in *Pneumocystis Carinii* pneumonia. Crit. Care Med. 18:21, 1990.

Heffner, J.E., Miller, K.S., and Sahn, S.A.: Tracheostomy in the intensive care unit. Part 1. Indications, technique, management. Chest 90:269, 1986a.

Heffner, J.E., Miller, K.S., and Sahn, S.A.: Tracheostomy in the intensive care unit. Part 2. Complications. Chest 90:430, 1986b.

Heinonen, J., Takki, S., and Tammisto, T.: Effect of the Trendelenburg tilt and other procedures on the position of endotracheal tubes. Lancet 1:850, 1969.

Horton, M.W., and Godley, P.J.: Continuous arteriovenous hemofiltration: An alternative to hemodialysis. Am. J. Hosp. Pharm. 45:1361, 1988.

Indeck, M., Peterson, S., Smith, J., and Brotman, S.: Risk, cost and benefit of transporting ICU patients for special studies. J. Trauma 28:1020, 1988.

Kalb, P.E., and Miller, D.H.: Utilization strategies for intensive care units. JAMA 261:2389, 1989.

Knaus, W.A., and Thibault, G.E.: Intensive care units today. *In* McNeil, B.J., and Cravalho, E.G.: Critical Issues in Medical Technology. Boston, Auburn House, 1982, p. 193.

Knaus, W.A., Draper, E.A., Wagner, D.P., and Zimmerman, J.E.: APACHE II: A severity of disease classification system. Crit. Care Med. 13:818, 1985.

Kronberg, F.G., and Goodwin, W.J.: Sinusitis in intensive care unit patients. Laryngoscope 95:936, 1985.

Matthay, M.A., and Chatterjee, K.: Bedside catheterization of the pulmonary artery: Risks compared with benefits. Ann. Intern. Med. 109:826, 1988.

Mayer-Oakes, S.A., Oye, R.K., Leake, B., and Brook, R.H.: The early effect of Medicare's prospective payment system on the use of medical intensive care services in community hospitals. JAMA 260:3146, 1988.

MayoSmith, M.F., Hirsch, P.J., Wodzinski, S.F., and Schiffman, F.J.: Acute epiglottis in adults. N. Engl. J. Med. 314:1133, 1986.

McHugh, T.J., Forrester, J.S., Adler, L., et al.: Pulmonary vascular congestion in acute myocardial infarction: Hemodynamic and radiologic correlations. Ann. Intern. Med. 76:29, 1972.

Milne, E.N., Pistolesi, M., Miniati, M., and Giuntini, C.: The radiologic distinction of cardiogenic and noncardiogenic edema. AJR 144:879, 1985.

Rosen, M.J., Cucco, R.A., and Teirstein, A.S.: Outcome of intensive care in patients with the acquired immunodeficiency syndrome. Journal of Intensive Care Medicine 1:55, 1986.

Shapiro, J., Eavey, R.D., and Baker, A.S.: Adult supraglottitis: A prospective analysis. JAMA 259:563, 1988.

Sibbald, W.J., Cunningham, D.R., and Chin, D.N.: Non-cardiac or cardiac pulmonary edema? A practical approach to clinical differentiation in critically ill patients. Chest 84:452, 1983.

Smith, R.C., Mann, H., Greenspan, R.H., et al.: Radiographic differentiation between different etiologies of pulmonary edema. Invest. Radiol. 22:859, 1987.

Sprung, C.L., Rackow, E.C., Fein, I.A., et al.: The spectrum of pulmonary edema: Differentiation of cardiogenic, intermediate, and noncardiogenic forms of pulmonary edema. Am. Rev. Respir. Dis. 124:718, 1981.

Taryle, D.A., Chandler, J.E., Good, J.T., Jr., et al.: Emergency room intubations—complications and survival. Chest 75:541, 1979.

Wachter, R.M., Luce, J.M., Lo, B., and Taffin, T.A.: Life-sustaining treatment for patients with AIDS. Chest 95:647, 1989.

Wagner, D.P., Knaus, W.A., and Draper, E.A.: Identification of low-risk monitor admissions to medical-surgical ICUs. Chest 92:423, 1987.

Wechsler, R.J., Steiner, R.M., and Kinori, I.: Monitoring the monitors: The radiology of thoracic catheters, wires, and tubes. Semin. Roentgenol. 23:61, 1988.

Weg, J.G., and Haas, C.F.: Safe intrahospital transport of critically ill ventilator-dependent patients. Chest 96:631, 1989.

Wiedemann, H.P., Matthay, M.A., and Matthay, R.A.: Cardiovascular-pulmonary monitoring in the intensive care unit (Part 2). Chest 85:656, 1984.

Zimmerman, J.E., (Ed.): APACHE III study design: Analytic plan for evaluation of severity and outcome. Crit. Care Med. 17:S169, 1989.

Zimmerman, J.E., Goodman, L.R., et al.: Effect of mechanical ventilation and PEEP on the chest radiograph. AJR 133:811, 1979.

Zimmerman, J.E., Goodman, L.R., St. Andre, A.C., and Wyman, A.C.: Radiographic detection of mobilizable lung water: The gravitational shift test. AJR 138:59, 1982.

SUPPORT AND MONITORING DEVICES

3

Pulmonary Support and Monitoring Apparatus

■

Lawrence R. Goodman

In the intensive care unit (ICU), various types of catheters, tubes, and support equipment are routinely used. Proper placement of this equipment is essential if it is to serve its purposes of monitoring and support. Many potential problems can be recognized on the radiograph and prevented before they occur. Other complications can be diagnosed soon after their occurrence, and corrective action can be taken before further damage is done. Each radiograph should be scanned for visible or *expected* catheters prior to evaluation for cardiopulmonary disease so that barely opaque or misplaced catheters are not overlooked. This chapter discusses the correct placement of pulmonary support and monitoring equipment and the early identification of complications associated with their use.

ENDOTRACHEAL TUBES

Normal Position and Appearance

Proper positioning of the endotracheal tube (orotracheal or nasotracheal tube) minimizes complications associated with intubation. Clinical evaluation of endotracheal tube position (bilateral breath sounds, symmetric thoracic expansion, and palpation of the tube in the suprasternal notch) does not detect the majority of malpositioned tubes (Birmingham et al., 1986; Brunel et al., 1989). Therefore, radiographs should be routinely obtained immediately after each intubation. Daily radiographs ensure that the tube has not been inadvertently displaced by the weight of the respirator apparatus, by the patient's coughing, or by other unforeseen events. Henschke and colleagues (1983), in a study of 611 consecutive portable chest radiographs of intubated patients, found that 12% of tubes were malpositioned.

Proper radiographic evaluation of the endotracheal tube position requires an estimate of the position of the tube tip in relation to the carina and a knowledge of the position of the head and neck during radiography. Most endotracheal tubes are opaque or have an opaque strip demarcating the tip of the tube (see Figs. 2–1 and 2–2). In some endotracheal tubes with reinforcing spiral wires used to prevent kinking, the opaque spiral ends several centimeters short of this tip. As a result, the depth of the tube may be underestimated (Gorback and Ravin, 1987) (Fig. 3–1).

The carina is most accurately located by following the inferior wall of the left main bronchus medially until it joins the right main bronchus. If the carina is not visible on a given radiograph, its position may be estimated in one of two ways: (1) It may be estimated from previous portable radiographs, because the carina maintains a relatively constant position in relation to the vertebral bodies. (2) It may be estimated in relation to the thoracic vertebral bodies. On the portable radiograph, the carina projects over T5, T6, or T7 in 95% of patients (Goodman et al., 1976) (Fig. 3–2). Therefore, if it is not visible, one should assume that the carina is at the level of the T4–T5 interspace. The vocal cords are usually at the level of C5–C6.

Flexion and extension of the head and neck cause considerable movement of the endotracheal tube tip in relation to the carina (Conrardy et al., 1976) (Fig. 3–3). Because the tube is fixed at the nose or mouth, only the distal tip is free to move with head and neck motion. Neck flexion from the neutral position causes approximately a 2-cm descent of the endotracheal tube. Similarly, neck extension from the neutral position causes a 2-cm ascent. This combined excursion of 4 cm is approximately one third the length of the trachea, which measures 12 cm in the average adult. Therefore, a tube that appears to be in good position

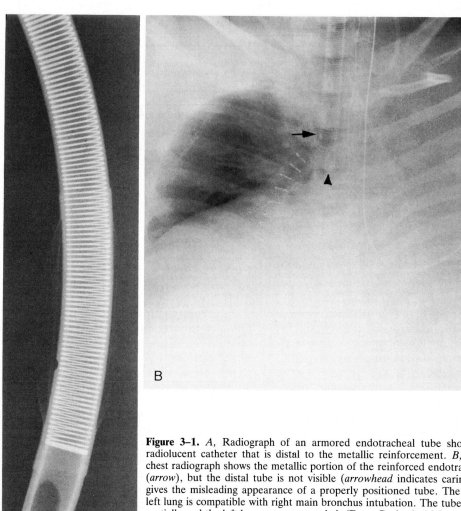

Figure 3–1. *A,* Radiograph of an armored endotracheal tube shows a relatively radiolucent catheter that is distal to the metallic reinforcement. *B,* Intraoperative chest radiograph shows the metallic portion of the reinforced endotracheal tube well (*arrow*), but the distal tube is not visible (*arrowhead* indicates carina). This image gives the misleading appearance of a properly positioned tube. The collapse of the left lung is compatible with right main bronchus intubation. The tube was withdrawn partially and the left lung was re-expanded. (From Gorback, M.S., and Ravin, C.E.: Reinforced endotracheal tube placement: Radiographic misdiagnosis. Radiology 162:579, 1987, with permission).

Figure 3–2. The position of the carina in relation to the vertebral bodies as shown on the portable chest radiograph (100 patients). (From Goodman, L.R., et al.: Radiographic evaluation of endotracheal tube position. AJR 127:433–434, 1976, with permission, © by American Roentgen Ray Society.)

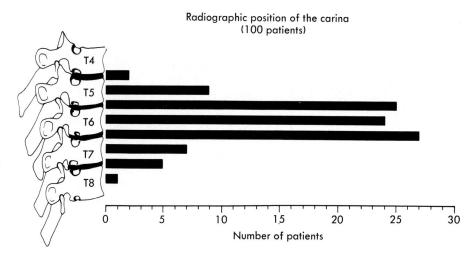

Radiographic position of the carina
(100 patients)

Number of patients

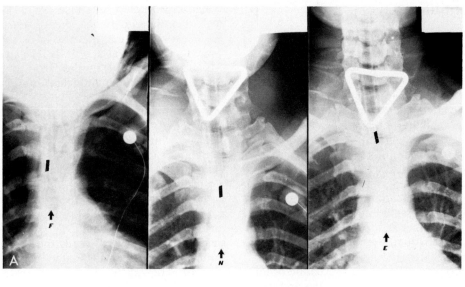

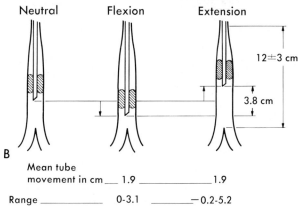

Figure 3–3. *A,* Effects of flexion and extension of the head and neck on endotracheal tube position (*arrows* indicate carina). The tube descends approximately 2 cm when the neck is flexed (F), and it ascends approximately 3 cm when the neck is extended (E). In the neutral position (N), the mandible is over the lower cervical spine. When the neck is flexed, the mandible is over the upper thoracic spine. When the neck is extended, the mandible is above C4, often off the film. *B,* Mean endotracheal tube movement with flexion and extension of the neck from the neutral position (in 20 patients). The mean tube movement is approximately one third the length of the normal adult trachea. (*B,* From Conrady, P. A., et al.: Alteration of endotracheal tube position: Flexion and extension of the neck. Crit. Care Med. 4:7–12, 1976, © by Williams & Wilkins Co., 1976.)

in the middle of the trachea when the head and neck are extended may lodge in the right main bronchus when the head and neck are flexed.

The position of the head and neck can usually be determined from the radiograph itself (Goodman et al., 1976). In the neutral position, the inferior border of the mandible projects over the lower cervical spine (C5–C6). In full flexion, the mandible is over the upper thoracic spine; in full extension, the mandible is above C4 (which is often off the film) (see Fig. 3–3*A*). Other alterations in position such as turning the head laterally, sitting, or assuming Trendelenburg's position cause only minor changes in the position of the endotracheal tube in relation to the carina (Alberti et al., 1967; Conrardy et al., 1976; Heinonen et al., 1969).

In summary, the following guidelines are suggested for evaluating endotracheal tube position:

1. When the head and neck are in the neutral position, the endotracheal tube tip is ideally in the mid-trachea, approximately 5 to 7 cm from the carina.

2. When the head and neck are flexed, the tube has descended maximally, so that it is ideally 3 to 5 cm from the carina.

3. When the head and neck are extended, the tube has ascended maximally, so that it is ideally 7 to 9 cm from the carina.

The ideal endotracheal tube as visualized on the radiograph is one half to two thirds the width of the trachea. Wider tubes are associated with an increased incidence of laryngeal injury, and narrower tubes have a significantly increased airway resistance. The inflated cuff should fill the tracheal lumen but not bulge the lateral tracheal walls. The cuff should not narrow the endotracheal tube nor deflect the tube bevel toward the lateral tracheal wall.

Potential Complications

In a prospective study of 226 endotracheal intubations, Stauffer and associates (1981) noted 268 complications. The most frequent problems were difficulty in sealing the airway (64 patients), self-extubation (29), right main bronchus intubation (21), and aspiration of gastric contents (17). Less frequent complications of radiographic importance included pharyngeal, laryngeal, or tracheal injuries, broken and aspirated teeth, esophageal intubation, and sinusitis.

Malposition. Approximately 10% to 20% of endotracheal tubes require repositioning after insertion, half for inadvertent intubation of the right main bronchus (Brunel et al., 1989; Pingleton, 1988; Stauffer et al., 1981; Zwillich et al., 1974). Following right main bronchial intubation, the left lung becomes atelectatic, and the right lung is hyperinflated. If radiography is performed early or if ventilation of the left lung continues via the side hole in the endotracheal tube, the radiograph merely demonstrates the aberrant catheter in the right main bronchus (Fig. 3–4). With time, the left lung becomes atelectatic, the mediastinum shifts to the left, and the right lung becomes hyperlucent (Fig. 3–5). The higher the inspired oxygen concentration, the more rapid the collapse of the left lung (see Fig. 3–1B). In mechanically ventilated patients, hyperdistension of the right lung leads to pneumothorax in as many as 15% of patients (Zwillich et al., 1974). Because the left main bronchus branches from the carina at a sharper angle, accidental left main bronchial intubation is uncommon.

If the endotracheal tube is inadvertently placed in the pharynx or is dislodged from the proximal trachea—owing to extension of the head and neck, coughing, or inadequate fixation—mechanical ventilation is disrupted, the stomach usually dilates, and gastric contents may be regurgitated (Fig. 3–6A). Reintubation, regardless of the cause, is associated with an increased incidence of aspiration pneumonitis and pneumonia (Rashkin and Davis, 1986). A tube placed just beyond the vocal cords may lead to vocal cord injury when the cuff is inflated between or just below the cords (Zwillich et al., 1974) (see Fig. 3–6B).

Inadvertent insertion of the endotracheal tube into the esophagus is an unusual but potentially life-threatening mishap that often goes undetected clinically (Birmingham et al., 1986). In a review of anteroposterior (AP) radiographs of six cases of esophageal intubation, Smith and co-workers (1990) noted that the endotracheal tube was lateral to the tracheal

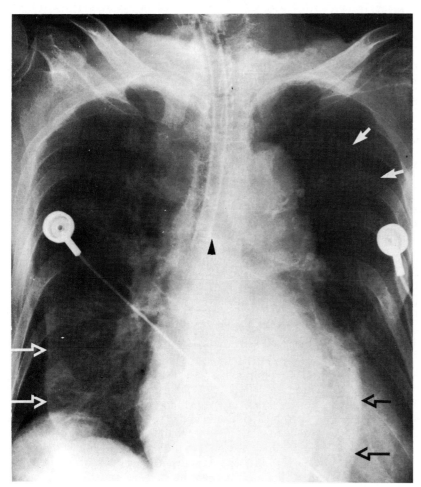

Figure 3–4. Film obtained immediately after intubation demonstrates endotracheal tube in the right main bronchus (*arrowhead* indicates carina). The effects of selective aeration are not yet evident. The density over the heart shadow (*black arrows*) is caused by the breast. A left upper skin fold (*closed white arrows*) and the right breast shadow (*open white arrows*) mimic a bilateral pneumothorax.

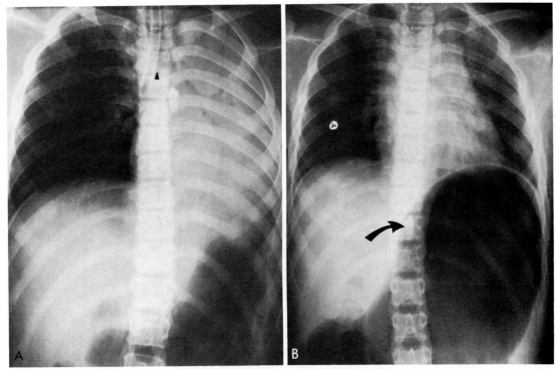

Figure 3–5. Right main bronchus intubation. *A,* The endotracheal tube is in the right main bronchus (*arrowhead* indicates carina). The left lung is completely opacified with marked atelectasis. To the left of the spine, the radiodensity represents a dislodged tooth in the esophagus. *B,* Twenty-four hours later, after the endotracheal tube has been repositioned, almost complete re-expansion of the left lung is evident. The mediastinum has returned to the midline. Marked gastric distention is noted. The swallowed tooth is now seen near the gastroesophageal junction (*arrow*). (From Goodman, L.R., and Putman, C.E.: Radiological evaluation of patients receiving assisted ventilation. JAMA 245:858, 1981, with permission. Copyright 1981, American Medical Association.)

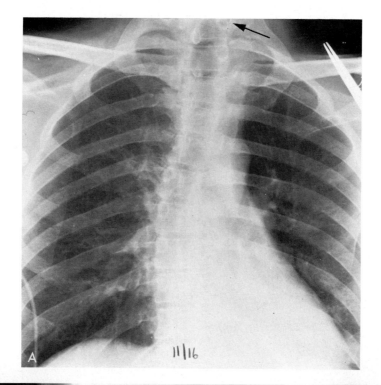

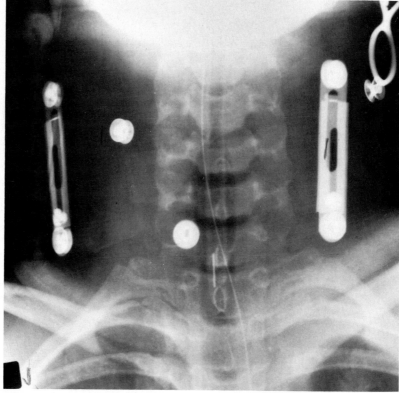

Figure 3–6. Endotracheal tube placed too high. *A*, The tip of the endotracheal tube (*arrow*) is above and to the left of the trachea, presumably in the pyriform sinus. Left lower lobe consolidation results from aspiration of gastric contents. *B*, Anteroposterior view of the neck of a different patient shows the endotracheal tube in the cervical trachea. The inflated cuff is between the vocal cords.

air shadow in five patients, that the stomach was dilated with air in four patients, that the esophagus was dilated with air in two patients, and that the trachea was displaced by the inflated cuff in one patient (Fig. 3–7A). In a subsequent study of 328 patients with both endotracheal and nasogastric tubes in appropriate position, the same authors demonstrated that turning the head to the right and turning the patient 25 degrees to the right threw the tracheal shadow to the right of the esophagus in more than 75% of patients. The opposite maneuver to the left superimposed the two structures in all patients. Thus, the right posterior oblique (RPO) positioning is useful, but not totally reliable, in confirming or refuting the possibility of esophageal intubation (see Fig. 3–7B).

Another uncommon but potentially serious complication of endotracheal intubation is tracheal or laryngeal laceration. Rollins and Tocino (1987) described the early radiographic signs of tracheal rupture in seven patients, five of whom had no history of blunt chest trauma. In all cases, the endotracheal tube tip was oriented to the right, and pneumomediastinum or subcutaneous emphysema was present on the first radiograph. In six of the seven patients, the tracheal cuff was greater than 2.8 cm (normal measurement is 2 to 2.5 cm), and the lower margin of the cuff was less than 1.2 cm from the tip of the tube (normal measurement is 2.5 cm). Four patients demonstrated pneumothorax on the initial film, and three showed development of pneumothorax on subsequent films. A combination of a deviated endotracheal tube and an enlarged cuff was present in six of the seven patients (Fig. 3–8). The large cuff was likely a result of the traumatic intubation, rather than the cause of the rupture, because none of the cuffs were inflated to excessive pressure. Other causes for enlarged tracheal balloons include inadvertent hyperinflation, intra-esophageal location, chronic intubation, and tracheomegaly.

Although superficial injury to the hypopharyngeal and laryngeal mucosa is common during intubation, perforation is not. When perforation occurs, it is usually through the pyriform sinus or the region of the cricopharyngeal muscle (Hirsch et al., 1978; Ward et al., 1985). The presence of subcutaneous emphysema, pneumomediastinum, or pneumothorax immediately after a difficult intubation suggests this diagnosis. Occasionally, the laceration may remain undiagnosed for days, until the patient develops fever or signs and symptoms of a mediastinal or cervical infection. Early diagnosis and treatment are associated with a greatly improved outcome. Therefore, the diagnosis should be pursued aggressively. Conventional radiographs may demonstrate mediastinal widening or air in the neck or mediastinum. Negative radiographs do not exclude the diagnosis. Computed tomography (CT) of the neck and upper mediastinum is considerably more sensitive than conventional imaging for the diagnosis of cervical or mediastinal infection. Computed tomography demonstrates air or fluid, or both, in the neck or mediastinum, often allows detection of the site of perforation, and allows documentation of the location of the endotracheal tube tip (Ward et al., 1985) (Fig. 3–9). A negative CT scan makes perforation extremely unlikely.

Secretions and Atelectasis. The clearance of pharyngeal, tracheobronchial, and pulmonary secretions is a serious problem for the intubated patient. Adequate coughing requires an intact, functioning glottis, functioning cilia, adequate respiratory muscles, and a vital capacity that is at least three times the tidal volume. Despite meticulous suctioning and physical therapy, atelectasis is the most frequent single cause of pulmonary consolidation in the intubated patient. Except for streaks of discoid atelectasis or major segmental or lobar collapse, definitive differentiation between atelectasis and other causes of parenchymal consolidation is usually difficult on the basis of a single radiograph. Rapid changes in the radiographic appearance over hours or days strongly suggest the diagnosis of atelectasis (see Chapter 5).

Tracheobronchial Obstruction. The most frequent cause of obstruction in the intubated patient is mucous plugs or blood clots, which are seldom recognized on the radiograph. Fillings, teeth, or broken dentures may be dislodged during intubation and either aspirated or swallowed. Symptoms are often unrecognized or absent in the obtunded patient. Well-penetrated AP radiographs usually allow detection of these opaque objects, but RPO radiographs may be necessary to separate an intratracheal from an upper esophageal location (see Fig. 3–5). Small endobronchial foreign bodies usually lodge in the gravity-dependent segments. Distal atelectasis is variable. A lateral radiograph, or even CT, may be necessary to localize the foreign body prior to bronchoscopy.

The endotracheal tube and cuff constitute another potential cause of airway obstruction. The high-volume, low-pressure cuff may cover the tip of the tube. This form of airway obstruction is most likely a consequence of partial withdrawal of the tube while the balloon is only partially deflated. Rarely, a hyperdistended cuff may pinch the catheter lumen, or eccentric dilatation of the cuff may deflect the tip laterally against the wall of the trachea (Sinfield et al., 1989). The cuff is usually visible and should therefore be evaluated on each radiograph.

Sinusitis. Nasotracheal intubation causes ipsilateral mucosal edema and obstruction in the majority of intubated patients. Fassoulaki and Pamouktsoglou (1989) performed CT scans on 16 intubated patients, 3 days and 8 days after intubation. By 3 days, six patients had evidence of mucosal thickening in the ipsilateral maxillary or sphenoid sinuses. By 8 days, 14 patients had evidence of mucosal thickening and fluid in at least one ipsilateral sinus. All CT scans cleared or improved without treatment within 8 days of extubation. Hansen and colleagues (1988) demonstrated CT changes in all of 12 neurosurgical patients 3 days after intubation. In seven patients, positive cultures were obtained from ipsilateral pu-

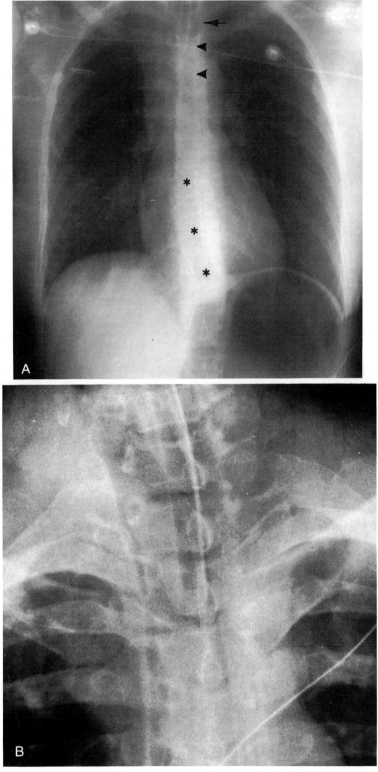

Figure 3–7. Esophageal intubation. *A,* The cuff of the endotracheal tube (*arrow*) is located to the left of the left wall of the trachea (*arrowheads*). Air distends the esophagus (*asterisks*) and the stomach. *B,* In a right posterior oblique projection of a different patient, the endotracheal tube in the esophagus projects to the left of the tracheal air column. (From Smith, G.M., et al.: Radiographic detection of esophageal malpositioning of endotracheal tubes. AJR 154:23–26, 1990, with permission, © by American Roentgen Ray Society.)

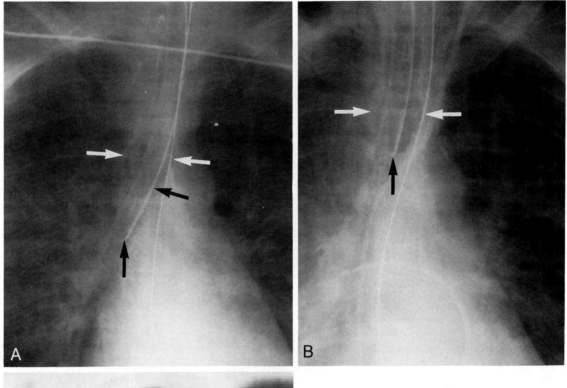

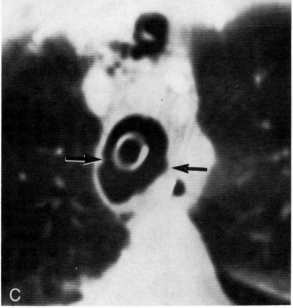

Figure 3–8. Tracheal rupture. *A,* After intubation, the endotracheal tube is in the right main bronchus with a balloon diameter of 3.2 cm (*white arrows*). The balloon-to-tip distance is 3.5 cm (*black arrows*). *B,* After repositioning, the overdistended balloon (*white arrows*) is now at the tip of the endotracheal tube (*black arrow*), and subcutaneous and mediastinal emphysema is now evident. *C,* Computed tomographic scan performed through trachea demonstrates tracheal laceration (*arrows*) with overdistended cuff in the mediastinum. Air is seen in the mediastinum. (From Rollins, R.J., and Tocino, I.: Early radiographic signs of tracheal rupture. AJR 148:695–698, 1987, with permission, © by American Roentgen Ray Society.)

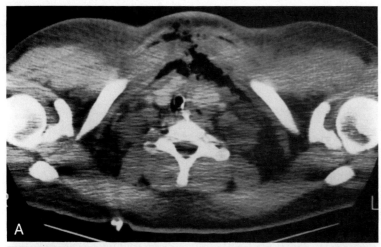

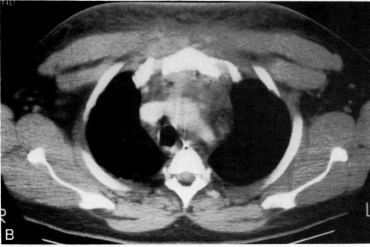

Figure 3–9. Patient developed a fever and a widened superior mediastinum several days after a difficult intubation. *A,* Computed tomographic scan at the base of the neck shows marked subcutaneous emphysema, edema, and the endotracheal tube within the tracheal lumen. *B,* Computed tomographic scan performed just above the aortic arch shows a large fluid collection in the anterior mediastinum as well as several small dots of air. The subcutaneous tissue is edematous. This abscess of the neck and substernal region was confirmed at surgery.

rulent nasal discharge. Conversely, Aebert and associates (1988) reported only a 2.3% incidence of purulent sinusitis based on clinical criteria and AP sinus radiographs.

From these diverse studies, one is left to conclude that mucosal edema and retained fluid are extremely common after nasal intubation but are usually self-limited and not associated with *clinical* sinus infection. Conversely, bedside sinus radiographs are not adequate to *exclude* fluid in the sinuses, especially in the sphenoid sinus. If sinusitis is suspected as a cause of an undetermined fever, and if the sinus radiographs are normal, CT allows determination of the presence or absence of mucosal thickening, fluid, or both. A negative scan essentially excludes sinusitis, but a positive scan requires bacteriologic evaluation.

TRACHEOSTOMY AND TRACHEOSTOMY TUBES

Normal Position and Appearance

Tracheostomy is rarely a primary procedure. It is usually performed 1 to 3 weeks after endotracheal intubation for patients who require long-term mechanical ventilation or tracheal suctioning, or in patients with upper airway obstruction. Because of the long-term risks of tracheostomy, the current trend is toward longer duration of endotracheal intubation, prior to tracheostomy (Heffner et al., 1986a, 1986b; Stauffer et al., 1981). The tracheostomy tube, which is inserted through a stoma at the level of the third tracheal cartilage, should sit with its tip several centimeters above the carina (Fig. 3–10). Unlike the endotracheal tube, motion of the head and neck has little influence on the position of the tube in relation to the carina. The ideal tube is one half to two thirds the width of the trachea. This width minimizes airway resistance and ensures that the tube is parallel to the tracheal lumen. The cuff should not distend to the tracheal wall.

After extubation, some patients who require further suctioning, or possibly re-intubation, are fitted with a short, straight tube that traverses the stoma and the anterior tracheal wall to hold the stoma open (Kistner's or Olympic button) (see Fig. 2–2B). Another transtracheal tube is the "mini-tracheostomy," a narrow-gauge tube used for transtracheal suctioning rather than respiration (Pedersen et al., 1988).

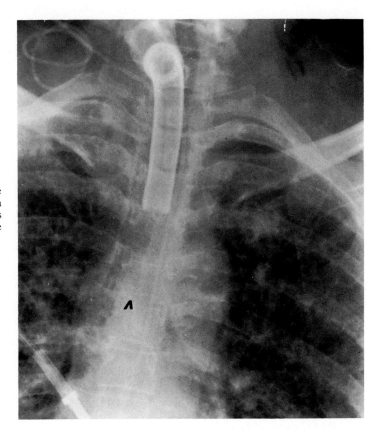

Figure 3–10. Ideally positioned tracheostomy tube. The tracheostomy tube is two thirds the width of the trachea and is parallel to the long axis of the trachea. The tip is located one half to two thirds the distance between the stoma and the carina.

Potential Complications

Complications of tracheostomy are usually divided into those occurring during the perioperative period, those occurring during intubation, and those occurring after extubation. With improved surgical techniques, significant perioperative complications such as major hemorrhage, injury to the adjacent structures, and cardiopulmonary arrest have decreased markedly (Stauffer et al., 1981; Stemmer et al., 1976; Stock et al., 1986).

Perioperative Complications. The immediate postoperative tracheostomy radiograph should be carefully evaluated for the position of the tracheostomy tube and for evidence of postoperative air leaks or hemorrhage. The tracheostomy tube should be parallel to the long axis of the trachea. An AP radiograph that shows that the internal and external ends of the tube appear to be in the same plane, or that the inner end is positioned more cephalad, indicates that the distal end of the tube has not successfully made the turn into the trachea (Fig. 3–11). This position may lead to accidental extubation, trauma to the posterior tracheal membrane, and obstruction to air flow. A kyphotic patient or a reverse lordotic radiograph causes a similar radiographic appearance. Rarely, the tube tip remains in the trachea, but the cuff lodges in the subcutaneous tissues. The radiograph demonstrates a cephalic tube tip and an enlarged cuff above the clavicles. Pneumomediastinum may also be present.

Persistent angulation of the tracheostomy tube within the trachea suggests that the tracheal stoma is eccentric, that the tube is narrow in relation to the trachea, or that the respirator tubing is tugging on the tracheostomy tube. Persistent anterior angulation is usually due to a low stoma. This may be associated with erosion into the innominate artery, which crosses anterior to the trachea. If the clinical situation or AP radiograph demonstrates a poorly positioned tube, a lateral film of the neck is often helpful (see Fig. 3–11).

Following tracheostomy, subcutaneous air in the neck and upper mediastinum is common and is usually an unimportant consequence of the surgery. Large or increasing air collections are most often due to air escaping around the tube into the subcutaneous tissues and being trapped beneath the skin by sutures or packing. Massive air collections are most often due to a paratracheal insertion of the tube or perforation of the trachea during surgery (Fig. 3–12). Pneumothorax immediately after tracheostomy is usually due to the inadvertent entry into the apical pleural space during surgery. This is most common in patients with chronic obstructive pulmonary disease, when the hyperinflated lung rises into the base of the neck. Tracheal perforation may also cause a pneumothorax.

Although high-volume, low-pressure (floppy) cuffs have decreased the incidence of tracheal ulceration and scarring, tracheal injury is still a serious complication of tracheostomy (Arola et al., 1981; Colice et al., 1989; Grillo and Mathisen, 1988). Mucosal ische-

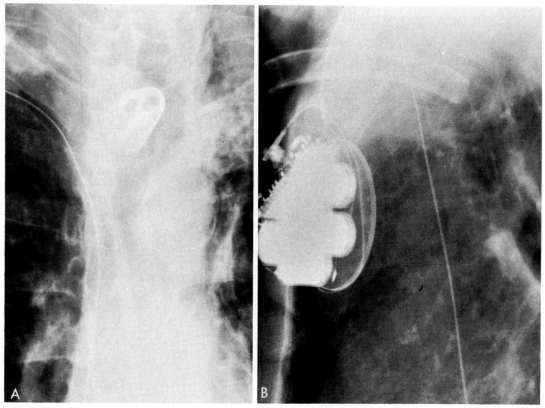

Figure 3–11. Poorly positioned tracheostomy tube. *A,* The proximal and distal ends of the tube are in the same plane. The tube does not appear to be parallel to the long axis of the trachea. Note benign pneumomediastinum after surgery. *B,* Lateral radiograph confirms that the tube has not made the turn into the trachea.

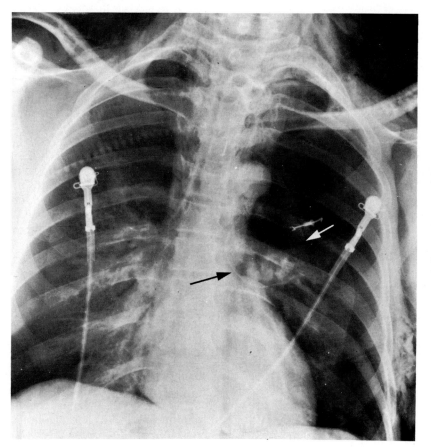

Figure 3–12. Post-tracheostomy pneumothorax. Large bilateral pneumothorax occurred with marked subcutaneous emphysema immediately following a tracheostomy. The initial tube insertion was paratracheal. The external pressure reservoir of the tracheostomy tube overlies the left hilum *(arrows).* This appearance of the reservoir should not be confused with a bulla or pneumatocele.

mia may be minimized by giving careful attention to the radiographic appearance of the cuff in relation to the trachea. The oval lucency of the cuff should fill, but not acutely dilate, the trachea. With prolonged intubation and positive-pressure therapy, gradual dilatation of the trachea may be unavoidable. Mild dilatation may not result in permanent damage. When the diameter of the cuff is more than one and one half times the diameter of the trachea (measured between the clavicles), however, severe mucosal ulceration or tracheostenosis occurs in approximately 30% of patients (Khan et al., 1976) (Fig. 3–13). As with endotracheal tubes, the cuff may occasionally cover the tip of the tube, pinch the tube, or deflect the tip laterally (Heffner et al., 1986a, 1986b; Sinfield et al., 1989).

Complications During Intubation

Infection. Colonization of the pharynx, larynx, and trachea with potential pathogenic bacteria occurs in the vast majority of seriously ill patients who have undergone tracheostomy or long-term endotracheal intubation. Tracheostomy causes cellulitis around the stoma in approximately one third of patients and purulent tracheobronchitis or pneumonia in approximately one half of patients (Heffner et al., 1986a, 1986b; Pingleton, 1988; Stauffer et al., 1981). These infections are usually due to gram-negative organisms and are often difficult to eradicate. Differentiation between pneumonia and other causes of pulmonary disease in the intubated patient is often difficult and is discussed in detail in Chapter 5.

Tracheal Ulceration or Perforation. The incidence of serious tracheal injuries has diminished significantly since the introduction of high-volume, low-pressure cuffs and more ingenious support devices for the respirator tubing (Bishop, 1989; Grillo and Mathisen, 1988; Heffner et al., 1986a, 1986b; Stauffer et al., 1981). Nonetheless, mucosal irritation from the tube and bacterial colonization lead to varying degrees of mucosal injury in virtually every patient. In only a small percentage of patients, however, does this injury progress to deep ulceration, which may eventually lead to cartilage necrosis and, rarely, erosion into the innominate artery, the esophagus, or the mediastinum. Tracheal–innominate arterial fistula is due to erosion through the right anterior tracheal wall, where the innominate artery crosses in front of the trachea. In two thirds of patients, massive, usually fatal, hemoptysis is the mode of presentation. In the remaining third, prodromal bleeding involving a small-to-moderate amount of arterial bleeding may precede massive hemoptysis by hours or days. In this latter group, aortography may be helpful in confirming the clinical suspicion of a tracheal–innominate artery connection (Conrad et al., 1977; Lane et al., 1975).

Erosion through the posterior tracheal membrane leads to tracheoesophageal, tracheopleural, or tracheomediastinal fistula in 0.5% of patients who have undergone tracheostomy (Harley, 1972; Heffner et al., 1986a, 1986b; Wechsler et al., 1982). Perforation occurs most often at the level of the tracheostomy

cuff, usually at the level of the manubrium sterni. Predisposing conditions include a hyperdistended cuff, a short tracheostomy tube causing posterior angulation, the presence of a nasogastric tube in the esophagus, and mediastinal malignancy (Fig. 3–14). In the majority of patients, perforation occurs during the second to fourth week of intubation. The gradual erosion of the posterior tracheal membrane causes an inflammatory welding between the trachea and the esophagus or pleura, which results in eventual direct tracheoesophageal or tracheopleural communication. Therefore, the absence of pneumomediastinum, mediastinal widening, or clinical evidence of mediastinal infection does not negate either diagnosis.

Both the symptoms and the radiographic presentation of a tracheoesophageal fistula depend on the relationship of the fistula to the tracheostomy cuff. If the fistula is below the cuff, signs and symptoms are due to reflux of gastric material, which then enters the lungs. Air from the trachea may dilate the esophagus or stomach. If the fistula is above the cuff, food or gastric contents accumulate in the upper trachea.

In the presence of a tracheal esophageal fistula, the AP radiograph may be normal, may demonstrate air distending the esophagus or stomach, may demonstrate evidence of basilar pneumonitis, or may demonstrate air or fluid in the mediastinum. Computed tomography may show air or fluid in the mediastinum or the tracheal esophageal connection itself. The judicious use of a dilute barium solution may facilitate visualization (Leeds et al., 1986). A fluoroscopically controlled barium-swallow study may also demonstrate the track. Lateral or extreme RPO videotaped or digital fluoroscopy may be necessary to demonstrate the small anteriorly placed connection. Aspiration from disordered swallowing, a common problem in the intubated patient, must be carefully differentiated from a tracheoesophageal fistula.

Erosion into the mediastinum or pleural space is extremely unusual. With mediastinal perforation, the radiograph may show air or mediastinal widening due to mediastinitis or abscess. These signs may be difficult to appreciate on portable radiograms; CT is considerably more sensitive in establishing or refuting the diagnosis. Direct erosion from the trachea into the pleural space or lung is usually a gradual process. Because tissue plains fibrose together, clinical and radiographic evidence of mediastinitis may be absent (Wechsler et al., 1982). The radiograph or the CT scan shows some combination of air or fluid in the pleural space or pneumonitis adjacent to the perforation.

SEQUELAE OF ENDOTRACHEAL INTUBATION AND TRACHEOSTOMY

After extubation, mucosal edema, erythema, and superficial ulcerations usually heal without significant functional impairment (Colice et al., 1989; Cooper

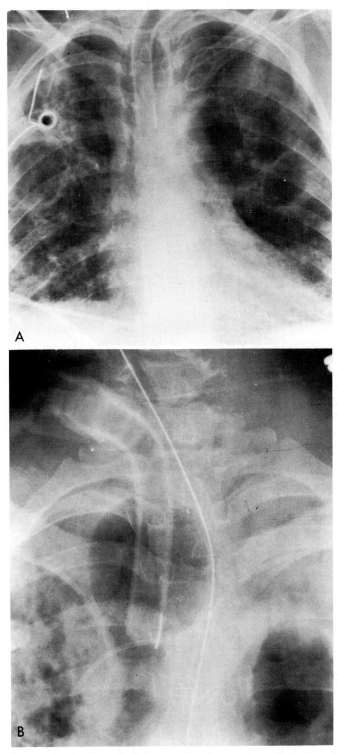

Figure 3–13. *A*, Mild dilatation of the trachea by the cuff. *B*, Same patient 6 weeks later demonstrated severe tracheal dilatation by the cuff. Autopsy showed destruction of the tracheal cartilage in this area.

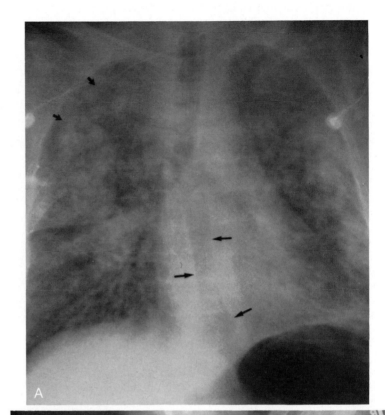

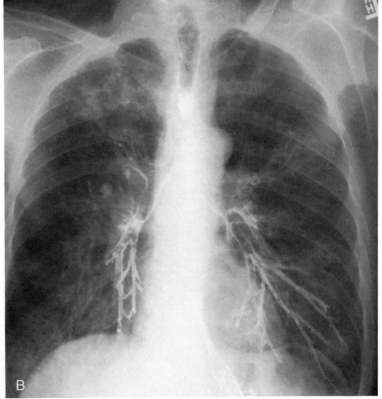

Figure 3–14. Tracheal esophageal fistula (two patients). *A,* Several days after initiation of radiation therapy for mediastinal Hodgkin's disease, the patient developed severe dyspnea and pneumonitis, necessitating intubation. This chest radiograph shows bilateral pulmonary opacities, air filling the lower esophagus (*lower arrows*), and marked gastric dilatation. A pneumothorax is also visible on the original radiograph (*upper arrows*). *B,* A 55-year-old man with esophageal tumor presented with bi-basal pneumonia and a history of dysphasia. A barium swallow showed a mass in the midesophagus, with no barium entering the trachea during the first few swallows. Suddenly, barium flooded the trachea bilaterally.

and Grillo, 1972; Stauffer et al., 1981). Deep ulcerations of the mucosa may result in permanent laryngeal scarring, tracheal stenosis, and tracheomalacia. Symptoms due to permanent airway compromise usually surface several weeks to many months after extubation. Recognition of the cause of the symptoms is often delayed because symptoms are often incorrectly attributed to the patient's underlying lung disease (Dane and King, 1975) (Fig. 3–15).

Laryngeal Injuries. In the vast majority of patients, the laryngeal edema or ulceration caused by endotracheal intubation subsides within 1 to 2 weeks (Colice et al., 1989). Permanent glottic damage is observed most often after prolonged orotracheal intubation. The most frequent permanent injuries include scarring of the posterior third of the glottis, fusion of the posterior commissure, arytenoid injury, and subglottic stenosis. Laryngeal injury due to a tracheostomy is uncommon.

Tracheostenosis. Because high-volume, low-pressure cuffs have replaced high-pressure round balloons, the incidence of symptomatic tracheal injury has fallen considerably from the previously reported levels of 8% to 20%. With the decrease in cuff-related injuries, stenosis at the level of the stoma and of the tube tip are relatively more frequent (Arola et al., 1981; Grillo and Mathisen, 1988; Stauffer et al., 1981). Lesions at the stoma are usually due to granulation tissue projecting into the lumen or to collapse and fibrosis of the anterior and lateral trachea where the cartilage has been removed or destroyed. Stenosis at the cuff site is usually a circumferential scar 1 to 4 cm long, starting approximately 1.5 cm below the

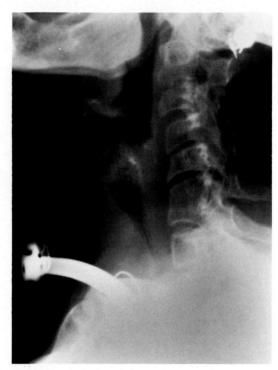

Figure 3–16. Proximal tracheostenosis. Over the last several years, the patient received endotracheal intubation several times for various cardiac problems. Note the severe, almost complete obliteration of the distal cervical trachea. A permanent tracheostomy was required to bypass the obstruction.

stoma. Other areas of obstruction include granulomas of the anterior wall at the site of the tube tip, and subglottic or glottic stenosis from a tracheostomy through the first tracheal ring (Fig. 3–16). Lesions may be multiple, and stenotic areas may have associated areas of tracheomalacia (Gamsu et al., 1980).

Tracheomalacia. Not all tracheal injuries result in stenosis, however. Deep ulceration of the mucosa and concomitant infection may cause dissolution of the supporting rings of cartilage. When the tracheal cartilage is destroyed, the trachea may lose its patency during the respiratory cycle. When the malacic segment is extrathoracic (affecting the cervical trachea), inspiration lowers the intratracheal pressure, and the mobile tissues are drawn in. The obstruction is relieved on expiration. Within the thorax, tracheal collapse occurs on expiration, when the intrathoracic pressure exceeds the intratracheal pressure (Gamsu et al., 1980). The area of malacia may be associated with an area of fixed stenosis as well.

Radiographic Evaluation. Following extubation, all radiographs should be studied for the possibility of laryngeal or tracheal narrowing. If an obstruction is suspected clinically, both the larynx and trachea should be radiographed and visualized endoscopically. Initial imaging evaluation requires high-kilovoltage posteroanterior (PA) and lateral chest radiographs and a lateral radiograph of the soft tissue of the neck. If the upper mediastinal trachea is not well visualized on the lateral radiograph, oblique radio-

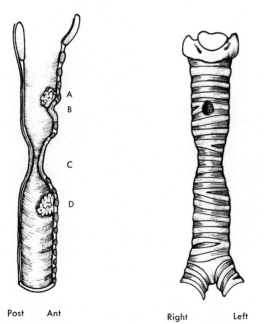

Post   Ant   Right   Left

Figure 3–15. Post-tracheostomy lesions. The four common sites of tracheal injury are polypoid granuloma above the stoma (A), posterior depression of the anterior tracheal wall at the stoma (B), circumferential narrowing of the trachea at the cuff site (C), and polypoid granuloma along the anterior wall at the tube tip (D).

graphs of the trachea are often helpful. Alternative techniques that improve contrast resolution or provide edge enhancement (computed radiography, phosphor-plate digital radiography, and xerography) may also aid in difficult cases. The inner tracheal walls should be parallel and sharply defined in their entire length. In most patients, the lumen is slightly narrowed or irregular at the stomal level after tracheostomy, but dyspnea is uncommon before a 50% to 75% decrease in tracheal diameter (Dane and King, 1975; Stauffer et al., 1981). (If a tracheostomy tube is still present, it must be removed to evaluate the trachea properly.)

Conventional tomography in both the AP and lateral projections may be required for further evaluation. The entire trachea from cords to carina must be studied, because lesions may be multiple (Muhm and Crowe, 1976) (Fig. 3–17). Videotaped fluoroscopy in which various respiratory maneuvers are used is necessary to evaluate cord movement and to check for tracheomalacia. In most cases, studies without contrast material adequately define the lesion or lesions. Positive-contrast tracheography is more accurate in defining the extent of both the stenosis and the malacia (Arola et al., 1981; Gamsu et al., 1980). This procedure should be performed with caution, however, because it may cause mucosal edema and narrow the lumen further. It should be reserved for the occasional case in which surgery is contemplated and the radiographic and endoscopic findings are inconclusive or at odds.

ASSISTED VENTILATION

The institution of positive-pressure therapy may markedly alter the appearance of the chest radiograph (McLoud et al., 1977; Zimmerman et al., 1979). Zimmerman and colleagues (1979) noted that the institution of mechanical ventilation, especially positive end-expiratory pressure (PEEP), improved lung inflation and either "cleared" or "diminished" the radiographic appearance of lung disease in over half their patients (see Fig. 2–3). Areas of consolidation disappeared, vessels became sharper and smaller, and areas of silhouetting disappeared. These radiographic changes, which reversed when the lung returned to prior inflation levels. This appeared to be most marked in patients with diffuse edema rather than other types of focal pulmonary consolidation (Fig. 3–18; see Figs. 2–3 and 2–4).

Gattinoni and associates (1988) studied the CT

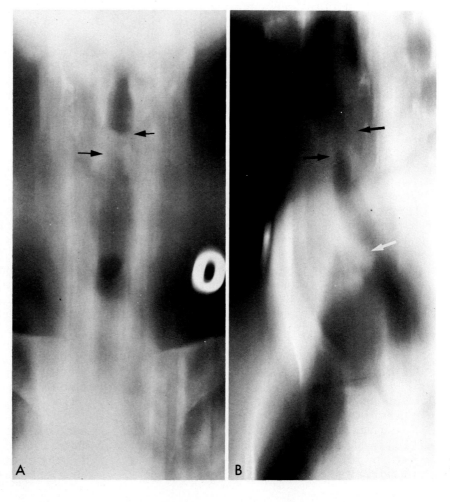

Figure 3–17. Suprastomal stenosis. The patient fractured her cervical spine and injured her upper trachea in an auto accident. A tracheostomy was performed shortly after admission. Several weeks later, she could not tolerate extubation. *A,* Anteroposterior tomogram shows complete occlusion of the trachea (*arrows*) several centimeters above the stoma (*lead marker*). The true and false cords on the right are thickened. *B,* Lateral tomogram confirms the complete obstruction of the upper trachea (*upper arrows*) and also demonstrates the polypoid granuloma at the level of the tracheostomy stoma (*lower arrow*).

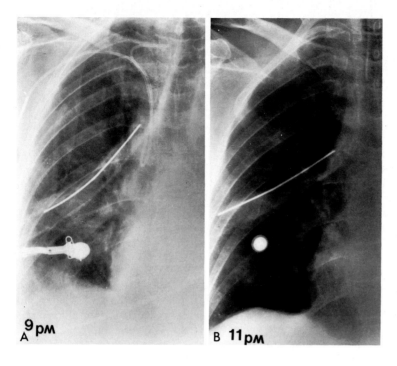

Figure 3–18. Effect of mechanical ventilation. *A,* Focal pulmonary consolidation is noted in the right middle and right lower lung fields. A central venous pressure (CVP) catheter is coiled in the superior vena cava. A chest tube is noted over the right midlung field. Note that both the opaque and nonopaque walls of the chest tube are visible. *B,* Two hours later, the CVP catheter has been removed, an endotracheal tube has been inserted, and positive pressure therapy has been instituted. Note the complete resolution of the atelectasis and better definition of the diaphragm.

appearance of adult respiratory distress syndrome in 22 patients receiving PEEP therapy. They showed that most of the parenchymal consolidation is located posteriorly in gravity-dependent segments and that the addition of PEEP causes re-aeration of many atelectatic areas. Increasing PEEP from 5 to 15 cm of water decreased the volume of totally consolidated lung tissue by about 15% and caused an equal increase in completely aerated tissue. The volume of the previously well-aerated lung did not increase significantly. The decreased consolidation was associated with decreased intrapulmonary shunting, increased blood oxygenation, decreased cardiac output, and decreased intrapulmonary blood volume. Thus, with diffuse atelectasis, the physiologic and radiographic improvement due to PEEP is caused by recruitment of atelectatic lung, rather than by hyperinflation of aerated lung.

Therefore, when reading radiographs of mechanically ventilated patients, one must know the relationship between the radiograph and the level of assisted ventilation. Otherwise, the paradoxical situation of increasing respiratory failure, increasing level of mechanical ventilation, and an "improving radiograph" cannot be explained. Conversely, as the patient improves and is gradually weaned, the appearance of the radiograph may appear to deteriorate.

Potential Complications

Barotrauma. Pulmonary injury and air leak due to mechanical ventilation occur in approximately 5% to 50% of patients, depending on the populations studied. Petersen and Baier (1983) found an 8% incidence in a general ICU population but a 50% incidence in mechanically ventilated patients with adult respira-

tory distress syndrome (ARDS). Other predisposing diseases include pulmonary fibrosis, obstructive lung disease, pulmonary necrosis (necrotizing pneumonia or aspiration), and lung laceration (de Latorre et al., 1977; Haake et al., 1987; Pierson et al., 1986). Uneven inflation of the lung also predisposes the patient to barotrauma. If the endobronchial tube is in a main bronchus, then that lung is hyperinflated and more likely to be injured. In patients with large asymmetric areas of consolidation, volume intended to ventilate the entire lung is delivered predominantly to the more compliant normal lung, injuring the normal lung (Altman and Johnson, 1979) (Fig. 3–19).

Barotrauma is also more frequent in patients on volume respirators and in patients receiving high peak airway pressures. Although no specific pressure is "safe," Petersen and Baier (1983) reported no cases of barotrauma below 50 cm of water, 8% of barotrauma cases between 50 and 70 cm of water, and 43% of cases with pressures exceeding 70 cm of water. Debate continues as to whether PEEP increases the incidence of barotrauma.

Barotrauma from mechanical ventilation develops when the alveoli are hyperdistended and rupture. The air, under pressure, dissects medially along the bronchovascular connective tissue to the mediastinum (Macklin and Macklin, 1944). As the pressure builds in the mediastinum, air can decompress cephalad into the visceral compartment of the neck or follow the esophagus caudad into the retroperitoneum (Maunder et al., 1984). Retroperitoneal gas may continue via the anterior and posterior perirenal space into the properitoneal fat, deep to the transversalis fascia. From here, it can track along the anterior abdominal wall, along the chest wall, and into the scrotum. In addition, air may rupture into the peritoneum.

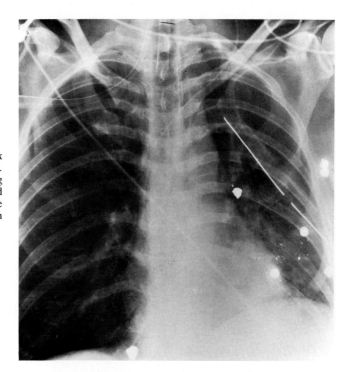

Figure 3–19. Radiograph of a young patient with pneumothorax and lung laceration following multiple gunshot wounds on the left. An atelectatic left lung and a markedly hyperinflated right lung are demonstrated. Films taken in expiration (*not shown*) showed normal deflation of the right lung with little or no excursion of the left lung. The rigid left lung and compliant right lung resulted in hyperventilation of the right lung.

If the above routes do not adequately decompress the mediastinum, air ruptures the mediastinal parietal pleura into the pleural space. Approximately two thirds of barotrauma-induced pneumothoraces occur under tension (Rohlfing et al., 1976; Zwillich et al., 1974). Pierson and co-workers (1986), in the study of the etiology of pneumothorax in 1700 ventilated patients, found that pneumothorax within the first 24 hours of intubation was observed almost exclusively in patients with blunt trauma. In this group, pneumothorax was probably due to pulmonary and pleural laceration and involved a mortality of 45%. Beyond the first day, pneumothorax occurred almost exclusively in severely ill patients with ARDS, pulmonary infections, and so forth and was associated with a mortality of 94%.

Steier and associates (1974) emphasized the importance of rapid diagnosis in respirator-induced pneumothorax. In their study of 74 pneumothoraces, 71 occurred under tension. In patients diagnosed at the bedside and treated immediately, mortality was 7%. In cases in which treatment was delayed one half to 8 hours, mortality increased to 31%. These investigators found that all 74 pneumothorax patients had palpable subcutaneous emphysema in the supraclavicular fossa or neck. Other signs present in the majority of patients included diminished breath sounds, hyperresonance, tachypnea, and hypotension. Clearly, therefore, a tension pneumothorax diagnosed clinically should be decompressed immediately. For equivocal cases requiring confirmation, radiography and evacuation should be performed without delay. In the mechanically ventilated patient, a pneumothorax first detected on a radiograph requires immediate notification of a responsible physician and appropriate treatment (see Chapter 8).

Meteorism. Following the insertion of an endotracheal or tracheostomy tube, the patient may swallow large amounts of air (Cooper and Malt, 1972). This phenomenon is most frequent when the inflated cuff exerts pressure on the esophagus, or when the patient is receiving positive-pressure therapy. Gastric dilatation is often associated with restlessness, and elevation of the left hemidiaphragm may be accompanied by diminished ventilation on that side. Gastric reflux and aspiration may follow. Marked gastric dilatation appearing on the chest radiograph should be noted so that appropriate therapeutic measures may be taken. If gastric dilatation persists, the possibility of inadvertent esophageal intubation, a tracheoesophageal fistula, or gastric outlet obstruction should be considered (see Figs. 3–5, 3–7A, and 3–14).

Isolated colonic ileus with marked cecal distention occasionally complicates mechanical ventilation. In these patients, the stomach may be dilated, the small bowel may be relatively normal, and the colon may be distended (Fig. 3–20). This condition is most likely due to a combination of aerophagia, normal small-bowel motility, and colonic ileus (Golden and Chandler, 1975). It may lead to cecal perforation if decompression is not performed. A nasogastric tube, colon tube, and reduced mechanical ventilation (if possible) usually constitute sufficient treatment. Cecostomy remains controversial but is probably indicated when the cecum is greater than 12 cm initially or cannot be decreased below 9 cm within 24 hours.

Bronchopulmonary Dysplasia. The lungs of patients on long-term mechanical ventilation are subject to many insults. Among these traumas is the constant hyperdistention caused by mechanical ventilation. Some evidence suggests that this form of barotrauma may lead to pathologic changes similar to broncho-

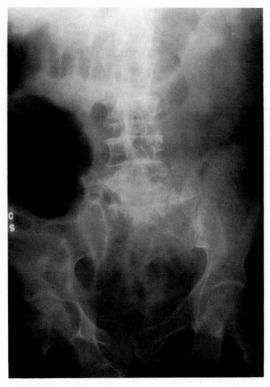

Figure 3–20. Cecal dilatation in patient receiving ventilatory assistance. Over several days, the cecum enlarged to 14 cm in diameter. The transverse colon is distended normally with air, and the remainder of the large and small bowel appears normal. No intrinsic lesion was visible during colonoscopy. Drainage of the cecum with a long tube was successful.

pulmonary dysplasia complicating respiratory distress of the newborn. Although the specific etiologic factors are difficult to delineate, this condition is usually associated with a combination of prolonged assisted ventilation, high inspiratory pressures, PEEP, and high inspired oxygen levels. As in the infant disease, bronchiolitis is present with dilatation of the terminal and respiratory bronchioles, and large cystic spaces form in the distal airways or the alveolar ducts (Churg et al., 1983; Pingleton, 1988; Slavin et al., 1982). In patients with long-standing ARDS, Churg and colleagues (1983) described a gradual change in the radiograph as bronchopulmonary dysplasia emerges. The classic ARDS appearance of diffuse ill-defined air space and interstitial thickening gradually changes to one of hyperinflation with multiple visible cysts.

PLEURAL DRAINAGE TUBES

In the bedridden patient, intrapleural air collects anteriorly, and intrapleural fluid collects posteriorly. The ideal position of the thoracostomy tube is therefore anterosuperior for pneumothorax and posteroinferior for hydrothorax. In reality, tubes in less than ideal position often function well in draining limited pneumothoraces and serous effusions. For large air leaks, loculated collections, or hemothorax, or for

empyemas, which rapidly become loculated, proper positioning is extremely important.

A thoracostomy tube placed in a major or minor fissure may cease to function properly when the pleural surfaces become apposed (Fig. 3–21). Although not every tube in the fissure is unsuccessful, Webb and LaBerge (1984) showed that eight of 12 tubes in the major fissure did not drain properly. The majority of major fissure tubes had been inserted laterally and on the radiograph appear to be straight or gently curved from an inferolateral to a superomedial direction. Correctly placed tubes usually have a gentle curve just within the thorax where the tube passes anteriorly or posteriorly in relation to the lung. Minor fissure tubes may appear to curve gently but pass directly medially. Despite the somewhat characteristic appearances, the majority of intrafissural tubes are not suspected on the initial AP radiograph (Maurer et al., 1982; Stark et al., 1983; Webb and LaBerge, 1984). A lateral radiograph should be part of the initial evaluation after every chest tube insertion. If a lateral radiograph was not obtained at the time of insertion, it is strongly indicated whenever one has a clinical reason to suspect suboptimal drainage (see Fig. 3–21).

A chest tube inserted too deeply may injure the mediastinal vessels or nerves (Fig. 3–22). If the tube is not inserted deeply enough, a side drainage hole is visible in the subcutaneous tissue (Fig. 3–23). Localized subcutaneous emphysema may be present. When a tube is mistakenly inserted into the subcutaneous tissues of the chest wall, rather than within the thorax, the malposition may not be apparent radiographically. Webb and Godwin (1980) have shown that the *nonopaque* wall of a properly positioned chest tube is usually visible on the radiograph, because air exists within the tube, and air exists outside the tube in the adjacent lung or pleural space (see Fig. 3–21). When the tube is positioned in the chest wall, the nonopaque outer wall is not visible against the soft tissue of the thorax.

For complex pleural/parenchymal disease or for multiloculated pleural fluid or air collections, conventional radiographs are frequently inadequate in documenting the relationship between the thoracostomy tube and the collection to be drained. If the chest tube is not functioning properly, CT performed early in the patient's course is often rewarding. It can document the presence or absence of residual loculated pockets and can demonstrate the relationship between that collection and the chest tube. The CT scan also serves as a guide for potential local percutaneous drainage of loculated collections. In cases of persistent air leaks, the CT occasionally documents the chest tube within the substance of the lung (Stark et al., 1983).

After removal of the tube, residual pleural lines often delineate the former tube position. They represent areas of pleural thickening around the tube track (Fig. 3–24A). They are rarely significant but may be confusing. On occasion, the dense pleural

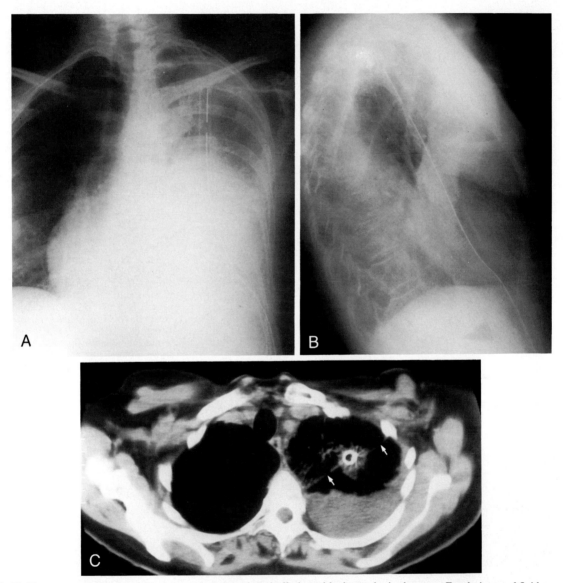

Figure 3–21. Thoracostomy tube in major fissure. *A,* Large pleural effusion with chest tube in the apex. For drainage of fluid, a posterior-inferior location is preferable. *B,* The tube traverses the expected course of the fissure. The fluid is shown posteriorly. The inner and outer walls of the nonopaque side of the tube are visible, indicating that they are surrounded by air. *C,* The tube in the fissure (*arrows*) and the fluid (shown posteriorly) are demonstrated by CT scan. A new tube had to be inserted to re-establish drainage.

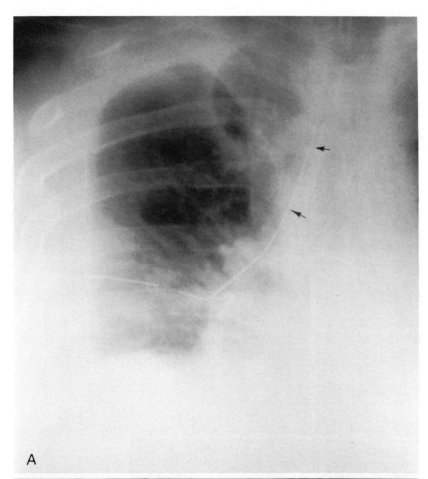

A

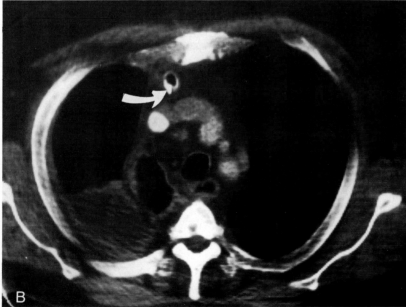

B

Figure 3–22. The chest tube was inserted for drainage for pleural effusion. *A,* The postero-anterior (PA) radiograph shows a large right effusion and a chest tube that is acutely angulated with its tip in a medial position (*arrows*). *B,* A CT scan shows the tip of the tube within the mediastinal fat (*arrow*) within 1 cm of the innominate vein. The tube was withdrawn without incident. (Case of Dr. David Smith, Zablocki Veterans Administration Hospital, Milwaukee, Wisconsin.)

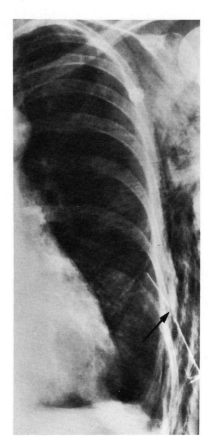

Figure 3–23. The side hole of the thoracostomy tube is in the subcutaneous tissue (*arrow*). Note the marked subcutaneous emphysema.

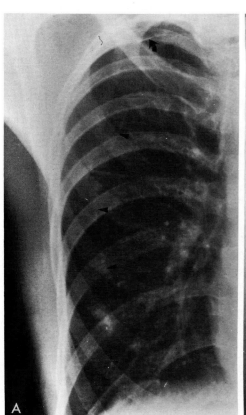
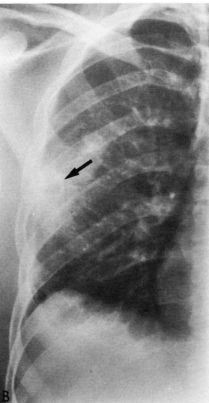

Figure 3–24. *A,* Tube track following the removal of a chest tube. A line of pleural thickening is seen along the path of the tube (*arrowheads*), simulating a pneumothorax. The density over the anterior fifth rib is the site of insertion of the tube. A small pneumothorax remains (*arrow*). *B,* Infected tube track (different patient). Fever and leukocytosis developed 2 days after removal of the chest tube. Note the diffuse pleural thickening plus the focal right midlung density with a central lucency (*arrow*). Purulent drainage was positive for *Staphylococcus aureus.*

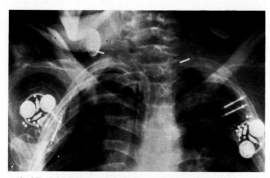

Figure 3–25. Diaphragmatic pacers. The platinum phrenic nerve electrodes are seen over the transverse processes of T1. A fine wire leads from each electrode to each receiver. (Case of Dr. Carl Ravin, Duke University, Durham, NC.)

stripe appears to be parallel to the lateral rib cage and may closely simulate a pneumothorax, which in fact it technically is. The thickened pleural space, when partially filled with fluid, may mimic an abscess and, when completely filled, may appear as a dense linear band. A review of previous films demonstrates the position occupied by the tube in relation to the line in question. These fluid collections usually decrease in size or disappear completely within days. An enlarging tube track in a patient with an unexplained fever suggests the possibility of empyema (see Fig. 3–24B).

DIAPHRAGMATIC PACING

Electrical pacing of the diaphragm is used occasionally in patients with chronic ventilatory insufficiency when the phrenic nerves, lung, and diaphragm are functional (for example, in quadriplegia or central alveolar hypoventilation). A radiofrequency receiver is implanted into the subcutaneous tissue of the anterior chest wall and is connected to a platinum electrode placed on the phrenic nerve behind the clavicle (Fig. 3–25). An external radiofrequency transmitter sends signals through the intact skin to the receiver, which sends an electrical signal to the phrenic nerve (Glenn, 1978; Nochomovitz et al., 1988). Complications of radiographic interest include infection around the implanted receiver and fracture of the electrode wire.

References

Aebert, H., Hünefeld, G., and Regel, G.: Paranasal sinusitis and sepsis in ICU patients with nasotracheal intubation. Intensive Care Med. 15:27, 1988.

Alberti, J., Hanafee, W., Wilson, G., et al.: Unsuspected pulmonary collapse during neuroradiologic procedures. Radiology 89:316, 1967.

Altman, A.R., and Johnson, T.H.: Roentgenographic findings in PEEP therapy: Indicators of pulmonary complications. JAMA 242:727, 1979.

Arola, M.K., Inberg, M.V., and Puhakka, H.: Tracheal stenosis after tracheostomy and after orotracheal cuffed intubation. Acta Chir. Scand. 147:183, 1981.

Birmingham, P.K., Cheney, F.W., and Ward, R.J.: Esophageal intubation: A review of detection techniques. Anesth. Analg. 65:886, 1986.

Bishop, M.J.: Mechanism of laryngotracheal injury following prolonged tracheal intubation. Chest 96:185, 1989.

Brunel, W., Coleman, D.L., Schwartz, D.E., et al.: Assessment of routine chest roentgenograms and the physical examination to confirm endotracheal tube position. Chest 96:1043, 1989.

Churg, A., Golden, J., Fligiel, S., and Hogg, J.C.: Bronchopulmonary dysplasia in the adult. Am. Rev. Respir. Dis. 127:117, 1983.

Colice, G.L., Stukel, T.A., and Dain, B.: Laryngeal complications of prolonged intubation. Chest 96:877, 1989.

Conrad, M.R., Cameron, J., and White, R.I., Jr.: The role of angiography in the diagnosis of tracheal-innominate artery fistula. AJR 128:35, 1977.

Conrardy, P.A., Goodman, L.R., Lainge, R., and Singer, M.M.: Alteration of endotracheal tube position: Flexion and extension of the neck. Crit. Care Med. 4:7, 1976.

Cooper, J.D., and Grillo, H.C.: Analysis of problems related to cuffs on intratracheal tubes. Chest 62(Suppl.):21S, 1972.

Cooper, J.D., and Malt, R.Q.: Meteorism produced by nasotracheal intubation and ventilatory assistance. N. Engl. J. Med. 287:652, 1972.

Dane, T.E.D., and King, E.G.: A prospective study of complications after tracheostomy for assisted ventilation. Chest 67:398, 1975.

de Latorre, F.J., Tomasa, A., Klamburg, J., et al.: Incidence of pneumothorax and pneumomediastinum in patients with aspiration pneumonia requiring ventilatory support. Chest 72:141, 1977.

Fassoulaki, A., and Pamouktsoglou, P.: Prolonged nasotracheal intubation and its association with inflammation of paranasal sinuses. Anesth. Analg. 69:50, 1989.

Gamsu, G., Borson, D.B., Webb, W.R., and Cunningham, J.H.: Structure and function in tracheal stenosis. Am. Rev. Respir. Dis. 121:519, 1980.

Gattinoni, L., Pesenti, A., Bombino, M., et al.: Relationships between lung computed tomographic density, gas exchange, and PEEP in acute respiratory failure. Anesthesiology 69:824, 1988.

Glenn, W.W.L.: Diaphragm pacing: Present status. PACE 1:357, 1978.

Golden, G.T., and Chandler, J.G.: Colonic ileus and cecal perforation in patients requiring mechanical ventilatory support. Chest 68:661, 1975.

Goodman, L.R., Conrardy, P.A., Laing, F., et al.: Radiographic evaluation of endotracheal tube position. AJR 127:433, 1976.

Gorback, M.S., and Ravin, C.E.: Reinforced endotracheal tube placement: Radiographic misdiagnosis. Radiology 162:579, 1987.

Grillo, H.C., and Mathisen, D.J.: Surgical management of tracheal strictures. Surg. Clin. North Am. 68:511, 1988.

Haake, R., Schlichtig, R., Ulstad, D.R., and Henschen, R.R.: Barotrauma—pathophysiology, risk factors and prevention. Chest 91:608, 1987.

Hansen, M., Poulsen, M.R., Bendixen, D.K., and Hattman-Andersen, F.: Incidence of sinusitis in patients with nasotracheal intubation. Br. J. Anaesth. 61:231, 1988.

Harley, H.R.: Ulcerative tracheo-eosophageal fistula during treatment by tracheostomy and intermittent positive pressure ventilation. Thorax 27:338, 1972.

Heffner, J.E., Miller, K.S., and Sahn, S.A.: Tracheostomy in the intensive care unit. Part 1. Chest 90:269, 1986a.

Heffner, J.E., Miller, K. S., and Sahn, S.A.: Tracheostomy in the intensive care unit. Part 2. Chest 90:430, 1986b.

Heinonen, J., Takki, S., and Tammisto, T.: Effect of the Trendelenburg tilt and other procedures on the position of endotracheal tubes. Lancet 1:850, 1969.

Henschke, C.I., Pasternack, G.S., Schroeder, S., et al.: Bedside chest radiography: Diagnostic efficacy. Radiology 149:23, 1983.

Hirsch, M., Abramowitz, H.B., Shapiro, S., and Barki, Y.: Hypopharyngeal injury as a result of attempted endotracheal intubation. Radiology 128:37, 1978.

Khan, F., Reddy, N., and Khan, A.: Cuff/trachea ratio as an indicator of tracheal damage. (Abstract.) Chest 70:431, 1976.

Lane, E.E., Temes, G.D., and Anderson, W.H.: Tracheal-innominate artery fistula due to tracheostomy. Chest 68:678, 1975.

Leeds, W.M., Morley, T.F., Zappasodi, S.J., and Giudice, J.C.: Computed tomography for diagnosis of tracheoesophageal fistula. Crit. Care Med. 14:591, 1986.

Macklin, M.T., and Macklin, C.C.: Malignant interstitial emphysema of the lungs and mediastinum as an important occult complication in many respiratory diseases and other conditions: An interpretation of the clinical literature in the light of laboratory experiment. Medicine 23:281, 1944.

Maunder, R.J., Pierson, D.J., and Hudson, L.D.: Subcutaneous and mediastinal emphysema. Arch. Intern. Med. 144:1447, 1984.

Maurer, J.R., Friedman, P.J., and Wing, V.W.: Thoracostomy tube in an interlobar fissure: Radiology recognition of a potential problem. AJR 139:1155, 1982.

McLoud, T.C., Barash, P.G., and Ravin, C.E.: PEEP: Radiographic features and associated complications. AJR 129:209, 1977.

Muhm, J.R., and Crowe, J.K.: The evaluation of tracheal abnormalities by tomography. Radiol. Clin. North Am. 14:95, 1976.

Nochomovitz, M.L., Peterson, D.K., and Stellato, T.A.: Electrical activation of the diaphragm. Clin. Chest Med. 9:349, 1988.

Pedersen, J., Schurizek, B.A., Melsen, N.C., and Juhl, B.: Minitracheotomy in the treatment of postoperative sputum retention and atelectasis. Acta Anaesthesiol. Scand. 32:426, 1988.

Petersen, G.W., and Baier, H.: Incidence of pulmonary barotrauma in a medical ICU. Crit. Care Med. 11:67, 1983.

Pierson, D.J., Norton, C.A., and Bates, P.W.: Persistent bronchopleural air leak during mechanical ventilation. Chest 90:321, 1986.

Pingleton, S.K.: Complications of acute respiratory failure. Am. Rev. Respir. Dis. 137:1463, 1988.

Rashkin, M.C., and Davis, T.: Acute complications of endotracheal intubation. Relationship to reintubation, route, urgency, and duration. Chest 89:165, 1986.

Rohlfing, B.M., Webb, W.R., and Schlobohm, R.M.: Ventilator-related extra-alveolar air in adults. Radiology 121:25, 1976.

Rollins, R.J., and Tocino, I.: Early radiographic signs of tracheal rupture. AJR 148:695, 1987.

Sinfield, A., DiVito, J., Jr., and Brandstetter, R.D.: Airway obstruction from overinflation and herniation of tracheostomy tube balloon. Heart Lung 18:260, 1989.

Slavin, G., Nunn, J.F., Crow, J., and Dore, C.J.: Bronchiolectasis—a complication of artificial ventilation. Br. Med. J. 185:931, 1982.

Smith, G.M., Reed, J.C., and Chaplin, R.H.: Radiographic detection of esophageal malpositioning of endotracheal tubes. AJR 154:23, 1990.

Stark, D.D., Federle, M.P., and Goodman, P.C.: CT and radiographic assessment of tube thoracostomy. AJR 141:253, 1983.

Stauffer, J.L., Olson, D.E., and Petty, T.L.: Complications and consequences of endotracheal intubation and tracheotomy: A prospective study of 150 critically ill adult patients. Am. J. Med. 70:65, 1981.

Steier, M., Ching, N., Roberts, E.B.R., et al.: Pneumothorax complicating continuous ventilatory support. J. Thorac. Cardiovasc. Surg. 67:17, 1974.

Stemmer, E.A., Oliver, C., Carey, J.P., and Connolly, J.E.: Fatal complications of tracheotomy. Am. J. Surg. 131:288, 1976.

Stock, M.C., Woodward, C.G., Shapiro, B.A., et al.: Perioperative complications of elective tracheostomy in critically ill patients. Crit. Care Med. 14:861, 1986.

Ward, M.P., Glazer, H.S., Heiken, J.P., and Spector, J.G.: Traumatic perforation of the pyriform sinus: CT demonstration. J. Comput. Assist. Tomogr. 9:982, 1985.

Webb, W.R., and Godwin, J.D.: The obscured outer edge: A sign of improperly placed pleural drainage tubes. AJR 134:1062, 1980.

Webb, W.R., and LaBerge, J.M.: Radiographic recognition of chest tube malposition in the major fissure. Chest 85:81, 1984.

Wechsler, R.J., Steiner, R.M., Goodman, L.R., et al.: Iatrogenic esophageal-pleural fistula: Subtlety of diagnosis in the absence of mediastinitis. Radiology 144:239, 1982.

Zimmerman, J.E., Goodman, L.R., and Shahvari, M.B.G.: Effect of mechanical ventilation and positive end-expiratory pressure (PEEP) on chest radiographs. AJR 133:811, 1979.

Zwillich, C.W., Pierson, D.J., Creagh, C.R., et al.: Complications of assisted ventilation: A prospective study of 354 consecutive episodes. Am. J. Med. 57:161, 1974.

4

Cardiovascular Monitoring Devices

■

Connie Mitchell Vail
Carl E. Ravin

Almost all critically ill patients have at least one central venous pressure (CVP) catheter. Such lines, with the exception of the femoral venous catheter, should be visible on routine chest radiographs, because veins of the neck and upper extremity are used to gain access to the central venous system. A knowledge of thoracic venous anatomy is therefore useful in determining the approach to use for catheter placement and, more important, in confirming optimal positioning of the catheter beyond the venous valves.

The subclavian veins drain the upper extremities and are a continuation of the axillary veins at a point demarcated by the lateral aspect of the first rib. They provide drainage of the shoulder, upper arm, and anterior thoracic wall. The vein courses posteriorly in relation to the clavicle and anteriorly in relation to the first rib. The location of the last valve in the subclavian vein is closely approximated by the position of the anterior first rib, as demonstrated on the chest radiograph (Ravin et al., 1976). This valve is located approximately 2 cm from the site at which the subclavian vein joins the internal jugular vein to form the brachiocephalic (innominate) vein (Williams et al., 1989). The internal jugular vein drains deep portions of the head and neck and also contains a valve approximately 2.5 cm from its junction with the subclavian vein. Despite the presence of this valve, malpositioned catheters from a subclavian approach commonly enter the internal jugular vein (Gilday, 1969) (Fig. 4–1). The external jugular vein and vertebral vein also contribute to the origin of the brachiocephalic vein.

The origin of the brachiocephalic vein is demarcated by the sternoclavicular joint. The right brachiocephalic vein is oriented vertically, while the left courses obliquely across the mediastinum, anterior to the great vessels, to join the right and form the superior vena cava. Because of the oblique orientation of the left brachiocephalic vein with respect to the right brachiocephalic vein, the appearance of catheters within each of these veins differs on the lateral chest radiograph. Catheters within the left brachiocephalic vein show an anterior curve not demonstrated on the right (Fig. 4–2). Neither brachiocephalic vein contains a valve.

The internal thoracic vein joins the brachiocephalic vein. The right internal thoracic vein is located centrally. On the lateral radiograph, anterior orientation of the catheter tip suggests that it has entered the right internal thoracic vein. The left pericardiophrenic vein drains the diaphragm, pericardium, and pleura. It may directly enter the left brachiocephalic vein near its origin or drain via the left internal thoracic vein or the left superior intercostal vein. The left superior intercostal vein drains the second through fourth posterior intercostal veins and arches anteriorly to join the left brachiocephalic vein. It courses along the aortic arch, variably forming a projection appearing on frontal chest radiographs that is referred to as the aortic nipple (Friedman et al., 1978; McDonald et al., 1970).

The superior vena cava is formed by the junction of the right and left brachiocephalic veins. A catheter location that is distal to this junction is preferred for measuring CVP and avoiding complications. This junction lies to the right of midline at the level of the first intercostal space. The superior vena cava is joined by the azygos vein posteriorly, just prior to entering the pericardium. Posterior orientation of the catheter tip suggests that it enters the azygos vein. Both the hemiazygos and accessory hemiazygos veins contribute to the azygos vein.

A left-sided superior vena cava is found in 0.3% of the normal population. It represents a persistent

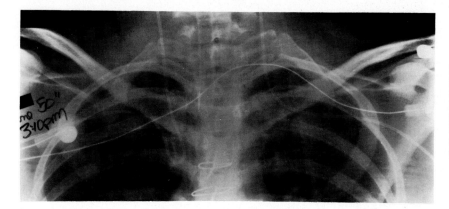

Figure 4–1. Bilateral central venous pressure (CVP) catheters inadvertently positioned in the internal jugular veins. True CVP cannot be monitored with this catheter position. (From Ravin, C.E., et al: Hazards of the ICU. AJR 126:423–431, 1976, with permission, © by American Roentgen Ray Society.)

communication of the left anterior and common cardinal veins. Eighty percent of these patients also have a right-sided superior vena cava (Cha and Khoury, 1972), and 60% have a left brachiocephalic vein connecting the right and left superior venae cavae. Both the right-sided superior vena cava and left brachiocephalic vein may be smaller than normal (Winter, 1954). The left-sided superior vena cava drains to the right atrium via the oblique vein of the left atrium (Marshall's oblique vein), the great cardiac vein, and the coronary sinus.

Catheters may occasionally enter the veins of the heart. In the case of the left superior vena cava, the cardiac veins represent an integral channel for systemic blood return to the right atrium. More frequently, however, the catheter enters the cardiac vein directly from the right atrium. On the frontal radiograph, the tip of the catheter or pacer lead points upward and laterally. Making this diagnosis may not be possible without lateral radiography (Fig. 4–3). This retrograde catheterization may be inadvertent or intentional for the purpose of atrial pacing and arrhythmia investigation.

The coronary sinus is approximately 2.5 cm in length and enters the right atrium at a site adjacent to the inferior vena cava. It is located in the posterior atrioventricular groove and drains the great, middle, and small cardiac veins as well as the oblique vein of the left atrium. These veins parallel the coronary arteries and are located in the epicardial fat. The great cardiac vein arises along the left anterior descending coronary artery in the anterior interventricular groove. It then joins the left atrial vein and runs posteriorly in the atrioventricular groove. The middle cardiac vein runs in the posterior interventricular groove. Pacing wires entering this vein may appear

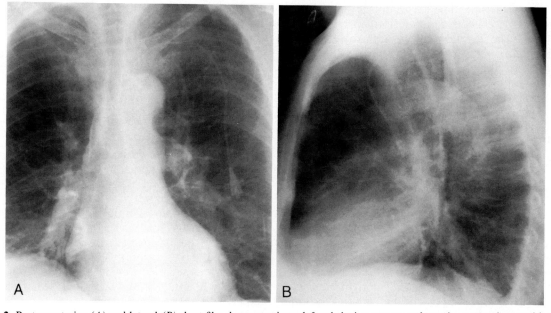

Figure 4–2. Posteroanterior *(A)* and lateral *(B)* chest film demonstrating a left subclavian venous catheter in appropriate position. On the lateral view, note the anterior curvature of the catheter high in the mediastinum as the left brachiocephalic vein crosses the mediastinum.

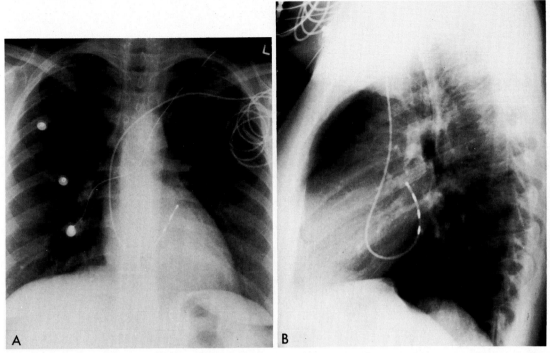

Figure 4–3. *A,* Radiograph shows upward direction of the catheter tip, which is positioned in the coronary sinus. The sinus runs in the posterior atrioventricular groove. *B,* The lateral view confirms positioning in the coronary sinus as evidenced by the posterior location of the catheter.

to have perforated the right ventricle and entered the pericardial space. The small cardiac vein arises in the right anterior atrioventricular groove.

SUBCLAVIAN AND CENTRAL VENOUS PRESSURE CATHETERS

A critical factor in the management of seriously ill patients is the maintenance of an optimal blood volume, that is, one that produces adequate circulation to critical organs without overloading cardiac pumping capabilities. Monitoring CVP via an intravenous (IV) catheter is one method by which this important relationship between intravascular blood volume and cardiac pumping capacity can be assessed (Wilson et al., 1962). In addition, these catheters serve as a secure route for IV administration of fluid. This route assures more consistent venous flow than does a route through the peripheral veins, which may vasoconstrict, particularly during periods of cardiovascular collapse, when access to the circulatory system is most needed.

The subclavian vein is now frequently used for rapid access to the central venous system (Fontenelle et al., 1971). Along with the internal jugular and femoral veins, it constitutes one of the three most common access sites for central venous catheter placement. Because of its large size and consistent anatomic location, the subclavian vein is readily available for venipuncture even when peripheral vessels are

not. Its size and rapid blood flow allow a catheter to be left in place for prolonged periods without significant risk of thrombosis, which is a great advantage in situations requiring hyperalimentation (Dudrick et al., 1969). Moreover, its proximity to the most central venous valves allows relatively short catheters to be used for the purpose of CVP monitoring. True CVP measurements can be obtained only within the true central venous system, beyond all the valves that interfere with direct transmission of right atrial pressure to the catheter. As stated previously, the most proximal of these valves are found in the subclavian and internal jugular veins approximately 2 cm from their junction with their respective brachiocephalic veins.

The internal jugular vein also provides rapid access to the central venous system and is used frequently by trained anesthesia personnel (Fig. 4–4). Because it drains the cerebral circulation and is smaller, however, the internal jugular vein is less acceptable to many investigators as a site for long-term catheter placement (Langston, 1971).

Ideal Position

In the ideal position, the tip of the subclavian catheter, internal jugular catheter, or CVP catheter of peripheral origin is central to the venous valves. Optimal placement of the tip for CVP measurements is even more central in the venous system, at the origin of the superior vena cava. This point is iden-

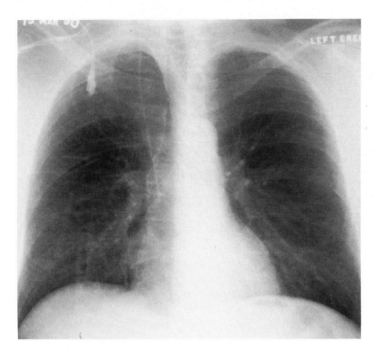

Figure 4–4. Frontal chest film demonstrating right internal jugular line in appropriate position.

tified on frontal chest radiographs at the level of the first anterior intercostal space.

Potential Complications

Aberrant Positioning

Prospective studies have shown that as many as one third of CVP catheters are incorrectly placed at the time of initial insertion (Langston, 1971). The most common aberrant locations include the internal jugular vein (see Fig. 4–1), the right atrium or ventricle, and various extrathoracic locations, including the upper extremities (Fig. 4–5) and the hepatic veins

(Fig. 4–6). Positions within the right atrium are undesirable for placement because of the increased incidence of cardiac perforation by the catheter (Huyghens et al., 1985). Continued infusion of fluid through the catheter into the pericardial space following perforation can rapidly produce fatal cardiac tamponade (Bone et al., 1973). Positioning distal to the tricuspid valve is more likely to cause cardiac arrhythmias because of irritation of the endocardium, but it can also cause perforation (Kline and Hofman, 1968). An important problem of all aberrant catheter positioning is that true CVP is not monitored; rather, some other pressure bearing no constant relationship to CVP is assessed. Such pressures can vary widely

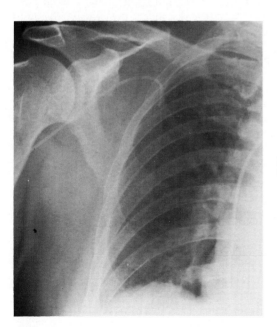

Figure 4–5. Central venous pressure catheter inserted into the basilic vein of the right upper extremity and terminating in an extrathoracic vein.

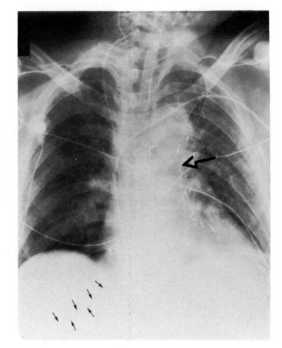

Figure 4–6. Central venous pressure catheter extending from the right internal jugular vein through the superior vena cava, the right atrium, and the proximal inferior vena cava to terminate in a hepatic vein *(solid arrows)*. The photograph has been retouched to enhance demonstration, but the catheter was easily visualized on the original radiograph. The Swan-Ganz catheter, inserted via the left subclavian vein, has its tip in the main pulmonary artery *(open arrow)*. (From Ravin, C.E., et al.: Hazards of the ICU. AJR 126:423–431, 1976, with permission, © by American Roentgen Ray Society.)

from the true CVP and provide erroneous information about the intravascular blood volume.

Additional complications of aberrant positioning are theoretically possible from infusion of potentially toxic substances (some antibiotics and hypertonic-hyperalimentation solutions) directly into the liver or heart rather than into the central venous system, where rapid dilution can take place (Daly et al., 1975). Finally, several reports have indicated the importance of recognizing a sharply curved catheter tip as a potential cause of venous perforation. The malpositioned catheter tip produces excessive pressure on a focal area of the vein, potentially leading to perforation and hydrothorax or hemothorax (Au and Badellino, 1988; Tocino and Watanabe, 1986) (see Fig. 4–9A).

Therefore, an attempt should be made to reposition catheters that are less than optimally placed. Fluoroscopy is helpful in making such adjustments, but unfortunately, it is not usually available in intensive care units. After any attempt at repositioning, the position of the catheter should be confirmed by appropriate radiographs.

Catheters frequently change position after initial placement because of patient motion, manipulation of the catheter by physicians or nursing personnel, or straightening or bending of the catheter itself within the vascular system. Position changes resulting from patient motion or from alterations of the catheter's course are more likely to occur if the catheter crosses a joint (especially the elbow) (Brandt et al., 1970), or follows a circuitous route to the central venous system. Therefore, the position of the catheter must be checked on each film obtained. One should not assume that because the catheter was correctly positioned on the initial examination it will remain so;

periodic radiographic confirmation of the catheter position is recommended.

Pneumothorax

The pleura covering the apex of the lung lies approximately 0.5 cm deep to the subclavian vein. Not surprisingly, therefore, pneumothorax represents one third of all major complications of subclavian venous catheterization and occurs in as many as 6% of cases (Gibson et al., 1985). This complication is often difficult to diagnose clinically; therefore, obtaining an upright chest film is strongly recommended whenever placement of a subclavian catheter has been attempted (Fig. 4–7). Should initial placement fail, a film must be obtained before placement is attempted on the opposite side, because failure to recognize a pre-existing pneumothorax may result in creation of bilateral pneumothoraces when contralateral placement is attempted (Fig. 4–8). Pneumothoraces occurring several days after line placement have also been reported (Sivak, 1986).

Ectopic Infusion

Another potential complication of subclavian and CVP catheterization is ectopic infusion of fluid into the mediastinum (Adar and Mozes, 1970) or pleural space (Aulenbacher, 1970). This complication occurs most frequently with catheters inserted via a subclavian approach, although it does occur with other central venous catheters. This finding probably reflects the greater chance of perivascular catheter placement with the subclavian approach. Infusion of fluid into mediastinal or pleural spaces produces a radiographic appearance suggestive of significant in-

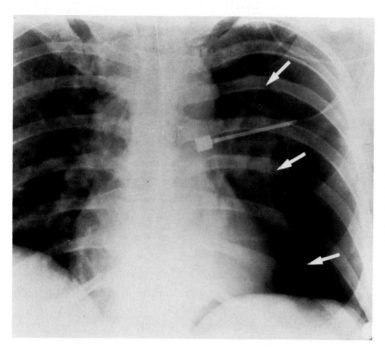

Figure 4–7. Anteroposterior (AP) portable chest film demonstrating a large left pneumothorax accompanied by complete collapse of the left lung *(arrows)*. This pneumothorax was not detected clinically, although the patient had been examined on several occasions before the film was obtained. Successful placement of the subclavian line had required several attempts, and the pneumothorax is thought to have resulted from one of the early unsuccessful attempts. (From Ravin, C.E., et al.: Hazards of the ICU. AJR 126:423–431, 1976, with permission, © by American Roentgen Ray Society.)

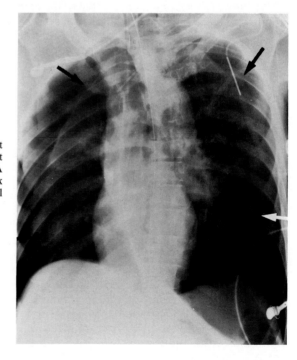

Figure 4–8. Bilateral pneumothoraces following an unsuccessful attempt at placement of a right subclavian catheter and several subsequent attempts at placement of a left subclavian catheter prior to successful positioning. A large pneumothorax appears on the right, and a tension pneumothorax *(arrows)*, evidenced by depression of the hemidiaphragm and contralateral shift of the mediastinal structures, appears on the left.

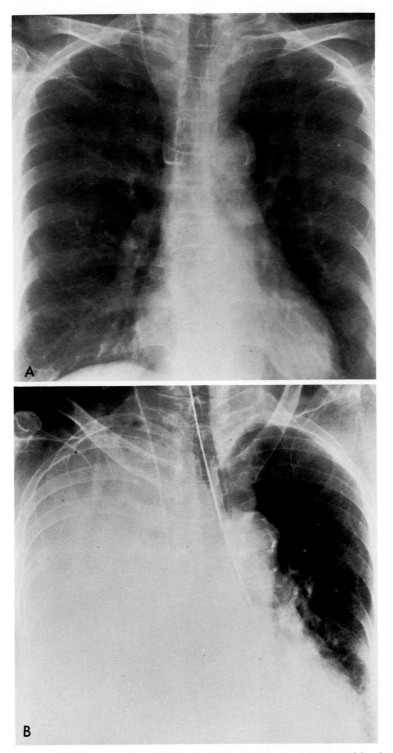

Figure 4–9. *A,* Posteroanterior radiograph demonstrating a CVP catheter inserted via the right internal jugular vein. The distal tip makes an unusual curve medially. *B,* Following intravenous administration of several liters of fluid through the catheter, complete opacification of the right hemithorax was noted. Diagnostic thoracentesis demonstrated the pleural fluid to be identical to that being infused through the catheter.

trathoracic bleeding (Fig. 4–9). In most cases, however, the rapid accumulation of such fluid after insertion of a subclavian catheter should suggest the diagnosis of ectopic infusion. This diagnosis can be confirmed by thoracentesis if the fluid is accumulating in the pleural space, or by injection of water-soluble contrast medium through the catheter itself, particularly if fluid is accumulating in the mediastinum. Confirmation of ectopic infusion by these methods avoids the more involved angiographic procedures required to exclude major arterial or venous bleeding. In general, mediastinal bleeding resulting from catheter injury tends to produce its own tamponade, and only rarely is surgical repair of the laceration required.

Catheter Embolization

Another potentially serious complication is that of catheter breakage and embolization. This problem can result from laceration of the catheter by the needle used to insert it, fracture at a point of stress, or detachment of the catheter from its hub. Following such an event, the catheter fragment may lodge in the superior or inferior vena cava, in the right side of the heart, or in the pulmonary artery and result in thrombosis, infection, or perforation (Blair et al., 1970). To facilitate detection of broken fragments, it is strongly recommended that only radiopaque catheters be employed in the ICU. Frequently, such radiopaque catheter fragments can be retrieved under fluoroscopic control, although occasionally thoracotomy is required (Blair et al., 1970).

Miscellaneous Complications

A multitude of other complications have been infrequently associated with the placement of central venous catheters, particularly when a subclavian approach is used. Of these complications, the most common is inadvertent puncture of the subclavian artery. In the vast majority of these cases, the resultant bleeding is of no clinical significance and is readily controlled by direct pressure. Local bleeding at the venipuncture site is usually not significant and is recognizable as a small, apical, extrapleural opacity

on the chest radiograph. Larger extrapleural opacities may signify more significant bleeding (possibly arterial), and on rare occasions surgical intervention is required to repair a lacerated subclavian artery (Gibson et al., 1985). Rarely, subclavian arterial catheterization occurs. Significant arcing of the catheter above the clavicle followed by midline or left-sided descent suggests cannulation of the subclavian artery (Dedhia and Schiebel, 1987).

Air embolization may occur and proves fatal in 29% to 36% of cases (Gibson et al., 1985). Air may enter the venous system via the original venipuncture needle or, more frequently, as a result of later line detachment. Radiographically, air may be visible in the main pulmonary artery. In addition, the phrenic nerve and nerves of the brachial plexus lie in close proximity to the subclavian vein and artery, and they may be injured during catheter placement. Clot frequently forms in the veins with prolonged catheterization; however, symptomatic venous obstruction (Bouffard et al., 1985) and pulmonary embolism are uncommon (Fig. 4–10). Experience and careful attention to technique can markedly reduce the incidence of complications resulting from catheter placement in the central venous system.

SWAN-GANZ CATHETERS

In 1970, the Swan-Ganz catheter was introduced as an alternative and complement to CVP recording devices. Pulmonary capillary wedge (PCW) pressures obtained from the Swan-Ganz catheter reflect left atrial pressure and left ventricular end-diastolic volume. Use of PCW pressure has allowed greater accuracy in maintenance of optimal blood volume of some critically ill patients, particularly those with

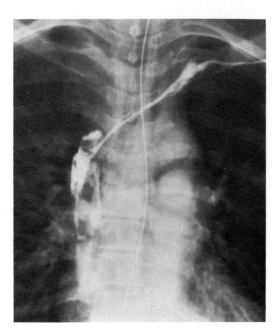

Figure 4–10. Superior vena cava (SVC) thrombosis after prolonged catheterization. Venogram through the offending catheter demonstrates a large clot in the SVC and innominate vein.

right ventricular infarction and adult respiratory distress syndrome (ARDS) with coexistent left ventricular dysfunction. Measurements of PCW pressure also aid in differentiating cardiogenic from noncardiogenic pulmonary edema (Brandstetter and Gitler, 1986).

The basic catheter consists of a central channel for pressure monitoring and a second channel connected to an inflatable balloon at the catheter tip (Swan and Ganz, 1975). At least one additional channel is now present on most catheters for determination of CVP and cardiac output (see Chapter 2). Pacing Swan-Ganz catheters have also been developed, with a lumen positioned in the right ventricle for the pacing wire (Colardyn et al., 1986). The catheter can be inserted at the bedside and "floated" to the pulmonary artery, generally without fluoroscopic monitoring. It is usually inserted from a subclavian approach through a sheath commonly referred to as the "cordis." This sheath allows easy advancement and withdrawal of the catheter as needed. It also serves as short-term venous access after the Swan-Ganz catheter has been removed. The radiographic appearance of the sheath is characteristic and should not be confused with routine central venous catheters. It is a barely opaque, short, wide-bore catheter.

Ideal Position

Ideally, the catheter is positioned so that it lies within the right or left main pulmonary artery (Swan and Ganz, 1975) (see Figs. 2–6 and 4–15). Inflation of the balloon causes the catheter to float downstream into a wedge position, and deflation of the balloon allows the catheter to recoil into the central pulmonary artery. Excessive intravenous or intracardiac slack enhances the likelihood of distal migration of the catheter, which increases the incidence of complication.

Potential Complications

Pulmonary Infarction

The most common significant complication associated with use of the Swan-Ganz catheter is pulmonary infarction distal to the catheter tip (Sise et al., 1981). Infarction occurs as a result of occlusion of the pulmonary artery by the catheter itself or as the result of clot formation in or about the catheter (McLoud and Putman, 1975; Ravin et al., 1976).

Another potential cause of thrombosis in situ is inadvertent failure to deflate the catheter balloon (Foote et al., 1974). The balloon appears radiographically as a 1-cm rounded radiolucency located at the tip of the catheter (Fig. 4–11). Because of its size, a persistently inflated balloon can potentially obstruct a major pulmonary artery and lead to significant pulmonary infarction. The radiographic patterns of pulmonary infarction are similar to those observed with infarction from other causes (McLoud and Putman, 1975). Most of these patterns consist of patchy airspace consolidation involving the area of the lung supplied by the pulmonary artery in which the catheter lies (Fig. 4–12). On occasion, a Hampton's hump configuration is identified (Fig. 4–13). Often, however, no definite radiographic manifestation of infarction is noted, although evidence of the infarction can be found at autopsy.

If recognized or suspected, pulmonary infarction is treated by removal of the Swan-Ganz catheter. Systemic heparinization is not required, because the source of the emboli and obstruction has been removed.

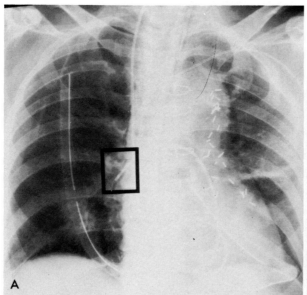
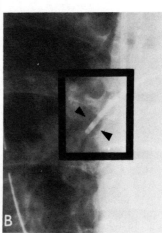

Figure 4–11. *A,* Anteroposterior portable radiograph demonstrating a Swan-Ganz catheter making several loops in the right ventricle. The area outlined in the box *(B)* shows that the balloon *(arrowheads)* at the tip of the catheter remains partially inflated, creating the potential for massive thrombosis. (From Ravin, C.E., et al.: Hazards of the ICU. AJR 126:423–431, 1976, with permission, © by American Roentgen Ray Society.)

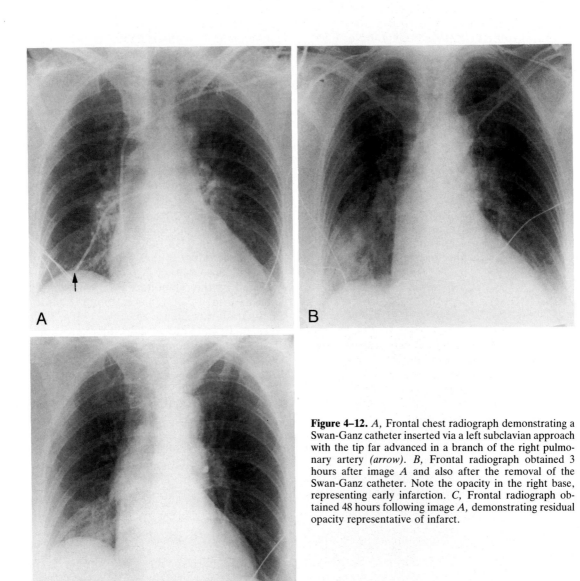

Figure 4–12. *A,* Frontal chest radiograph demonstrating a Swan-Ganz catheter inserted via a left subclavian approach with the tip far advanced in a branch of the right pulmonary artery *(arrow). B,* Frontal radiograph obtained 3 hours after image *A* and also after the removal of the Swan-Ganz catheter. Note the opacity in the right base, representing early infarction. *C,* Frontal radiograph obtained 48 hours following image *A,* demonstrating residual opacity representative of infarct.

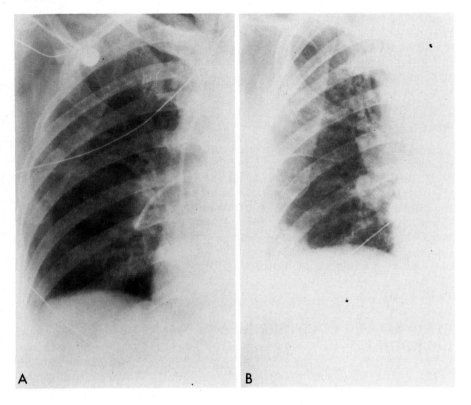

Figure 4–13. *A,* Swan-Ganz catheter positioned in a basilar segmental artery of the right lower lobe. *B,* Follow-up examination 2 days later, demonstrating a pleural-based density in the right costophrenic angle with a convex upper border consistent with pulmonary infarction. (From Ravin, C.E., et al.: Hazards of the ICU. AJR 126:423–431, 1976, with permission, © by American Roentgen Ray Society.)

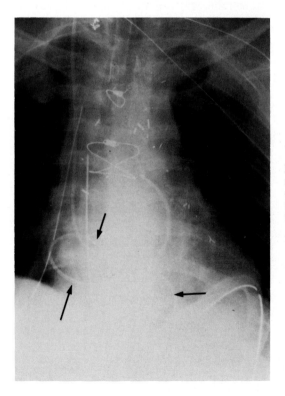

Figure 4–14. Inadvertent insertion of an excessive length of Swan-Ganz catheter resulted in coiling of loops in the right atrium and right ventricle *(arrows).* This condition frequently produces arrhythmias that are refractory to drug therapy; these are readily corrected, however, by straightening the catheter. The tip of the catheter is in the right main pulmonary artery.

Arrhythmias

Passage of Swan-Ganz catheters through the right side of the heart has been associated with both atrial and ventricular arrhythmias, as well as with complete heart block. In addition, insertion of an excessive length of catheter can lead to coiling or redundancy in the right side of the heart, resulting in irritation of the conducting bundle and production of premature ventricular contractions (Fig. 4–14).

Miscellaneous Complications

Rare instances of pulmonary arterial rupture, pulmonary arterial pseudoaneurysm formation (Dieden et al., 1987), pulmonary to bronchial tree fistulae (Rubin and Puckett, 1979), intracardiac knotting of the catheter (Lipp, et al., 1971), and balloon rupture (Swan et al., 1970) have been reported with use of the Swan-Ganz catheter. Most of these complications can be avoided, however, if the recommendations for use and for positioning of the catheter are strictly followed.

INTRA-AORTIC COUNTERPULSATION BALLOON

The intra-aortic counterpulsation balloon (IACB) is employed with increasing frequency to improve cardiac function in the setting of cardiogenic shock or high-risk cardiac surgery. The device consists of a fusiform inflatable balloon that is approximately 26 to 28 cm in length and that surrounds the distal end of a centrally placed catheter. The balloon is inflated with approximately 40 ml of gas, usually helium, during diastole and is forcibly deflated during systole.

Inflation-deflation timing is linked to the electrocardiogram and can vary from assistance on every cardiac cycle to assistance on every third or fourth cycle. Inflation during diastole increases diastolic pressure in the proximal aorta, thereby increasing perfusion of the coronary arteries and increasing oxygen delivery to the myocardium. The pattern of balloon deflation is such that it starts the column of aortic blood moving distally, thereby decreasing the afterload, against which the left ventricle must eject its stroke volume, and diminishing left ventricular work and oxygen requirements. The overall effect of balloon pumping, therefore, is increased oxygen delivery to the myocardium and decreased left ventricular work, resulting in overall improvement in cardiac function (Dunkman et al., 1972). Radiographically, the device appears as a catheter surrounded at its distal end during diastole by an oblong, gas-filled balloon (Figs. 4–15 and 4–16). During systole, the balloon is deflated and is not visualized radiographically. A radiopaque marker defines the tip of the catheter.

Ideal Position

Intra-aortic balloon pumps are placed percutaneously via the common femoral artery and are then advanced in a retrograde manner to the thoracic aorta. Ideally, the tip of the catheter is just distal to the left subclavian artery (see Figs. 4–15 and 4–16). This location allows maximal augmentation of diastolic pressures in the proximal aorta and decreases the risk of embolization of the cerebral vessels. In clinical practice, the tip of the device is placed so that it projects at the level of the aortic arch on the frontal radiograph. Despite appropriate positioning in the aortic arch, the mesenteric and renal artery ostia are

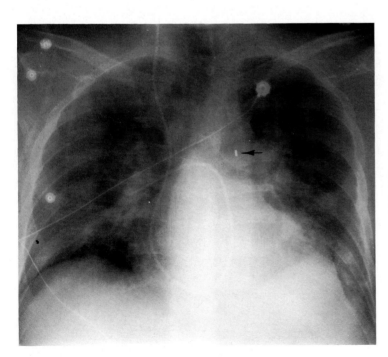

Figure 4–15. Frontal radiograph demonstrating the tip of a Swan-Ganz catheter in the right interlobar pulmonary artery. Intra-aortic balloon pump is shown with the balloon deflated in the descending thoracic aorta. Note the intra-aortic balloon pump marker tip just above the left main bronchus *(arrow).*

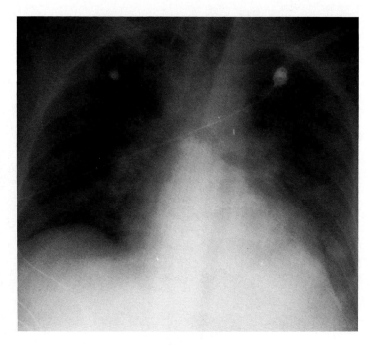

Figure 4–16. Frontal radiograph of the same patient as in Figure 4–15, again demonstrating a Swan-Ganz catheter. The inflated balloon (diastole) is visible to the left of the spine.

crossed, owing to the length of the balloon (Vail et al., 1988). Unless they are placed intraoperatively, most intra-aortic balloon pumps are placed at the bedside. Post-procedure chest radiography is imperative to confirm appropriate positioning of the catheter. Subtle changes in the appearance of the radiopaque marker tip should be sought as an indicator of inappropriate position.

Potential Complications

Aberrant Positioning

If the catheter is advanced too far, it either may enter and obstruct the left subclavian artery or may be positioned in the aortic arch, increasing the risk of cerebral embolus. More often, the aorta is more tortuous than anticipated and the balloon does not reach the level of the aortic arch, but is positioned more distally, resulting in less effective counterpulsation.

Aortic Dissection

Another potential complication of the intra-aortic balloon pump is dissection into or through the aortic wall at the time of insertion. Several cases have been described in which such dissection occurred but was of no clinical consequence (Dunkman et al., 1972). In other instances, however, dissection has been followed by death (Pace et al., 1977). A history of difficulty in inserting the device or complaints of pain by the patient during the procedure should alert the radiologist to this potential complication. In addition, loss of definition of the descending thoracic aorta on the chest radiograph following placement of the

IACB may occasionally be an early clue to intramural positioning (Hyson et al., 1977) (Fig. 4–17). Aortography or contrast-enhanced computed tomography (CT) scanning is usually required to confirm this ectopic location. The angiographer should be aware that patients undergoing balloon pumping are fully heparinized, and that performance of arteriography is therefore more complicated and the risk of post-procedure bleeding increased.

Miscellaneous Complications

Other risks associated with use of the intra-aortic balloon pump include reduction of platelets, red blood cell destruction, emboli, balloon rupture with gas embolus, renal failure, and vascular insufficiency of the catheterized limb. Most of these complications are not recognized radiographically, although confirmation of vascular insufficiency may require arteriography.

HICKMAN, INFUSAPORT, AND OTHER SURGICALLY IMPLANTED CATHETERS

The institution of bone marrow and organ transplantation services has increased the number of long-term intensive care unit patients and, hence, the use in the ICU of catheters designed for long-term venous access. The most commonly used catheters for this purpose include the Hickman, Infusaport, and Portacath catheters. Each of these catheters is placed surgically, usually into the subclavian vein. The Hickman catheter provides external access (Fig. 4–18 A), whereas the other catheters have a subcutaneous access port identifiable radiographically.

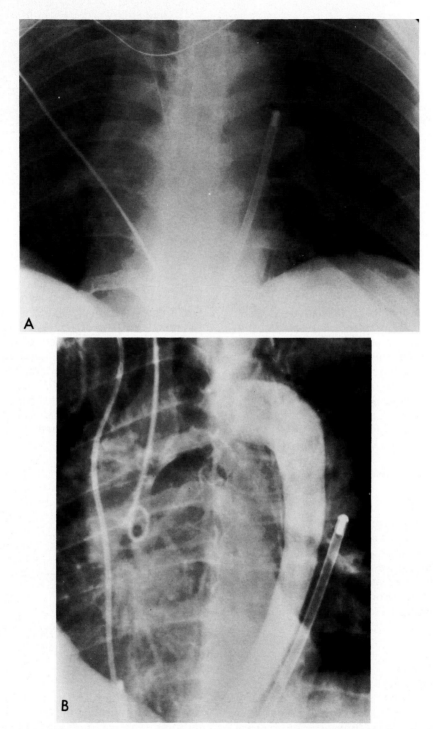

Figure 4–17. *A,* Following treatment of an intra-aortic counterpulsation balloon (IACB), the border of the descending aorta is indistinct. The patient complained of pain at the time of insertion. *B,* Aortogram demonstrating the extraluminal position of the IACB. (From Hyson, E.A., et al.: The intra-aortic counterpulsation balloon: Radiographic considerations. AJR 128:915–918, 1977, with permission, © by American Roentgen Ray Society.)

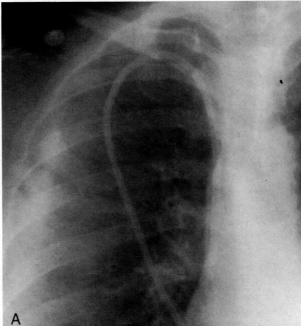

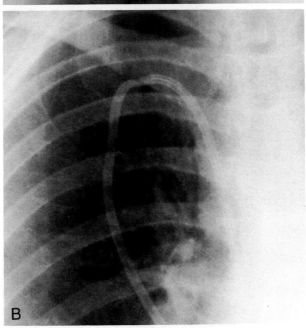

Figure 4–18. *A*, Frontal radiograph demonstrating Hickman catheter in the distal SVC in a patient with breast carcinoma. *B*, Frontal radiograph demonstrating "pinching" of the catheter between the clavicle and the first rib. The catheter did not function with the arm at the side.

Ideal Position

As with other central venous catheters, the optimal position of the catheter tip is within the distal superior vena cava or proximal right atrium. This location provides the greatest dilution of infused substances without the risk of significant cardiac complications.

Potential Complications

Because of the subcutaneous ports and long subcutaneous tracks used by these catheters, the risk of infection is decreased in relation to that of percutaneously placed catheters. In a small but significant

number of patients, the catheter becomes pinched between the clavicle and the first rib. This pinching results in difficult infusion when the arms are down, thrombosis, and occasional fraying and embolization of the catheter (Hinke et al., 1990) (see Fig. 4–18*B*). Other potential complications, such as aberrant positioning and vessel perforation, occur as described previously for subclavian and CVP catheters.

TRANSVENOUS PACEMAKERS

Since its introduction in the late 1950s, transvenous endocardiac pacing has become the method of choice for maintaining cardiac rhythm in patients with heart block or bradyarrhythmias (Chung, 1976). The pacemaker electrode catheter is inserted into the cephalic or subclavian vein and is directed under fluoroscopic control to the apex of the right ventricle.

Ideal Position

Ideally, the catheter is positioned in the apex of the right ventricle and is wedged beneath the cardiac trabeculae to ensure stability as well as intimate contact with the endocardium. Sharp angulation in the course of the catheter from the pulse generator unit to the distal tip should be avoided, because such areas are under increased mechanical stress and may fracture (McHenry and Grayson, 1970). Gentle curves of the catheter through the veins and heart are also desirable to help avoid catheter recoiling. Radiographs in both frontal and lateral projections are required to assess positioning completely (Fig. 4–19). On the frontal view, the catheter should project at the apex of the ventricle, and on the lateral view, the tip of the catheter should lie 3 to 4 mm beneath the epicardial fat stripe (Ormond et al., 1971). Catheter positions that are anterior to this point suggest the possibility of myocardial perforation.

Potential Complications

Aberrant Positioning

The most common abnormality recognized radiographically is malpositioning. Common aberrant lo-

cations include the coronary sinus (see Fig. 4–3), the right atrium, the pulmonary outflow tract, and the pulmonary artery (Fig. 4–20). Of these locations, the coronary sinus is the most difficult in which to assess radiographically the malpositioning of a pacemaker electrode catheter. In this location, the catheter often appears to be ideally positioned on the frontal projection, but is directed posteriorly rather than anteriorly on the lateral projection. If only a frontal view can be obtained, however, a clue to ectopic placement in the coronary sinus is an upward deflection of the catheter tip as it follows the sinus around the posterior atrioventricular groove (see Fig. 4–1). The pacing wire may also enter the middle cardiac vein via the coronary sinus.

On occasion, pacemakers are intentionally placed in the coronary sinus to achieve atrial rather than ventricular pacing. This placement is performed primarily in the investigation of various bradyarrhythmias and tachyarrhythmias (Hewitt et al., 1981). For the most part, however, such investigations are not carried out in the intensive care unit; thus, positioning in the coronary sinus should be viewed with suspicion in this setting.

Myocardial Perforation

Another potential complication is perforation of the myocardium by the catheter itself. This problem may be difficult to recognize unless the catheter clearly projects outside the myocardium (Fig. 4–21) or anteriorly in relation to the epicardial fat stripe. Although hemopericardium accompanied by cardiac

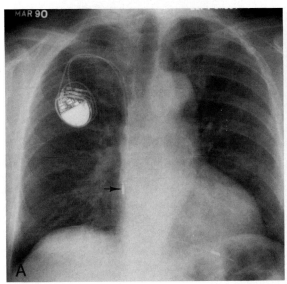

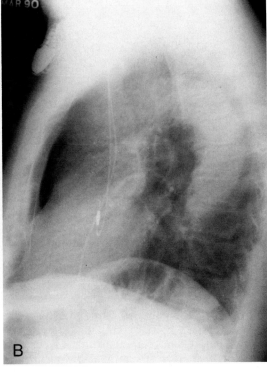

Figure 4–19. *A,* Frontal radiograph demonstrating a permanent atrioventricular pacemaker. Note the upward curvature of the atrial pacer tip. The tip is preferably directed medially to enter the right atrial appendage *(arrow). B,* Lateral radiograph in the same patient, demonstrating the atrioventricular pacing leads.

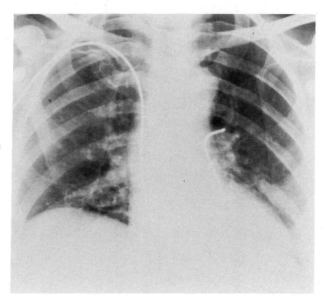

Figure 4–20. Transvenous pacer wire inadvertently advanced to the left pulmonary artery.

tamponade can occur, the majority of such perforations are not of great clinical significance, because withdrawal of the catheter corrects the position and does not cause significant bleeding (Sorkin et al., 1976).

Mechanical Problems

In the clinical setting of inadequate pacing, the radiologist must also be alert to the possibility of fracture of the electrode wires or detachment of the pacemaker wires from the pulse unit. Although detachment can be readily recognized, electrode frac-

ture (Fig. 4–22) may be more difficult to define because the insulating sheath can hold the broken ends close enough together to escape detection (Hall and Rosenbaum, 1971). Fluoroscopy, when available, is sometimes useful in evaluation of pacemaker electrodes for fracture.

Inadequate pacing may also result from failure of the pulse generator due to battery failure. Although initial reports enthusiastically outlined radiographic criteria by which battery failure could be determined, such techniques are difficult to apply in actual practice. Thus, an easier method of determining battery failure, particularly in the intensive care unit, involves

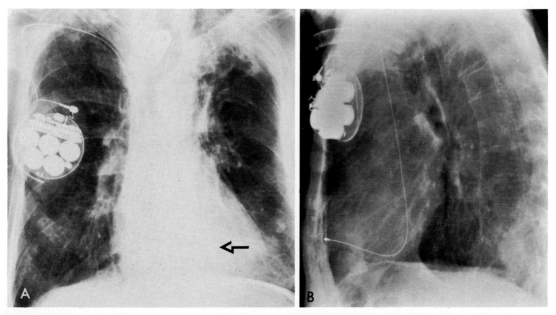

Figure 4–21. *A,* Posteroanterior chest radiograph of a patient with a transvenous pacemaker who developed a pneumomediastinum following tracheostomy. The tip of the pacing electrode is barely visible, projecting over the right ventricle *(arrow).* *B,* Lateral view showing the pacemaker tip extending beyond the myocardium and into the pericardial space. This problem had not been clinically suspected before the patient developed a pneumomediastinum. Note that the tracheostomy tube is poorly positioned in the trachea.

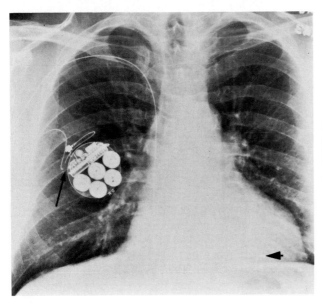

Figure 4–22. Posteroanterior chest radiograph in a patient who had symptoms of congestive failure and demonstrated unsatisfactory pacing. The pacer wire is fractured *(arrow)* just beyond the pacer unit. The electrode tip projects over the apex of the right ventricle *(arrowhead)*.

direct measurement of the electronic output of the pacer.

AUTOMATIC IMPLANTABLE CARDIOVERTER DEFIBRILLATOR ("PATCH" DEFIBRILLATOR)

The use of the automatic implantable cardioverter defibrillator (AICD) ("patch" defibrillator) for prophylaxis against fatal ventricular tachyarrhythmias became widespread in the 1980s. Because of the prevalence of sudden cardiac death, unassociated with acute myocardial infarction, and the limited effectiveness of antiarrhythmic drugs in this setting, AICD therapy is considered by some to be the emerging "gold standard" for prophylaxis against fatal ventricular tachyarrhythmias (Lehmann et al., 1988). The AICD is composed of a fine titanium mesh placed on the surface of the heart, but only the nonfunctioning peripheral marking wires are visible radiographically (Fig. 4–23). Crumpling of these wires has been suggested as a sign of pericardial fibrosis or infection

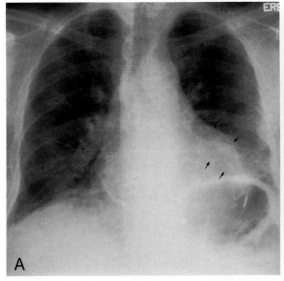

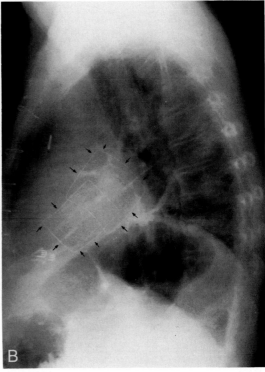

Figure 4–23. Frontal *(A)* and lateral *(B)* radiographs demonstrating automatic implantable cardioverter defibrillator *(arrows)*. The anterior patch is not visible over the spine on the frontal view. The marker wires delineate the margins of the titanium mesh pad. The leads near the inferior aspect of the heart with coiled tips represent sensing electrodes.

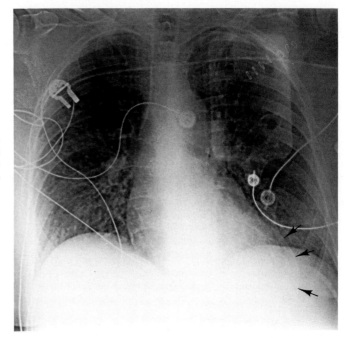

Figure 4–24. Frontal radiograph demonstrating Zoll's transcutaneous pacing unit. In this particular unit, the rectangular pad appearing over the left lung apex is placed posteriorly. The circular pad that is placed anteriorly over the cardiac apex is barely visible *(arrows)*.

(Goodman et al., 1989). Other complications and considerations include lead fracture, rare traumatic or inflammatory effects of the epicardial patch, and limited generator longevity (18 to 24 months) (Lehmann et al., 1988).

TRANSCUTANEOUS PACERS

Transcutaneous temporary pacing was first successfully introduced in 1983 (Falk et al., 1983). Known for its inventor, the Zoll noninvasive temporary pacemaker is now in widespread use, particularly in situations requiring emergency cardiac pacing, such as bradycardia or asystole (Zoll et al., 1985). Pacing is achieved with two electrodes, one placed over the lower left thorax near the sternum and the other placed posteriorly below the left scapula or anterolaterally along the anterior axillary line.

The electrodes are large (16 cm in diameter) but only moderately radiopaque and may be difficult to identify on radiographs (Fig. 4–24). Complications have been limited to pain requiring sedation or analgesics, prominent chest wall muscle contractions, and the potential for tachyarrhythmia induction (Peters, 1986).

SUMMARY

Although development of various cardiovascular monitoring and assist devices during the past 10 to 15 years has contributed significantly to improved management of seriously ill patients, the devices are not without potential complications. Many of these complications are difficult, if not impossible, to detect clinically but are readily apparent on standard radiographs. Knowledge of the purpose of the device and its ideal position and potential complications facilitates better interpretation of radiographs obtained in the intensive care unit and leads to early detection of complications.

References

Adar, R., and Mozes, M.: Hydromediastinum. JAMA 214:372, 1970.

Au, F.C., and Badellino, M.: Significance of a curled central venous catheter tip. Chest 93:890, 1988.

Aulenbacher, C.E.: Hydrothorax from subclavian vein catheterization. JAMA 214:372, 1970.

Blair, E., Hunziker, R., and Flanagan, M.E.: Catheter embolism. Surgery 67:457, 1970.

Bone, D.K., Maddrey, W.C., Eagan, J., and Cameron, J.L.: Cardiac tamponade: A fatal complication of central venous catheterization. Arch. Surg. 106:868, 1973.

Bouffard, Y., Bouletreau, P., and Motin, J.: Deep venous thrombosis with clinical signs after catheterization of the superior vena cava system. Acta Anaesthesiol. Scand. 81:65, 1985.

Brandstetter, R.D., and Gitler, B.: Thoughts on the Swan-Ganz catheter. Chest 89:5, 1986.

Brandt, R.L., Foley, W.J., Fink, G.H., et al.: Mechanism of perforation of the heart with production of hydropericardium by a venous catheter and its prevention. Am. J. Surg. 119:311, 1970.

Cha, E.M., and Khoury, G.H.: Persistent left superior vena cava. Radiology 103:375, 1972.

Chung, E.K.: Artificial cardiac pacing. Postgrad. Med. 59:83, 1976.

Colardyn, F., Vandenborgaerde, J., DeNiel, C., and Jordaens, L.: Ventricular pacing via a Swan-Ganz catheter: A new mode of pacemaker therapy. Acta Cardiol. 41:23, 1986.

Daly, J.M., Ziegler, B., and Dudrick, S.J.: Central venous catheterization. Am J. Nurs. 75:820, 1975.

Dedhia, H.V., and Schiebel, F.: What is wrong with this chest roentgenogram? Chest 92:921, 1987.

Dieden, J.D., Friloux III, L.A., and Renner, J.W.: Pulmonary artery false aneurysms secondary to Swan-Ganz pulmonary artery catheters. AJR 149:901, 1987.

Dudrick, S.J., Wilmore, D.W., Vars, H.M., et al.: Can intravenous feeding as the sole means of nutrition support growth in the child and restore weight loss in an adult? An affirmative answer. Ann. Surg. 169:974, 1969.

Dunkman, W.B., Leinbach, R.C., Buckley, M.J., et al.: Clinical and hemodynamic results of intra-aortic balloon pumping and surgery for cardiogenic shock. Circulation 46:465, 1972.

Falk, R.H., Zoll, P.M., and Zoll, R.H.: Safety and efficacy of noninvasive cardiac pacing. N. Engl. J. Med. 309:1166, 1983.

Fontenelle, L.T., Dooley, B.N., and Cuello, L.: Subclavian venipuncture and its complications. Ann. Thorac. Surg. 11:331, 1971.

Foote, G.A., Schabel, S.I., and Hodges, M.: Pulmonary complications of the flow-directed balloon-tipped catheter. N. Engl. J. Med. 290:927, 1974.

Friedman, A.C., Chambers, E., and Sprayregen, S.: The normal and abnormal left superior intercostal vein. AJR 131:599, 1978.

Gibson, R.N., Hennessy, O.F., Collier, N., and Hemingway, A.P.: Major complications of central venous catheterization: A report of five cases and a brief review of the literature. Clin. Radiol. 36:205, 1985.

Gilday, D.L.: The value of chest radiography in the localization of central venous pressure catheters. Can. Med. Assoc. J. 101:363, 1969.

Goodman, L.R., Almassi, G.H., Troup, P.J., et al.: Complications of automatic implantable cardioverter defibrillators: Radiographic, CT, and echocardiographic evaluation. Radiology 170:447, 1989.

Hall, W.M., and Rosenbaum, H.B.: The radiology of cardiac pacemakers. Radiol. Clin. North Am. 9:343, 1971.

Hewitt, M.J., Chen, J.T.T., Ravin, C.E., and Gallagher, J.J.: Coronary sinus atrial pacing: Radiographic considerations. AJR 136:323, 1981.

Hinke, D.H., Zandt-Stastny, D., Goodman, L.R., et al.: Pinch-off syndrome: A complication of implantable subclavian venous access devices. Radiology 177:353, 1990.

Huyghens, L., Sennesael, J., Verbeelen, D., et al.: Cardiothoracic complications of centrally inserted catheters. Acute Care 11:53, 1985.

Hyson, E.A., Ravin, C.E., Kelley, M.J., et al.: The intra-aortic counterpulsation balloon: Radiographic considerations. AJR 128:915, 1977.

Kline, I.K., and Hofman, W.I.: Cardiac tamponade from CVP catheter perforation. JAMA 206:1794, 1968.

Langston, C.S.: The aberrant central venous catheter and its complications. Radiology 100:55, 1971.

Lehmann, M.H., Steinman, R.T., Schuger, C.D., and Jackson, K.: The automatic implantable cardioverter defibrillator as antiarrhythmic treatment modality of choice for survivors of cardiac arrest unrelated to acute myocardial infarction. Am. J. Cardiol. 62:803, 1988.

Lipp, H., O'Donoghue, K., and Resnekov, L.: Intracardiac knotting of a flow-directed balloon catheter. N. Engl. J. Med. 284:220, 1971.

McDonald, C.J., Castellino, R.A., and Blank, N.: The aortic "nipple." Radiology 96:533, 1970.

McHenry, M.M., and Grayson, C.E.: Roentgenographic diagnosis of pacemaker failure. AJR 109:94, 1970.

McLoud, T.C., and Putman, C.E.: Radiology of the Swan-Ganz catheter and associated pulmonary complications. Radiology 116:19, 1975.

Ormond, R.S., Rubenfire, M., Anbe, D.T., et al.: Radiographic demonstration of myocardial perforation by permanent endocardial pacemakers. Radiology 98:35, 1971.

Pace, P.D., Tilney, N.L., Lesch, M., and Couch, N.P.: Peripheral arterial complications of intra-aortic balloon counterpulsation. Surgery 82:685, 1977.

Peters, R.W.: Temporary transcutaneous pacing. AORN J. 44:245, 1986.

Ravin, C.E., Putman, C.E., and McLoud, T.C.: Hazards of the ICU. AJR 126:423, 1976.

Rubin, S.A., and Puckett, R.P.: Pulmonary artery–bronchial fistula: A new complication of Swan-Ganz catheterization. Chest 75:515, 1979.

Sise, M.J., Hollingsworth, P., Brimm, J.E., et al.: Complications of the flow-directed pulmonary artery catheter: A prospective analysis of 219 patients. Crit. Care Med. 9:315, 1981.

Sivak, S.L.: Late appearance of pneumothorax after subclavian venipuncture. Am. J. Med. 80:323, 1986.

Sorkin, R.P., Schuurmann, B.J., and Simon, A.B.: Radiographic aspects of permanent cardiac pacemakers. Radiology 119:281, 1976.

Swan, H.J.C., and Ganz, W.: Use of a balloon flotation catheter in critically ill patients. Surg. Clin. North Am. 55:501, 1975.

Swan, H.J.C., Ganz, W., Forrester, J., et al.: Catheterization of the heart in man with use of a flow-directed balloon-tipped catheter. N. Engl. J. Med. 283:447, 1970.

Tocino, I.M., and Watanabe, A.: Impending catheter perforation of superior vena cava: Radiographic recognition. AJR 146:487, 1986.

Vail, C., Chiles, C., Coblentz, C., and Carroll, B.: Radiologic evaluation of intra-aortic balloon pumps. RSNA, 1988.

Williams, P.L., Warwick, R., Dyson, M., and Bannister, L.H.: Gray's Anatomy, ed. 37. New York, Churchill Livingstone, 1989.

Wilson, J.N., Grow, J.B., Demong, C.V., et al.: Central venous pressure in optimal blood volume maintenance. Arch. Surg. 85:563, 1962.

Winter, F.S.: Persistent left superior vena cava. Angiology 5:90, 1954.

Zoll, P.M., Zoll, R.H., Falk, R.H., et al.: External noninvasive temporary cardiac pacing: Clinical trials. Circulation 71:937, 1985.

ACUTE PULMONARY DISEASE

PART III

5

Acute Inflammatory Disease

∎

Lawrence R. Goodman

Although acute cardiopulmonary problems encountered in the intensive care unit (ICU) are not unique to this setting, several factors make radiographic evaluation difficult and at times impossible. Portable radiographs do not provide the resolution and reproducibility achieved by stationary equipment. The lung and cardiac abnormalities visualized are frequently the result of more than one disease process. The acute process may be superimposed on a chronic lung disease (e.g., chronic obstructive pulmonary disease [COPD]) or on an underlying systemic disorder (e.g., diabetes or immunosuppression), which alter the appearance of the acute cardiopulmonary disease. The heart or lung may be one of several failing organ systems, and the changes on the chest radiograph may be more a reflection of extrathoracic disease (renal failure or sepsis) than one of primary cardiopulmonary disease. In addition, various support and monitoring devices, as well as therapeutic maneuvers, may alter the appearance of the radiograph.

The next six chapters review the major cardiopulmonary disorders encountered in the ICU. Many of the radiographic changes are nonspecific and require careful attention to the time of onset, speed of progression, and distribution of the lesions. Serial radiographs must be viewed for day-to-day changes as well as for general trends. An ongoing and timely dialogue between the radiologist and the referring physician is vital for optimal interpretation.

PULMONARY INSUFFICIENCY

Acute respiratory failure is the sudden inability of the respiratory system to provide adequate arterial oxygenation and adequate carbon dioxide elimination for the patient's metabolic level. Usually, the arterial oxygen pressure (Pa_{O_2}) is less than 50 mm Hg, and the arterial carbon dioxide pressure (Pa_{CO_2}) is greater than 50 mm Hg. Carbon dioxide retention is most frequently due to inadequate ventilation (mechanics

of breathing), whereas hypoxia is usually secondary to impaired gas exchange. These disorders are seldom present as completely separate conditions, however. Respiratory insufficiency is frequently associated with underlying chronic cardiopulmonary disease or multiorgan failure, which further complicates diagnosis and treatment and increases both mortality and morbidity.

Potentially life-threatening pulmonary insufficiency may be present despite a normal radiograph. This situation suggests several diagnostic possibilities. In patients with central nervous system disease, neuromuscular disorders, and most drug overdoses, the initial and subsequent radiographs are normal unless a secondary complication, such as aspiration pneumonitis or atelectasis, develops. Patients with severe COPD frequently have potentially fatal pulmonary insufficiency with little or no radiographic evidence of an acute process superimposed on the emphysema. In such disorders as pulmonary embolus, sepsis, smoke inhalation, and adult respiratory distress syndrome (ARDS), the speed at which the radiograph becomes "positive" may help confirm or refute the initial impression (Fraser et al., 1991) (Fig. 5–1).

ATELECTASIS

The most frequent chest radiographic abnormality in the ICU is atelectasis. Various factors, sometimes multiple in a given case, lead to atelectasis in the critically ill or postoperative patient. Hypoventilation due to central depression, general anaesthesia, or splinting from trauma or thoracic or abdominal surgery leads to progressive decrease in alveolar volumes, which is most pronounced at the lung bases. The lack of alveolar distention reduces surfactant, which leads to further atelectasis. This process causes "micro-" or peripheral atelectasis within minutes to hours and causes hypoxia from intrapulmonary shunting (Pierce and Robertson, 1977). At this point, the

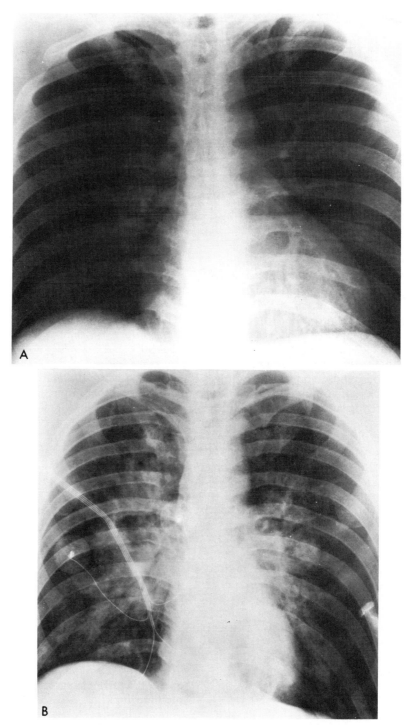

Figure 5–1. Smoke inhalation. *A,* Initial radiograph (approximately 2 hours after the patient inhaled large amounts of burning electrical insulation fumes) appears normal. *B,* Approximately 8 hours later, severe bilateral alveolar edema is evident. The patient died of pulmonary insufficiency within 36 hours of admission.

radiograph is normal or shows minimal linear atelectasis or increased basilar density. Westcott and Cole (1985b) have shown that in autopsied lungs, peripheral atelectasis is considerably more extensive than is radiographically apparent. Morimoto and associates (1989) and Strandberg and colleagues (1986) have shown that experimentally induced hypoventilation in humans and rabbits rapidly results in gravity-dependent atelectasis, which is visible on computed tomography (CT) scans but is probably not visible radiographically. Most of the clinical and experimental changes are reversible with hyperventilation.

Retained tracheobronchial secretions may also cause atelectasis. Inflammatory lung disease or edema causes increased production of secretions at a time when mobilization is impaired. Tracheal intubation decreases the ability to cough and diminishes mucociliary clearance. Inadequate humidification thickens secretions and makes mobilization more difficult as well.

The radiographic appearance of atelectasis varies markedly from that of clear lungs to one of total consolidation and volume loss. As discussed previously, the radiograph may appear normal or show only mild basilar shadowing or linear atelectasis when significant intrapulmonary shunting is occurring. In the case of broad bands of platelike atelectasis or segmental or lobar consolidation with volume loss, the radiographic diagnosis is usually apparent, and the physiologic changes are understandable (Figs. 5–2 and 5–3). The most direct evidence of volume loss is shifting of normally visible structures (e.g., minor

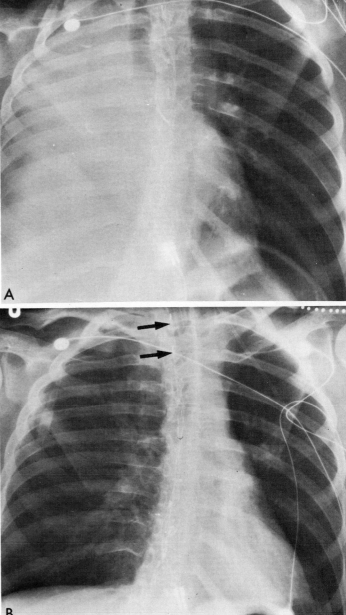

Figure 5–2. Right lung atelectasis. This young quadriplegic entered the hospital with increasing shortness of breath and a low-grade fever. *A,* The anteroposterior (AP) radiograph reveals total opacification of the right hemithorax with no visible air bronchograms. The mediastinum is shifted to the right, and the left lung is hyperinflated. *B,* Fiberoptic bronchoscopy revealed tenacious secretions in all the large airways. This radiograph, obtained 14 hours after bronchoscopy and suctioning, reveals almost total re-expansion of the right lung. Incidentally noted is flattening of the upper margins of the third, fourth, and fifth posterior ribs on the right due to pressure from the scapula, a common finding in long-standing quadriplegia. The electrodes noted over the first and second thoracic vertebrae are those of the dorsal column stimulator, used for intractable pain *(arrows).*

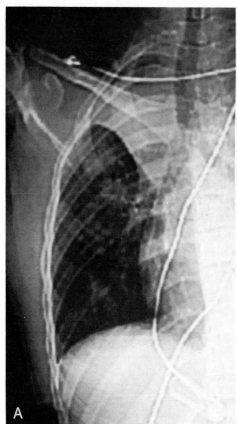

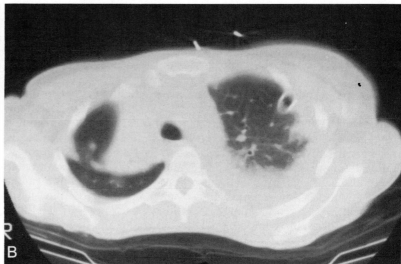

Figure 5–3. *A,* Acute right upper lobe collapse after surgery for left lung decortication. The minor fissure is elevated, the right upper lobe is opaque, and there are no visible air bronchograms. The initial postoperative radiograph showed a normal right lung. *B,* A representative axial scan through the right upper lobe shows complete collapse of the right upper lobe with no air bronchograms. Multiple plugs were found at bronchoscopy, and the chest radiograph obtained the following day was normal.

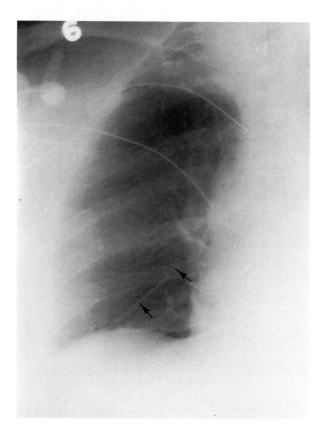

Figure 5–4. Right middle and right lower lobe atelectasis. One day after coronary artery surgery, the major fissure is visible on the frontal radiograph *(arrows)*. The minor fissure is barely visible on the original radiograph, 1.5 cm above the elevated right hemidiaphragm. These findings were not present on the preoperative radiographs nor on a subsequent radiograph obtained several days later.

fissure, pulmonary vessels, or granulomas). Normally, the major fissure is not visible on the frontal radiograph. With partial or complete lower lobe atelectasis, the fissure may assume a sagittal orientation and become visible (Fig. 5–4). Fisher (1981) found this sign to be three times more frequent in the right lung than in the left lung. She also found that fluid in an incomplete fissure, lordotic positioning, and right upper lobe consolidation, with or without atelectasis, may also account for visualization of the fissure on the frontal radiograph.

Another consequence of airway obstruction or hypoventilation is pulmonary consolidation without significant volume loss. The radiographic appearance may vary from patchy local consolidation to opacification of a whole lobe and be difficult to differentiate from that of significant lung disease (e.g., pneumonia or infarct) on the basis of a single radiograph (Fig. 5–5). Serial radiographs often show substantial change over a short time span, or improvement from the use of mechanical maneuvers to mobilize secretions or facilitate ventilation. Once the secretions are removed, the lung may appear normal. Although the secretions often contain pathogens, this occurrence is usually due to colonization rather than to established infection. The foregoing findings frequently lead to the overdiagnosis of pneumonia (see the next section).

Atelectasis is most frequent and most severe at the left lung base. In a study of 200 consecutive ICU patients, Shevland and co-workers (1983) found that 15 of 17 cases of lobar collapse occurred in the left lower lobe (Fig. 5–6). Although occurrence of this phenomenon after cardiac and left upper quadrant surgery is well known, it was also more frequent in patients with medical illnesses and trauma. The investigators postulate that in the supine bedridden patient, the heart may press on the left lower lobe bronchus, impeding drainage. In addition, blind suctioning of the left lower lobe bronchus is more difficult than that of the right lower lobe bronchus (Freedman et al., 1982).

The radiographic diagnosis of left lower lobe atelectasis may be difficult through the cardiac silhouette. On a well-penetrated radiograph, one may see an air bronchogram in the retrocardiac area, silhouetting of the diaphragm or the lateral border of the descending aorta, and increased retrocardiac density with loss of the retrocardiac vessels. Lower lobe volume loss is detected by crowded retrocardiac vessels or air bronchograms, by elevation of the diaphragm, by shift of the mediastinum, or by depression of the left hilum. The left upper lobe may be hyperlucent.

Several potential pitfalls are encountered in diagnosing left lower lobe consolidation or atelectasis. If

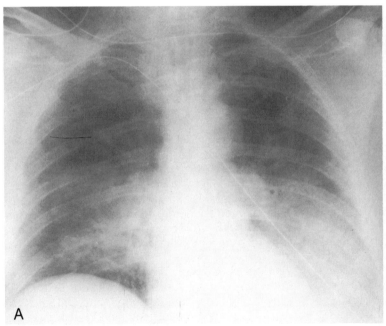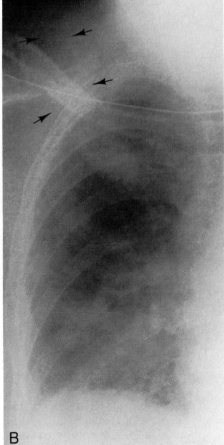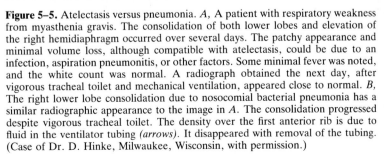

Figure 5–5. Atelectasis versus pneumonia. *A,* A patient with respiratory weakness from myasthenia gravis. The consolidation of both lower lobes and elevation of the right hemidiaphragm occurred over several days. The patchy appearance and minimal volume loss, although compatible with atelectasis, could be due to an infection, aspiration pneumonitis, or other factors. Some minimal fever was noted, and the white count was normal. A radiograph obtained the next day, after vigorous tracheal toilet and mechanical ventilation, appeared close to normal. *B,* The right lower lobe consolidation due to nosocomial bacterial pneumonia has a similar radiographic appearance to the image in *A.* The consolidation progressed despite vigorous tracheal toilet. The density over the first anterior rib is due to fluid in the ventilator tubing *(arrows).* It disappeared with removal of the tubing. (Case of Dr. D. Hinke, Milwaukee, Wisconsin, with permission.)

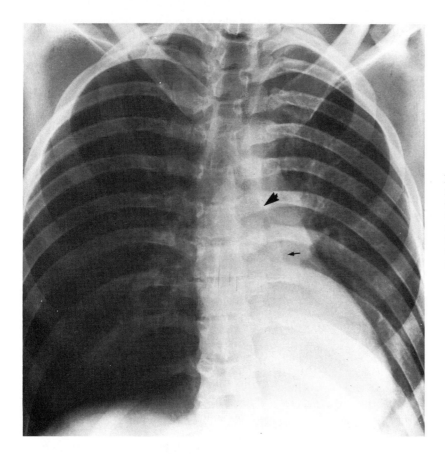

Figure 5–6. Left lower lobe collapse. The mediastinum is shifted to the left. The left diaphragm is elevated and obscured. The descending aorta cannot be visualized. A homogeneous density appears in the retrocardiac area, and the left main bronchus *(upper arrow)* and left lower bronchus *(lower arrow)* are depressed and moved medially.

the radiograph is not adequately penetrated for visualization of the spine, the foregoing signs may not be visible or may be falsely attributed to consolidation. If the x-ray beam is angled cephalad (lordotic projection), the diaphragm may be indistinct. Zylak and co-workers (1988) demonstrated in a study of one phantom and 10 patients that as little as 10 degrees of cranial beam angulation causes "pseudo-consolidation" of the left lower lobe or the appearance of a pleural effusion. Angulation toward the feet does not cause a similar problem. They demonstrated that the diaphragm becomes indistinct because the beam is no longer parallel to the dome of the diaphragm and the anterior extrapleural fat is projected upward over the lung base. With partial left lower lobe atelectasis, a pleural effusion may collect medially in relation to the lung, causing a triangular density that may also simulate total collapse of the lower lobe. In questionable cases of left lower lobe disease, an overpenetrated anteroposterior (AP) or slight right posterior oblique (RPO) radiograph, or "high" KUB radiograph, demonstrates the retrocardiac area more clearly. A right lateral decubitus radiograph causes hyperinflation of the left lung and causes fluid to shift medially, facilitating retrocardiac evaluation (Lerner, 1978).

The presence or absence of air bronchograms may indicate the cause of atelectasis, the approximate site of obstruction, and the appropriate course of therapy. Air bronchograms that are clearly visualized within a focal, segmental, or lobar consolidation strongly sug-

gest that the atelectasis or consolidation is not due to an endobronchial obstruction (e.g., mucous plug, clot, or tumor). Conversely, the *absence* of an air bronchogram in an area of consolidation suggests endobronchial obstruction. The more proximal the defect, the larger the occluded airway. On a supine or semi-erect radiograph, poor definition of a main bronchus may signify pooling of fluid posteriorly and collection of air anteriorly in a partially filled bronchus (Harris, 1985). Marini and associates (1979) showed that ICU patients demonstrating absence of air bronchograms did have large airway secretions and benefited markedly from bronchoscopy, whereas those with air bronchograms showed minimum benefit from bronchoscopy (see Fig. 5–2 and Fig. 5–3).

At times, mucous plugging may be surprisingly acute, may or may not cause distal consolidation and collapse, and may mimic a pulmonary embolus clinically. Pham and colleagues (1987) reported eight patients who had dyspnea, hypoxia, shunting, and diminished carbon dioxide partial pressure (P_{CO_2}) and therefore were suspected of having pulmonary emboli. Three had normal chest radiographs, and five demonstrated radiographic evidence of lobar collapse. All had complete or nearly complete absence of ventilation and partially diminished perfusion on isotopic evaluation. All were eventually proved to have major airway secretions as a cause of their clinical, radiographic, and ventilation/perfusion abnormalities.

INFECTION

Pneumonia

The majority of pulmonary infections found in the ICU are hospital acquired and they differ significantly from community-acquired infections. Hospital-acquired or nosocomial infections are defined as infections occurring more than 72 hours after admission. Although nosocomial urinary tract and wound infections are much more common, pneumonia is the leading infectious cause of death in the hospital. The incidence of nosocomial pulmonary infection is 1% in the general hospital population and considerably higher in the ICU. The pneumonia rate is estimated to be 8% to 12% in medical and surgical ICUs, and as high as 60% among patients with ARDS. In the critical care setting, the mortality from nosocomial pneumonia is estimated to be 20% to 35%. This estimate rises to 50% in patients with ARDS and to greater than 90% when nosocomial pneumonia is associated with multi-organ failure. Gram-negative bacillary nosocomial pneumonia is twice as lethal as gram-positive pneumonia (Bamberger, 1987; Bartlett et al., 1986; Pingleton, 1988; Ruiz-Santana et al., 1987; Toews, 1986).

Numerous factors contribute to the high incidence of infection in the ICU. Almost every ICU patient can be considered a "compromised host." The patient's primary disease (e.g., malignancy, diabetes, or chronic obstructive pulmonary disease [COPD]) may increase susceptibility to infection. Prolonged hospitalization and debility are associated with gradual alterations of normal pharyngeal flora to one that is rich in gram-negative organisms (Sanford and Pierce, 1979). Previous antibiotic therapy or administration of steroids accelerates colonization. Normal physical barriers to infection may be bypassed by various tubes and catheters. Most patients with intratracheal tubes develop tracheal colonization within several days of intubation. Finally, drugs that elevate the gastric pH promote bacterial overgrowth in the stomach. This material is frequently regurgitated and serves as an additional endogenous source of infection. In the past, respirator tubing, humidifiers, and so forth were major sources of respiratory tract infection. Improved equipment and disinfecting techniques have markedly diminished this source of infection.

The majority of community-acquired infections are due to viruses, *Mycoplasma* organisms, or gram-positive cocci. Usually, a single infecting agent is involved, and most infections are either self-limited or readily treatable with antibiotics. Nosocomial infections differ from community-acquired infections in several ways. The majority are due to gram-negative aerobes, such as *Klebsiella* or *Pseudomonas* species, or to anaerobic gram-negative rods. Gram-positive organisms are cultured in less than 20% of infections. In at least half the patients, more than one pathogen is cultured (Bartlett et al., 1986; Ruiz-Santana et al., 1987; Toews, 1986). Nonbacterial infections, such as viral and fungal infections, are uncommon in the general ICU population but quite common in patients with specific immune problems such as acquired immunodeficiency syndrome (AIDS) and organ transplantation. The immunocompromised patient is discussed in Chapter 10. Gram-negative or polymicrobial infections are associated with higher complication rates (e.g., abscess, empyema, and bronchopleural fistula) and are more likely to be resistant to antibiotics.

Despite its frequency, nosocomial pneumonia is often extremely difficult to diagnose (Tobin and Grenvik, 1984). The signs traditionally used to diagnose pneumonia—fever, leukocytosis, sputum production, positive sputum cultures, and radiographic abnormalities—frequently have other causes in the critically ill patient or may be absent in a significant number of patients with proven pneumonia. Fever may have an infectious or noninfectious cause unrelated to pneumonia. Fever is present in at least 50% of patients having atelectasis and no infection (Roberts et al., 1988). Similarly, leukocytosis may be due to extrathoracic inflammation or infection. Both fever and leukocytosis may be absent in pneumonia patients who are severely debilitated, immunocompromised, or receiving anti-inflammatory medication.

Sputum production may not be readily apparent in critically ill patients, or sputum production may be secondary to tracheobronchitis rather than pneumonia. Sputum cultures may be misleading because they are often contaminated with pharyngeal or tracheal flora that may or may not predict the underlying infection. Conversely, cultures from bronchoscopy samples may be negative in a significant minority of established pulmonary infections. In a large, multi-institutional study of nosocomial infection, a confident bacteriologic diagnosis was established in fewer than 40% of patients (Ruiz-Santana et al., 1987). The radiographic evaluation and limitations of radiography in diagnosis of pneumonia are discussed later in this section.

Several studies highlight the difficulties of documenting the presence or absence of pulmonary infection in the critically ill. In a study of 60 patients who were believed by their primary physician to have pneumonia, Bryant and colleagues (1973) found approximately two thirds of the diagnoses to be in error. Misdiagnosis was based on transient fevers or abnormalities of physical or chest radiographic examination. In 58 of 60 patients, a potential pathogen was recovered from the sputum. In an autopsy study of 24 patients who died of ARDS, Andrews and associates (1981) found that 14 patients (58%) had histologic evidence of infection. The clinical diagnosis of pneumonia had been correctly made in only nine (64%) of those patients with proven infection. Two of the ten uninfected patients were thought to be infected. Overall, the misdiagnosis rate was 29%. The vast majority of patients of both groups had fever, elevated or depressed white blood counts, and positive sputum cultures. The infected patients were

Table 5–1. ADULT RESPIRATORY DISTRESS SYNDROME: DIAGNOSIS OF PNEUMONIA

Sign	Pneumonia (n = 14)	No Pneumonia (n = 10)
Fever	100%	80%
Altered white blood count	100%	80%
Positive sputum culture	86%	70%
Asymmetric chest radiograph	57%	30%

Adapted from Andrews, C. P., et al.: Diagnosis of nosocomial bacterial pneumonia in acute diffuse lung disease. Chest 80:254, 1981.

twice as likely as the uninfected patients to have focal, asymmetric consolidation on their radiographs (Table 5–1).

Mock and co-workers (1988) approached pneumonia from the radiographic perspective to determine whether one could separate patients who had colonization from patients who had pulmonary infection. Radiographs of 80 patients with positive sputum cultures were rated on the "probability of pneumonia." Radiographic criteria used were (1) acinar shadows, (2) air bronchograms, (3) segmental consolidation, (4) asymmetric consolidation, and (5) ipsilateral pleural effusion and the absence of (6) volume loss, (7) a large heart or (8) a large hilum. Patients whose radiographs demonstrated moderate or high probability of pneumonia were more likely to have positive blood or pleural cultures, polymicrobial cultures, *Escherichia coli* or *Pseudomonas* cultures, and multiorgan failure, and to show improvement with antibiotic therapy. These radiographic criteria did not correlate with differences in fever, white blood cell count, presence of respiratory failure, or mortality. From these studies, one can conclude that the chest radiograph is a modest predictor of pulmonary infection, but at least on a par with, if not superior to, many other traditional clinical and laboratory investigations.

Medical lore indicates that established pneumonia may not be visible radiographically in a dehydrated patient until that patient is rehydrated. This concept is difficult to prove or disprove, as one must separate the normal progression of pneumonia from the effects of dehydration or overhydration. Caldwell and associates (1975) infected four dehydrated and four control dogs with pneumococci to study the effects of dehydration and rehydration on the clinical, radiologic, and pathologic appearances of the lung. No differences were noted. In dogs with established pneumococcal infection, Colligan and colleagues (1982) infused fluids until the pulmonary capillary wedge pressure reached 10 cm of water. At autopsy, the infected lobe was found to be much heavier in the infused dogs than in the euhydrated control dogs. Noninfected lobes, however, were also found to be heavier in the infused dogs. Hall and Simon (1987) presented a clinical case of an 84-year-old woman demonstrating clinical evidence of pneumonia and a negative radiograph who developed severe right upper lobe opacification within hours of modest rehydration.

From the scanty literature, one can only conclude that dehydration masking radiographic evidence of pneumonia is uncommon. Infection or inflammation, however, does increase capillary permeability, which causes subsequent exudation of fluid if the patient's hydrostatic pressure increases.

The radiographic diagnosis of pneumonia is difficult. Atelectasis and artifacts (see Fig. 5–5B) are common and easily attributed to pneumonia. Although radiographic patterns may suggest a particular infection, they are not a substitute for bacterial confirmation. The majority of nosocomial infections are bacterial in origin and most likely to appear as areas of focal consolidation with or without evidence of volume loss. Progressive, patchy opacification is observed most often in gravity-dependent areas and is

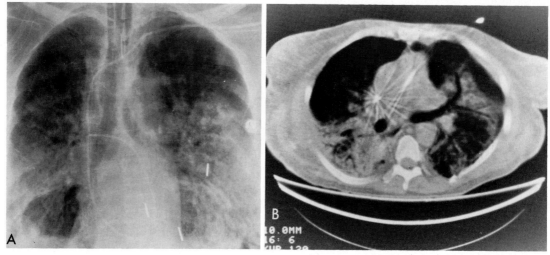

Figure 5–7. *Pseudomonas* pneumonia. *A,* Diffuse bilateral asymmetric infiltrates are noted in the lower two thirds of both lungs. The heart does not appear enlarged. The wedge pressure was normal. Cultures repeatedly grew *Pseudomonas* organisms. *B,* After some initial improvement, the patient's condition worsened. Clinically and radiographically, a right-sided empyema could not be excluded. The CT scan shows diffuse parenchymal infiltrates. Little or no pleural effusion is noted. No empyema is present.

often difficult to distinguish from atelectasis or aspiration. Less frequently, viral, pneumocystic and gram-negative infections, such as those involving *Pseudomonas* organisms and *E. coli*, rapidly spread to involve the entire lung (Joffe, 1969; Renner et al., 1972). Their symmetric appearance, mixed interstitial and air-space pattern, and rapid progression may simulate pulmonary edema (Fig. 5–7). In gram-negative infections, small lucencies may represent the uninvolved lung or focal areas of air trapping and may simulate micro-abscesses. Nodules may coalesce to become true abscesses (Figs. 5–8 and 5–9).

A negative radiograph does not totally exclude significant infection. Computed tomography has been particularly helpful in demonstrating focal consolidation not visible on the AP radiograph, and high-resolution CT may demonstrate diffuse interstitial pneumonia or small nodules in immunocompromised patients before their appearance on the radiograph. Positive results of gallium lung scans may also precede those of the radiograph. In severely neutropenic patients, significant infection may exist with minimal inflammatory reaction and therefore negative imaging examinations (Zornoza et al., 1976).

Complications of Pneumonia

Pleural effusion, empyema, bronchopleural fistula, and abscess frequently complicate nosocomial infections. Pleural effusions associated with gram-negative or polymicrobial infections are more likely to represent empyema than are those associated with a community-acquired infection. Lung abscesses appear as one or more cavities with or without air–fluid levels.

Differentiation between lung abscess and loculated empyema can usually be made by a combination of clinical history and review of serial radiographs. In general, pleural air–fluid collections occur along the posterior chest wall. Therefore, on the AP radiograph, they appear to have a long air–fluid level that is not dense, which is a reflection of the long, oval configuration of most intrapleural collections. On the lateral radiograph, the air–fluid level is relatively short and dense (Fig. 5–10). The air–fluid level usually touches the chest wall (Baker and Stein, 1986; Friedman and Hellekant, 1976; Schachter et al., 1976). Lateral loculations are broad in their AP diameter and narrow in their lateral dimension. An air–fluid level crossing a fissure also indicates a pleural collection. Abscesses tend to be thick-walled and spherical and therefore have air–fluid levels of equal lengths in the posteroanterior (PA) and lateral views. With abscesses, the air–fluid level does not reach the chest wall and usually does not cross fissures (Fig. 5–11).

In cases of extensive pleural or parenchymal disease or loculated collections, distinguishing these various components is often difficult on conventional radiographs. When the diagnosis based on conventional

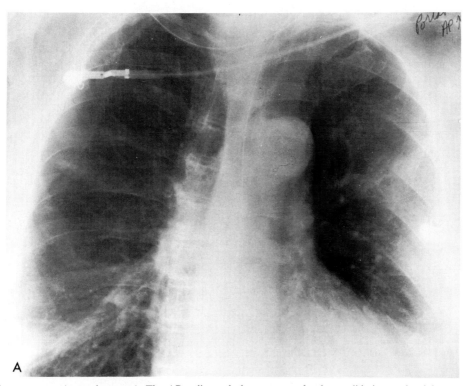

A

Figure 5–8. *Pseudomonas aeruginosa* abscess. *A,* The AP radiograph demonstrates focal consolidation at the right costophrenic angle and diffuses haziness at the left costophrenic angle, suggesting a left effusion.

Illustration continued on following page

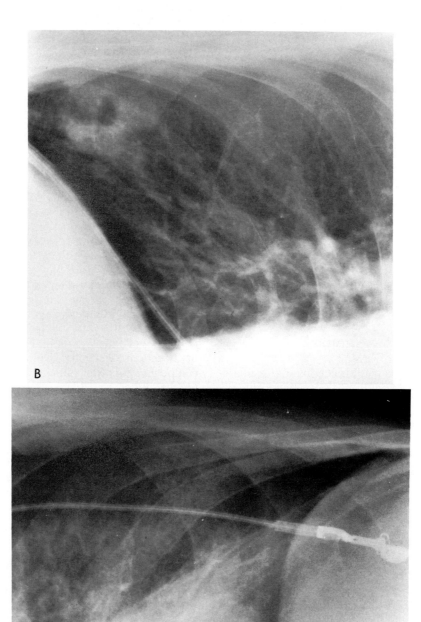

Figure 5–8 *Continued B,* Left lateral decubitus film. For technical reasons, the left side was not well visualized. The right side, however, shows an air–fluid level in the lateral infiltrate, indicating an abscess. *C,* Right lateral decubitus film. The left costophrenic angle appears to be clear, indicating that the density on the AP film is due to a pleural effusion.

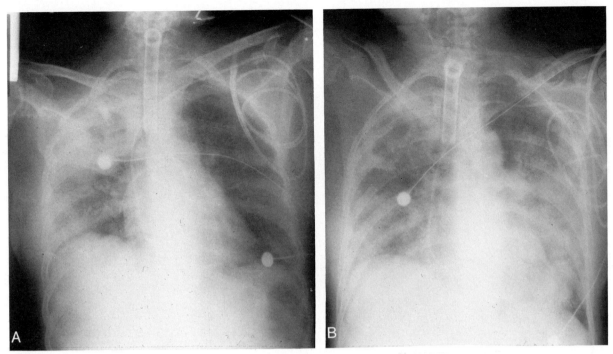

Figure 5–9. Hospital-acquired infection in a comatose trauma patient. Two weeks after admission, the patient developed some minimal consolidation in his right upper and right lower lobes. *A,* The consolidation rapidly progressed to right upper lobe consolidation, volume loss, and cavitation or pneumatocele formation. Scattered patchy consolidation is present elsewhere in the right middle lobe. Protected bronchial brushes revealed gram-positive cocci, gram-positive rods, and gram-negative rods on smear. Cultures grew *Staphylococcus aureus,* and *Pseudomonas* and *Serratia* organisms, and yielded coagulase-positive results. *B,* Over the next 2 days, the pneumonia spread to involve both lungs. This condition eventually led to the patient's demise.

radiographs is uncertain, the early use of CT is often rewarding for documenting the presence, distribution, and extent of both pulmonary and pleural disease and for planning appropriate therapy. On CT examination, a free fluid collection is crescentic and separates the visceral and parietal pleura (Bressler et al., 1987; Stark et al., 1983; Waite et al., 1990). When empyema is present, the pleura is almost always thickened and enhanced by intravenous contrast. The soft tissue between the parietal pleura and chest wall is usually thickened and of increased density (Fig. 5–12). These changes are uncommon with noninfected or malignant effusions (Waite et al., 1990).

Loculated fluid collections, which may be more difficult to distinguish from lung abscesses, tend to be oval and form obtuse angles with the chest wall whereas abscesses tend to form acute angles. Bronchovascular markings are displaced by pleural collections but usually continue directly into an abscess (see Fig. 5–12). The walls of pleural collections tend to be smooth and thin, whereas abscesses tend to be ragged (see Fig. 5–11). When pleural collections are loculated, CT demonstrates the loculations and the relationship of the chest tubes to the loculation, and it helps determine the most direct strategy for drainage. Drainage of loculated collections under imaging guidance is usually more successful and less traumatic than conventional thoracostomy tube placement (Westcott, 1985).

Hematogenous Infection

Systemic infection may affect the lung in several ways: (1) focal septic emboli (e.g., staphylococci), (2) diffuse hematogenously spread lung infection (e.g., *Pseudomonas* organisms or miliary tuberculosis), and (3) capillary permeability edema associated with sepsis syndrome and ARDS. Septic emboli most often arise from infectious phlebitis (e.g., drug abuse or infected indwelling catheters) or from a focus of infection elsewhere in the body (e.g., a wound infection or endocarditis). The classic radiographic appearance of multiple basilar nodules, with or without cavitation, is present in fewer than 50% of patients. Often, however, the radiograph contains one or more ill-defined opacities that may be unilateral or otherwise may not suggest the diagnosis.

Two recent studies have examined the role of CT in the diagnosis of septic emboli (Huang et al., 1989; Kuhlman et al., 1990). Computed tomography demonstrates nodules in approximately three quarters of patients and pleural-based densities in two thirds of patients. The majority of lesions have evidence of frank cavitation or central necrosis. A feeding vessel leading directly to the opacity strengthens the diagnosis but is observed in only a minority of patients. With intravenous contrast administration, the peripheral margins of the pleural-based densities may be enhanced. Both studies indicate that in one third to

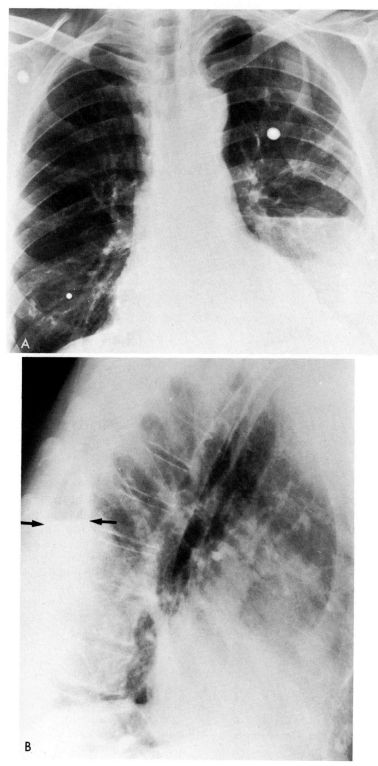

Figure 5–10. Bronchopleural fistula. *A,* The AP upright film demonstrates an air–fluid level across the entire hemithorax. In this case, it does not quite reach the lateral chest wall. A fluid collection is also noted over the left scapula. *B,* Lateral radiograph demonstrates a sharp air–fluid level running the entire length of the lesion *(arrows).* The lesion is long and flat, and the margins taper because of its intrapleural location.

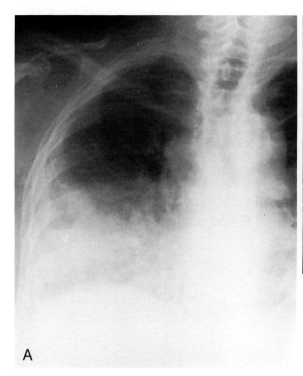

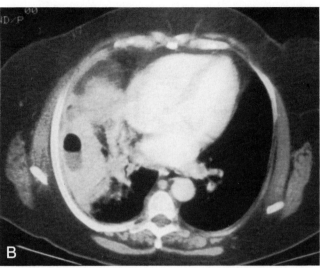

Figure 5–11. Pneumonia and lung abscess. *A,* The chest radiograph, several days after admission, shows dense consolidation in the right middle and right lower lobe. An air–fluid level that does not reach the chest wall is present laterally. A lateral pleural effusion is suggested. *B,* A CT scan through the air–fluid collection shows it to be within the lung parenchyma. Only a small amount of fluid is present in the lateral pleural space.

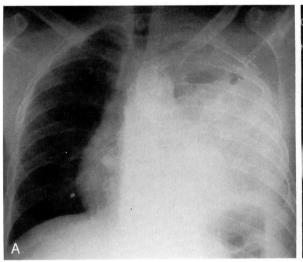

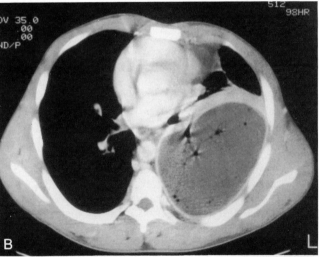

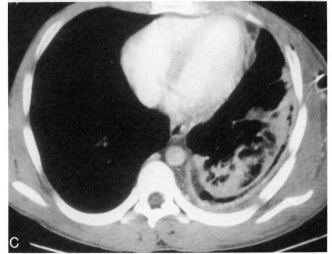

Figure 5–12. Pneumonia and empyema. *A,* The AP radiograph shows a dense left hemithorax with multiple lucencies within it. The left heart border and aortic knob are visible, indicating at least partial aeration of the lingula and upper lobe. *B,* A CT scan at the level of the left atrium shows anterior displacement of the lung and a large intrapleural fluid collection with multiple dots of air. Mild thickening and enhancement of the parietal pleura are shown. *C,* Two days later, after chest tube drainage, a CT scan 3 cm lower shows diffuse pneumonitis, as well as the drained pleural space. The parietal pleura is thicker and shows more enhancement. The extra pleural space is thickened and is of water rather than fat density.

one half of cases, CT surpasses conventional radiographic detection of septic emboli, and that in several cases, the CT diagnosis preceded either the clinical or the radiographic suspicion of septic emboli.

Diffuse pulmonary infection due to hematogenous dissemination of hospital-acquired infection is associated with high mortality and morbidity. Frequent sources of infection include the urinary tract, infected wounds, the lungs, and intra-abdominal abscess (Norwood and Civetta, 1987). The radiographs show either patchy areas of consolidation that rapidly expand to include much of the lung or diffuse ill-defined mixed pattern consolidation that worsens rapidly. These changes may be so rapid that they seem to suggest edema rather than infection (capillary leak edema and ARDS are discussed in Chapters 6 and 7).

ASPIRATION SYNDROMES

Another frequent cause of pulmonary inflammation in the ICU is "aspiration pneumonitis." The clinical and radiographic course depends on the nature of the material aspirated. Bartlett and Gorbach (1975) divided aspiration into three separate syndromes: (1) aspiration of toxic fluids, (2) aspiration of bland fluids or particles, and (3) aspiration of infected material. Although this division is helpful in understanding the various patterns caused by aspiration, overlap may occur (Bartlett and Gorbach, 1975; Wynne, 1982). The only common denominator is the breakdown of the normal protective mechanisms of the pharynx and larynx.

Factors predisposing a patient to aspiration include conditions that reduce consciousness (e.g., general anesthesia, alcohol), conditions that cause dysphagia (e.g., neuromuscular disorders, esophageal disease), and mechanical devices that alter esophageal function (e.g., nasogastric tubes, intratracheal tubes). Both nasogastric tubes and intratracheal tubes, which, a priori, should reduce aspiration, may in fact cause regurgitation and aspiration. Nasogastric tubes alter esophageal sphincter function and may serve as a wick for gastric secretions. Endotracheal tubes and tracheostomy tubes cause disordered swallowing, making it more difficult for the patient to handle secretions and regurgitated material, and they also diminish ciliary activity in the tracheobronchial tree (Fig. 5–13).

Aspiration of Toxic Fluids

The most frequently aspirated toxic fluid is gastric juice (Mendelson's syndrome). When the pH of the gastric contents is 2.5 or less, severe bronchospasm and inflammatory lung changes occur within minutes of aspiration. As the pH of the gastric contents increases, the severity of the lung reaction decreases. The presence of food particles may add to the inflam-

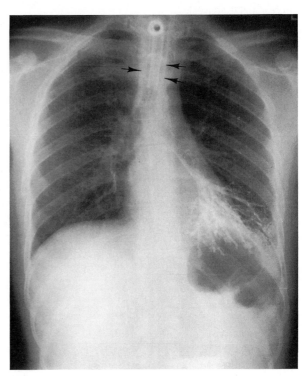

Figure 5–13. Barium aspiration around a tracheostomy tube. This radiograph is a dramatic illustration of the inability of a cuffed tube *(arrows)* to prevent aspiration.

matory changes at higher pH levels (Wynne, 1982). Other liquids, such as hydrocarbons, animal fats, alcohol, and water-soluble contrast agents can also induce chemical pneumonitis.

The signs and symptoms of aspiration pneumonitis often surface within a matter of minutes. Cough, dyspnea, tachypnea, rales, and wheezing are almost universal. When massive aspiration occurs, hypotension, shock, and apnea may follow. Fever and elevated white count are present in approximately one half of patients (Bartlett and Gorbach, 1975; Bynum and Pierce, 1976; Le Frock et al., 1979; Wynne, 1982). Although signs and symptoms subside within 1 to 2 days in the majority of patients, a significant percentage progress to either respiratory insufficiency or focal lung infection.

The radiographic appearance of chemical pneumonitis is quite variable, but some basic patterns are discernible (Landay et al., 1978). In general, the *first* radiograph shows evidence of pulmonary consolidation, which often increases for the first day or so (Fig. 5–14). Over the next 24 to 48 hours, the pneumonitis either stabilizes or begins to clear. If no lung disease is visible on the radiograph within the first 24 hours, that episode is unlikely to lead to significant chemical pneumonitis.

The initial radiographic pattern may be interstitial, air-space, or mixed. It tends to favor the perihilar and basilar areas; consolidation is bilateral in approximately two thirds of patients and is frequently asymmetric. Extensive aspiration may result in a bilateral, rapidly progressing air-space consolidation similar to those of other forms of capillary permeability edema (see Fig. 5–14). Other somewhat atypical appearances include upper lobe disease, unilateral disease, and predominantly left-sided disease. Volume loss is not an early feature. The vast majority of radiographs show some evidence of clearing by the third day, and complete clearing may require 1 to 2 weeks (Fig. 5–15; see Fig. 5–14).

In approximately one quarter of patients, the chemical pneumonitis is complicated by bacterial infection, and abscess or empyema formation is frequent. Infection usually appears as a reversal of the patient's recovery. Fever, leukocytosis, or change in the character of the sputum may recur. The radiograph tends to stabilize or worsen, and volume loss, abscess formation, or pleural effusion may be evident (see Fig. 5–14C). Focal volume loss suggests the possibility of retained secretions or food particles obstructing the bronchus. As with other nosocomial infections, multiple gram-negative organisms, such as those of *Klebsiella, Pseudomonas,* and *Proteus,* and *Escherichia coli,* are frequently cultured.

Repeated small aspirations of gastric contents (silent aspirations) frequently occur at night and are more difficult to diagnose. In older or obtunded patients, recurrent bouts of lower lobe atelectasis, pneumonitis, or cavitation without apparent cause should lead one to consider this possible diagnosis. Cultures from these patients often yield mixed flora whose significance is difficult to ascertain.

Aspiration of Bland Fluids or Solids

Fluids such as blood, water, barium, and neutralized gastric contents do not cause chemical pneumonitis. Transient respiratory distress is either due to the volume of aspirated fluid (asphyxiation) or due to bronchospasm caused by the foreign substance (Bartlett and Gorbach, 1975). The radiograph is normal unless a large volume of fluid was aspirated. If pulmonary consolidation is present, it rapidly disappears following coughing, suctioning, or positive-pressure therapy.

The aspiration of food particles or blood clots usually elicits a bout of coughing, owing to direct bronchial irritation. A large inoculum may cause wheezing, dyspnea, or cyanosis. The initial radiograph may be normal or may demonstrate areas of atelectasis or focal hyperinflation (Fig. 5–16). Blood clots usually lyse and are coughed up, whereas food particles may remain in the bronchi despite cessation of acute symptoms. When clinical evidence of focal wheezing or radiographic evidence of persistent consolidation suggests a retained foreign body, bronchoscopic removal prevents delayed infection.

Aspiration of Infected Secretions

The clinical and radiographic appearances of pneumonia due to aspirated infected secretions depend on the circumstances surrounding the event. In the community, patients with poor dentition or sinusitis tend to aspirate small volumes of heavily infected material repeatedly into the gravity-dependent segments (posterior segment of the upper lobes, and superior and posterior segments of the lower lobes). The clinical course varies from fulminant pneumonia to indolent pneumonia, abscess, or empyema (Fig. 5–17). The majority of infections are polymicrobial and are frequently due to anaerobic gram-positive bacilli. In the hospitalized patient, colonization of the pharynx and airway often causes infection of the lung as a result of a more generalized dispersion of less heavily infected material. The course and difficulties of diagnosis have been described within the previous discussion of nosocomial pneumonia.

ACUTE SMOKE INHALATION

Following smoke inhalation, respiratory tract injury may be due to direct thermal burns or to chemical irritation from noxious gases. Significant airway burns are usually confined to the mouth and larynx and result in edema, which may lead to upper airway obstruction. Tracheobronchial injuries, which are due to chemical agents, cause mucosal edema, ulceration, and sloughing, which may lead to cough, bronchospasm, and airway obstruction (Herndon et al., 1987; Peitzman et al., 1989). Lung injuries are due to the effects of various chemicals on the alveolar epithelium and the alveolar capillaries. The severity of the chemical pneumonitis depends on the volume of the inhaled smoke and its chemical composition. Closed compartment inhalation and the inhalation of smoke from manmade materials (e.g., plastics) produce the most lethal results.

The percentage of body burn remains a major prognostic factor, but because of the improving techniques for treating burns, pulmonary complications are now the leading cause of death. Herndon and associates (1987) estimated that only 20% of skin burn victims die, whereas 60% of patients with pulmonary complications die. The reported incidence of pulmonary complications varies from 10% to 70% (Haponik et al., 1986; Michael and O'Connell, 1988).

Conflicting evidence is found in the literature regarding the role of the radiograph in the diagnosis of lung injuries. Putman and colleagues (1977) studied patients with only respiratory injury and no body burns. The majority had either normal chest radiographs or focal consolidation believed to be due to atelectasis. In those patients who developed pneumonitis, the radiographs were often normal for the first 24 hours. The investigators found little correlation between the chest radiograph and the blood oxygen and carbon monoxide levels and concluded that the radiograph is not a sensitive indicator of airway or parenchymal damage.

Several recent studies of patients with more severe exposure suggest that the radiograph may be more

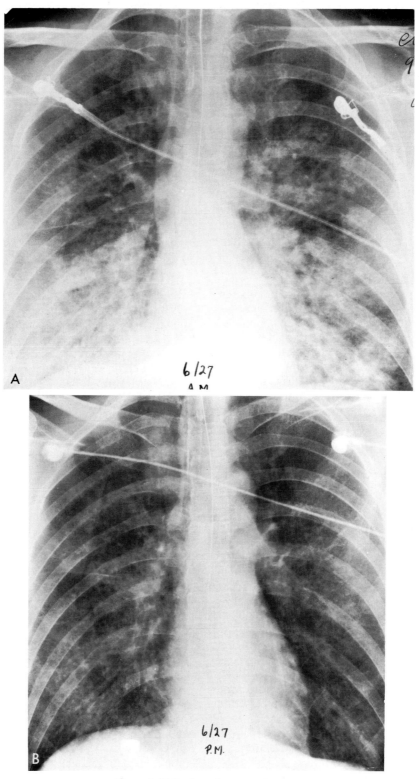

Figure 5–14 *See legend on opposite page*

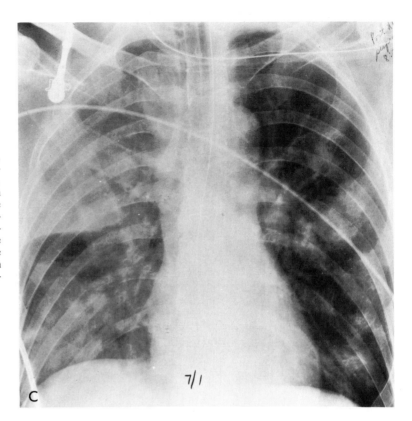

Figure 5–14. Aspiration pneumonitis. *A,* Diffuse, fluffy, bilateral air-space consolidation is demonstrated several hours after gastric acid aspiration. The rapid onset and the radiographic distribution suggest pulmonary edema, but the cardiac silhouette is small. *B,* Eighteen hours later, considerable clearing has occurred. (Part of the improvement is undoubtedly due to greater inflation caused by positive end-expiratory pressure.) *C,* Four days later, diffuse patchy consolidation, as well as lobar consolidation of the right upper lobe, is present. *Klebsiella* organisms were cultured from the sputum.

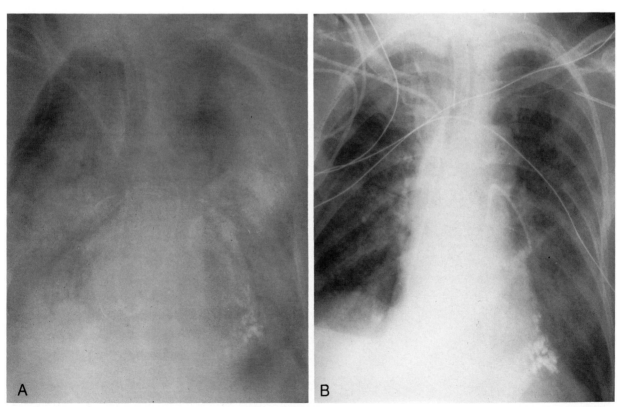

Figure 5–15. Massive aspirations. *A,* Severe air-space consolidation following massive aspiration. The heart is mildly enlarged. Barium is visible in the left lower lobe from a remote aspiration. The radiographic appearance and rapidity of onset suggest severe congestive heart failure as an alternative etiologic mechanism. The wedge pressure was normal. *B,* Four days later, clearing is almost complete.

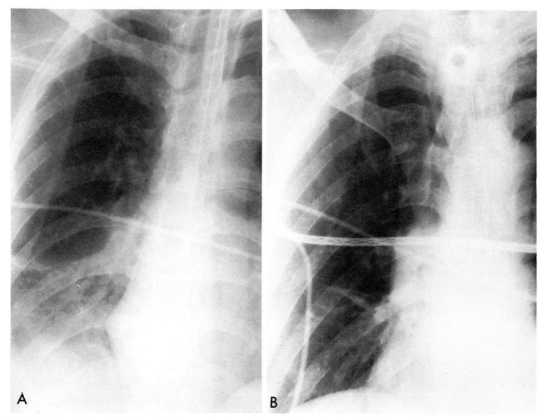

Figure 5–16. Aspiration of blood. *A,* Consolidation and volume loss are shown in the right lower lobe. The patient was aspirating blood from multiple facial fractures. *B,* A tracheostomy was performed to protect the trachea and to facilitate suctioning. Film taken 18 hours later shows almost complete clearing of the right lower lobe infiltrate and atelectasis.

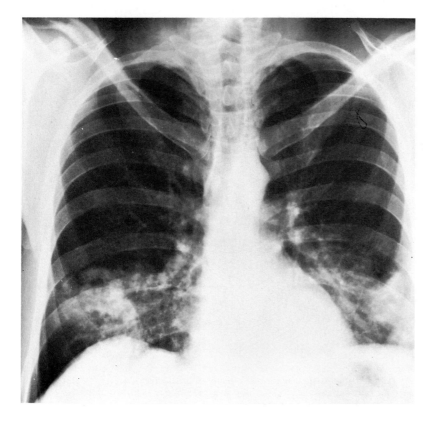

Figure 5–17. Aspiration of infected secretions. Bilateral lower lobe infiltrates and cavities are due to aspiration of infected secretions. Cultures repeatedly grew mixed flora.

useful than previously reported. Michael and O'Connell (1988), reviewing radiographs of a group of 45 patients obtained within an hour of the patients' being removed from a fire, found 33 abnormal radiographs (29 with bronchial wall thickening, 13 with subglottic narrowing, and two with perihilar or upper lung edema). Five additional cases of lung edema were visible within 24 hours (see Fig. 5–1). All 18 patients who eventually developed pneumonia had an abnormal radiograph within 24 hours. Beyond the first day, no abnormal examinations followed normal examinations.

Teixidor and associates (1983) studied 56 patients believed to have smoke inhalation injuries. Thirty-one radiographs were abnormal within 24 hours, and four additional abnormalities were found by 48 hours. The investigators found nine cases of peribronchial or perivascular edema, five cases of diffuse alveolar edema, and 21 cases with mixed patterns (see Fig. 5–1). Upper and perihilar areas were most often involved. Beyond the first 3 days, radiographic abnormalities were due to complications of the burns, such as pneumonia, aspiration, and congestive heart failure. These authors believe also that interstitial edema is a potentially early sign of lung injury. Peitzman and co-workers (1983) studied a severely ill group of patients and graded their radiographs from +1 (perivascular edema) to +4 (diffuse consolidation). A strong correlation was found between the radiographic grade and extravascular lung water, intrapulmonary shunting, and compliance. Seventy-two percent of patients with normal examinations had no or minor pulmonary function abnormalities, whereas 93% with +2 to +4 chest radiographs had abnormal pulmonary function tests.

A major problem in the management of skin burns is determination of the appropriate levels of fluid replacement. Excess crystalloid fluid administration,

coupled with a low colloid oncotic pressure from surface protein loss, contributes to delayed pulmonary edema. Haponik and associates (1986) measured the pulmonary vascular pedicle (i.e., the width across the mediastinum at the level of the left brachiocephalic artery) to determine whether this "monitor of intravascular blood volume" could predict the development of pulmonary edema. Within 24 hours, 12 of the 18 patients who eventually developed pulmonary edema showed an increase in their pulmonary vascular pedicles by at least 1 cm above baseline (Fig. 5–18). Only one of 26 nonedema patients showed a 1-cm increase. Thus, widening of the pedicle presaged significant hypervolemia in three quarters of the cases, with only a 4% false-positive rate.

Air trapping in the first few days after smoke inhalation is usually due to a combination of edema, sloughing, and retained secretions. Xenon-133 (^{133}Xe) ventilation scanning is a relatively sensitive indicator of air trapping and, therefore, of lung injury.

To summarize these divergent reports, the radiograph is a helpful but imperfect screening tool. The early signs of lung injury include subglottic edema, thickening of the trachea and bronchi, and edema around the vessels and small airways. Bronchial thickening or perivascular edema is an early indicator of lung injury and often precedes diffuse edema or infection. Edema, which results from the chemical pneumonitis, is usually present within 24 hours. Focal areas of consolidation in the first 48 hours suggest atelectasis from sloughed mucosa and retained secretions. Beyond the third day, focal and multifocal consolidation suggests infection, which complicates more than one half of respiratory injuries. Widening of the vascular pedicle indicates overhydration and a strong likelihood of subsequent edema. Diffuse edema is often multifactorial, and contributing factors include fluid overload, high cardiac output due to a

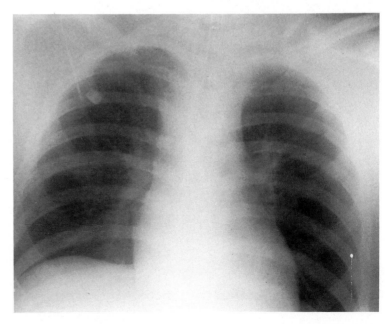

Figure 5–18. Severe volume overload after burns. The patient suffered 90% body burn and was inadvertently markedly overhydrated during his first 3 days in the hospital. This radiograph, obtained 3 days after admission, shows a 7-cm pulmonary vascular pedicle, an increase of approximately 1.8 cm from the admission examination. The upper lobe vessels are distended and slightly indistinct when compared with the admission film. Subsequent reassessment revealed that the patient had approximately a 20-liter excess of fluids. The radiograph returned to normal after several days of diuresis and fluid restriction.

hypermetabolic state, decreased oncotic pressure (protein loss and crystalloid fluid replacement), and increased capillary permeability (chemical pneumonitis and systemic sepsis).

NEAR DROWNING

Drowning is defined as death within 24 hours that is due to asphyxiation from submersion, whereas near drowning indicates survival for at least 24 hours. Submersion accidents are the third leading cause of death in young and teenage children and are exceeded only by motor vehicle accidents and cancer (Orlowski, 1987; Sarnaik and Vohra, 1986). The process of drowning can be broken down into three stages. In Stage 1, the aspiration of a small amount of liquid causes laryngeal spasm for 1 to 2 minutes. In Stage 2, panic and struggling cause increased hypoxia, and a significant amount of water is swallowed. In Stage 3, a large volume of liquid is aspirated into the lungs. In 10% to 15% of cases, laryngeal spasm recurs or persists, preventing flooding of the lung ("dry drowning") (Orlowski, 1987). In such cases, pulmonary damage is most likely due to hypoxia alone. Vomiting and aspiration of gastric contents or the aspiration of sand, mud, and so forth may add to the pulmonary damage.

Animal studies have shown that in salt-water drowning, the hypertonic sea water causes intravascular water to be drawn into the lung, causing pulmonary edema and hemoconcentration. In freshwater drowning, the hypotonic water is rapidly absorbed from the lung and results in hemodilution. In human drowning, however, the physiologic differences between salt-water and fresh-water drowning in patients who survive long enough to reach the hospital are *minor*.

A major physiologic consequence of drowning is hypoxia. In addition to the mechanical effects of asphyxiation, the water damages both the alveoli and the capillaries, resulting in capillary-permeability edema. Fresh water appears to alter the function of surfactant as well, resulting in atelectasis and intrapulmonary shunting (Orlowski, 1987). Although the lungs are the immediate focus of attention, long-term sequelae are usually due to hypoxic central nervous system damage.

As one would expect from the variable volume and composition of the aspirated fluid, the radiographic appearance of the lungs in near drowning is variable as well. Hunter and Whitehouse (1974) reported that in milder clinical cases, patients demonstrated either a normal chest radiograph or mild perihilar edema, whereas in more severe clinical cases, patients tended to have denser, more diffuse alveolar edema (Fig. 5–19). Putman and colleagues (1975) reported that the radiographic pattern varied from diffuse irregular infiltrates (50%) to segmental lobar and basilar consolidation (see Fig. 6–21). As in Hunter and Whitehouse's series, some patients with severe hypoxia had normal or relatively normal radiographs. Putman and colleagues (1975) found less correlation between the radiographic and clinical status and also cautioned that the radiograph may be normal for 24 to 48 hours before the appearance of significant pulmonary disease. Clearing usually commences several days after the aspiration, and clearing is often quite rapid. Delayed clearing or reversal of clearing may be due to nosocomial infection, ARDS, or complications due to aspiration of other substances.

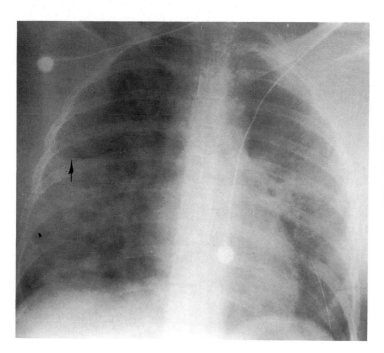

Figure 5–19. Near drowning. The patient was found face down in a bathtub in an apparent suicide attempt. A patchy, somewhat nodular consolidation appears in the right lung, and a more homogeneous ground-glass appearance is shown on the left. Incidentally noted is some air outlining the minor fissure *(arrow)*. Subsequent radiographs showed a right pneumothorax and then tension pneumothorax.

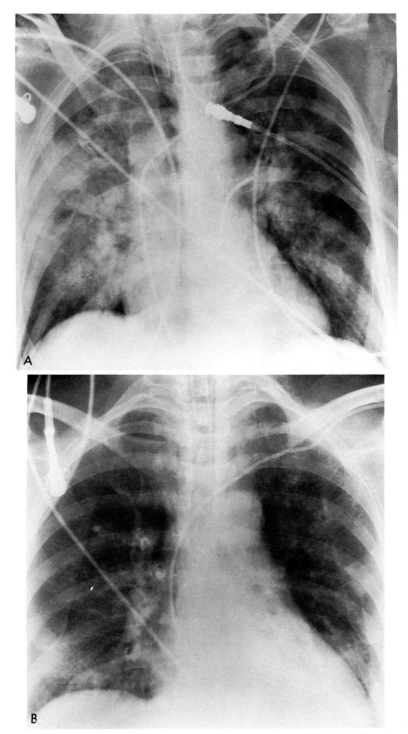

Figure 5–20. Pulmonary hemorrhage. *A,* Diffuse patchy air-space disease developed over 24 hours in this patient with renal failure. During this same period, the hematocrit dropped several points, and the patient was found to be thrombocytopenic. Three days later, considerable clearing has occurred. A small residual infiltrate is seen at both bases.

HEMOPTYSIS

Bloody sputum may be due to tracheobronchial disease, parenchymal disease, or extrathoracic disease (e.g., of the nose or stomach). Blood-streaked sputum is usually tracheobronchial in origin and most often due to tracheobronchitis or mucosal abrasion from intubation or suctioning. Brisk arterial bleeding in a tracheostomized patient suggests a tracheo-innominate fistula from erosion of the tube into the innominate artery. When the bleeding is massive, the hemorrhage is usually controlled manually at the bedside, and the patient is taken to the operating room. On occasion, several short premonitory bouts of bleeding precede the massive bleeding. Angiography confirms or refutes the diagnosis.

Parenchymal bleeding has many possible causes (Table 5–2). On occasion, the radiograph may demonstrate a specific abnormality, such as a mycetoma, cancer, or foreign body, but it is usually nonspecific, and the primary disease may be difficult to distinguish from aspirated blood in the lung.

Evaluation is also difficult in the patient with known chronic inflammatory disease (cystic fibrosis, sarcoidosis, or tuberculosis) who presents with brisk or recurrent hemorrhage that requires localization for potential therapeutic intervention. A chest radiograph may not show changes from a prior film, or determination of whether new consolidation is due to active disease or simply to blood in the alveoli may be difficult. The role of bronchoscopy and arteriography in both the diagnosis and therapy for this group of patients is discussed in Chapter 16.

In patients with coagulation disorders, Goodpasture's syndrome, or vasculitis, or in patients receiving anticoagulant therapy, pulmonary parenchymal hemorrhage occurs at the microvascular level. The hemorrhage usually occurs with the triad of anemia, hemoptysis, and pulmonary consolidation. The radiographic pattern varies from mild interstitial thickening to nodulation to air-space disease. Most often, progression is rapid, and when the disorder is bilateral, it may mimic pulmonary edema. Shadowing tends to spare the apices and periphery (Albelda et al., 1985; Bowley et al., 1979; Palmer et al., 1978) (Fig. 5–20).

Within a few days, the radiograph stabilizes and gradually regresses as a reticular interstitial pattern replaces the alveolar consolidation. The interstitial thickening gradually subsides and returns to normal over the following 1 to 2 weeks. Repeated bouts of hemorrhage cause hemosiderin-induced interstitial fibrosis.

On occasion, severe pulmonary hemorrhage may occur with little or no hemoptysis. Therefore, the absence of hemoptysis does not exclude the diagnosis. When the clinical or radiographic appearance suggests hemorrhage, further investigation is required. The demonstration of hemosiderin-laden macrophages in bronchial lavage samples supports the diagnosis (Finley et al., 1975).

Table 5–2. HEMOPTYSIS

Trauma
Tracheal intubation, suctioning, etc.
Tracheostomy tube: tracheal innominate fistula?
Blunt trauma
Penetrating trauma

Infections
Tracheobronchitis
Parenchymal infection: pneumonia, abscess
Bronchiectasis
Mycetoma

Inflammation
Aspiration pneumonitis
Inhalation injuries

Endobronchial Neoplasm

Systemic Disorders
Vasculitis
Goodpasture's syndrome
Hemosiderosis
Coagulation abnormality

Miscellaneous Lung Disease
Broncholith
Foreign body

Cardiovascular Disease
Increased pulmonary venous pressure: congestive heart failure, mitral stenosis
Vascular anomalies: arteriovenous malformations, aneurysms
Pulmonary embolus and infarction

Extrathoracic Source

References

Albelda, S.M., Gefter, W.B., Epstein, D.M., and Miller, W.T.: Diffuse pulmonary hemorrhage: A review and classification. Radiology 154:289, 1985.

Andrews, C.P., Coalson, J.J., Smith, J.D., and Johanson, W.G.: Diagnosis of nosocomial bacterial pneumonia in acute diffuse lung disease. Chest 80:254, 1981.

Baker, S.R., and Stein, H.D.: Radiologic consultation: Its application to an acute care surgical ward. AJR 147:637, 1986.

Bamberger, D.M.: Nosocomial pneumonia. In Farber, B.F. (ed.): Infection Control in Intensive Care. London, Churchill Livingstone, 1987.

Bartlett, J.G., and Gorbach, S.L.: The triple threat of aspiration pneumonia. Chest 68:560, 1975.

Bartlett, J.G., O'Keefe, P., Tally, F.P., et al.: Bacteriology of hospital-acquired pneumonia. Arch. Intern. Med. 146:868, 1986.

Bowley, N.B., Steiner, R.E., and Chin, W.S.: The chest x-ray in antiglomerular basement membrane antibody disease (Goodpasture's syndrome). Clin. Radiol. 30:419, 1979.

Bressler, E.L., Francis, I.R., Glazer, G.M., and Gross, B.H.: Bolus contrast medium enhancement for distinguishing pleural from parenchymal lung disease: CT features. J. Comput. Assist. Tomogr. 11:436, 1987.

Bryant, L.R., Mobin-Uddin, K., Dillon, M.L., et al.: Misdiagnosis of pneumonia in patients needing mechanical respiration. Arch. Surg. 106:286, 1973.

Bynum, L.J., and Pierce, A.K.: Pulmonary aspiration of gastric contents. Am. Rev. Respir. Dis. 114:1129, 1976.

Caldwell, A., Glauser, F.L., Smith, W.P., et al.: The effects of dehydration on the radiologic and pathologic appearance of experimental canine segmental pneumonia. Am. Rev. Respir. Dis. 112:651, 1975.

Colligan, T., Light, R.B., Wood, L.D.H., and Mink, S.N.: Plasma volume expansion in canine pneumococcal pneumonia: Its effect on respiratory gas exchange and pneumonia size. Am. Rev. Respir. Dis. 126:86, 1982.

Finley, T.N., Aronow, A., Cosentino, A.M., and Golde, D.W.: Occult pulmonary hemorrhage in anticoagulated patients. Am. Rev. Respir. Dis. 112:23, 1975.

Fisher, M.S.: Significance of a visible major fissure on the frontal chest radiograph. AJR 137:577, 1981.

Fraser, R.G., et al.: Diagnosis of Diseases of the Chest, ed. 3, vol. IV. Philadelphia, W.B. Saunders, 1991, p. 2974.

Freedman, A.P., and Goodman, L.R.: Suctioning of the left bronchial tree in the intubated adult. Crit. Care Med. 10:43, 1982.

Friedman, P.J., and Hellekant, A.C.G.: Diagnosis of air-fluid levels in the thorax: Radiologic recognition of bronchopleural fistula. Am. Rev. Respir. Dis. 113(Suppl.):159, 1976.

Hall, F., and Simon, M.: Occult pneumonia associated with dehydration: Myth or reality. AJR 148:853, 1987.

Haponik, E.F., Adelman, M., Munster, A.M., and Bleecher, E.R.: Increased vascular pedicle width preceding burn-related pulmonary edema. Chest 90:649, 1986.

Harris, R.S.: The importance of proximal and distal air bronchograms in the management of atelectasis. Can. Assoc. Radiol. J. 36:103, 1985.

Herndon, D.N., Langer, F., Thompson, P., et al.: Pulmonary injury in burned patients. Surg. Clin. North Am. 67:31, 1987.

Huang, R.M., Naidich, D.P., Lubat, E., et al.: Septic pulmonary emboli: CT-radiographic correlation. AJR 153:41, 1989.

Hunter, T.B., and Whitehouse, W.M.: Fresh-water near-drowning: Radiological aspects. Radiology 112:51, 1974.

Joffe, N.: Roentgenologic aspects of primary *Pseudomonas aeruginosa* pneumonia in mechanically ventilated patients. AJR 107:305, 1969.

Kuhlman, J.E., Fishman, E.K., and Teigen, C.: Pulmonary septic emboli: Diagnosis with CT. Radiology 174:211, 1990.

Landay, M.J., Christensen, E.E., and Bynum, L.J.: Pulmonary manifestations of acute aspiration of gastric contents. AJR 131:587, 1978.

Le Frock, J.L., Clark, T.S., Davies, B., and Klainer, A.S.: Aspiration pneumonia: A ten-year review. Am. Surg. 45:305, 1979.

Lerner, M.A.: Inspiration chest radiography by lateral recumbency. Clin. Radiol. 29:155, 1978.

Marini, J.J., Pierson, D.J., and Hudson, L.D.: Acute lobar atelectasis: A prospective comparison of fiberoptic bronchoscopy and respiratory therapy. Am. Rev. Respir. Dis. 149:971, 1979.

Michael, J.L., and O'Connell, D.J.: The plain chest radiograph after acute smoke inhalation. Clin. Radiol. 39:33, 1988.

Mock, C.N., Burchard, K.W., Hasan, F., and Reed, M.: Surgical intensive care unit pneumonia. Surgery 104:494, 1988.

Morimoto, S., Takeuchi, N., Imanaka, H., et al.: Gravity-dependent atelectasis: Radiologic, physiologic, and pathologic correlation in rabbits on high-frequency oscillation ventilation. Invest. Radiol. 24:522, 1989.

Norwood, S.H., Civetta, J.M.: Evaluating sepsis in critically ill patients. Chest 91:137, 1987.

Orlowski, J.P.: Drowning, near-drowning and ice water submersions. Pediatr. Clin. North Am. 34:75, 1987.

Palmer, P.E., Finley, T.N., Drew, W.L., and Golde, D.W.: Radiographic aspects of occult pulmonary haemorrhage. Clin. Radiol. 29:139, 1978.

Peitzman, A.B., Shires III, G.T., Teixidor, H.S., et al.: Smoke inhalation injury: Evaluation of radiographic manifestations and pulmonary dysfunction. J. Trauma 29:1232, 1989.

Pham, D.H., Huang, D., Korwan, A., and Greyson, N.D.: Acute unilateral pulmonary nonventilation due to mucous plugs. Radiology 165:135, 1987.

Pierce, A.K., and Robertson, J.: Pulmonary complications of general surgery. Annu. Rev. Med. 28:211, 1977.

Pingleton, S.: Complications of acute respiratory failure. Am. Rev. Respir. Dis. 137:1463, 1988.

Putman, C.E., Loke, J., Matthay, R.A., and Ravin, C.E.: Radiographic manifestations of acute smoke inhalation. AJR 129:865, 1977.

Putman, C.E., Tummillo, A.M., Myerson, D.A., and Myerson, P.J.: Drowning: Another plunge. AJR 125:543, 1975.

Renner, R.R., Coccaro, A.P., Heitzman, E.R., et al.: *Pseudomonas* pneumonia: A prototype of hospital-based infection. Radiology 105:555, 1972.

Roberts, J., Barnes, W., Pennoch, M.H.S., and Browne, G.: Diagnostic accuracy of fever as a measure of postoperative pulmonary complications. Heart Lung 17:166, 1988.

Ruiz-Santana, S., Garcia, J.A., Esteban, A., et al.: ICU pneumonias: A multi-institutional study. Crit. Care Med. 15:930, 1987.

Sanford, J.P., and Pierce, A.K.: Lower respiratory tract infection. *In* Bennett, J.R., and Bachman, S. (eds.): Hospital Infection. Boston, Little Brown, 1979.

Sarnaik, A.P., and Vohra, M.P.: Near-drowning: Fresh, salt, and cold water immersion. Clin. Sports Med. 5:33, 1986.

Schachter, E.N., Kreisman, H., and Putman, C.: Diagnostic problems in suppurative lung disease. Arch. Intern. Med. 136:167, 1976.

Shevland, J., Hirleman, M.T., Huang, K.A., and Kealey, G.P.: Lobar collapse in the surgical intensive care unit. Br. J. Radiol. 56:531, 1983.

Stark, D.D., Federle, M.P., Goodman, P.C., et al.: Differentiating lung abscess and empyema: Radiography and computed tomography. AJR 141:163, 1983.

Strandberg, A., Tokics, L., Brismar, B., et al.: Atelectasis during anesthesia and in the postoperative period. Acta Anaesthesiol. Scand. 30:154, 1986.

Teixidor, H.S., Rubin, E., Novick, G.S., and Alonso, D.R.: Smoke inhalation: Radiologic manifestations. Radiology 149:383, 1983.

Tobin, M.J., and Grenvik, A.: Nosocomial lung infection and its diagnosis. Crit. Care Med. 12:191, 1984.

Toews, G.B.: Nosocomial pneumonia. Am. J. Med. Sci. 291:355, 1986.

Waite, R.J., Carbonneau, R.J., Balikian, J., et al.: Parietal pleural changes in empyema: Appearances at CT. Radiology 175:145, 1990.

Westcott, J.L.: Percutaneous catheter drainage of pleural effusion and empyema. AJR 144:1189, 1985.

Westcott, J.L., and Cole, S.: Plate atelectasis. Radiology 155:1, 1985.

Wynne, J.W.: Aspiration pneumonitis: Correlation of experimental models with clinical disease. Clin. Chest Med. 3:25, 1982.

Zornoza, J., Goldman, A.M., Wallace, S., et al.: Radiographic features of gram-negative pneumonias in the neutropenic patient. AJR 127:989, 1976.

Zylak, C.J., Littleton, J.T., and Durizch, M.L.: Illusory consolidation of the left lower lobe: A pitfall of portable radiography. Radiology 167:653, 1988.

6

Cardiac and Noncardiac Edema: Radiologic Approach

■

Charles E. Putman

PULMONARY EDEMA

Diffuse alveolar opacities indicative of pulmonary edema are a common finding in the intensive care unit. Excluding atelectasis, pulmonary edema—both cardiogenic and noncardiogenic—is the most frequent cause of decreased oxygenation as well as of the sudden appearance of an abnormal chest radiograph.

The clinical assessment of patients with pulmonary edema may be difficult because physical examination may be unreliable and because invasive techniques have both theoretic and practical limitations. Many recent articles attest to the controversy regarding the validity and overall accuracy of these techniques and their ability to determine the mechanisms responsible for extravascular water accumulation (Anderson et al., 1979; Chinard, 1975; Fein et al., 1979; Glauser et al., 1974; Hayes et al., 1982; Petty et al., 1979). The three main varieties of pulmonary edema are (1) cardiac edema, resulting from myocardial or endocardial heart disease, (2) overhydration, caused by excess fluid administration or renal failure, and (3) increased capillary permeability, resulting from various injuries to the pulmonary microvasculature.

Three basic mechanisms of pulmonary edema are (1) increased hydrostatic pressure generated across the capillary membrane, (2) a diminished oncotic pressure gradient across the membrane, and (3) increased capillary permeability due to damage to the endothelial cell junctions, which permits leakage of fluid and proteins from the microvasculature. In the intensive care unit, one or *more* mechanisms may be responsible for the pulmonary edema pattern; thus, distinguishing cardiogenic from noncardiogenic edema is often difficult.

The lung parenchyma is essentially a three-compartment structure consisting of the alveolar space, the vascular space, and the interstitium (Crandall et al., 1983; Heitzman, 1973a; Pattle, 1958). The integrity of these units is preserved essentially by the endothelium and epithelial layers of the alveolar capillary membrane. The normal exchange of oxygen, carbon dioxide, water, and micromolecules moving across the alveolar capillary membrane can be altered by a variety of local or systemic agents that damage the cell layers of the two membranes.

As defined by Starling's equation, damage to the epithelium increases the permeability of the capillary membrane to water and protein and represents the basic pathophysiologic basis of noncardiac edema (Crandall et al., 1983). An increase in pulmonary capillary pressure (e.g., from left heart failure) causes the accumulation of excess lung water by increasing the hydrostatic pressure between the capillary and interstitium. The integrity of both the epithelium and endothelium provides the interface for the transfer of water and the retention of proteins. The alveolar epithelium also contributes significantly to the development and resolution of alveolar edema and is the limiting membrane that prevents the sudden movement of fluid and proteins into the alveolar spaces (Crandall et al., 1983).

For the optimal treatment of critically ill patients who have pulmonary edema, hydrostatic or high-pressure edema must be differentiated from the edema resulting from noncardiac mechanisms. Techniques for detection and quantification of lung water—including advanced imaging techniques—are briefly reviewed in the following sections. Reviewing these techniques along with the ubiquitous portable chest radiograph allows the utility and efficacy of each to be understood. This chapter first reviews the radiologic findings in cardiogenic and noncardiogenic edema and then reviews other invasive and noninvasive tests of lung water.

Chest Radiography

Serial portable chest radiographs are routinely used to evaluate patients with pulmonary edema. The ability of these radiographs to demonstrate and monitor changes in pulmonary edema in critically ill patients remains controversial. The sensitivity and specificity of the portable radiograph in determining the presence or absence of edema, and in distinguishing cardiac from noncardiac edema, are still subjects of debate (Greenbaum and Marshall, 1982; Halperin et al., 1985; Pistolesi and Giuntini, 1978; Pistolesi et al., 1982; Sivak et al., 1983; Van de Water et al., 1970).

In the critical care unit, many factors are responsible for the transudation of water into the interstitium and alveolar spaces of the lung. One must learn the common patterns of edema and be aware that many unusual patterns of pulmonary edema—inhomogeneous, focal, and asymmetric—can be confusing. This atypical distribution of the edema often leads to the erroneous radiographic diagnosis of pneumonitis, hemorrhage, and less likely, a drowned lung (Finley et al., 1964). (Airless lung tissue peripheral to a totally obstructed bronchus may produce pulmonary edema.) Underlying chronic obstructive pulmonary disease, lung contusion, pulmonary embolism, pneumonia, and drug toxicity alter the characteristic radiographic pattern of pulmonary edema.

A radiograph of the patient in an erect position is ideal but often not possible. The supine anteroposterior (AP) radiograph precludes the use of more traditional radiographic determinants of cardiogenic pulmonary edema, such as borderline cardiomegaly and redistribution of pulmonary blood flow. Pleural effusions are difficult to identify and to quantitate. Therefore, semi-erect radiographs, decubitus views, and serial daily radiographs should be employed judiciously and to their fullest potential benefit. Rapid improvement of a focal or diffuse alveolar opacity almost always indicates excess lung water. Lobar collapse and drowned lung should not pose a problem in the differential diagnosis of pulmonary edema, but obviously, these two entities may also show rapid clearance with appropriate treatment.

Zimmerman and associates (1982) reported the use of the gravitational shift test by exposing bedside frontal films before and after prolonged lateral decubitus positioning. Excess lung water was identified by detection of a shift in the opacity to the dependent lung while the opposite side cleared or remained stable. This test was highly accurate in determining that the cause of the majority of the opacities involved mobilizable lung water.

In our experience, this test has also been highly reliable and has improved the diagnosis of pulmonary edema. The appearance of shifting opacities has facilitated diagnosis of edema and has properly distinguished transudates (e.g., edema) from exudates (e.g., pneumonia) in complex cases. In patients receiving positive end-expiratory pressure (PEEP), a change in ventilatory pressure also tends to cause much more alteration in opacities, when the disease causes transudates rather than exudates (Gittinoni et al., 1988). Patients with edema from acute obliterating bronchiolitis with terminal bronchiolar mucous plugging, or patients with acute parenchymal hemorrhage, may occasionally have false-positive results of the gravitational shift test or a false-positive response to PEEP. Some patients with acute alveolar inflammation, such as that occurring from inhalation injury, may also show some improvement in the opacities with positional change. In these cases, most of the opacity is due to epithelial damage and resultant transudation of water into the interstitium and adjacent air spaces.

Chest radiography remains the most commonly used noninvasive technique for assessing the presence or absence of pulmonary edema in critically ill patients. Recent reviews on the detection of extravascular lung water have emphasized that the chest radiograph is still the standard method for assessing patients with pulmonary edema and has a sensitivity that cannot be attained by other techniques of measurement (Milne and Pistolesi, 1990; Milne et al., 1985; Miniati et al., 1988; Pistolesi and Giuntini, 1978; Pistolesi et al., 1985). Many of the methods to be discussed differentiate between cardiogenic and noncardiogenic pulmonary edema and have been aimed largely toward the detection of increased capillary permeability. Recent studies have indicated that the chest radiograph is able to define and quantify extravascular lung water accumulation. Objective criteria able to distinguish patients who have edema from cardiogenic mechanisms from those developing edema from overhydration, capillary permeability, or both have been established (Milne et al., 1985; Pistolesi et al., 1985).

These criteria for elucidating the status of edema are discussed, and the literature containing conflicting viewpoints is summarized.

Cardiogenic vs. Noncardiogenic Edema: Radiographic Distinction

The ability of chest radiography to detect interstitial pulmonary edema prior to the onset of clinical symptoms has been demonstrated. In two different series of patients with acute myocardial infarction, left-sided heart failure was detected radiographically in 24% to 38% of the patients when a clinical diagnosis was not possible (Harrison et al., 1971; Logue et al., 1963) (Fig. 6–1). Pistolesi and Giuntini (1978) also convincingly demonstrated an excellent correlation, in both acute and chronic cardiac patients, between extravascular lung water measured by the modified indicator dilution method and radiographic criteria used to grade pulmonary interstitial edema.

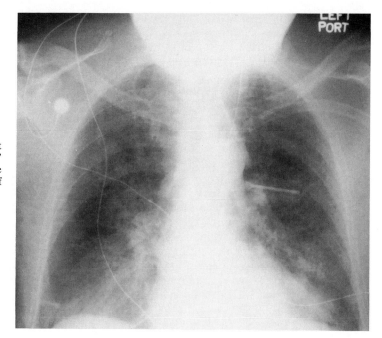

Figure 6–1. An anteroposterior (AP) radiograph in patient with elevated "wedge" pressure. Bilateral perihilar "haze" with peribronchial wall thickening is noted. Findings are consistent with edema even though clinical evidence of cardiac decompensation was minimal.

The relationship between cardiac hemodynamics and the chest radiograph in patients with left-sided cardiac failure has been well documented. Positive correlations have been found between pulmonary venous pressures and radiographic findings of pulmonary venous hypertension and edema (Hamosh and Cohen, 1971; McHugh et al., 1972; Sjoegren, 1970). The radiographs used in these studies were of high quality and were obtained in the posteroanterior (PA) projection in an erect or semi-erect position. An important feature of cardiac failure, particularly chronic cardiac failure, is a redistribution of blood flow (from base to apex), with distention and recruit-

ment of upper lobe vessels (Pistolesi and Giuntini, 1978).

The use of the Swan-Ganz catheter has provided clinicians with a more timely and reliable physiologic determinant of cardiac function. The "wedge" pressure is not in itself reflective of the extent of pulmonary edema, however, nor is there a direct correlation with the radiographic findings of edema (Fig. 6–2). Likewise, false readings may occur, owing to failure to wedge the catheter appropriately, clotting within the lumen of the catheter, kinking of the catheter, failure to place the tip of the catheter in the third zone (lung bases), alteration in lung compliance due

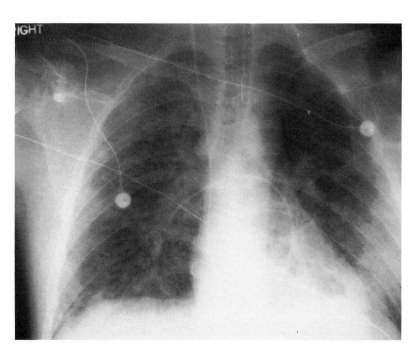

Figure 6–2. An AP radiograph in patient with normal wedge pressure. Persistent patchy edema is present with confluent opacity in the left lower lobe. Wedge pressure and radiograph were compatible with heart failure 72 hours prior to this radiograph, which represents a delay in resorption of edema after the reversal of the heart failure.

to severe chronic obstructive lung disease or to adult respiratory distress syndrome (ARDS), or the effects of high levels of PEEP (Eaton et al., 1983; Lefcoe et al., 1979; Milne et al., 1985).

Other discrepancies between the pulmonary wedge pressure and the radiographic manifestations of edema have been reported. Two such discrepancies have been termed the "preclinical failure" and "post-therapeutic phase lag" phenomena (McHugh et al., 1972; Rotman et al., 1974; Sjoegren, 1970). The term preclinical failure is used to describe those patients with no radiographic evidence of edema in the presence of an elevated pulmonary wedge pressure, which is usually rapid in onset. The preclinical failure phenomenon is unusual in our experience, but we have observed a few cases in which an apparent transient increase in left ventricular filling pressure was not followed by the development of any radiographically detectable edema. Any persistent elevation of wedge pressure associated with a totally normal chest radiograph suggests an erroneous left atrial pressure measurement, because this phenomenon occurs so infrequently.

The post-therapeutic lag phenomenon is not unusual, particularly in the patient with recurrent left-sided heart failure. When the wedge pressure returns to normal, it may take hours to days before the lymphatics can resorb large amounts of extravascular water (Nakahara et al., 1983) (see Fig. 6–2). The persistence of radiographic signs of edema is a more accurate index of extravascular lung water than is the hemodynamic measurement.

Several authors have suggested that some correlation exists between the size of the azygos vein, the circulating blood volume, and the right atrial pressure (Heitzman, 1973b; Milne, 1973). Milne, Pistolesi, and their associates were the first to actually quantify

these measurements, using the "vascular pedicle" (the width of the mediastinum just above the aortic arch) to estimate circulating blood volume (Milne et al., 1984; Pistolesi et al., 1984). The right border of the vascular pedicle, formed by the right brachycephalic vein and the superior vena cava, is venous and distensible, whereas the left border formed above the aorta by the subclavian artery is arterial and much less compliant. The measurement of the vascular pedicle in healthy subjects averages 48 mm ± 5 mm. The pedicle widens approximately 10% to 40% in the supine position. Therefore, comparison of the vascular pedicle on successive films should be made with the patient in the same position. Increased intrathoracic pressure from Valsava's maneuver or from PEEP diminishes the width of the pedicle. Milne and co-workers reported that in cardiac failure, 60% of their patients showed a vascular pedicle width greater than 53 mm, and 40% showed widths in the normal range. Of the renal or overhydration patients, 85% revealed a wide pedicle and only 15% showed normal pedicles. Of patients with capillary permeability edema, 35% had a narrowed pedicle, and 60% had a normal pedicle (Milne et al., 1985) (Fig. 6–3).

Aberle, Smith, and their colleagues were unable to confirm the observation made by Milne and co-workers that the vascular pedicle width helped to distinguish cardiac patients from those with overhydration renal failure, permeability edema, or both (Aberle et al., 1988; Smith et al., 1987). Their patients tended to have more severe edema, and fewer were able to be radiographed in the upright position. An increase in circulating blood volume does not imply that it has any direct correlation with the pathogenesis of the edema, unless it is accompanied by an increase in right or left ventricular diastolic pressure.

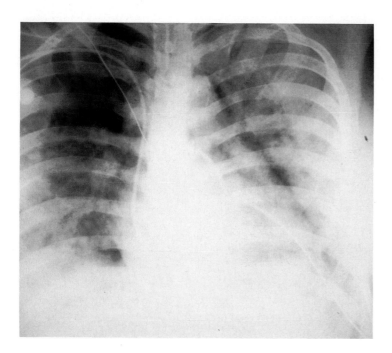

Figure 6–3. An AP radiograph in patient with permeability edema. The peripheral opacities and lack of pleural effusion are consistent with the diagnosis. The vascular "pedicle" width is increased, but cardiac decompensation and overhydration are *not* present.

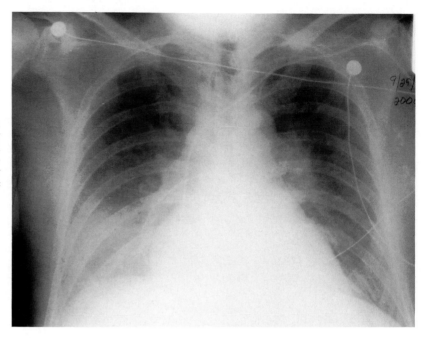

Figure 6–4. An AP radiograph in patient with renal failure. The wedge pressure is slightly elevated, and the heart is enlarged. The bilateral edema is both central and peripheral. The pulmonary vessel caliber is normal. The vascular pedicle is wide. This radiograph is characteristic of overhydration edema.

Our observations indicate that overhydration edema is relatively unusual as an isolated event. Left ventricular dysfunction, either acute or chronic, occurs with a high frequency in patients who also have overload edema. The condition of patients with so-called renal edema is also complex. Their cardiac output is rarely completely normal, and their capillaries may be leaky. True overhydration edema rarely involves the interstitium of the lung and often mimics permeability edema (Fig. 6–4). Pure overhydration is rare in the intensive care unit (see Fig. 5–18). In most cases, it is a combination of permeability and hydrostatic forces, worsened by the overload state.

Milne and co-workers also emphasized the importance of determining pulmonary blood volume (pulmonary vascular engorgement) in distinguishing cardiac from noncardiac edema (Milne et al., 1985). Capillary permeability edema, in their experience, demonstrated normal pulmonary vascular size unless the vessels were decreased as a result of the effects of PEEP (Fig. 6–5). Normal pulmonary blood volume was more common in patients with cardiac edema and usually increased in patients with overhydration or renal edema. As with redistribution of pulmonary blood flow, assessment of the size of the pulmonary vessels can be extremely difficult in the presence of extensive alveolar edema. Correlation between redistribution and pulmonary blood volume is essentially impossible to demonstrate on the supine radiograph. Thus, these measurements are often difficult to apply in many of the patients routinely being evaluated within intensive care units.

In cardiac failure, edema fluid is a transudate, low in protein. The first site of accumulation of edema is in the connective tissues surrounding the blood vessels and airways (Staub et al., 1967). This tissue is continuous around vessels and bronchi, and into the inter-

lobular septa and the subpleural space. Fluid in these spaces is visualized on the radiograph as peribronchial cuffing, Kerley's lines, and subpleural fluid accumulation (accentuation of fissures). These signs are characteristic features of hydrostatic edema (Fig. 6–6). The excess water accumulated in the interstitium is resorbed and flows centrally through the lymphatics, which carry the fluid back to the systemic veins. Staub (1980) has suggested that an osmotic pressure gradient from the periphery of the lung, where the

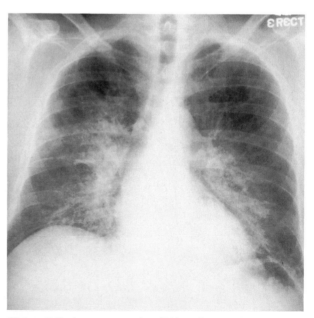

Figure 6–5. A posteroanterior (PA) radiograph in patient with noncardiac edema. The findings of central edema, which is primarily interstitial, and engorged central vessels are *not* characteristic findings of permeability edema. The radiograph revealed diffuse alveolar edema 24 hours later.

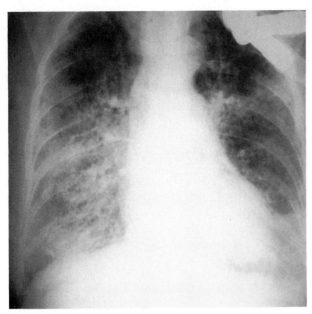

Figure 6–6. An AP radiograph demonstrating classic signs of hydrostatic edema. Kerley's A lines, fissure thickening, peribronchial cuffing, and confluent areas of alveolar edema are present.

pressure is low, to the center of the lung, where the osmotic pressure is high, is at least partially responsible for the distribution of the edema (Staub, 1980). As fluid progressively accumulates within the perivascular space, the interstitium becomes "saturated," and alveolar edema may quickly develop.

In contradistinction, patients with permeability edema have protein-rich edema fluid, which accumulates in the extravascular space as a consequence of increased microvascular permeability (Bachofen and Weibel, 1982). Because of the high protein osmotic pressure of the extravasated proteins, water

may not flow from the extravasation site toward the loose connective tissue but may flood the alveolar space. Alveolar flooding increases when concomitant epithelial injury occurs (Bachofen and Weibel, 1982). Also the clearance of protein-rich exudate is slower than that of nonproteinaceous fluid (Matthay et al., 1980). Milne and colleagues (1985) believe that the inability of this proteinaceous edema to migrate centrally explains the absence of peribronchial cuffs, the absence of Kerley's lines, and the infrequent occurrence of pleural effusions in patients with permeability edema (Fig. 6–7).

Unlike cardiac patients, whose radiographs often feature a generalized increase in lung density, the increased lung density in patients with permeability edema is often patchy and with a peripheral distribution (Fig. 6–8). This patchy peripheral distribution has been confirmed in an oleic acid canine model by the use of computed tomography (CT) (Hedlund et al., 1982b). Numerous studies have shown that interstitial edema does form in capillary-leak edema but is masked radiographically by alveolar edema (Malo et al., 1984; Vreim and Staub, 1976; Wegenius et al., 1984) (Fig. 6–9). Milne and colleagues (1985) confirm this experience in that the persistence of the peripheral distribution of permeability edema is a poor prognostic sign, whereas central migration of the edema pattern seems to be an indicator of injury resolution or remodeling of the lung architecture.

In a series of patients with cardiac and noncardiac edema, Smith and co-workers (1987) were able to distinguish permeability from nonpermeability edema in 83% of cases. They applied the following criteria: if the heart size is enlarged, or if the heart size is normal and Kerley's lines are present, cardiogenic edema is diagnosed (Fig. 6–10). If heart size is normal and Kerley's lines are absent, permeability edema is

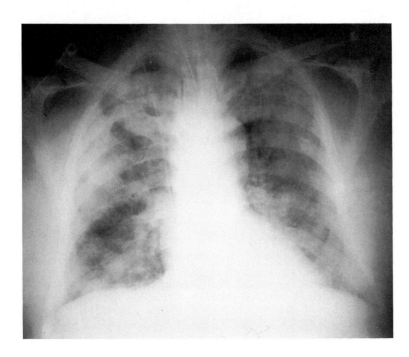

Figure 6–7. An AP radiograph in patient with diffuse edema. Vascular pedicle and pulmonary artery size are normal. Absence of Kerley's A lines, of pleural effusion, and of peribronchial cuffs is characteristic of permeability edema.

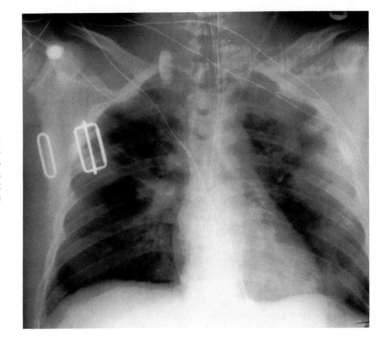

Figure 6–8. An AP radiograph in patient with acute decompensation following surgery. Numerous tubes and a metallic brace are in place. The asymmetric edema is primarily alveolar. Note the indistinct right hilum, which indicates focal edema in the superior segment of the right lower lobe. No distinct interstitial signs are present. These features indicate permeability edema.

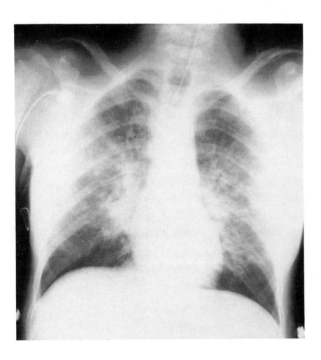

Figure 6–9. An AP radiograph in patient with probable neurogenic edema. Note hyperdistention of the cuff of the endotracheal tube. The perihilar haze, acinar edema, and peribronchial cuffs are signs of permeability and hydrostatic edema. No pleural effusion is present, and the heart is of normal size.

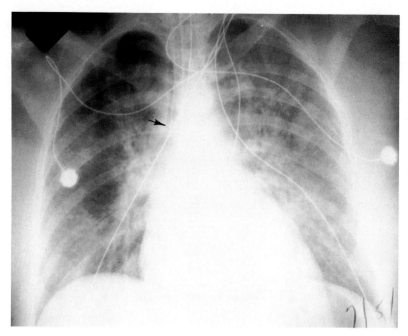

Figure 6–10. An AP radiograph in patient with acute heart failure. Perihilar haze, peribronchial cuffs, and central edema predominate. The tip of the endotracheal tube is near the right main bronchus (arrow).

diagnosed (Fig. 6–11). The presence of Kerley's lines, particularly Kerley's A lines, almost always indicates cardiac or concomitant hydrostatic edema in the setting of the intensive care unit. Kerley's lines may also be seen in respiratory compromised patients with overwhelming influenzal viral pneumonitis and in patients with lymphatic obstruction due to central nodal enlargement or lymphohematogenous metastasis to the lung (Fig. 6–12).

The distribution of edema may change with the use of PEEP ventilation. Malo and associates (1984) reported that PEEP shifted alveolar air-space edema to the interstitium in a morphologic study of acute pulmonary edema in dogs. Wegenius and Modig (1985) reported that increased permeability edema commonly appeared to be interstitial in patients receiving positive-pressure ventilation. According to the hypothesis presented by Aberle and associates (1988), with expansion of the collapsed fluid-filled spaces, margination of the edema in the air spaces may occur and thereby simulate an interstitial pattern on radiographs.

The controversy in the literature concerning the radiographic appearance of edema may be more reflective of the differences in patient population than the actual debate regarding the precise pathogenesis

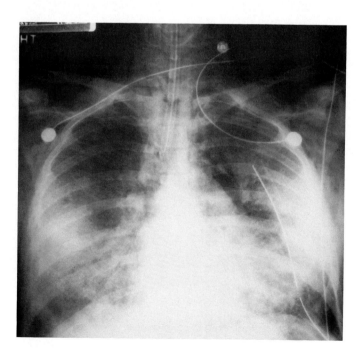

Figure 6–11. An AP radiograph in patient with noncardiac edema and adult respiratory distress syndrome (ARDS). Note the left pneumothorax that is secondary to barotrauma and requires a chest tube. The peripheral alveolar opacities and air bronchograms are classic patterns of permeability edema.

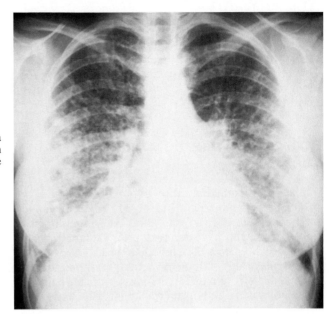

Figure 6–12. A PA radiograph in a young nurse with acute influenza pneumonia. Perihilar indistinctness, bronchial wall thickening with cuffs, and prominent Kerley's lines are noted. The opacities are predominantly acinar.

of edema formation. The application of animal models is not altogether reasonable in some cases of induced pulmonary edema, and quantification of the extent of overall lung injury and classification of the edema are difficult (Aberle et al., 1988). The state of the underlying lung, the presence or absence of sepsis, and modifications of treatment account for some of the differences reported within the clinical literature.

In summary, patients with noncardiac edema are *usually* characterized by a normal heart size, and infrequent Kerley's lines, peribronchial cuffs, and pleural effusions (Figs. 6–13 and 6–14). Peribronchial cuff thickening may also indicate luminal bronchial

wall edema or inspissated mucus. Therefore, in patients maintained on ventilators, the bronchi may appear thickened for reasons other than increased lung water.

Our ability to determine the cause of edema radiographically is enhanced by the use of those parameters and observations that have been adequately assessed by well-controlled clinical trials. Conventional radiog-

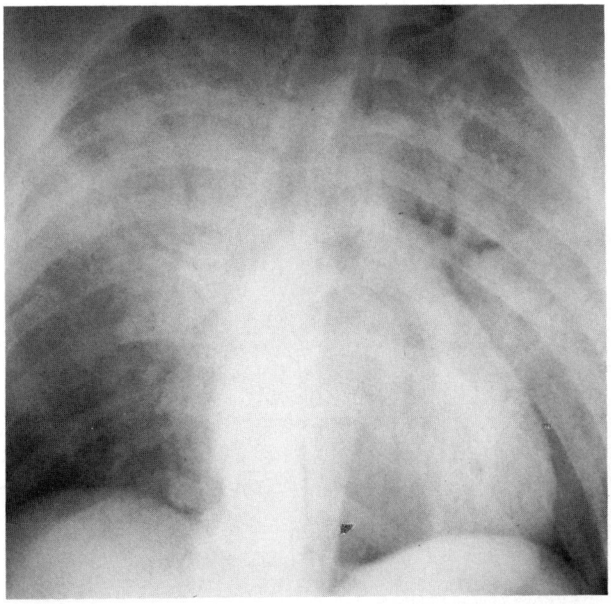

Figure 6–13. An AP radiograph in patient with permeability edema. Extensive alveolar opacities with air bronchograms are evident. Pleural effusion and Kerley's lines are absent.

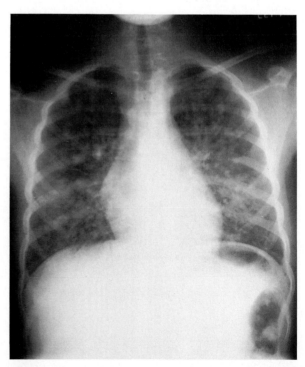

Figure 6–14. A PA radiograph in patient with acute mitral insufficiency. The vascular pedicle is wide, Kerley's lines are present centrally, bronchial cuffs are present, and the inhomogeneous edema spares the peripheral zones. Contrast this radiograph with that of Figure 6–13.

raphy offers acceptable sensitivity for the detection of pulmonary edema. In select cases, conventional radiography can distinguish between cardiac and noncardiac edema, but the overall specificity is low. Overall diagnosis requires the appropriate use of other clinical and physiologic data for a more precise diagnosis (Table 6–1).

Atypical Patterns of Pulmonary Edema

The most common cause of atypical pulmonary edema is concomitant acute or chronic obstructive pulmonary disease. Patients who have subtle interstitial fibrosis, who have received prior radiation treatment, or who are in the immediate post-thoracotomy period may also exhibit a nonuniform pulmonary edema pattern. Likewise, patients with chronic or acute pulmonary embolism, or patients who may have other perfusion-ventilation defects, may have focal or asymmetric pulmonary opacities that suggest atelectasis or pneumonia rather than pulmonary edema (Fraser and Paré, 1970; Heitzman, 1973a). Hemodynamic measurements, confirmatory clinical information, and modification of the pulmonary opacities following therapeutic trial usually confirm the source of the opacity as a simple transudate.

In a recent unpublished series of cases from our institution, we observed that unilateral cardiac edema usually occurred in the right lower and right middle lobes. The diagnosis was usually not difficult because other radiographic signs of congestive heart failure were present. When the additional radiographic findings were not observed, the radiologist would frequently interpret these opacities as representative of pneumonia. In the same study, we noted that pleural

Table 6–1. RADIOGRAPHIC CRITERIA DISTINGUISHING CARDIAC FROM NONCARDIAC EDEMA

Signs	Cardiac	Noncardiac
Major		
Kerley's lines	Present	Unusual
Pleural effusions	Present	Unusual
Cardiomegaly	Present	Unusual
Opacities	Diffuse	Patchy and peripheral
Minor		
Air bronchograms	Rare	Often present
Hilar haze	Present	Infrequent
Peribronchial cuffs	Present	Unusual

effusions in congestive heart failure were usually bilateral, and unilateral small effusions were just as frequent on the left side as on the right side. The large left pleural effusion suggests a diagnosis other than simple congestive heart failure.

Gurney and Goodman recently reported a pulmonary edema pattern that is localized to the right upper lobe and accompanies mitral regurgitation (Gurney and Goodman, 1989). We have confirmed this finding in an additional five patients with mitral insufficiency (Fig. 6–15). The pathogenesis of the isolated right upper lobe alveolar pulmonary edema is related to the vector of blood flow across the incompetent mitral valve, which may be targeted at the pulmonary vein of the right upper lobe. This causes a local increase in pulmonary venous pressure and accentuates the formation of edema.

The Waterston shunt for tetralogy of Fallot creates an anastomosis between the ascending aorta and the right pulmonary artery and may be responsible for unilateral edema resulting from hyperperfusion (Mutchler et al., 1974). The Blalock-Taussig anasto-

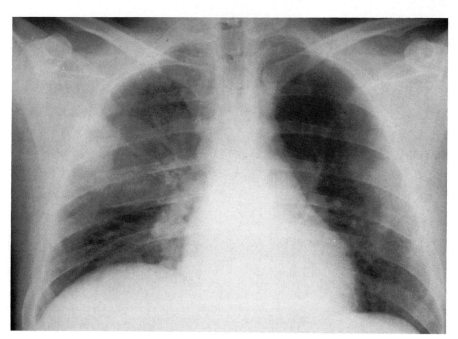

Figure 6–15. An AP radiograph in patient with mitral insufficiency and heart failure. Signs of pulmonary venous hypertension are present. The predominant edema pattern is in the right upper lobe.

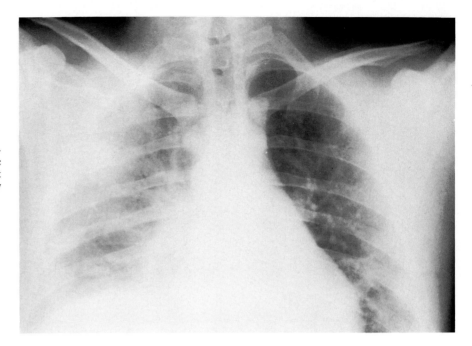

Figure 6–16. An AP radiograph in patient with splenic surgery and cardiac failure. Patient was positioned on right side following surgery. Pulmonary edema is primarily in the right lung.

mosis also produces right-sided edema, whereas Potts procedure results in left-sided edema. In either case, the etiologic factor is high hydrostatic pressure due to increased blood flow, which in turn results in an increase in venous pressure combined with pulmonary capillary damage, which produces the high surface tension.

Gravity has also been implicated as a major cause of unilateral pulmonary edema and may be a particular problem in patients within the intensive care unit (Leeming, 1973; Zimmerman et al., 1982). Gravity raises the hydrostatic pressure in the dependent lung, impairing circulation, and if this increased pressure is prolonged, it may lead to capillary damage. This process has been shown in patients on a mechanical ventilator, who may be positioned on one side to promote bronchial drainage, or in patients with chest injuries or a recent surgical procedure, who prefer to lie on their nontraumatized side (Leeming, 1973) (Fig. 6–16).

Asymmetric or unilateral edema has numerous other noncardiac causes. The most common cause of unilateral pulmonary edema within the critical care unit is the aspiration of gastric contents (Newman et al., 1982a). Direct irritation of the alveolar epithelium occurs, and rapid desquamation of the membrane exposes the capillaries to the highly acidic irritant (Pattle, 1958). The volume of aspirate may have little bearing on the extent of pulmonary edema that develops. Gastric aspiration may be responsible for unilateral edema or generalized edema, which mimics hydrostatic pulmonary edema (Fig. 6–17) (see Chapter 5). Aspiration must be distinguished from congestive heart failure. In the patient who has aspirated acidic fluid, pulmonary edema diminishes blood volume, and inappropriate use of diuretic therapy may prove to be fatal.

Edema induced by drugs such as heroin, methadone or cocaine may also be unilateral, because the patient may be unconscious and lying on one side (Wilen et al., 1975) (Fig. 6–18). In addition to a rise in hydrostatic pressure, surface tension increases as a result of hypoxemia, which produces a combination of hydrostatic and nonhydrostatic edema. Neurogenic as well as cardiac manifestations of drug toxicity may also be responsible for typical or atypical edema patterns (Calenoff et al., 1978).

Inhomogeneous edema may occur peripherally

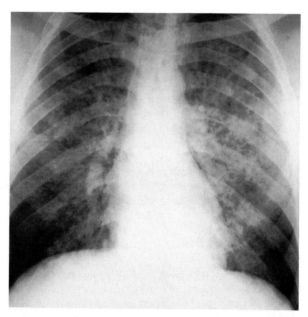

Figure 6–17. An AP radiograph in patient with gastric aspiration. The asymmetric edema often resembles congestive heart failure. Pleural effusion is rare with aspiration.

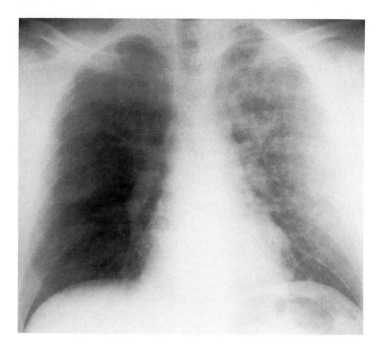

Figure 6–18. An AP radiograph in patient with cocaine toxicity. The patient was discovered lying on his left side. No evidence of aspiration was obvious. Regardless of the mechanism of edema, the opacity is uniform and unilateral.

when a central venous pressure catheter is misdirected into a peripheral pulmonary artery. The rapid infusion of dilute crystalloid is postulated to stimulate neural reflexes and a release of vasoactive substances, which leads to increased capillary permeability (Royal et al., 1975). The rapid removal of large amounts of pleural fluid or air may be followed by unilateral pulmonary edema (Trapnell and Thurston, 1970). This edema usually occurs immediately after thoracentesis and is due to the rapid re-expansion of the compressed lung with a sudden increase in hydrostatic pressure and persistence of high surface tension. The rapid return of pulmonary blood flow caused by the sudden rise in negative intrapleural pressure produces the edema (Ziskind et al., 1965).

Childress and colleagues have suggested that in addition to rapid re-expansion of a collapsed lung, a bronchus must be occluded by mucus or other material to produce edema (Childress et al., 1971). The same phenomenon is responsible for lobar pulmonary edema (drowned lung) following acute bronchial obstruction and is probably secondary to focal hypoxia and increased epithelial membrane permeability.

The other major causes of atypical or unilateral pulmonary edema are related to congenital or acquired perfusion abnormalities. Congenital absence of the pulmonary artery, Swyer-James-McCloud syndrome, or other destructive mechanisms affecting the pulmonary vascular bed result in the formation of edema only in areas that are normally perfused (Saleh et al., 1974). Following lobectomy, the remaining lung becomes overexpanded and thus unevenly perfused. This phenomenon may be responsible for development of either no edema or an inhomogeneous alveolar pattern with congestive heart failure.

Lung collapse due to pneumothorax or a large pleural effusion causes diminished perfusion in the ipsilateral lung. If heart failure occurs during lung compression, edema often develops only in the contralateral lung. The same phenomenon may occur in neonatal respiratory distress syndrome. The lung that is protected may be the lung that is underperfused initially.

Kohen and colleagues (1986) reported several unusual patterns occurring in patients with uremic pulmonary edema. We, too, have reviewed edema in chronic renal patients requiring dialysis treatment. Alwall (1960) noted twice the mortality in patients with uremia and pulmonary edema compared with patients having uremia alone. The focal and diffuse alveolar opacities (edema pattern) in patients with uremia are more characteristic of exudates than of transudates; their pattern and distribution may be more inhomogeneous and lobar than the classic "butterfly" description (Fig. 6–19). Focal opacities occurring in the uremic patient tend to recur in the same location. One must not confuse these focal opacities with opportunistic infection or underlying vasculitis.

Atypical pulmonary edema frequently simulates other acute pulmonary disorders. A detailed understanding of pathophysiologic events as well as an adequate and up-to-date assessment of the clinical situation is mandatory for an accurate differential diagnosis. An isolated and uninformed interpretation often leads to misdiagnosis in cases of atypical cardiac or noncardiac edema.

ADULT RESPIRATORY DISTRESS SYNDROME

The term *adult respiratory distress syndrome* (ARDS) is used to describe a heterogeneous group of patients with respiratory insufficiency who develop

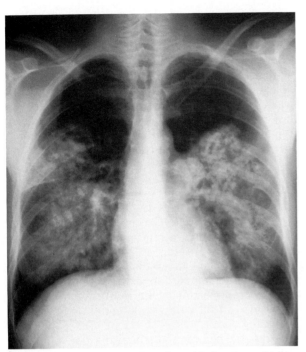

Figure 6–19. A PA radiograph in patient with chronic renal failure. The "butterfly" distribution of edema is infrequent and usually signifies hydrostatic edema.

such as aspiration pneumonia, fluid overload, or congestive heart failure (Fig. 6–20). The first definite radiographic abnormality usually appears about 24 hours after the initial insult, but the more fulminant the injury, the shorter the latent period.

The initial radiograph shows a bilateral perihilar haze with ill-defined linear opacities extending from the hilum, which is consistent with interstitial edema. These signs may be masked by portable radiographs of suboptimal quality and by shallow inspiration. Low lung volume demonstrated by radiography may be the only manifestation of the diminished lung compliance of early ARDS. The linear opacities coalesce rapidly and resemble focal areas of alveolar edema or pneumonitis (Fig. 6–21). At this time, differentiation between ARDS and congestive heart failure or diffuse pneumonitis is almost impossible. Other radiographic signs of cardiac edema, such as cardiomegaly, pulmonary vascular redistribution, and pleural effusion, are either absent or difficult to assess with only the supine radiograph. The radiographs should be correlated with physiologic data, such as central venous pressure (CVP) or pulmonary capillary wedge (PCW) pressures.

Serial radiographs reveal rapid progression of the disease, from localized confluent opacities to a complete alveolar filling pattern within 24 hours following

a characteristic clinical, pathophysiologic, and radiographic pattern hours to days after a severe local or systemic insult.

In addition to the primary disease, many therapeutic maneuvers appear to contribute to the clinical, pathologic, and radiographic appearance. Overzealous use of intravenous (IV) fluids, prolonged ventilatory treatment, high oxygen concentrations, and excessive use of respiratory depressants aggravate pulmonary insufficiency. Therapeutic errors of omission have also been implicated, especially inadequate control of sepsis, poor control of blood filtration, and suboptimal pulmonary management. Pathophysiologic, clinical, and therapeutic aspects of ARDS are discussed in Chapter 7.

Radiographic Features

Because both clinical and radiographic features of ARDS are not specific, radiologists must be aware of the complete clinical course of a patient suspected of having ARDS (Curtis, 1988; Greene et al., 1983; Putman et al., 1972). Films must be interpreted in a serial fashion, because the initial abnormalities may change from hour to hour and then stabilize after 48 to 72 hours. Serial radiographs may suggest ARDS by demonstrating this progression of abnormalities.

The chest radiographic findings correspond closely to the described pathologic abnormalities. The radiograph is usually normal for the first 12 to 24 hours. An abnormal chest radiograph during the first 8 to 12 hours is usually due to some complicating factors

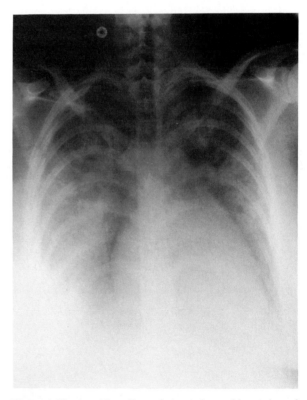

Figure 6–20. An AP radiograph in patient with sepsis and a consumptive coagulopathy. This radiograph was obtained 6 hours after systemic hypotension. The wide vascular pedicle, bilateral effusions, and homogeneous edema are due to concomitant cardiac decompensation rather than to capillary leak.

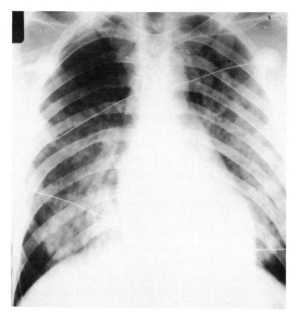

Figure 6–21. An AP radiography in patient 36 hours after near drowning. The initial radiograph was normal. The confluent alveolar opacities with scattered air bronchograms mask any interstitial changes. Absent pleural effusion and normal heart size with this edemalike pattern suggest ARDS.

the onset of pulmonary symptoms (Fig. 6–22). After the pattern of pulmonary edema develops, little alteration may appear in the radiograph for several days (Fig. 6–23). The radiographic appearance may be dramatically altered, however, by treatment. Therapy-related changes may be due to overhydration, barotrauma, or infection. Most notable is the apparent improvement in aeration following the use of PEEP. Over a period that may vary from several days to several weeks, the radiograph may return to

a normal baseline or may show focal areas of scarring consistent with interstitial fibrosis (Table 6–2).

Thin walled cysts, suggesting bronchopulmonary dysplasia, may appear during the chronic phase.

Patients with underlying chronic obstructive pulmonary disease or congestive heart failure who also have ARDS often demonstrate radiographic changes more in keeping with the primary disease process. Asymmetric consolidation raises the possibility of superimposed pneumonia (see Chapter 5).

Differential Diagnosis

In cases of acute respiratory insufficiency and a radiograph demonstrating a diffuse alveolar or interstitial process, the diagnosis of ARDS is one of exclusion. Edema, aspiration pneumonia, drug toxicity, severe infection, lung contusion, pulmonary embolism, and fat emboli may mimic ARDS radiographically (Joffe, 1974; Putman, 1988). In many instances, the clinical and laboratory data allow adequate differentiation. A discussion of pulmonary embolism and fat embolism, which may be confused with ARDS, follows.

Pulmonary embolism is a frequent diagnostic consideration early in the course of ARDS. In both conditions, the patient has a rapid onset of respiratory insufficiency and a normal or minimally abnormal chest radiograph. The diffuse parenchymal infiltrates that develop in ARDS, however, are rarely observed in pulmonary embolism. The presence of a pleural effusion strongly suggests pulmonary embolism rather than ARDS. A special problem is encountered when the condition of a patient with known ARDS significantly worsens, which raises the possibility of a superimposed pulmonary embolism. In such cases, a

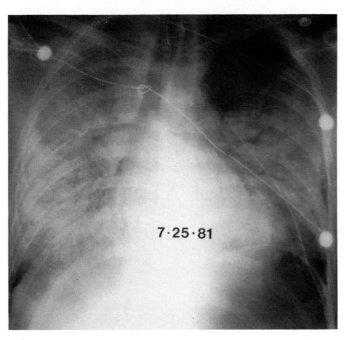

7·25·81

Figure 6–22. An AP radiograph in patient with progressive pulmonary insufficiency. The pattern is extensive alveolar consolidation 48 hours after severe hypoxemia. The stomach is distended with air. Air bronchograms and absent pleural effusion are characteristic of ARDS.

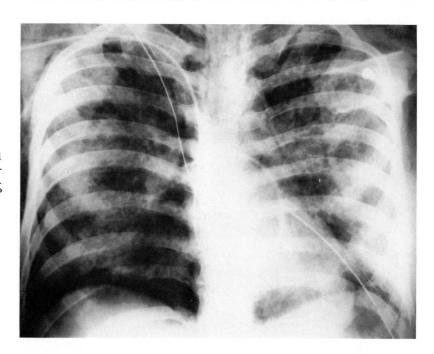

Figure 6–23. An AP radiograph in patient 1 week following the diagnosis of ARDS. Peripheral asymmetric opacities are usual at this time. The left pneumothorax is secondary to PEEP and barotrauma.

perfusion lung scan or pulmonary angiogram may be required for confirmation or exclusion of pulmonary embolism (see Chapter 9).

In ARDS, the lung scan is normal or diffusely abnormal with multiple subsegmental defects (Newman et al., 1982b) (Fig. 6–24). Adult respiratory distress syndrome alone does not cause segmental defects. When uncertainty persists, pulmonary angiography is required. Four types of angiographic abnormality have been ascribed to the vascular occlusion sometimes present in ARDS: (1) intraluminal filling defects in vessels 1 to 3 mm in diameter, (2) absent filling of small arterial side branches, (3) vascular deformities, and (4) altered microvascular background opacification (Greene et al., 1983). These angiographic findings are usually distinct from those described in classic thromboembolism.

Regardless of whether pulmonary vascular occlu-

sion in ARDS is a primary or a secondary event, the resulting underperfused lung contributes to endothelial injury. The primary and secondary changes within the pulmonary circulation contribute to a diminished cardiac output. Thus, in the later stages of severe ARDS, right- and left-sided heart failure may be apparent radiographically.

In patients with fat embolism, both the clinical and the radiographic appearances may occasionally simulate those of ARDS. Fat embolism syndrome consists of the triad of neurologic dysfunction, respiratory insufficiency, and petechiae following major orthopedic trauma or manipulation. As in ARDS, a latent period between the trauma and the clinical syndrome often occurs.

Our experience suggests the occurrence of three clinical, pathologic, and radiographic patterns of response to the embolic fat (Curtis et al., 1979). The

Table 6–2. SEQUENCE OF EVENTS IN ADULT RESPIRATORY DISTRESS SYNDROME

Findings	Phase 1 (12–24 hr)	Phase 2 (24–36 hr)	Phase 3 (36–72 hr)	Phase 4 (72 hr–6 wk)
Clinical	Negative	Tachypnea, dyspnea, decreased O_2, decreased CO_2	Respiratory and metabolic acidosis; increased alveolar-arterial P_{O_2} gradient	Progressive respiratory failure or complete recovery with variable signs of pulmonary disease
Pathologic (gross)	Edema with or without petechiae	Increased edema, congestion	Hepatization	Further hepatization, fibrosis, or normal findings
Microscopic	Microemboli, periarteriolar hemorrhage	Interstitial and intra-alveolar edema	Congestive atelectasis, intra-alveolar hemorrhage, hyaline membranes	Interstitial fibrosis or nonspecific findings
Radiographic	Negative or fulminant edema	24 hr: perihilar haze, interstitial edema; 36 hr: alveolar edema	Little change in radiograph after 36 hr; secondary problems (e.g., infection)	Little change after 72 hr or focal-diffuse fibrosis; barotrauma

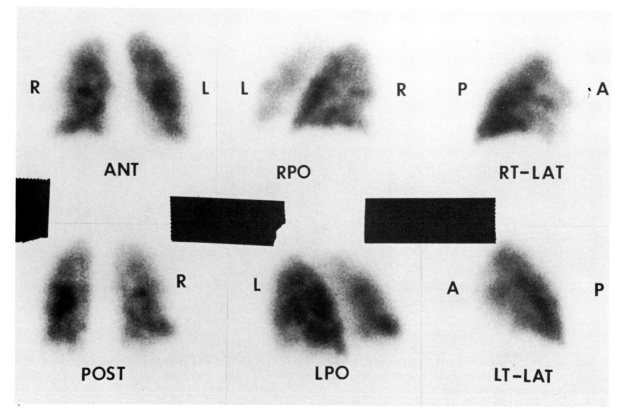

Figure 6–24. Perfusion lung scan in patient described in Figure 6–23. This scan reveals the classic pattern described in patients with diffuse lung disease. The scan shows multiple subsegmental defects ("Swiss-cheese" pattern).

classic pattern is characterized by equivocal chest radiographs, which are often borderline abnormal and rarely progress to an interstitial or alveolar pattern. Histologic examination shows microscopic fat emboli within capillaries, and arterioles with areas of interstitial and alveolar edema. With ventilatory support, most of these patients have an uneventful recovery.

The second pattern of response to the embolic fat is characterized by consistently abnormal chest radiographs, progressing from normal to diffuse alveolar consolidation within 24 to 48 hours. Histologic examination demonstrates multiple fat emboli surrounded by fibrin and platelet aggregates, and both interstitial and alveolar hemorrhage, which can progress to hyaline membrane formation and, eventually, to pulmonary fibrosis. This type of response, therefore, is indistinguishable clinically, pathologically, and radiographically from ARDS (Fig. 6–25).

The third pattern involves those patients who have massive fat embolism and die within the first 24 hours. These patients usually have evidence of right-to-left shunting. This condition is due to sudden rises in right ventricular pressure accompanied by paradoxical embolization, through a patent foramen ovale or through other cardiac defects. This hyperacute form is rarely unrecognized while the patient is alive, and death results from sudden changes in right-sided

pressure accompanied by terminal arrhythmias. Usually, these radiographs remain normal.

OTHER MEASURES OF LUNG WATER

Thermal-Dye–Dilution Technique

In the thermal-dye–dilution method, the modification of the double-indicator–dilution technique, two indicators are injected into the superior vena cava or right atrium and are sampled from the femoral artery (Allison et al., 1985; Effros, 1985). One of the two indicators diffuses extravascularly, and the other remains intravascular. The method estimates the volume of distribution of the two indicators and, by calculation of the difference, the volume of extravascular water. In the thermal-dye–dilution method, heat and indocyanine green are the diffusible and intravascular indicators. With the characteristic diffusing nature of heat, the thermal-dye–dilution method estimates a thermal volume (extravascular thermal volume), which includes not only lung water, but also contributions of fluid and blood from the heart and great vessels.

Studies measuring gravimetric estimates of lung water have demonstrated an excellent correlation between the data obtained by the in vivo and in vitro methods (Gray et al., 1984). The thermal-dye–dilu-

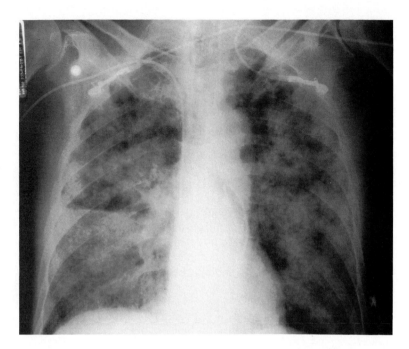

Figure 6–25. An AP radiograph in patient with extensive fat embolism. Swan-Ganz catheter tip is in the right ventricle. The diffuse alveolar opacities are indistinguishable from any condition causing noncardiac edema.

tion technique has been used in several clinical studies to compare extravascular lung water with radiographic, hemodynamic, and other physiologic parameters, to define and follow the course of acute lung injury (Baundendistel et al., 1982; Laggner et al., 1984). Because this technique is invasive, the application is confined essentially to patients in the intensive care unit. In patients with normal lungs, thermal-dye measurements overestimate gravimetric water content by inclusion of extrapulmonary tissue. More important, the delivery of the heat indicator to the lung tissues depends solely on the distribution of pulmonary blood flow, and many patients with complex pulmonary and systemic disease have markedly uneven lung perfusion (Effros, 1985).

The probability that hemodynamic changes may affect the thermal-dilution measurements in the absence of significant alterations in the extravascular lung water content is particularly significant in critically ill patients, who are often hemodynamically unstable (Rice and Miller, 1981). Published data indicate that PEEP can increase the thermal-dilution values for lung water, although this increase may reflect a redistribution of lung perfusion (Carlile et al., 1986). Giuntini and associates (1987) also emphasized that although chest radiographs may not provide precise estimates of lung water, they have at least three advantages over any indicator-dilution technique: (1) The radiograph does not depend on perfusion of edematous lung regions. (2) The radiograph can detect focal or regional edema. (3) The radiograph helps to determine the nature of an opacity exclusive of edema.

Soluble Inert Gas Technique

With the soluble inert gas technique, an inhaled soluble inert gas (e.g., acetylene) equilibrates instan-

taneously within the pulmonary tissues (Cander and Forster, 1959). The remaining alveolar inert gas is slowly subtracted by the pulmonary capillary blood. The rate of disappearance of the inert gas from the alveoli is estimated through use of a rebreathing technique (Sackner et al., 1975). Values for tissue volume reflect lung water content, and acceptable correlations between lung tissue volume measurement and gravimetric extravascular lung water have been demonstrated (Freidman et al., 1980).

The potential for clinical applications of the soluble inert gas technique is good because the technique is noninvasive, its measurements are rapid and reproducible, and in addition to allowing determination of lung tissue volume, it can be used to determine pulmonary capillary blood flow (Cutillo, 1987). The problem with the technique is that it measures not only extravascular lung water but also a fraction of intravascular water. The delivery of the gas to the alveoli depends on the distribution of ventilation; therefore, the presence of any ventilation defect causes significant errors in the measurement of lung tissue volume (Petrini et al., 1978). Although its sensitivity is questionable when used for severe pulmonary edema or other parenchymal conditions associated with significant alteration in ventilation-perfusion, the soluble inert gas technique does have some clinical application, particularly in patients who have medical complications and are prone to development of pulmonary edema.

Qualitative and Quantitative Densitometric Measurements

Lung density, which is normally low, increases significantly with the accumulation of water (Simon et al., 1979). Lung density has been estimated in animals and in humans through the use of x-ray densitometry, Compton scattering densitometry, CT and positron-emission tomography (Gamsu et al., 1979; Hedlund et al., 1983; Rhodes et al., 1981; Simon et al., 1979). Values for spatial frequency distributions of lung density have also been obtained through the use of CT in animals with experimentally induced pulmonary edema and in humans with a variety of acute lung injuries. The heart and pulmonary vessels can be excluded from the densitometric measurements by using a modified subtraction technique available with CT (Hedlund et al., 1982).

Topographic information obtained by CT reveals that cardiogenic edema and renal pulmonary edema tend to be associated with a perihilar and gravitational distribution, whereas permeability edema tends to be distributed in the peripheral and dependent portions of the lung (Hedlund et al., 1982b; Schuster et al., 1986) (Figs. 6–26 and 6–27). These observations have led to a better understanding of the distinguishing characteristics of cardiac and noncardiac pulmonary edema as visualized by conventional radiography. Only the Compton scattering technique can be used at the bedside, but thus far its clinical application remains limited.

Positron-Emission Tomography

Positron-emitting isotopes have proved to be suitable for radioactive labeling of indicators for extravascular and intravascular water measurements, partially owing to the fact that the water molecule itself

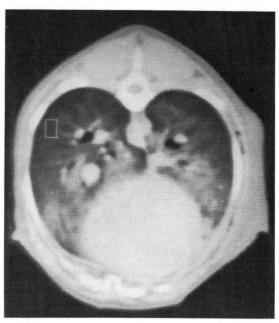

Figure 6–27. A CT scan in prone dog with elevation of left atrial pressure. Note the prominence of the central vessels compared with those of the oleic acid model (see Fig. 6–26). The increased lung density developed centrally and primarily in the dependent areas in contrast to the distribution of oleic acid edema.

can be labeled with the positron-emitting isotope oxygen-15 (^{15}O). Meyer and colleagues (1984) described a technique for measuring the volume of extravascular lung water in which the constant infusion of radioactive water is used to label the water pool, and in which carbon-11 (^{11}C)–labeled carbon monoxide is subsequently inhaled to label the blood pool. Schuster and colleagues described a technique for measuring the volume of extravascular lung water by the injection of a bolus of radioactive water followed by equilibration of the tracer. A good correlation was found between gravimetric measurements and values for extravascular lung water calculated by positron-emission tomography (Schuster et al., 1986).

In these studies and others, the tomographic technique tended to underestimate the volume of extravascular lung water. A major advantage of positron-emission tomography is the ability to quantitate accurately the regional distribution of fluid in pulmonary edema. Wollmer and associates (1987) reported the use of positron-emission tomography to study patients with acute cardiogenic pulmonary edema. In patients with radiologic evidence of interstitial pulmonary edema and moderately elevated pulmonary vascular pressure, extravascular lung density was uniformly increased throughout the lungs. In patients with radiographic evidence of air-space edema and significantly elevated pulmonary vascular pressure, extravascular lung density was significantly increased in dependent regions. Because it is expensive and available in only a few clinical centers, positron-

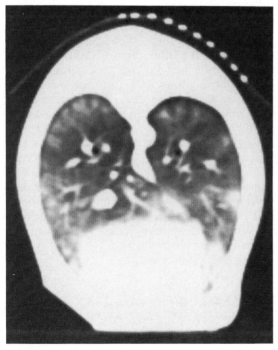

Figure 6–26. A CT scan in prone dog 75 minutes after oleic acid infusion. Note the patchy opacities, especially in the periphery. The vessels are of normal caliber.

emission tomography as used in the evaluation of pulmonary edema remains an investigative technique.

Magnetic Resonance Imaging

Studies based on various experimental animal models have demonstrated that magnetic resonance imaging (MRI) techniques can detect and quantify pulmonary edema. Shioya and co-workers (1985) correlated gravimetric data, data regarding bronchial alveolar lavage, and histologic data and found an increase in T_1 (nuclear spin relaxation time) associated with water accumulation during the acute stage of epithelial injury. Several investigators have shown the potential of MRI (proton density) for assessing water distribution in normal and edematous lungs (Carroll et al., 1985; Wexler et al., 1985). Recent studies indicate the possibility that T_1 and T_2 measurements may complement the proton density information, thus providing a more accurate assessment of lung water and pulmonary edema. Determination of T_1, T_2, or both, in addition to proton density, might be valuable in differentiating lung edema from other causes of increased proton density (Mathur-De Vré, 1984; Podgorski et al., 1986).

Magnetic resonance imaging techniques are particularly attractive because unlike other methods for measuring lung water, they are not invasive. At present, however, MRI techniques cannot discriminate between intravascular and extravascular lung water. The use of sodium imaging, in combination with proton imaging and the administration of an intravascular paramagnetic agent, has been suggested as a possible means of assessing the distribution of lung water between the two compartments (Montgomery et al., 1987). These and other potential solutions are still at a preliminary stage of experimentation and need further testing. Lack of mobility and the effects of the magnetic field on monitoring instruments and support equipment currently restrict the use of MRI in patients who are at high risk for edema.

Measurement of Lung Epithelial Permeability—Technetium-99m DTPA

The permeability of the pulmonary epithelium can be evaluated by measuring the rate of absorption of inhaled tracer particles from the alveolar to the vascular space (Newhouse et al., 1987). Most investigators use technetium-99m(^{99m}Tc)–labeled diethylene-triaminepenta-acetic acid (DTPA) as the tracer molecule. Because the clearance from the alveoli of small hydrophilic particles is limited primarily by diffusion rather than by perfusion, pulmonary blood flow is unlikely to have a significant effect on lung epithelial permeability measurements. The rate of absorption of ^{99m}Tc-labeled DTPA usually increases in the presence of lung injury or inflammation (Rees et al., 1985). The proven sensitivity of this technique may allow the early identification of lung epithelial damage and monitoring of the response to recovery. Further clinical investigation is warranted to determine the usefulness of this rather noninvasive technique for quantifying the extent of epithelial damage.

CONCLUSION

No optimal method of classifying and quantifying global and regional lung water has yet been found. The ideal method to be used within intensive care units should have the following characteristics: (1) accuracy and reproducibility, (2) sensitivity, (3) noninvasiveness, (4) simplicity of operation, and (5) low cost. Obviously, none of the methods previously mentioned meets all of these criteria, and this fact is in part responsible for the limited application of these techniques in clinical medicine. Improvements and modification of the principles employed with many of these advanced imaging techniques will undoubtedly be made in the future. At present, however, chest radiography remains the acceptable technique for the assessment of lung water, and its complementary role within the overall clinical assessment of these critically ill patients deserves emphasis.

References

Aberle, D.R., Wiener-Kronish, J.P., Webb, R.W., and Matthay, M.: Hydrostatic versus increased permeability pulmonary edema: Diagnosis based on radiographic criteria in critically ill patients. Radiology 168:73, 1988.

Allison, R.C., Carlile, P.V., Jr., and Gray, B.A.: Thermodilution measurement of lung water. Clin. Chest Med. 6:439, 1985.

Alwall, N.: Pathogenesis and therapy in edema. In Gigon, A. (ed.): Proceedings of the 6th International Congress of Internal Medicine. Basel, Benno Schwabe, 1960, p. 107.

Anderson, R.R., Sibbald, W.J., Holliday, R.L., et al.: Documentation of pulmonary capillary permeability in human adult respiratory distress syndrome (ARDS) secondary to sepsis. Am. Rev. Respir. Dis. 119:669, 1979.

Bachofen, M., and Weibel, E.R.: Structural alterations of lung parenchyma in the adult respiratory distress syndrome. Clin. Chest Med. 3:35, 1982.

Baundendistel, L., Shields, T.B., and Kaminski, D.L.: Comparison of double indicator thermodilution measurements of extravascular lung water (EVLW) with radiographic estimation of lung water in trauma patients. J. Trauma 22:983, 1982.

Calenoff, L., Kruglik, G., and Woodruff, A.: Unilateral pulmonary edema. Radiology 126:19, 1978.

Cander, L., and Forster, R.E.: Determination of pulmonary parenchymal tissue volume and pulmonary capillary blood flow in man. J. Appl. Physiol. 14:541, 1959.

Carlile, P.V., Lowery, P.D., and Gray, B.A.: Effect of PEEP and type of injury on thermal-dye estimation of pulmonary edema. J. Appl. Physiol. 60:22, 1986.

Carroll, F.E., Loyd, T.E., Nolop, K.B., et al.: NMR imaging parameter in the study of lung H$_2$O: A preliminary study. Invest. Radiol. 20:381, 1985.

Childress, M.E., Moy, G., and Mottram, M.: Unilateral pulmonary edema resulting from treatment of spontaneous pneumothorax. Am. Rev. Respir. Dis. 104:119, 1971.

Chinard, F.D.: Estimation of extravascular lung water by indicator dilution techniques. Circ. Res. 37:137, 1975.

Crandall, E.D., Staub, N.C., Goldberg, H.I., and Effros, R.M.: Recent developments in pulmonary edema. Ann. Intern. Med. 99:808, 1983.

Curtis, A.M.: Adult respiratory distress syndrome. *In* Putman, C.E., and Ravin, C.E. (eds.): Textbook of Diagnostic Imaging. Philadelphia, W.B. Saunders, 1988.

Curtis, A.M., Knowles, G.D., Putman, C.E., et al.: The three syndromes of fat embolism: Pulmonary manifestations. Yale J. Biol. Med. 52:149, 1979.

Cutillo, A.: The clinical assessment of lung water. Chest 92:795, 1987.

Eaton, R.J., Taxmian, R.M., and Avioli, L.V.: Cardiovascular evaluation of patients treated with PEEP. Arch. Intern. Med. 143:1958, 1983.

Effros, R.M.: Lung water measurements with the mean transit time approach. J. Appl. Physiol. 59:673, 1985.

Fein, A., Grossman, R.F., Jones, J.G., et al.: The value of edema fluid protein measurement in patients with pulmonary edema. Am. J. Med. 67:32, 1979.

Finley, T.N., Tooley, W.H., Swenson, E.W., et al.: Pulmonary surface tension in experimental atelectasis. Am. Rev. Respir. Dis. 89:372, 1964.

Fraser, R.G., and Paré, J.A.P.: Diagnosis of Diseases of the Chest. An Integrated Study Based on the Abnormal Roentgenogram. Philadelphia, W.B. Saunders, 1970, pp. 199, 855, 958.

Freidman, M., Kaufman, S.H., and Wilkins, S.A.: Analysis of rebreathing measurements of pulmonary tissue volume in pulmonary edema. J. Appl. Physiol. 48:66, 1980.

Gamsu, G., Kaufman, L., Swann, S.J., and Brito, A.C.: Absolute lung density in experimental canine pulmonary edema. Invest. Radiol. 14:261, 1979.

Gittinoni, L., Pesent, S., Baglioni, G., et al.: Inflammatory pulmonary edema and positive end-expiratory pressure: Correlations between imaging and physiologic studies. J. Thorac. Imaging 313:59, 1988.

Giuntini, C., Pistolesi, M., and Miniati, M.: Extravascular lung water. Eur. J. Nucl. Med. 13:63, 1987.

Glauser, F.L., Wilson, A.F., Hoshiko, M., et al.: Pulmonary parenchymal tissue (Yt) changes in pulmonary edema. J. Appl. Physiol. 36:648, 1974.

Gray, B.A., Beckett, R.C., Allison, R.C., et al.: Effect of edema and hemodynamic changes on extravascular thermal volume of the lung. J. Appl. Physiol. 56:878, 1984.

Greenbaum, D.M., and Marshall, K.E.: The value of routine daily chest x-rays in intubated patients in the medical intensive care unit. Crit. Care Med. 10:29, 1982.

Greene, R., Jantsch, H., Boggis, C., and Strauss, W.: Respiratory distress syndrome with new consideration. Radiol. Clin. North Am. 21:699, 1983.

Gurney, J.W., and Goodman, L.R.: Pulmonary edema localized in the right upper lobe accompanying mitral regurgitation. Radiology 171:397, 1989.

Halperin, B.D., Feeley, T.W., Milhan, F.O., et al.: Evaluation of the portable chest roentgenogram for quantitating extravascular lung water in critically ill adults. Chest 88:649, 1985.

Hamosh, P., and Cohen, J.N.: Left ventricular function in acute myocardial infarction. J. Clin. Invest. 50:523, 1971.

Harrison, M.O., Conte, P.J., and Heitzman, E.R.: Radiological detection of clinically occult cardiac failure following myocardial infarction. Br. J. Radiol. 44:265, 1971.

Hayes, C.E., Case, T.A., Acilion, D.C., et al.: Lung water quantitation by nuclear magnetic resonance imaging. Science 216:1313, 1982.

Hedlund, L.W., Volk, P., and Effmann, E.L.: Computed tomography of the lung: Densimetric studies. Radiol. Clin. North Am. 21:755, 1983.

Hedlund, L.W., Anderson, R.F., Goulding, P.L., et al.: Two methods for isolating the lung area of a CT scan image for density and volume information. Radiology 144:353, 1982a.

Hedlund, L.W., Effmann, E.L., Bates, W.M., et al.: Pulmonary edema: A CT study of regional changes in lung density following oleic acid injury. J. Comput. Assist. Tomogr. 6:939, 1982b.

Heitzman, E.R.: The Lung: Radiologic-Pathologic Correlations. St. Louis, C.V. Mosby 1973a, p. 11.

Heitzman, E.R.: Radiologic appearance of the azygos vein in cardiovascular disease. Circulation 47:628, 1973b.

Joffe, N.: The adult respiratory distress syndrome. AJR 122:719, 1974.

Kohen, J.A., Opsahl, J., and Kjellstrand, C.M.: Deceptive patterns of uremic pulmonary edema. Am. J. Kidney Dis. 7:456, 1986.

Laggner, A., Kleinberger, G., Haller, J., et al.: Bedside estimation of extravascular lung water in critically ill patients: Comparison of the chest radiograph and the thermal dye technique. Intensive Care Med. 10:309, 1984.

Leeming, B.W.A.: Gravitational edema of the lungs observed during assisted respiration. Chest 64:719, 1973.

Lefcoe, M.S., Sibbald, W.J., and Holiday, R.L.: Wedged balloon catheter angiography in the critical care unit. Crit. Care Med. 7:449, 1979.

Logue, B.R., Rogers, J.V., and Gay, B.B.: Subtle roentgenographic signs of left heart failure. Am. Heart J. 65:464, 1963.

Malo, J., Ali, J., and Wood, L.D.H.: How does positive end-expiratory pressure reduce shunt in canine pulmonary edema? J. Appl. Physiol. 57:1002, 1984.

Mathur-De Vré, R.: Biomedical implications of the relaxation behaviour of water related to NMR imaging. Br. J. Radiol. 57:955, 1984.

Matthay, M.A., Landolt, C.C., Bhattacharya, J., and Staub, N.L.: Alveolar fluid removal from the lungs of sheep. (Abstract.) Clin. Res. 28:9A, 1980.

McHugh, T.J., Forrester, J.L., Adler, L., et al.: Pulmonary vascular congestion in acute myocardial infarction: Hemodynamic and radiologic correlations. Ann. Intern. Med. 76:29, 1972.

Meyer, G.J., Schober, O., Bossaller, C., et al.: Quantification of regional extravascular lung water in dogs with positron emission tomography, using constant infusion of ^{15}O-labeled water. Eur. J. Nucl. Med. 9:220, 1984.

Milne, E.N.: Correlation of physiological findings with chest roentgenology. Radiol. Clin. North Am. 11:17, 1973.

Milne, E.N., and Pistolesi, M.: Pulmonary edema—cardiac and noncardiac. *In* Putman, C.E. (ed.): Diagnostic Imaging of the Lung. New York, Marcel Dekker, 1990.

Milne, E.N., Pistolesi, M., Miniati, M., and Giuntini, C.: The radiographic distinction of cardiogenic and noncardiogenic edema. AJR 144:879, 1985.

Milne, E.N., Pistolesi, M., Miniati, M., and Giuntini, C.: The vascular pedicle of the heart and the vena azygos. Part I: The normal subject. Radiology 152:1, 1984.

Miniati, M., Pistolesi, M., Paoletti, P., et al.: Objective radiographic criteria to differentiate cardiac, renal and injury lung edema. Invest. Radiol. 23:433, 1988.

Montgomery, A.B., Paajanen, H., Brasch, R.C., et al.: Aerosolized gadolinium DTPA enhances the magnetic resonance signal of extravascular lung water. Invest. Radiol. 22:377, 1987.

Mutchler, R.W., Jr., Rose, J.S., Garzon, A.A., et al.: Localized pulmonary edema following surgically created left-to-right shunts. AJR Radium Ther. Nucl. Med. 122:807, 1974.

Nakahara, K., Nanjo, S., Maeda, M., et al.: Dynamic insufficiency of lung lymph from the right lymph duct with acute infiltration edema. Am. Rev. Respir. Dis. 127:67, 1983.

Newhouse, M., Jordana, M., and Dolovich, M.: Evaluation of lung epithelial permeability. Eur. J. Nucl. Med. 13:S58, 1987.

Newman, G.E., Effman, E.L., and Putman, C.E.: Pulmonary aspiration complexes in adults. Curr. Probl. Diagn. Radiol. 11:1, 1982a.

Newman, G.E., Sullivan, D.E., Gottschalk, A., and Putman, C.E.: Scintigraphic perfusion patterns in patients with diffuse lung disease. Radiology 143:227, 1982b.

Pattle, R.E.: Properties, function and origin of the alveolar lining layer. Proc. R. Soc. Lond. [Biol.] 148:217, 1958.

Petrini, M.F., Peterson, B.T., and Hyde, R.W.: Lung tissue volume and blood flow by rebreathing theory. J. Appl. Physiol. 44:795, 1978.

Petty, T.L., Silver, G.W., Paul, G.W., et al.: Abnormalities in lung elastic properties and surfactant function in adult respiratory distress syndrome. Chest 75:571, 1979.

Pistolesi, M., and Giuntini, C.: Assessment of extravascular lung water. Radiol. Clin. North Am. 16:551, 1978.

Pistolesi, M., Miniati, M., Milne, E.N., and Giuntini, C.: The chest roentgenogram in pulmonary edema. Clin. Chest Med. 6:315, 1985.

Pistolesi, M., Miniati, M., Ravell, V., and Giuntini, C.: Injury versus hydrostatic lung edema: Detection by chest x-ray. Ann. NY Acad. Sci. 384:364, 1982.

Pistolesi, M., Milne, E.N., Miniati, M., et al.: The vascular pedicle of the heart and the vena azygos. Part II: Acquired heart disease. Radiology 152:9, 1984.

Podgorski, G.T., Carroll, F.E., and Parker, R.E.: NMR evaluation of pulmonary interstitial and intravascular fluids. Invest. Radiol. 21:478, 1986.

Putman, C.E.: Infectious pneumonias including aspiration states. In Putman, C.E., and Ravin, C.E. (eds.): Textbook of Diagnostic Imaging. Philadelphia, W.B. Saunders, 1988.

Putman, C.E., Minagi, H., and Blaisdell, F.W.: Roentgen appearance of disseminated intravascular coagulation (DIC). Radiology 109:13, 1972.

Rees, P.J., Shelton, D., Chan, T.B., et al.: Effects of histamine on lung permeability in normal and asthmatic subjects. Thorax 40:603, 1985.

Rhodes, C.G., Wollmer, P., Fazio, F., and Jones, T.: Quantitative measurement of regional extravascular lung density using positron emission and transmission tomography. J. Comput. Assist. Tomogr. 5:783, 1981.

Rice, D.L., and Miller, W.C.: Flow-dependence of extravascular thermal volume as an index of pulmonary edema. Intensive Care Med. 7:269, 1981.

Rotman, M., Chen, J.T., Seningen, R.P., et al.: Pulmonary arterial diastolic pressure in acute myocardial infarction. Am. J. Cardiol. 33:357, 1974.

Royal, H.D., Shields, J.B., and Donati, R.M.: Misplacement of central venous pressure catheters and unilateral pulmonary edema. Arch. Intern. Med. 135:1502, 1975.

Sackner, M.A., Greeneltch, D., Heiman, M.S., et al.: Diffusing capacity, membrane diffusing capacity, capillary blood volume, pulmonary tissue volume, and cardiac output measured by a rebreathing technique. Am. Rev. Respir. Dis. 111:157, 1975.

Saleh, M., Miles, A.I., and Lasser, R.P.: Unilateral pulmonary edema in Swyer-James syndrome. Chest 66:594, 1974.

Schuster, D.P., Markin, G.F., Minutin, M.A., et al.: PET measurement of regional lung density. J. Comput. Assist. Tomogr. 10:723, 1986.

Shioya, S., Haida, M., Ohta, Y., et al.: Detection of oxygen lung injury by NMR methods. Kokyu To Junkan 33:603, 1985.

Simon, D.S., Murray, J.F., and Staub, N.C.: Measurement of pulmonary edema in intact dogs by transthoracic x-ray attenuation. J. Appl. Physiol. 47:1228, 1979.

Sivak, E.D., Richmond, B.J., O'Donovan, P.B., and Borkowski, G.P.: Value of extravascular lung water measurements vs. portable chest x-ray in the management of pulmonary edema. Crit. Care Med. 11:498, 1983.

Sjoegren, A.: Left heart failure in acute myocardial infarction: A clinical hemodynamic and therapeutic study. Acta Med. Scand. 188(Suppl. 510):1, 1970.

Smith, R.C., Mann, H., Greenspan, R.H., et al.: Radiographic differentiation between different etiologies of pulmonary edema. Invest. Radiol. 22:859, 1987.

Staub, N.C.: The pathogenesis of pulmonary edema. Prog. Cardiovasc. Dis. 23:53, 1980.

Staub, N.C., Nagano, H., and Pearce, M.L.: Pulmonary edema in dogs, especially the sequence of fluid accumulation in lungs. J. Appl. Physiol 22:227, 1967.

Trapnell, D.H., and Thurston, J.G.B.: Unilateral pulmonary edema after pleural aspiration. Lancet 1:1367, 1970.

Van de Water, J., Sheh, J.M., O'Connor, N.E., et al.: Pulmonary extravascular water volume: Measurement and significance in critically ill patients. J. Trauma 10:440, 1970.

Vreim, C.E., and Staub, N.C.: Protein composition of lung fluids in acute alloxan edema in dogs. Am. J. Physiol. 230:376, 1976.

Wegenius, G., Erikson, V., Borg, T., et al.: Value of chest radiography in adult respiratory distress syndrome. Acta Radiol. (Diagn.) (Stockh.) 25:177, 1984.

Wegenius, G., and Modig, J.: Determinants of early adult respiratory distress syndrome with special reference to chest radiography: A retrospective analysis of 220 patients with major skeletal injuries. Acta Radiol. [Diagn.] (Stockh.) 26:649, 1985.

Wexler, H.R., Nicholson, R.L., Prato, F.S., et al.: Quantitation of lung water by nuclear magnetic resonance imaging: A preliminary study. Invest. Radiol. 20:583, 1985.

Wilen, S.B., Ulreich, S., Rabinowitz, J.G.: Roentgenographic manifestations of methadone-induced pulmonary edema. Radiology 114:51, 1975.

Wollmer, P., Rhodes, C.G., Deanfield, J., et al.: Regional extravascular density of the lung in patients with acute pulmonary edema. J. Appl. Physiol. 63:1890, 1987.

Zimmerman, J.E., Goodman, L.R., St. Andre, A.C., Wyman, A.C.: Radiographic detection of mobilizable lung water: The gravitational shift test. AJR 138:59, 1982.

Ziskind, M.N., Weill, H., and George, R.A.: Acute pulmonary edema following the treatment of spontaneous pneumothorax with excessive intrapleural pressure. Am. Rev. Respir. Dis. 92:632, 1965.

7

Adult Respiratory Distress Syndrome: Clinical Perspective

■

Frank Casty
Roger C. Bone

Adult respiratory distress syndrome (ARDS) is a dramatic, often catastrophic series of events that represents the final common pathway of acute lung injury secondary to a variety of initial insults (Andreadis and Petty, 1985; Sibbald and Bone, 1987). First described in 1967 by Ashbaugh and co-workers, ARDS remains an important clinical entity, with an estimated 150,000 cases per year, and a mortality greater than 60 percent (Andreadis and Petty, 1985). Clinical and pathologic aspects are remarkably similar, despite a variety of etiologic factors. Hypoxemia, diffuse bilateral infiltrates, and decreased lung compliance characterize the clinical manifestations, while atelectasis, hyaline membranes, and capillary engorgement represent common pathologic findings (Andreadis and Petty, 1985; Ashbaugh et al., 1967; Murray, 1977; Petty, 1982; Pontoppidan et al., 1972).

Although much has been learned about ARDS since 1967, most notably the appreciation of concurrent multi-organ dysfunction and the identification of mediators of lung injury, the precise mechanism of lung injury remains unknown (Bell et al., 1983; Decamp and Demling, 1988; Petty, 1990). Treatment remains primarily supportive, and prognosis has not changed essentially over the last 20 years (Ashbaugh et al., 1967).

HISTORICAL ASPECTS

The earliest descriptions of fulminant respiratory failure date back to the early 1900s, when, during World War I, physicians described progressive pulmonary failure that was subsequent to battlefield injuries (Simeone, 1968). Osler reported similar experiences when he wrote in his text *The Principles and Practice of Medicine* (1927) that "uncontrolled septicemia leads to frothy pulmonary edema." These early cases of respiratory collapse were usually terminal.

With the advent of blood banking and the salvage of patients with massive blood loss during World War II, renal failure was described as a major cause of late mortality (Bywaters, 1944). Soon after World War II, Jenkins and colleagues (1950) described what is known today as "shock lung."

During the Vietnam War, rapid helicopter evacuation and the availability of arterial blood gas analysis resulted in a description of shock lung. With the earlier initiation of supportive care, and of ventilation when necessary, the likelihood of survival improved.

In 1967, Ashbaugh and colleagues reported 12 patients with a syndrome similar to infantile respiratory distress syndrome, but with a variety of etiologic factors, including trauma, infection, drug ingestion, hemorrhagic pancreatitis, and shock. Because the clinical and pathologic findings were similar among the patients, the term "adult respiratory distress syndrome" was coined. Emphasis at that time was focused primarily on the pulmonary complications that occurred after a variety of both direct and indirect insults to the lungs' gas-exchanging membrane.

Subsequent retrospective and prospective studies have expanded our understanding of this disorder. Adult respiratory distress syndrome now appears to be a systemic disorder not fully defined by hypoxemic respiratory failure and noncardiogenic pulmonary edema (Bell et al., 1983). Indeed, the sepsis syndrome accounts for the greatest fraction of mortality from ARDS (Bell et al., 1983; Montgomery et al., 1985). Currently, the management of ARDS patients has been directed toward improving peripheral microcirculatory flow, improving oxygen availability at a cellular level, and preventing the occurrence of multiple organ system failure (Pine et al., 1983; Showmaker, 1985).

DEFINITION

Adult respiratory distress syndrome results from a variety of both direct and indirect insults to the lung, causing cell injury and interstitial and alveolar edema and inflammation (Table 7–1). Hypoxemia, diffuse pulmonary infiltrates, and reduced lung compliance have remained essential to the diagnosis of ARDS.

Many clinicians and investigators have used pulmonary capillary wedge pressure (PCWP) measurements greater than 12 to 19 mm Hg as a means of excluding the diagnosis of ARDS (Bone et al., 1987; Fowler et al., 1983; Pepe et al., 1982; Pontoppidan et al., 1972). In fact, previous reports may have underestimated the incidence of ARDS because of strict PCWP criteria for inclusion in their studies, thus failing to identify patients with ARDS *and* a simultaneous hydrostatic contribution to the clinical condition. Because elevated PCWP measurements do not exclude the diagnosis of ARDS, we do not consider them to be critical to the definition of ARDS. If wedge pressure is increased, however, some of the pulmonary edema observed could be cardiogenic.

Table 7–1. ETIOLOGY OF ARDS

Aspiration	**Inhalation**
Gastric contents	Ammonia
Near drowning	Cadmium
Drug	Chlorine
Chlordiazepoxide	Nitrogen dioxide
Colchicine	Ozone
Cyclosporine	Phosgene
Dextran 40	Smoke
Ethchlorvynol	**Trauma**
Fluorescein	Burns
Heroin	Fat embolism
Leukoagglutinin reaction	Fractures
Methadone	Head trauma
Paraquat	Pulmonary contusion
Propoxyphene	Nonthoracic trauma
Salicylates	Shock
Thiazides	**Miscellaneous**
Tricyclic antidepressants	Amniotic fluid embolism
	Bowel infarction
Hematologic	Carcinomatosis
Multiple transfusions	Cardiopulmonary bypass
Disseminated intravascular	Dead fetus
coagulation	Diabetic ketoacidosis
Thrombotic	Eclampsia
thrombocytopenic	High altitude
purpura	Pancreatitis
Leukemia	Pulmonary edema
	Radiation
Infectious	Uremia
Sepsis syndrome	
Pneumonia	
Bacteria	
Fungus	
Mycoplasma virus	
Pneumocystis carinii	
Tuberculosis	

Appreciation of the protean manifestations of ARDS has prompted many investigators to call for a new, expanded definition of the syndrome (Rocker et al., 1989; Sibbald and Bone, 1987). Murray and associates (1988) proposed a broader, more refined definition that takes into account an acute lung injury score, identification of the etiologic factor, and the multi-organ failure that is known to occur with ARDS. The lung injury score is based on four factors: ratio of arterial oxygen pressure (Pa_{O_2}) to fractional inspired oxygen (FIO_2), chest radiograph (scoring based on type and location of infiltrates), compliance, and level of positive end-expiratory pressure (PEEP). The factors are scored, and the total serves as a measure of the level of lung injury.

The second criterion of the Murray scoring scheme regards the underlying disorder. The thought that the pathogenesis of ARDS is important to its understanding is not new. Previous workers have agreed that identification of the etiologic mechanism is important both for understanding of pathogenesis and for the impact on clinical trials (Fowler et al., 1983; Pepe et al., 1982). This part of the Murray definition correctly identifies ARDS resulting from the fat embolism syndrome as having a good prognosis, and those cases due to sepsis often having a poor prognosis (Kaplan et al., 1979; Pepe et al., 1982; Schonfeld et al., 1983).

Murray's third criterion considers nonpulmonary organ dysfunction, including renal, hepatic, cardiovascular, acid-base, and central nervous system (CNS) abnormalities. This new criterion should make diagnosis, as well as future studies, more discriminating with regard to severity, etiology, and end-organ failure. For these reasons, it has been eagerly accepted both as a refinement of definition and for its usefulness in future studies (Petty, 1988).

EPIDEMIOLOGY AND RISK FACTORS

Two large prospective studies have identified several important risk factors that increase the risk of developing ARDS (Fowler et al., 1983; Pepe et al., 1982). Fowler and colleagues followed a total of 993 patients who had one or more of eight conditions believed to be risk factors for ARDS. Adult respiratory distress syndrome occurred subsequently in 68 (6.8%) of these patients. With the exception of aspiration, the incidence rates were higher in patients with multiple risk factors (24.6%) than in those with a single risk factor (5.8%) (Fowler et al., 1983).

Pepe and co-workers (1982) identified the sepsis syndrome as a major predisposing condition, resulting in ARDS in 38% of cases. They were also able to report in detail the dramatic increase in occurrence when additional risk factors were present in a given patient (Table 7–2). Other major risk factors identified were aspiration of gastric contents (30%), multiple emergency transfusions (24%), and pulmonary contusion (17%) (Pepe et al., 1982).

Both studies confirmed original data stating that

Table 7–2. INCIDENCE OF ARDS OCCURRING WITH SINGLE AND MULTIPLE RISK FACTORS

Condition	Fowler et al (1983)	Pepe et al. (1982)	With One Other Condition	With Two Other Conditions	Total
Sepsis					
Sepsis syndrome	—	5/13 (38)	2/4	2/2	9/19 (47)
Bacteremia	9/239 (4)	—	—	—	—
Aspiration of gastric contents	16/45 (36)	7/23 (30)	3/9 (33)		10/32 (31)
Multiple transfusions	9/197 (5)	4/17 (24)	3/11 (27)	12/24 (50)	19/42 (45)
Pulmonary contusion	—	5/29 (17)	7/12 (58)	7/9 (78)	19/50 (38)
Fractures	2/3 (67)	1/12 (8)	4/10 (40)	10/12 (83)	15/34 (44)
Near drowning	—	2/3	1/1		3/4
Pancreatitis	—	1/1			1/1
Prolonged hypotension	—	0/1	0/1	2/2	2/4
Disseminated intravascular coagulation	2/9 (22)	—	—	—	—
Pneumonia in intensive care unit	1/84 (1)	—	—	—	—
Burn	2/87 (2)	—	—	—	—
Cardiopulmonary bypass	4/237 (2)	—	—	—	—

All data are expressed as n (%).

90% of patients identified to be at risk for ARDS require endotracheal intubation within 72 hours of the onset of the risk factor (Ashbaugh et al., 1967).

PATHOPHYSIOLOGY OF LUNG INJURY

Although the precise mechanism of acute lung injury in ARDS remains unknown, much has been learned in the past 20 years about the potential mediators of injury. Pathologically, three phases of injury are said to occur (Bachofen and Weibel, 1977). The acute phase is typically described as being characterized by accumulation of a protein-rich pulmonary fluid with large numbers of neutrophils in the interstitium of the lungs. Microscopic examination of patients dying during this phase has consistently shown endothelial cell injury as well (Bachofen and Weibel, 1982). Presumably, this injury results in capillary leakage and increased permeability leading to interstitial pulmonary edema. The occurrence of significant epithelial cell injury is well known, however (Bachofen and Weibel, 1977; Lamy et al., 1976). Cellular debris and protein-rich edematous fluid that forms hyaline membranes are characteristically found in the air spaces in this phase of injury. Size selectivity for proteins traversing alveolar membrane is lost with injury. This loss results in inundation of alveolar spaces with this protein-rich edematous fluid and causes impairment of the gas exchange (Holter et al., 1986). Indeed, one study has suggested that sequential pulmonary edema protein concentrations may reflect epithelial function and may be a useful prognostic indicator (Wiener-Kronish and Matthay, 1989).

In the subacute phase, occurring at 5 to 10 days, proliferation of Type II epithelial cells occurs, presumably in response to destruction of Type I epithelial cells. Growth factors, possibly released by alveolar macrophages, stimulate epithelial cell proliferation, as well as proliferation of fibroblasts, which results in formation of collagen (Clark and Greenberg, 1987).

The chronic phase occurs after 2 to 3 weeks of illness and is characterized by intense fibrosis, with lung destruction and emphysema (Bachofen et al., 1977, 1982).

Considerable evidence implicates the neutrophil as key in initiating acute lung damage and increased capillary permeability (Tate and Repine, 1983). This finding is not surprising, because large numbers of neutrophils are found in the air spaces and interstitium in acutely injured lungs (Bachofen et al., 1977; Weiland et al., 1986). Clinical studies examining the bronchoalveolar lavage fluid of ARDS patients, and of those at risk for ARDS have shown significantly greater numbers of neutrophils compared with controls (Weiland et al., 1986). The extent of gas-exchange abnormalities and lung-protein permeability has been directly correlated to the number of neutrophils recovered (Weiland et al., 1986). In addition, neutrophil products capable of causing lung injury (e.g., collagenase, myeloperoxidase) were recovered (Weiland et al., 1986; Zheatlin et al., 1986).

Neutrophil activation and adhesion to endothelial cells by particular agents (e.g., complement, endotoxin, chemotactic agents) have been proposed as constituting an important aspect of lung injury (Harlan, 1985; Klausner et al., 1988). These agents may act independently to activate neutrophils or as priming factors in the presence of one another, as may be the case with endotoxin and complement (Parsons et al., 1989). These activated neutrophils may be the source of vasoactive mediators, toxic oxygen radicals, or proteases capable of causing injury.

The role of the neutrophil, however, is by no means clear. How, for instance, can one explain the occurrence of ARDS in neutropenic patients? Furthermore, intrapulmonary sequestration of neutrophils has not been shown to result in lung injury in animal models (Maunder et al., 1986; Shaw and Henson, 1982). Clearly, the role of the neutrophil is not yet well defined and may not even be necessary to the development of lung injury.

Numerous agents that may contribute significantly

to acute lung injury have been identified. These agents include those capable of causing vasoconstriction, vascular damage, or bronchoconstriction, such as complement, fatty acids, fibrin split products, histamine, kinins, lysosomes, platelet-activating factor (PAF), platelets, prostaglandins, proteolytic enzymes, serotonin, and leukotrienes.

Quantitative and qualitative surfactant abnormalities have been recognized in ARDS patients since early descriptions (Petty et al., 1977, 1979). These abnormalities likely result from damage to Type II epithelial cells, the source of surfactant, as well as to the damaging effects of oxidative enzymes on surfactant already present in the air spaces (Baldwin et al., 1986; Cochrane et al., 1983). Recognition of these surfactant alterations has led to investigations of surfactant replacement therapy as a potential early intervention in acute lung injury (Richman et al., 1987).

Only when we understand more fully the mechanism of this inflammation and the various mediators involved can we be able to block the reaction and, possibly, improve survival.

CLINICAL COURSE AND PROGNOSIS

Four stages characterize the course of progressive respiratory insufficiency: (1) injury, (2) apparent stability, (3) respiratory insufficiency, and (4) the terminal stage. The injury phase occurs up to 6 hours after an inciting event, during which time the clinical and radiographic findings are absent. The phase of apparent stability is typified by hyperventilation and abnormalities appearing on physical examination and the chest radiograph. By the time the respiratory insufficiency phase occurs, the chest radiograph usually shows diffuse bilateral alveolar and interstitial infiltrates, the patient is tachypneic, and rales are present on examination. Finally, the terminal phase is identified by persistent hypoxemia (despite high FIO_2) and carbon dioxide retention.

The primary reason for hypoxemia is intrapulmonary shunting that occurs when air spaces are perfused but not ventilated. Increased physiologic dead space as a consequence of ventilation without perfusion of alveoli also results. The functional residual capacity (FRC) is decreased in ARDS, owing to microatelectasis and edema. This decrease in FRC has important therapeutic implications. Lung compliance, the change in volume per unit of applied pressure, is also decreased.

Ploysongsang and colleagues (1986) found that at least 50% of patients with ARDS had airway abnormalities. The ARDS patient has increased air-flow resistance as well as increased responsiveness to inhaled β-agonists (Simpson et al., 1978; Wright and Bernard, 1989). Animal studies have shown that *Escherichia coli* endotoxemia causes significant bronchoconstriction, which is mediated by thromboxane

and blocked by indomethacin or meclofenamate sodium (Snapper et al., 1983).

Pleural involvement has recently been established in ARDS patients (Wiener-Kronish et al., 1988a, 1988b). Previously, the absence of pleural effusions was necessary for the diagnosis of ARDS, but ultrasound studies have shown that moderate-sized effusions commonly occur, and that supine, portable chest radiographs frequently fail to identify them. These effusions may act as drains via lymphatics for as much as 25% of the water of pulmonary edema (Wiener-Kronish et al., 1988a).

Mortality rates have remained essentially unchanged since the earliest descriptions of ARDS (Ashbaugh et al., 1967). Fowler and Pepe, along with their associates, reported mortality rates of 64.8% and 61%, respectively (Fowler et al., 1983; Pepe et al., 1982). Median survival was 13.3 days, with only 35.2% of patients surviving 6 months after extubation (Fowler et al., 1983). Within 14 days of the onset of ARDS, 90% of deaths occurred, as shown in Figure 7–1 (Fowler et al., 1983).

Patients with ARDS are not likely to die from direct pulmonary causes attributable to injuries to the lung's gas-exchange mechanism. Montgomery and associates (1985) showed that early deaths (within the first 3 days) were usually due to the underlying illness that initiated ARDS. Late deaths were overwhelmingly the result of the sepsis syndrome. Sepsis syndrome occurred in ARDS patients six times more frequently than in a control group of critically ill patients without ARDS (Montgomery et al., 1985; Sibbald and Bone, 1987). Seidenfeld and colleagues (1986) recognized the increased risk of sepsis in ARDS patients and showed that the use of empiric, prophylactic antibiotics in the absence of clinical infection did not decrease mortality.

Fowler and associates (1985) also emphasized nonpulmonary causes of death in ARDS patients and identified "systemic aberrations" as predictors of sur-

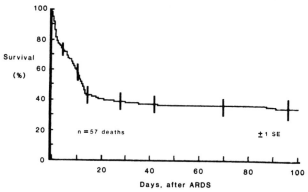

Figure 7–1. Survival of patients with the adult respiratory distress syndrome (ARDS). Median survival time of the 88 patients was 13.3 days after onset of the syndrome. (Reproduced, with permission, from Fowler, A.A., et al.: Adult respiratory distress syndrome: Risk with common predispositions. Ann. Intern. Med. 98:593, 1989.)

vivorship and mortality. Their study identified the presence of low pH, low bicarbonate, and less than 10% bands to be significantly associated with increased mortality.

The sepsis syndrome may be both an etiologic factor and a sequela of ARDS (Bell et al., 1983; Montgomery et al., 1985; Seidenfeld et al., 1986). Mortality from ARDS and sepsis is often related to the multi-organ system failure that ensues (Bell et al., 1983; DeCamp and Demling, 1988; Kaplan et al., 1979). Recently, the relationship of multi-organ system failure and ARDS has been studied in an attempt to find common etiologic factors and possible predictors of survival. In particular, hepatic dysfunction has been implicated as having a key role in the development of multi-organ system failure and may represent a major determinant of survival (Matuschak and Rinaldo, 1989; Schwartz et al., 1989). One study showed that elevations of serum bilirubin and alkaline phosphatase levels that occurred initially and during the first week of respiratory failure correlated with a significant increase in mortality (Schwartz et al., 1989). The healthy liver may protect the lung by eliminating mediators of lung injury via the reticulo-endothelial system. When this clearance mechanism is impaired—that is, when hepatic microvascular permeability is increased (perhaps by means similar to that found in the injured pulmonary microvasculature)—such a protective effect is compromised (Matuschak and Rinaldo, 1989).

Clinical and physiologic impairment of survivors of ARDS is variable. Earlier studies reported mild to moderate symptoms in 10% of survivors (Douglas and Downs, 1977; Downs and Olsen, 1974). More recently, smaller studies have shown that as many as 30% of survivors have mild to moderate symptoms, but symptoms do not necessarily reflect the degree of physiologic abnormalities in survivors (Ghio et al., 1989; Peters et al., 1989). Restrictive lung abnormalities are most common, with decreased forced vital capacity (FVC) and diffusion capacity (DL_{CO}) being the most typical (Lakshminarayan and Hudson, 1978). Nonspecific hyperactivity of airways, even in patients without a history of asthma or smoking, is also found (Simpson et al., 1978). Overall, the majority of ARDS survivors return to nearly normal lung function within 1 year of onset and typically lead normal lives (Bywaters, 1944; Ghio et al., 1989; Jenkins et al., 1950; Peters et al., 1989).

TREATMENT OF ACUTE RESPIRATORY FAILURE

Regardless of the etiologic mechanism, the primary therapeutic goal of treatment of acute respiratory failure is supportive care until the lung's gas-exchange mechanism is restored. Efforts are directed primarily to improving gas exchange and cardiac output, thereby enhancing oxygen delivery to tissues.

The use of mechanical ventilation is often necessary for support of hypoxemic patients. Because alveolar collapse and atelectasis contribute to hypoxemia, PEEP is used to distend and recruit alveoli. This action increases FRC and prevents further atelectasis, allowing adequate oxygenation at a lower FIO_2. The use of PEEP, however, is not without complications. Reduced venous return and decreased cardiac output may result in hypotension and inadequate oxygen delivery. Barotrauma is another serious consequence of PEEP (see Chapters 3 and 8). Positive end-expiratory pressure should be used to attain a therapeutic goal of a partial pressure of oxygen (P_{O_2}) greater than 60 mm Hg, particularly when an FIO_2 greater than 50% is necessary. Although earlier studies suggested improved survival when PEEP was used prophylactically, more recent prospective trials have shown no improvement (Pepe et al., 1984; Schmidt et al., 1976; Weigelt et al., 1979).

Additional treatment includes maintenance of blood volume, correction of factors that decrease oxygen transport, antibiotics when clinically warranted, and adequate nutritional support.

Initially, the use of corticosteroids was appealing, because of their known anti-inflammatory effects. Schumer reported favorable results in patients with septic shock treated with steroids (Schumer, 1976). Other studies suggested that microvascular injury was reduced in ARDS patients treated with steroids and that multi-organ failure was less likely (Sibbald et al., 1981; Sprung et al., 1984). However, recent multicenter trials have shown no benefit to ARDS patients treated with steroids (Bernard et al., 1987; Bone et al., 1987a, 1987b; Luce et al., 1988). Indeed, one large study showed that mortality was increased in patients with septic shock that were treated with steroids (Bone et al., 1987b). The use of corticosteroids, therefore, cannot be recommended in the treatment of either septic shock or ARDS.

FUTURE TREATMENT

Future treatment of patients with ARDS will require manipulation of one of the many known mediators of acute lung injury. Such manipulation has recently been attempted through studies of prostaglandins of the E series (PGE 1). In these studies, PGE 1 was reported to inhibit neutrophil adherence to endothelium and to diminish macrophage toxic oxygen radical production (Gee et al., 1986b; Gordon et al., 1976). It was also reported to reduce pulmonary artery pressures and increase arterial oxygen content and cardiac output in patients with ARDS (Holcroft et al., 1986; Melot et al., 1989; Shoemaker and Appel, 1986). In two clinical studies of small numbers of patients improved survival rates were reported in patients with ARDS (Holcroft et al., 1986; Shoemaker and Appel, 1986). A large multicenter trial, however, has shown no evidence that PGE 1 was effective in improving survival in patients with ARDS (Bone et al., 1989).

Animal models of the sepsis syndrome, in which endotoxin was used as a mediator of injury, have shown encouraging results with oxygen radical scavengers such as n-acetylcysteine and ibuprofen (Bernard et al., 1984; Gee et al., 1985). Ibuprofen has been found to be effective in modifying endothelial injury; it may prevent free radical release and may act as a free radical scavenger (Gee et al., 1985, 1986a, 1986b). Ibuprofen also interferes with some of the physiologic consequences of endotoxin infusion by preventing increases in airway resistance and decreases in pulmonary compliance (Jacobs et al., 1981).

Therapy directed toward inhibiting the inflammatory effects of cytokines on neutrophils is being investigated with pentoxifylline (Mandell, 1988). This agent decreases neutrophil adherence to endothelial cells and decreases superoxide release when neutrophils have been incubated with cytokines, possibly by a mechanism that activates adenosine receptors and increases cyclic adenosine monophophate (cAMP) concentrations (Rose et al., 1988; Sullivan et al., 1988).

A renewed interest in extracorporeal membrane oxygenation (ECMO) and carbon dioxide removal is being explored after uncontrolled studies in Europe have shown encouraging results of the use of different dialysis techniques and low-frequency ventilation (Gattinoni et al., 1986, 1988). The original ECMO studies compared that technique with conventional mechanical ventilation and PEEP, and no difference in survival was found between the two groups (Zapol et al., 1979). A randomized, controlled, prospective study of the newer technique is currently being performed (Petty, 1990).

Surfactant replacement has offered the hope of a therapy in which the ultimate outcome of acute lung injury is altered by opening of the atelectatic areas of lung. This technique has been effective in infants with the infantile form of respiratory distress syndrome and has been shown to improve compliance and gas exchange in the adult form (Davis et al., 1988; Horbar et al., 1989; Lachman, 1988; Merritt et al., 1986; Richman et al., 1987). Ongoing trials are under way.

Although no agent has yet been shown to change the outcome of ARDS, the future holds promise, as more continues to be learned about this devastating entity. The importance of multicenter trials for study of the pathophysiology of ARDS and its sequelae, particularly the multi-organ system failure that often ensues and contributes to the continued high mortality rates, cannot be overemphasized.

References

Andreadis, N., and Petty, T. L.: Adult respiratory distress syndrome: Problems and progress. Am. Rev. Respir. Dis 132:1344, 1985.

Ashbaugh, D. G., Bigelow, D. B., Petty, T. L., et al.: Acute respiratory distress in adults. Lancet 2:319, 1967.

Bachofen, M., and Weibel, E. R.: Alterations of the gas exchange apparatus in adult respiratory insufficiency associated with septicemia. Am. Rev. Respir. Dis. 116:589, 1977.

Bachofen, M., and Weibel, E. R.: Structural alterations of lung parenchyma in the adult respiratory distress syndrome. Clin. Chest Med. 3:35, 1982.

Baldwin, S. R., Simon, R. H., Grum, C. M., et al.: Oxidant activity in expired breath of patients with adult respiratory distress syndrome. Lancet 1:11, 1986.

Bell, R. C., Coalson, J. J., Smith, J. D., et al.: Multiple organ system failure and infection in adult respiratory distress syndrome. Ann. Intern. Med. 99:293, 1983.

Bernard, G. R., Luce, J. M., Sprung, C. L., et al.: High-dose corticosteroids in patients with the adult respiratory distress syndrome. N. Engl. J. Med. 317:1565, 1987.

Bernard, G. R., Lucht, W. D., Niedermeyer, M. E., et al.: Effect of N-acetylcysteine on the pulmonary response to endotoxin in awake sheep and upon in vitro granulocyte function. J. Clin. Invest. 73:1772, 1984.

Bone, R. C., Fisher, C. J., Clemmer, T. P., et al.: Early methylprednisolone treatment for septic syndrome and the adult respiratory distress syndrome. Chest 92:1032, 1987b.

Bone, R. C., Fisher, P., Clemmer, T. P., et al.: Controlled clinical trial of high-dose methylprednisolone in the treatment of severe sepsis and septic shock. N. Engl. J. Med. 317:653, 1987a.

Bone, R. C., Slotman, G., Maunder, R., et al.: Randomized double-blind multicenter study of prostaglandin E₁ in patients with the adult respiratory distress syndrome. Chest 96:114, 1989.

Bywaters, E. G.: Ischemic muscle necrosis: A type of injury seen in air raid casualties following burial beneath debris. JAMA 124:1103, 1944.

Clark, J. G., and Greenberg, J.: Modulation of the effects of alveolar macrophages on lung fibroblast collagen production rate. Am. Rev. Respir. Dis. 135:52, 1987.

Cochrane, C. G., Spragg, R., and Revak, S. D.: Pathogenesis of the adult respiratory distress syndrome: Evidence of oxidant activity in bronchoalveolar lavage fluid. J. Clin Invest. 71:754, 1983.

Davis, J. M., Veness-Meehan, K., Notter, R. H., et al.: Changes in pulmonary mechanics after the administration of surfactant to infants with respiratory distress syndrome. N. Engl. J. Med. 319:476, 1988.

DeCamp, M. M., and Demling, R. H.: Post-traumatic multisystem organ failure. JAMA 260:530, 1988.

Douglas, M. E., and Downs, J. B.: Pulmonary function following severe acute respiratory failure and high levels of positive end-expiratory pressure. Chest 71:18, 1977.

Downs, J. B., and Olsen, G. N.: Pulmonary function following adult respiratory distress syndrome. Chest 65:92, 1974.

Fowler, A. A., Hamman, R. F., Good, J. T., et al.: Adult respiratory distress syndrome: Risk with common predispositions. Ann. Intern. Med. 98:593, 1983.

Fowler, A. A., Hamman, R. F., Zerbe, G. O., et al.: Adult respiratory distress syndrome: Prognosis after onset. Am. Rev. Respir. Dis. 132:472, 1985.

Gattinoni, L., Pesenti, A., and Marcolin, R.: Extracorporeal support in acute respiratory failure. Intensive Care World 5:42, 1988.

Gattinoni, L., Pesenti, A., Mascheroni, D., et al.: Low-frequency positive pressure ventilation with extracorporeal CO₂ removal in severe acute respiratory failure. JAMA 256:881, 1986.

Gee, M. H., Margiotta, M., Tahamont, M. V., et al.: Role of free radical generation in complement-induced pulmonary dysfunction in sheep. In Matalin, S., and Taylor, A. (eds.): Physiology of Oxygen Radicals. Bethesda, MD, American Physiological Society (Clinical Physiology Series), 1986a, p. 187.

Gee, M. H., Tahamont, M. V., Margiotta, M., et al.: Effect of prostaglandin E in neutrophil-dependent acute lung injury in sheep. Semin. Resp. Med. 8:16, 1986b.

Gee, M. H., Tahamont, M. V., Perkowski, S. Z., et al.: Eicosanoids, leukocytes, and lung injury. In Lefer, A. M., Gee, M. H. (eds.): Leukotrienes in Cardiovacular and Pulmonary Functions. New York, Alan R. Liss, 1985, p. 237.

Ghio, A. J., Elliott, C. G., Crapo, R. O., et al.: Impairment after adult respiratory distress syndrome: An evaluation based on American Thoracic Society recommendations. Am. Rev. Respir. Dis. 139:1158, 1989.

Gordon, D., Bray, M., and Morley, J.: Control of lymphokine secretion by prostaglandins. Nature 262:401, 1976.

Harlan, J. M.: Leukocyte-endothelial interactions. Blood 65:513, 1985.

Holcroft, J. W., Vassar, M. J., and Wever, C. J.: Prostaglandin E1 and survival in patients with the adult respiratory distress syndrome. Ann. Surg. 203:371, 1986.

Holter, J. F., Weiland, J. E., Pach, E. R., et al.: Protein permeability in the adult respiratory distress syndromes. J Clin. Invest. 78:1513, 1986.

Horbar, J. D., Soll, R. F., Sutherland, J. M., et al.: A multicenter, randomized, placebo-controlled trial of surfactant therapy for respiratory distress syndrome. N. Engl. J. Med. 320:959, 1989.

Jacobs, E. R., Soulsby, M.E., Bone, R. C., et al.: Ibuprofen in canine endotoxin shock. J. Clin. Invest. 70:536, 1981.

Jenkins, M. T., Jones, R. F., Wilson, B., et al.: Congestive atelectasis: A complication of the intravenous infusion of fluids. Ann. Surg. 132:327, 1950.

Kaplan, R. L., Sahn, S. A., and Petty, T. L.: Incidence and outcome of the adult respiratory distress syndrome in gram-negative sepsis. Arch. Intern. Med. 139:867, 1979.

Klausner, J. M., Kobzik, L., and Valeri, C. R.: Selective lung leukosequestration after complement activation. J. Appl. Physiol. 65:80, 1988.

Lachman, B.: Surfactant treatment for lung diseases other than the infant respiratory distress syndrome. In Jobe, A. H., and Taeusch, H. W. (eds.): Surfactant Treatment of Lung Diseases. Columbus, OH, Ross Laboratories, 1988, p. 123.

Lakshminarayan, S., and Hudson, L. D.: Pulmonary function following the adult respiratory distress syndrome. Chest 74:489, 1978.

Lamy, M., Fallat, R., Koeniger, E., et al.: Pathologic features and mechanisms of hypoxemia in adult respiratory distress syndromes. Am. Rev. Respir. Dis. 114:267, 1976.

Luce, J. M., Montgomery, A. B., Marks, J. D., et al.: Ineffectiveness of high-dose methylprednisolone in preventing parenchymal lung injury and improving mortality in patients with septic shock. Am. Rev. Respir. Dis. 138:62, 1988.

Mandell, G. L.: ARDS, neutrophils, and pentoxifylline. Am. Rev. Respir. Dis. 138:1103, 1988.

Matuschak, G. M., and Rinaldo, J. E.: Organ interactions in the adult respiratory distress syndrome during sepsis: Role of the liver in host defense. Chest 94:400, 1989.

Maunder, R. J., Hackman, R. C., Riffi, E., et al.: Occurrence of the adult respiratory distress syndrome in neutropenic patients. Am. Rev. Respir. Dis. 133:313, 1986.

Melot, C., Lujeunc, P., Leeman, M., et al.: Prostaglandin E1 in the adult respiratory distress syndrome. Am. Rev. Respir. Dis. 139:106, 1989.

Merritt, T. A., Hallman, M., Bloom, B. T., et al.: Prophylactic treatment of very premature infants with human surfactant. N. Engl. J. Med. 315:785, 1986.

Montgomery, A. B., Stager, M. A., Carrico, C. J., et al.: Causes of mortality in patients with the adult respiratory distress syndrome. Am. Rev. Respir. Dis. 132:485, 1985.

Murray, J. F.: Mechanisms of acute respiratory failure. Am. Rev. Respir. Dis. 115:1071, 1977.

Murray, J. F., Matthay, M. A., Luce, J., et al.: An expanded definition of the adult respiratory distress syndrome. Am. Rev. Respir. Dis. 138:720, 1988.

Osler, W.: The Principles and Practice of Medicine, ed. 10. New York, D. Appleton, 1927.

Parsons, P. E., Worthen, G. S., Moore, E. E., et al.: The association of circulating endotoxin with the development of the adult respiratory distress syndrome. Am. Rev. Respir. Dis. 140:294, 1989.

Pepe, P. E., Hudson, L. D., and Carrico, C. J.: Early application of positive end-expiratory pressure in patients at risk for the adult respiratory-distress syndrome. N. Engl. J. Med. 311:281, 1984.

Pepe, P. E., Potkin, P. T., Reus, P. H., et al.: Clinical predictors of the adult respiratory distress syndrome. Am. J. Surg. 144:124, 1982.

Peters, J. I., Bell, R. C., Prihoda, T. J., et al.: Clinical determinants of abnormalities in pulmonary functions in survivors of the adult respiratory distress syndrome. Am. Rev. Respir. Dis. 139:1163, 1989.

Petty, T. L.: Adult respiratory distress syndrome: Definition and historical perspective. Clin. Chest Med. 3:3, 1982.

Petty, T. L.: ARDS: Refinement of concept and redefinition. Am. Rev. Respir. Dis. 138:724, 1988.

Petty, T. L.: Adult respiratory distress syndrome. Dis. Mon. 36:1, 1990.

Petty, T. L., Reiss, O. K., Paul, G. W., et al.: Characteristics of pulmonary surfactant in adult respiratory distress syndrome associated with trauma and shock. Am. Rev. Respir. Dis 115:531, 1977.

Petty, T. L., Silvers, G. W., Paul, G. W., et al.: Abnormalities in lung elastic properties and surfactant function in adult respiratory distress syndrome. Chest 75:571, 1979.

Pine, R. W., Wertz, M. J., Lennard, E. S., et al.: Determinants of organ malfunction or death in patients with intra-abdominal sepsis. Arch. Surg. 118:242, 1983.

Ploysongsang, Y., Rashkin, M., Rossi, A., et al.: Lung mechanics in adult respiratory distress syndrome (Abstract). Am. Rev. Respir. Dis. 133:266, 1986.

Pontoppidan, H., Geffin, B., and Lowenstein, E.: Acute respiratory failure in the adult (first of three parts). N. Engl. J. Med. 287:690, 1972.

Richman, P. S., Spragg, R. G., Merritt, T. A., et al.: Administration of bovine lung surfactant to humans with adult respiratory distress syndrome and initial experience (Abstract). Am. Rev. Respir. Dis. 135:A5, 1987.

Rocker, G. M., Pearson, D., Wiseman, M. S., et al.: Diagnostic criteria for adult respiratory distress syndrome: Time for reappraisal. Lancet 1:120, 1989.

Rose, R. F., Hirschhorn, R., Weissmann, G., and Cronstein, B. N.: Adenosine promotes neutrophil chemotaxis. J. Exp. Med. 167:1186, 1988.

Schmidt, G. B., O'Neill, W. W., Kobt, K., et al.: Continuous positive airway pressure in the prophylaxis of the adult respiratory distress syndrome. Surg. Gynecol. Obstet. 143:613, 1976.

Schonfeld, S. A., Ploysongsang, Y., DiLisio, R., et al.: Fat embolism prophylaxis with corticosteroids. Ann. Intern. Med. 99:438, 1983.

Schumer, W.: Steroids in the treatment of clinical septic shock. Ann. Surg. 184:333, 1976.

Schwartz, D. B., Bone, R. C., Balk, R. A., and Szidon, J. P.: Hepatic dysfunction in the adult respiratory distress syndrome. Chest 95:871, 1989.

Seidenfeld, J. J., Pohl, D. F., Bell, R. C., et al.: Incidence, site, and outcome of infections in patients with the adult respiratory distress syndrome. Am. Rev. Respir. Dis. 134:12, 1986.

Shaw, J., and Henson, P.: Pulmonary sequestration of activated neutrophils: Failure to induce light-microscopic evidence of lung injury in rabbits. Am. J. Pathol. 108:17, 1982.

Shoemaker, W. C., and Appel, P. L.: Effects of prostaglandin E1 in adult respiratory distress syndrome. Surgery 99:275, 1986.

Showmaker, W. C.: Controversies in the pathophysiology and fluid management of postoperative adult respiratory distress syndrome. Surg. Clin. North Am. 65:931, 1985.

Sibbald, W. J., and Bone, R. C.: The adult respiratory distress syndrome in 1987: Is it a systemic disease? SCCM, Crit. Care, State of the Art 8:279, 1987.

Sibbald, W. J., Anderson, R. R., Reid, B., et al.: Alveo-capillary permeability in human septic ARDS. Chest 79:133, 1981.

Simeone, F. A.: Pulmonary complications of nonthoracic wounds: A historical perspective. J. Trauma 8:625, 1968.

Simpson, D. L., Goodman, M., Spector, S. L., and Petty, T. L.: Long-term follow-up and bronchial reactivity testing in survivors of the adult respiratory distress syndrome. Am. Rev. Respir. Dis. 117:449, 1978.

Snapper, J. R., Hutchison, A. A., Ogletre, M. L., et al.: Effects of cyclo-oxygenase inhibitors on the alterations in lung mechanics caused by endotoxemia in the unanesthetized sheep. J. Clin. Invest. 72:63, 1983.

Sprung, C. L., Caralis, P. V., Marcial, E. H., et al.: The effects of high-dose corticosteroids in patients with septic shock: A prospective, controlled study. N. Engl. J. Med. 311:1137, 1984.

Sullivan, G. W., Carper, H. T., Novick, W. J., and Mandell, G. L.: Inhibition of the inflammatory action of interleukin-1 and tumor necrosis factor (alpha) on neutrophil function by pentoxifylline. Infect. Immun. 56:1722, 1988.

Tate, R. M., and Repine, J. E.: Neutrophils and the adult respiratory distress syndrome. Am. Rev. Respir. Dis. 128:552, 1983.

Weigelt, J. A., Mitchell, R. A., and Snyder, W. H.: Early positive end-expiratory pressure in the adult respiratory distress syndrome. Arch. Surg. 114:497, 1979.

Weiland, J. E., David, W. B., Holter, J. F., et al.: Lung neutrophils in the adult respiratory distress syndrome: Clinical and pathophysiological significance. Am. Rev. Respir. Dis. 133:218, 1986.

Wiener-Kronish, J. P., and Matthay, M. A.: Sequential measurements of pulmonary edema protein concentrations provide a reliable index of alveolar epithelial function and prognosis in patients with the adult respiratory distress syndrome. Clin. Res. 37:165A, 1989.

Wiener-Kronish, J. P., Goldstein, R., and Matthay, M. A.: Pleural effusions are frequently associated with the adult respiratory distress syndrome. Am. Rev. Respir. Dis. 137:227A, 1988b.

Wiener-Kronish, J. P., Broaddus, V. C., Albertine, K. H., et al.: The relationship of pleural effusions to increased permeability pulmonary edema in sheep. J. Clin. Invest. 82:1422, 1988a.

Wright, P. E., and Bernard, G. R.: The role of airflow resistance in patients with the adult respiratory distress syndrome. Am. Rev Respir. Dis. 139:1169, 1989.

Zapol, W. M., Snider, M. T., Hill, S. D., et al.: Extracorporeal membrane oxygenation in severe acute respiratory failure: A randomized prospective study. JAMA 242:2193, 1979.

Zheatlin, L. M., Jacobs, E. R., Hanley, M. E., et al.: Plasma elastase levels in the adult respiratory distress syndrome. J. Crit. Care 1:39, 1986.

8

Abnormal Air and Pleural Fluid Collections

■

Irena Tocino

One of the most common life-threatening events in the clinical course of critically ill patients is the development of extra-alveolar air (EAA) collections. While the reason for the sudden deterioration of the patient's condition may not be apparent at the bedside, the portable supine radiograph offers the necessary information concerning the location and severity of the abnormal air collections. Knowledge of the subtle and early radiographic findings of extra-alveolar air and prompt communication with the attending medical staff minimize the deleterious effect that EAA has on the critically ill.

Other than direct blunt chest trauma, most abnormal air collections in patients in the intensive care unit (ICU) follow diagnostic or therapeutic maneuvers (Westcott and Cole, 1983), mainly intubation (Zwilich et al., 1974), central venous catheterization (Bernard et al., 1971), and mechanical ventilation (Bone, 1982; Bone et al., 1976; Leeming, 1968; Nash et al., 1967; Rohlfing et al., 1976). The incidence of EAA in the ICU patient is difficult to estimate because most reports focus on the presence of pneumomediastinum and pneumothorax and lack any reference to pulmonary interstitial emphysema (PIE) or even subcutaneous emphysema. The incidence of pneumothorax after central venous catheterization is estimated at 6% (Bernard et al., 1971), and less than 1% of tracheal intubations lead to pneumomediastinum and deep cervical fascia emphysema as a result of lacerations of the tracheal wall (Zwilich et al., 1974).

Abnormal air collections are most often the result of mechanical ventilation. The incidence of barotrauma in mechanically ventilated patients has been reported to be between 4% and 15% (Westcott and Cole, 1983; Zwilich et al., 1974), although higher numbers can be expected when underlying lung disease, such as pneumonia, is present (Latorre et al., 1977). In 1974, Steier and associates reported a 45%

increase in the yearly incidence of pneumothorax related to the use of mechanical ventilation. Factors associated with barotrauma included excessive tidal volumes, peak inspiratory pressures above 46 cm of water, the use of positive end-expiratory pressure (PEEP), underlying chronic lung disease, and percutaneous subclavian catheterization during pressure breathing. Most recent studies have identified peak airway pressures above 40 cm of water as the single most important contributing factor in the development of barotrauma (Woodring, 1985). Whether higher peak pressures are truly a cause of barotrauma or merely a reflection of the severe alveolar wall damage already present has not been established. Similarly, the presence of extra-alveolar air does not necessarily suggest a worse prognosis for the patient with adult respiratory distress syndrome (ARDS); rather, it is another manifestation of the severity of the lung damage.

The inability to improve mortality for ARDS patients has encouraged research efforts in the field of mechanical ventilation, suggesting new ventilatory modes capable of obtaining adequate oxygenation while minimizing the risks of barotrauma. Specifically, pressure-controlled, inverse-ratio ventilation (Lain et al., 1989) and extracorporeal carbon dioxide removal are being evaluated in prospective randomized studies as alternatives to conventional methods (Gattinoni et al., 1986). Whether these new techniques will result in a decrease in incidence of barotrauma is still unclear.

The immediate effect of sudden as well as sustained increased intra-alveolar pressure is rupture of the alveolar wall. When the pressure within the air cysts resulting from alveolar wall rupture exceeds the pressure within the surrounding interstitium, air dissects along the peribronchovascular sheaths and the interlobular septa. Interstitial emphysema can progress toward the hila, to produce pneumomediastinum and pneumothorax, or peripherally, to produce subpleural blebs and eventually pneumothorax (Macklin and Macklin, 1944). Direct rupture of alveoli into the pleural space can certainly produce a pneumothorax without recognizable pulmonary interstitial emphysema or pneumomediastinum.

PULMONARY INTERSTITIAL EMPHYSEMA

The presence of air in the interstitium of newborn babies with hyaline membrane disease is a well-recognized sign of barotrauma (Avery, 1968; Campbell, 1970). Its occurrence in the adult respiratory distress syndrome (ARDS) has received attention only within the last 15 years (Johnson and Altman, 1979; McLoud et al., 1977; Ovenfors and Hedgcock, 1979; Pratt, 1982; Westcott and Cole, 1974, 1983; Woodring, 1985). Radiographic recognition of pul-

monary interstitial emphysema (PIE) requires radiographs of optimal quality, knowledge of the anatomy of the interstitium, and close clinical correlation to establish an adequate index of suspicion. A significant amount of alveolar consolidation is also necessary to visualize PIE in its early phase prior to the formation of air cysts.

The first radiographic sign of PIE is the sudden development of lucent streaks radiating from the hila to the periphery of the lung in a disorganized fashion (Table 8–1). Unlike air bronchograms, these lucencies do not branch or decrease in caliber as they progress toward pleural surfaces. They represent air in the peribronchovascular loose connective tissue or axial interstitium (Fig. 8–1). Closely related to this phenomenon are the perivascular halos as described by Ovenfors (1964), a definite but uncommon sign of PIE. Air within the interlobular septa also contributes to the streaky appearance of the chest radiograph in PIE. Studies of the interlobular septa by Heitzman

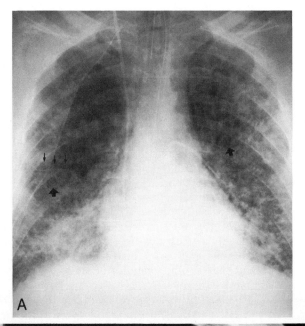

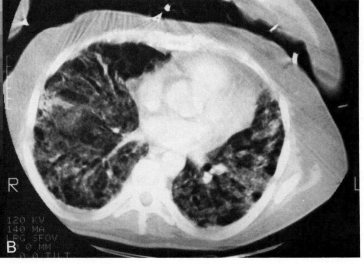

Figure 8–1. Interstitial emphysema. *A,* Portable radiograph in patient with severe adult respiratory distress syndrome (ARDS). Mottled appearance of infiltrates and streaked lucencies are combined with small air cysts *(arrowheads).* The minor fissure is accentuated by subpleural air *(small arrows). B,* Computed tomography (CT) confirms the perivascular nature of the lucent streaks and the presence of air cysts.

Table 8–1. RADIOGRAPHIC SIGNS OF
PULMONARY INTERSTITIAL EMPHYSEMA

Lucent streaks
Mottled radiolucencies
Vascular rings
Air cysts
Pneumatoceles
Subpleural air

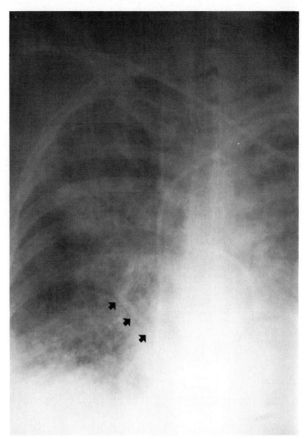

Figure 8–2. Perivascular air. Air outlines an inferior pulmonary vein *(arrowheads)* in patient with ARDS.

(1984) complement previous descriptions of the peripheral interstitium by Reid (1959) and emphasize the presence of septa not only in anteromedial surfaces of the lung, but posteriorly and laterally, corresponding to the radiographic Kerley's A and B lines. In fact, air in the interstitium can be described as a negative image of the Kerley's line spectrum. The random arrangement of secondary pulmonary lobules explains the disorganized nature of the streaky lucencies of PIE (Heitzman, 1984).

Some investigators have suggested that air dissects more easily around the pulmonary veins and lymphatics (interlobular septa) than around the pulmonary arteries, which perhaps provides an explanation for the uncommon incidence of perivascular halo sign in PIE (Fig. 8–2).

Air cysts of up to 5 mm in size can be recognized in perihilar and subpleural distribution, giving the lungs a mottled appearance. When compared with previous radiographs, radiographs of extensive parenchymal disease now appear more radiolucent. These air cysts are difficult to differentiate from underlying emphysema and from the microabscesses that complicate nosocomial infections, which are often present in patients with a prolonged course of ARDS. The cysts may not be radiographically apparent until they become confluent, under pleural surfaces—the so-called blebs—or until they outline the fissures with a sharp radiolucent band, much as subpleural edema renders the fissures more apparent.

The blebs, or subpleural air cysts, are directly related to the presence of air in the peripheral interstitium (the interlobular septa) and account for the development of pneumothorax. While any radiographic manifestation of PIE should be considered a precursor for pneumothorax, subpleural air cysts represent the finding most likely to progress to pneumothorax. Conversely, central pneumatoceles, which may become quite large, can persist through the course of the disease without resulting in pneumothorax. We have observed two cases in which the pneumatoceles continued to grow, occupying most of the lungs; both patients succumbed to respiratory failure (Fig. 8–3). Unlike traumatic pneumatoceles, which often become infected, the pneumatoceles of barotrauma seldom display air–fluid levels or other signs of complications. As a general rule, they progressively decrease in size and eventually disappear.

In contrast with the rapid changes in appearance and resolution of PIE reported previously, the picture of PIE in our ICU patients has been often monoto-

nous and persisting for days, even weeks, with neither improvement nor development of air-leak phenomena. In spite of this stable picture, we consider early recognition of PIE fundamental to the management of the ventilatory care of the patient and monitor this progression with daily chest radiographs correlated with clinical information. We have also taken advantage of the fact that most critically ill patients undergo body or head computed tomography (CT) during the course of their disease, and we include three or four CT sections through the lung bases. These additional images often demonstrate unsuspected pneumothoraces and pleural fluid collections and reveal barotrauma before it becomes apparent on the chest radiograph. This information allows the ICU clinician to change the ventilator settings to minimize progression of PIE and development of pneumothorax (Fig. 8–4).

PNEUMOMEDIASTINUM

Air in the mediastinum of the critically ill patient is often due to barotrauma, but other etiologic factors, including rupture of the airway, the esophagus, or an intra-abdominal hollow viscus, should be strongly considered in the appropriate clinical setting (Cyrlak et al., 1984). In patients with facial fractures,

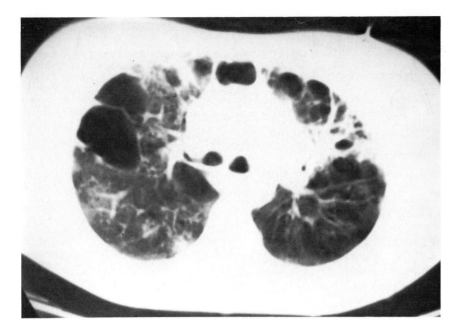

Figure 8–3. Pneumatoceles. In this young patient, ARDS progressed into large subpleural pneumatoceles, accounting for as much as 80% dead space.

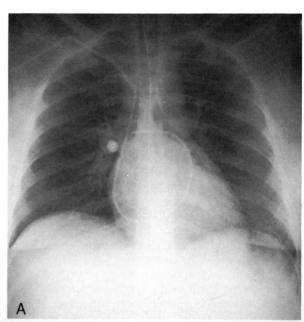

Figure 8–4. Early detection of pulmonary interstitial emphysema (PIE). *A,* The admission chest radiograph showed diffuse infiltrates but no signs of barotrauma. *B,* Images of lung bases on the same morning in which abdominal CT scan was performed demonstrate air cysts in both lungs.

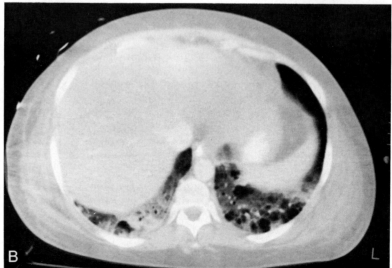

air can also dissect from the soft tissues of the face and neck into the mediastinum (Switzer et al., 1976). Pneumomediastinum is a common finding after blunt chest trauma. A sudden increase in intra-alveolar pressure with rupture of alveolar walls is the most likely explanation for the pneumomediastinum in trauma, asthma, severe coughing, the stress of labor, and diabetic ketoacidosis (Toomey and Chinnock, 1975).

In the presence of interstitial emphysema, air-leak phenomena are common. Thirty-eight percent of patients with PIE in Woodring's (1985) study developed pneumomediastinum, while pneumothorax occurred in 77% of patients. Air in the axial interstitium of the lung dissects the bronchovascular bundles toward the hila, resulting in pneumomediastinum. As with other manifestations of barotrauma, pneumomediastinum is a clinically silent event, except for a few instances in which a retrosternal crunch can be heard. Rarely, a mediastinal air collection becomes large enough to compromise hemodynamic functions, much like a tension pneumothorax. In fact, in some patients, both clinical and radiographic differentiation between pneumomediastinum and pneumothorax may be difficult. Decubitus radiographs or CT may be necessary to make the distinction.

Pneumomediastinum is detectable on the radiograph when air outlines the edges of anatomic structures not normally visible (Cimmino, 1967; Cyrlak et al., 1984). A pneumopericardium or anteromedial pneumothorax may have a similar appearance. An optical illusion—the so-called Mach effect—may also mimic a pneumomediastinum (Lane et al., 1976). To be certain of the presence of pneumomediastinum, one must then recognize abnormal air in regions of the mediastinum not enhanced by the Mach effect. Specifically, air dissecting the medial border of the superior vena cava, left subclavian artery, left common carotid artery, and right innominate artery, and the continuation of the dissection along these vessels into the neck, are pathognomonic signs of pneumomediastinum (Fig. 8–5). The visualization of the azygos vein or the superior intercostal vein previously obscured by mediastinal fat can be accepted as evidence for pneumomediastinum. Air can be seen around the central pulmonary arteries (ring around the artery) (Hammond, 1984) and ascending aorta, and it can be seen dissecting pericardial fat pads.

Because of the continuity of right and left sides of the mediastinum, air can outline the central portion of the diaphragm (Levin, 1973) under the cardiac silhouette, as opposed to subpulmonic pneumothoraces, which do not cross the midline. Also, because the mediastinum is continuous with the retroperitoneum, a posterior pneumomediastinum can cross the diaphragm to outline retroperitoneal structures. This is one route of extra-alveolar air into the peritoneum in patients with barotrauma (Fig. 8–6). Posteromedial pneumomediastinum may be present in spontaneous esophageal rupture. A V-shaped lucency representing air between the costophrenic angle and the diaphragm

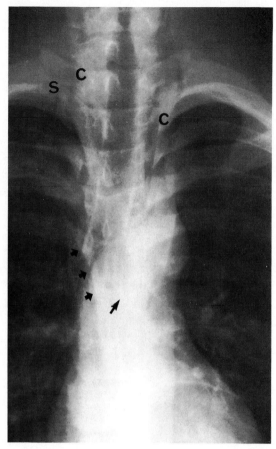

Figure 8–5. Pneumomediastinum. Air dissects the azygos vein in patient with azygos lobe *(small arrowheads)* and dissects the common carotid arteries (C). In addition, it emphasizes the wall of the left main bronchus and carina *(arrow)*. Air is also present in soft tissues of the neck. S, Superior vena cava.

was described by Naclerio (1957) as a pathognomonic sign of esophageal rupture.

The posteromedial segment of the major fissure in the left hemithorax (Cyrlak et al., 1984) and the azygos lobe fissure in the right hemithorax may cause confusion and occasionally lead to an erroneous diagnosis of pneumothorax. In these and other uncertain circumstances, the concomitant presence of subcutaneous emphysema provides confirmation of the presence of pneumomediastinum.

SUBCUTANEOUS EMPHYSEMA

From the mediastinum, air can travel along fascial planes into the subcutaneous tissue of the neck and chest wall, as well as of the abdominal wall. The presence of air in the chest wall in patients receiving mechanical ventilation is often the first radiographic sign of barotrauma, because the underlying pneumothorax may be impossible to detect in the supine portable radiograph. Air in the soft tissues of the

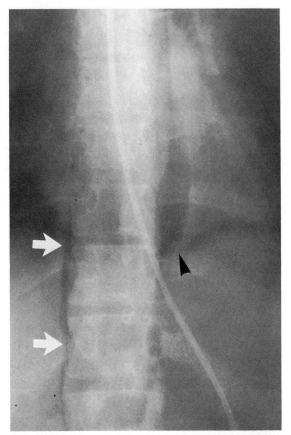

Figure 8–6. Pneumomediastinum extends below the diaphragm as pneumoretroperitoneum outlining the right crus of diaphragm *(arrows)*. On the left hemithorax, a posteromedial pneumothorax stops at the costovertebral sulcus *(arrowhead)*. (From Tocino, I.M.: Pneumothorax in the supine patient: Radiographic anatomy. Radiographics, 5:557–586, 1985, with permission.)

neck in the absence of pneumomediastinum signifies possible injury to the upper airway during intubation or during blind attempts at placement of a feeding tube (Kassner et al, 1977; Woodall et al, 1987).

Although it presents a dramatic clinical picture, subcutaneous emphysema is a benign event that resolves as pneumomediastinum and pneumothorax improve. A continuous increase in the amount of subcutaneous air close to a chest tube site indicates malfunctioning of the thoracostomy tube or improper wound dressing (Pasternak and O'Cain, 1983). The radiograph of the patient with subcutaneous emphysema looks as alarming as that of the puffed-up patient and limits the amount of information obtainable regarding parenchymal and pleural disease. Air dissecting muscular bundles can mimic alveolar infiltrates or may obscure true parenchymal disease. Some air bubbles in the soft tissues can also mimic parenchymal infiltrates with cavitation. Conversely, true pulmonary cavities and pneumatoceles may be obscured by the subcutaneous emphysema. The lucent lines may mimic pneumothorax, and any attempts to confirm its presence by obtaining cross-table lateral views or decubitus films involve the same limitations. Computed tomography of the chest can add important information regarding the presence of pneumothorax and parenchymal disease in patients with severe subcutaneous emphysema, particularly in cases of blunt chest trauma (Tocino and Miller, 1987) (Fig. 8–7).

PNEUMOTHORAX

Air may reach the pleural space following pneumomediastinum or may enter directly into the pleural space from rupture of alveoli or pneumatoceles. Pneumothorax due to barotrauma is probably the most common emergency in patients supported by mechanical ventilation. Incidence rates as high as 25% have been reported (Greene et al., 1977). Pneumothorax can also be a complication of invasive procedures, such as central venous catheterization, endotracheal intubation, and feeding tube placement. The incidence of such complications is greater in the mechanically ventilated patient, and the chances for progression to a tension pneumothorax are also greatly increased in this population. Blunt chest trauma may result in pneumothorax even in the absence of rib fractures, probably as a result of a sudden increase in intra-alveolar pressure and concomitant closing of the glottis. Pneumothorax often follows certain surgical procedures, such as coronary artery bypass surgery, particularly in patients with pericardial defects in which the pericardium and the pleural space are in anatomic continuity (Broadbent et al., 1966). Esophageal perforation may cause hydropneumothorax, or if rupture occurs at the level of the inferior pulmonary ligament, a paramediastinal air collection develops within the leaves of the ligament.

A spontaneous pneumothorax may complicate the course of infections, such as *Pneumocystis carinii* pneumonia (Sherman et al., 1986; Tocino, 1985) and cavitary pneumonias (e.g., staphylococcal pneumonia, *Klebsiella* pneumonia, invasive aspergillosis and *Candida* pneumonia).

Unfortunately, in the ICU and emergency department, only supine and cross-table radiographs can be obtained on severely injured and severely ill patients and patients with known or suspected spinal injuries. The radiographic diagnosis of pneumothorax in the supine patient requires a detailed knowledge of the anatomy of the pleural recesses and mediastinal structures (Tocino, 1985) and an understanding of the forces governing the movement of pleural air, that is, gravity and lung compliance (Lams and Jolles, 1982).

The distribution of pneumothorax in the supine radiograph has been studied in 88 ICU patients, and anteromedial (AM) and subpulmonary (SBP) pneumothoraces appear to represent the majority of the air collections (Tocino et al, 1985). Apicolateral (APL) pneumothorax is relatively uncommon be-

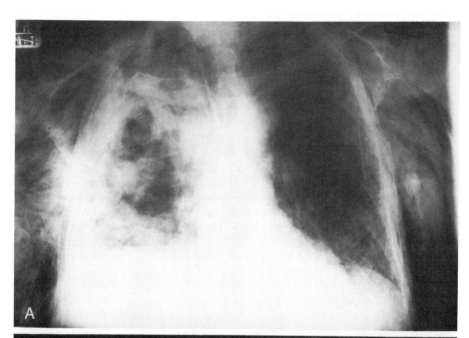

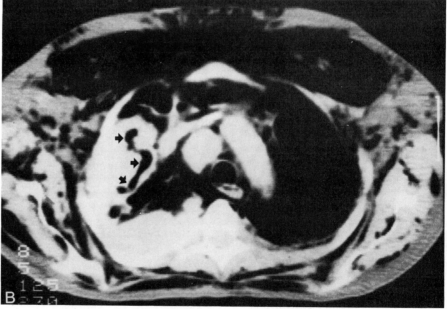

Figure 8–7. Subcutaneous emphysema. *A,* After blunt chest trauma, subcutaneous emphysema obscures pleural and parenchymal disease. *B,* The CT scan illustrates parenchymal laceration within the lung contusion. Pneumothorax was also seen at different lung windows, as were subpleural hematomas *(arrows).* (Reprinted from Tocino, I.M., and Miller, M.H.: Computed tomography in blunt chest trauma. Journal of Thoracic Imaging, Vol. 2, No. 3, p. 57, with permission of Aspen Publishers, Inc., © 1987.)

Table 8–2. RADIOGRAPHIC SIGNS OF
ANTEROMEDIAL PNEUMOTHORAX

Suprahilar anteromedial pneumothorax
   Sharp delineation of:
     Superior vena cava
     Azygos vein
     Left subclavian artery
     Anterior junction line
     Superior pulmonary vein
Infrahilar anteromedial pneumothorax
   Sharp outline of:
     Heart border
     Inferior vena cava
   Deep anterior cardiophrenic sulcus
   Outline of medial diaphragm under heart silhouette
   Unusually sharp delineation of pericardial fat pad

cause the air moves preferentially to the less dependent pleural spaces. On a supine radiograph, the presence of APL pneumothorax suggests that a large volume of pleural air has already accumulated and has displaced the visceral pleura medially so that it becomes tangential to the x-ray beam (Moskowitz and Griscom, 1976).

Not only is calculation of the size of a pneumothorax on the basis of the supine radiograph impossible, but it is also superfluous, because the size of the pneumothorax in the ICU patient correlates poorly with its clinical significance. Hence, all pneumothoraces discovered in the chest radiograph should be promptly evaluated for the need for treatment.

Anteromedial Pneumothorax

In the supine position, air preferentially accumulates in front of the lung and surrounds the anterior mediastinal structures (Moskowitz and Griscom, 1976). The pulmonary hilum divides the space into a superior and inferior pleural recess, which accounts for a spectrum of radiographic findings (Tocino, 1985) (Table 8–2). Sharp visualization of the superior vena cava and azygos vein on the right (Fig. 8–8) and of the left subclavian artery as it curves over the apex of the left lung are initial signs of anteromedial (AM) pneumothorax. Recognition of the left superior intercostal vein and the superior pulmonary veins (Fig. 8–9), on the right or left side, may be the only sign of pneumothorax when small amounts of air are present

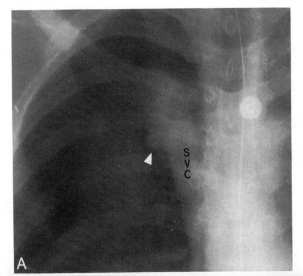

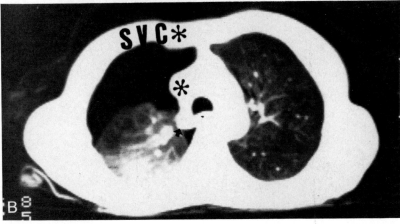

Figure 8–8. Anteromedial pneumothorax. *A,* The superior vena cava (SVC) and azygos vein *(arrowhead)* are outlined by air in the medial pleural space. *B,* In a different patient, the superior vena cava *(asterisk)* and azygos vein *(arrowhead)* are in contact with right pneumothorax. (From Tocino, I.M.: Pneumothorax in the supine patient: Radiographic anatomy. Radiographics, 5:557–586, 1985, with permission.)

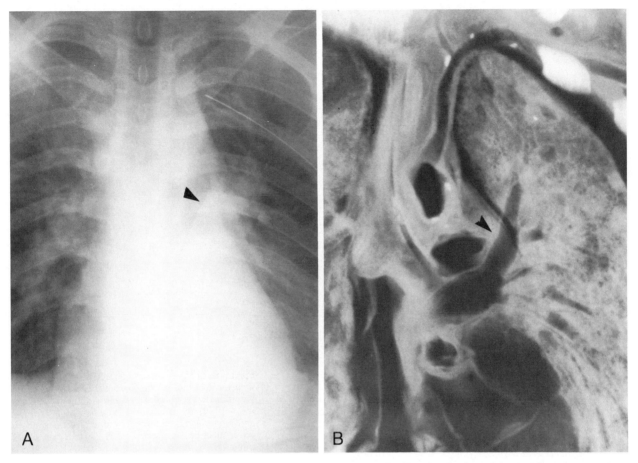

Figure 8–9. Anteromedial pneumothorax. Radiographic visualization *(A)* of the left superior pulmonary vein *(arrowhead)* corresponds to same structure in anatomic specimen *(B)*. *(B,* From Heitzman, E.R.: The Lung: Radiologic-Pathologic Correlations. St. Louis, C.V. Mosby, 1984, p. 50, with permission.)

in the medial pleural space. The anterior junction line becomes sharply outlined (Markowitz, 1988), and even displaced to the opposite hemithorax, a common finding in CT scans of patients with pneumothorax (Fig. 8–10).

Infrahilar AM pneumothorax accounts for a sharp delineation of the heart border and a deep, lucent cardiophrenic sulcus. The pericardial fat pad is well outlined (Ziter and Westcott, 1981), mimicking a mass or even segmental collapse to the inexperienced observer (Fig. 8–11). The inferior vena cava may become apparent as it enters the right atrium. If the amount of AM air is large, the affected hemithorax may appear hyperlucent when compared with the opposite side. Confirmation can be obtained through cross-table lateral or decubitus views (Hoffer and Ablow, 1984).

Subpulmonary Pneumothorax

The diagnosis of subpulmonary (SBP) pneumothorax may be difficult unless the radiograph includes the upper abdomen. This positioning can be easily accomplished by obtaining all supine radiographs with the cassette in vertical orientation. A combination of faulty technique and a lack of knowledge of radiographic anatomy of this space probably accounts for the high rate of failure to diagnose SBP pneumothorax (Tocino et al., 1985).

In SBP pneumothorax, a hyperlucent upper quadrant of the abdomen with visualization of the superior surface of the diaphragm can be expected (Kurlander and Helmen, 1966) (Table 8–3). The diaphragm is visible only to the midline, whereas in pneumomediastinum and pneumoperitoneum, the central portion of the diaphragm is outlined by air. Other signs of SBP pneumothorax are a deep costophrenic sulcus (Gordon, 1980), a sharp hemidiaphragm despite lower lung parenchymal disease, and visualization of the inferior surface of the consolidated lung. Placement of chest tubes in SBP pneumothorax may require knowledge of the location of the air collection on the lateral view. When SBP pneumothorax occupies the anterior space, air outlines the anterior structures surrounding the costophrenic sulcus. A posterior SBP pneumothorax merges with the costovertebral sulcus and the paraspinal line. Also, the

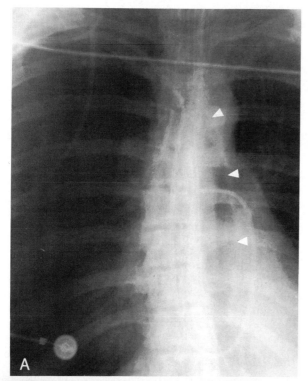

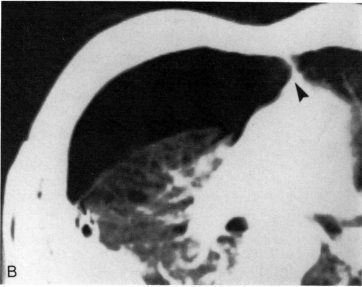

Figure 8–10. Anteromedial pneumothorax. *A,* The anterior junction line *(arrowheads)* is outlined by right anteromedial pneumothorax and is displaced, indicating tension. *B,* The CT scan in patient with ARDS and bilateral pneumothoraces, demonstrating the anterior junction line *(arrowhead).* (From Tocino, I.M.: Pneumothorax in the supine patient: Radiographic anatomy. Radiographics, 5:557–586, 1985, with permission.)

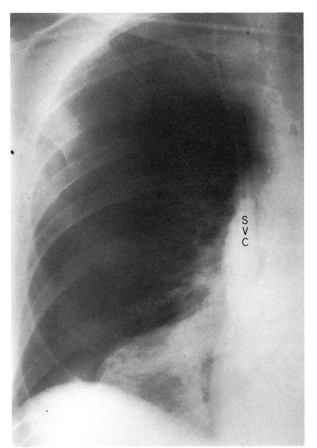

Figure 8–11. Anteromedial pneumothorax. Pericardial fat pad and superior vena cava (SVC) outlined by air. The fat pad could easily be mistaken for a collapsed lower lobe.

configuration of the anterior diaphragmatic sulcus and its more superior position can be easily distinguished from the posterior diaphragmatic surface (Rhea et al., 1979). Occasionally, both surfaces are present in subpulmonic pneumothorax, which gives rise to a double-diaphragm sign (Ziter and Westcott, 1981). A horizontal-beam view can be helpful in this analysis of SBP pneumothorax.

Apicolateral Pneumothorax

The conventional radiographic description of an apicolateral (APL) pneumothorax often does not apply to the appearance of APL pneumothorax in the ICU. Visualization of a thin, white pleural line with no lung markings beyond it, and a radiolucent

Table 8–3. RADIOGRAPHIC SIGNS OF
SUBPULMONARY PNEUMOTHORAX

Hyperlucent upper quadrant
Deep costophrenic sulcus
Sharp diaphragmatic outline
Visualization of anterior and posterior diaphragmatic sulci
Visualization of inferior vena cava

space close to the chest wall, have been considered the main signs of APL pneumothorax. A pleural line may not always be visible, because visualization of the line requires normal aerated lung and air in the pleura. Many ICU patients have parenchymal disease, which may obscure a pleural line. Similarly, a concomitant pleural effusion renders a pneumothorax more dense than expected (Fig. 8–12). Because of the difference in compliance of the lung parenchyma when randomly affected by pneumonia or ARDS, segments of the lung may collapse under a pneumothorax, while others more severely involved are seen beyond the pneumothorax. Hence, the presence of lung markings beyond a pleural line does not exclude pneumothorax in an ICU patient (Fig. 8–13A). Focal pleural adhesions may cause a similar effect.

When the amount of air accumulated is small, the first sign of APL pneumothorax is a lack of contact between the minor fissure and the chest wall. This finding is helpful in patients with pleural or subpleural fluid, in whom the fissures are readily apparent. Progressive accumulation of air further displaces the pleura medially, rendering it tangential to the x-ray beam in a longer segment, which makes the pneumothorax easier to diagnose.

Skinfolds, which are often seen in emaciated patients, or as a normal morphologic feature associated with the scapula, can mimic APL pneumothorax. As a differential point, skinfolds may cross the midline or the chest wall, are usually present in pairs, and

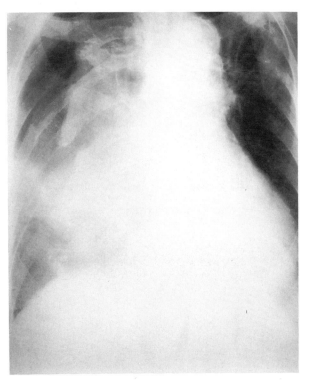

Figure 8–12. Pneumothorax and pleural effusion. The severity of this pneumothorax may be less apparent because of the absence of hyperlucency and of the pleural line, which is obliterated by the fluid in the right hemithorax.

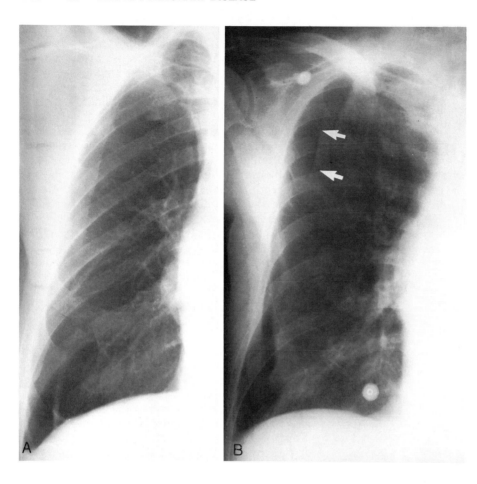

Figure 8–13. Lateral pneumothorax versus skinfolds. *A,* The variations in lung recoil of diseased lung segments account for different degrees of collapse in the presence of pneumothorax. *B,* Skinfolds. The lack of pleural line and the multiple interfaces enhanced by negative Mach effect signal skinfolds *(arrows).*

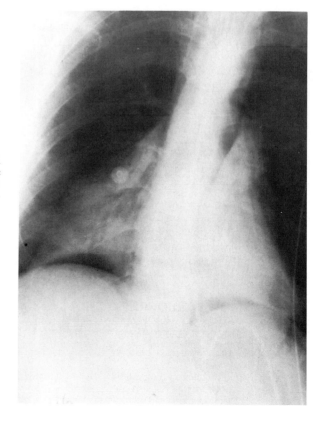

Figure 8–14. Posteromedial pneumothorax. In the presence of bilateral lower lobe collapse, air collects posteromedially and in subpulmonic distribution. (From Tocino, I.M.: Pneumothorax in the supine patient: Radiographic anatomy. Radiographics, 5:557–586, 1985, with permission.)

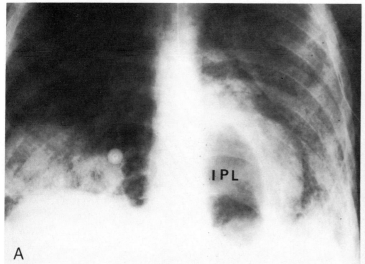

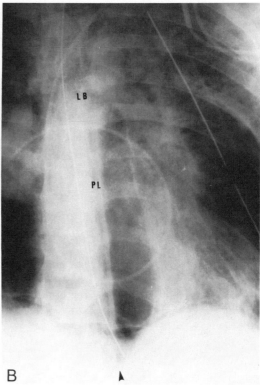

Figure 8–15. Air in the inferior pulmonary ligament (IPL). *A,* Paramediastinal air collection with convex configuration, presumably within IPL. *B,* Twelve days later, the air collection ruptured into the posteromedial pleural space. (PL, paraspinal line; LB, left main bronchus.)

tend to disappear suddenly, having no association with a pleural line (Tocino and Armstrong, 1988). A negative Mach effect or black edge, enhancing the skinfolds can often be recognized (see Fig. 8–13*B*).

Posteromedial Pneumothorax

In the presence of lobar collapse, air preferentially surrounds the surfaces of the abnormal lung, often seeming to defy the laws of gravity. Posteromedial (PM) pneumothorax is associated with volume loss, lower lobe parenchymal disease (a common occurrence in the ICU patient), or both (Proto and Tocino, 1980). The posterior mediastinal structures, paraspinal line, descending aorta, and costovertebral sulcus become apparent. The medial surface of the lower lobe also appears to be displaced away from the midline (Fig. 8–14).

Radiographic differentiation of PM pneumothorax and pneumomediastinum is possible because air in the mediastinum often continues into the retroperitoneum, and PM pneumothorax remains above the diaphragm, ending at the costovertebral sulcus. A more challenging exercise is the differentiation of PM pneumothorax from air within the inferior pulmonary ligament (IPL) (Elyaderani and Gabriele, 1979; Volberg et al., 1979) (Fig. 8–15). Whereas PM pneumothorax maintains a triangular shape with the apex at the hilum, air in the IPL has a balloon-like configuration and does not outline the posterior costovertebral sulcus or the diaphragm, because it is contained

within two layers of serosa. The lower lobe may be normally aerated in IPL air collections, and a cross-table lateral view shows air in the midchest, while the air of PM pneumothorax is paraspinal. Even when PM pneumothorax is not loculated, it does not rise to less dependent pleural surfaces, but always surrounds the abnormal collapsed lower lung.

Air in the Fissures

Just as fluid may collect within interlobular fissures, air can dissect the fissures, giving the appearance of pneumatoceles or air–fluid collections within the lung. Anatomic knowledge of fissural planes explains these unusual air collections (Nightingale and Flower, 1984; Spizarny and Goodman, 1986) (Fig. 8–16).

Tension Pneumothorax

A pneumothorax is considered under tension when the pressure in the pleural space equals atmospheric pressure. This diagnosis is clearly a clinical judgment and not a radiographic diagnosis, because the respiratory and hemodynamic consequences of tension pneumothorax do not have a radiographic equivalent in most circumstances. Because most pneumothoraces in mechanically ventilated patients progress to tension pneumothorax, therapeutic decisions are made regardless of the size of the pneumothorax seen on the

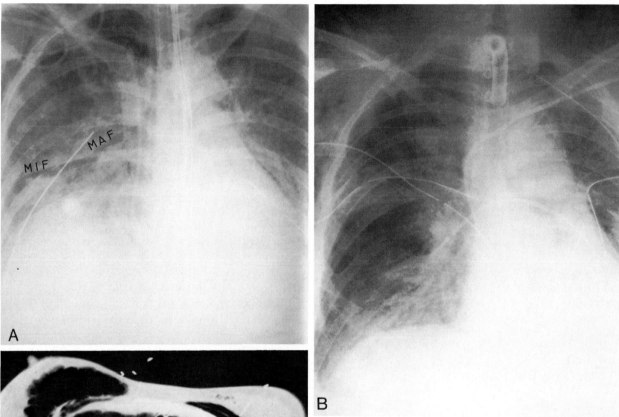

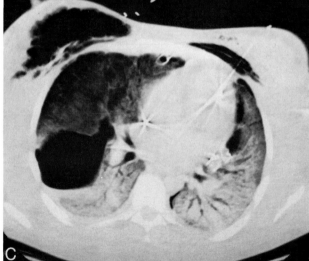

Figure 8–16. Air in fissures. *A,* The planes of the right minor and major fissures are outlined by air. (MIF, minor fissure; MAF, major fissure.) *B,* In a different patient, a large amount of air is loculated in the minor fissure. *C,* A CT scan in same patient shows exact location of air, which is difficult to evaluate in the conventional radiograph because of the associated subcutaneous emphysema.

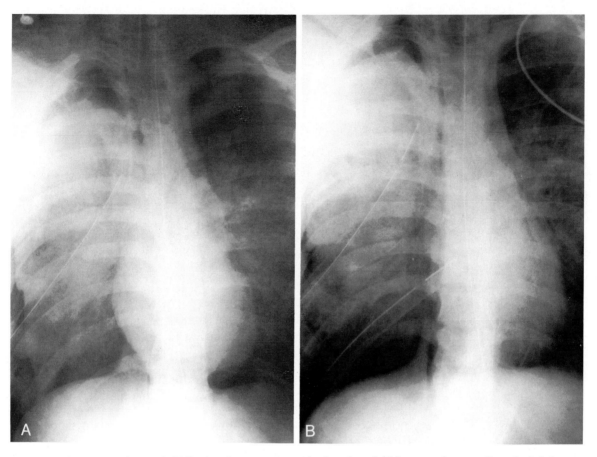

Figure 8–17. Tension pneumothorax. *A,* Following chest trauma, a subpulmonic and AM pneumothorax outlines the inferior vena cava. Note the superior vena cava outline. *B,* Severe hypotension necessitated an additional chest tube placement, which prompted this radiograph. The inferior vena cava and heart border are flat, indicating severe compromise to venous return from tension pneumothorax. (From Tocino, I.M.: Pneumothorax in the supine patient: Radiographic anatomy. Radiographics, 5:557–586, 1985, with permission.)

radiograph. Furthermore, because of pleural adhesions, a small loculated collection of air can be the source of tension even while concomitant ipsilateral pneumothorax is being drained by a thoracostomy tube.

Because of pleural adhesions and because of the stiffness of lung parenchyma in ARDS, total lung collapse and mediastinal shift may be absent in the presence of a tension pneumothorax. More often, the diaphragm is inverted, or the anterior junction line is displaced to the contralateral side. Displacement of the azygo-esophageal recess is also a good sign of tension. Perhaps the most specific sign of tension pneumothorax, and one that correlates with clinical findings, is the flattening of the heart border and other vascular structures, including the superior and inferior vena cava. This sign is a radiographic reflection of the impairment to the normal venous return that occurs in tension pneumothorax (Gobien et al., 1982; Tocino, 1985) (Fig. 8–17).

Occult Pneumothorax

Even an exhaustive knowledge of radiographic signs of pneumothorax cannot lead to detection of all pleural air collections. In the supine position, certain pneumothoraces, not necessarily small ones, may escape detection. Because they may also be unsuspected clinically, other radiographic projections, such as erect, decubitus, or cross-table lateral views, may not be requested. These pneumothoraces may be discovered during the course of CT examinations—for example, of the abdomen (Wall et al., 1983) or chest (Tocino et al., 1984)—as incidental findings. They are not inconsequential, however, because many of these patients may later undergo mechanical ventilation, inhalational anesthesia, or both. As in other manifestations of barotrauma, such as those found in the diagnosis of PIE, chest CT is an invaluable tool in the diagnosis and, often, treatment of pneumothorax. It should be used judiciously but aggressively in the acutely ill patient (Fig. 8–18). Digitized portable chest radiographs with edge enhancement may in the future improve detection of small pneumothoraces, but further evaluation of this technique is needed (Goodman et al., 1988).

A discussion of pneumothorax is incomplete without a word of caution regarding radiographic artifacts that may simulate pneumothorax. These artifacts include dressings, tubing, bags (Shapiro and Gerzof, 1987), other paraphernalia in the surface of the chest,

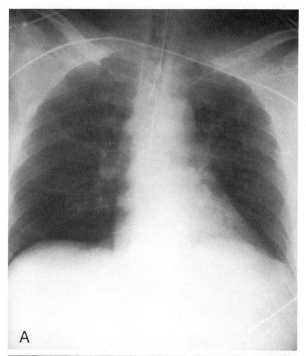

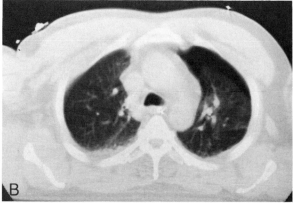

Figure 8–18. Occult pneumothorax. *A,* Initial radiograph following blunt chest trauma does not disclose pneumothorax. *B,* A CT scan reveals unexpected left pneumothorax.

fingernail damage of the film prior to processing, and tracks of previous chest tubes. Not only can these artifacts mimic pneumothorax, but they may also obscure a real pneumothorax. Care must be taken when obtaining chest radiographs to remove all artifacts, wires, and tubing with the assistance of the ICU nurses to minimize potential misdiagnosis (see Fig. 3–12).

PNEUMOPERICARDIUM

Pneumopericardium as a sign of barotrauma is more commonly observed in the pediatric population (Grosfeld et al., 1970; Sagel et al., 1973). In the adult ICU patient, air in the pericardium is frequently found after coronary artery bypass surgery. Segmental air collections are easier to identify as pneumo-

pericardium, because pneumomediastinum and AM pneumothorax may result in delineation of the heart border, which is indistinguishable from pneumopericardium.

When the superior pericardial reflection around the great vessels is outlined by air, pneumopericardium is easily diagnosed. Visualization of the main pulmonary artery and undivided right pulmonary artery, although uncommon, can signal pneumopericardium.

PNEUMOPERITONEUM AND PNEUMORETROPERITONEUM

Air dissects from the mediastinum to the retroperitoneum through the diaphragmatic hiatus. This mechanism explains most intra-abdominal air collections in patients with barotrauma. After coronary artery bypass surgery, air is often observed under the diaphragm, probably owing to inadvertent transdiaphragmatic insertion of retrosternal mediastinal drainage tubes. In either situation, correlation with clinical evaluation is crucial so that a life-threatening explanation for the pneumoperitoneum, such as perforation of a hollow viscus, is not overlooked (Andrew and Milne, 1980).

The diagnosis of pneumoretroperitoneum is made when the psoas muscle, pararenal fascia, or diaphragmatic crura, is outlined by air. Pneumoperitoneum may be difficult to diagnose on the basis of the supine radiograph. Right upper quadrant air collections and visualization of the inferior surface of the diaphragm and lateral edge of the liver are classic signs. In patients with subpulmonary pneumothorax, visualization of both sides of the diaphragm is evidence of concomitant pneumoperitoneum (Fig. 8–19). When the wall of the bowel appears as a thin line, a pneumoperitoneum is invariably present. Other signs of supine pneumoperitoneum, such as the football sign and visualization of the falciform ligament, are seldom seen (Levine et al., 1991). Air may dissect the bowel wall, producing pneumatosis cystoides intestinalis. This sign is also present in extensive bowel ischemia, and the differential diagnosis should be performed in consideration of the clinical history (see Chapter 17).

PLEURAL FLUID

Pleural effusions are commonly present in the ICU patient but may go undetected because of the difficulty of recognizing small, or even moderate-sized, fluid collections in the supine chest radiograph. Perhaps the most common reason for pleural effusions in the ICU is congestive heart failure. Patients with ARDS can also have pleural effusions in the absence of congestive heart failure, as a manifestation of increased capillary permeability (Wiener-Kronish and Matthay, 1988). Pulmonary embolism, pneumonia, pancreatitis, and intra-abdominal disease cause pleural effusions. Following abdominal surgery, 50%

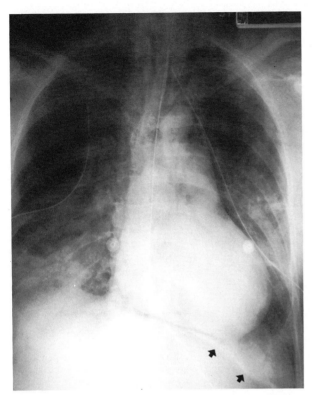

Figure 8–19. Pneumoperitoneum and pneumothorax. The diaphragm is seen as a white line outlined by air in the peritoneum *(arrowheads)* as well as in the subpulmonic pleural space. The patient also has pneumomediastinum and subcutaneous emphysema.

of patients develop small pleural effusions (Light and George, 1976). A hydrothorax occurring after placement of central venous catheters may be the result of superior vena cava perforation (Tocino and Watanabe, 1986) (see Chapter 4).

The radiographic appearance of pleural effusions as described by Fleischner (1963) and by Raasch (1982a) emphasizes the importance of forces of gravity and lung recoil ("form elasticity") in the distribution of pleural fluid. In the supine position, the most dependent pleural spaces are the apex of the hemithorax and the posterior basilar space. Fluid in these locations may be difficult to detect.

In an analysis of 34 supine radiographs performed by Ruskin and associates in 1987, 12 of 36 pleural effusions present in decubitus films could not be identified in the corresponding supine radiograph. The presence of fluid in the posterior basilar pleural space is first reflected by a homogeneous increase in density of the lower hemithorax, without obliteration of the normal bronchovascular markings, in the absence of radiographic signs of parenchymal disease or collapse such as air bronchograms, or reorientation of hilar or mediastinal structures (Woodring, 1984) (Figs. 8–20 and 8–21). Blunting of the costophrenic angle, decreased visibility of the lower lobe vessels behind the density of the diaphragm, loss of the diaphragmatic contour, and elevation of the diaphragm are helpful radiographic signs of pleural effusion in the erect posteroanterior (PA) radiograph. Technical factors in the supine radiograph, however, including poor centering, rotation, underpenetration, respiratory motion, small lung volumes, and the common presence of lower lobe parenchymal disease often explain the difficulty in diagnosing pleural fluid. A careful analysis of the radiographic findings and detection of fluid in other locations, such as the paraspinal region, fissures, and apex of the hemithorax, increase the predictive value of the initial observation.

Fluid in the apex of the hemithorax is promptly recognized as a pleural cap. Owing to the relatively small capacity of the pleural apex, fluid soon collects in the lateral as well as the medial apical pleura. The lateral fluid produces a pleural interface tangential to the x-ray beam, while the medial fluid obliterates the mediastinal contours and raises the question of mediastinal widening, particularly in patients with trauma. A radiograph in the sitting position resolves this uncertainty, provided the patient's clinical condition allows the change in position (Tocino and Miller, 1987) (Fig. 8–22). Ultrasound in the bedridden patient may demonstrate the paramediastinal space (Lewandowski and Winsberg, 1982).

As CT studies have shown, subpulmonary effusion is frequently present in the ICU patient, even when the fluid cannot be recognized in the supine chest radiograph. The common occurrence of atelectasis in the lung bases in supine ICU patients explains the preferential collection of fluid in subpulmonic space, just as posteromedial pneumothorax occurs in patients with lower lobe collapse. Extension of fluid into the paramediastinal gutter accounts for the triangular configuration of the paraspinal interface. Large subpulmonic collections can displace the gastric air bubble and splenic flexure of the colon inferiorly. Fluid in the fissure renders them more apparent in the chest radiograph, or brings to view segments of the fissures not visible in the normal radiograph. Fluid tracking up in the major fissure may cause the diaphragm to fade gradually into the lung. On occasion, the superior margin of the major fissure is visualized as an arcuate line approximately parallel to the fifth or sixth posterior rib.

The appearance of intrafissural fluid depends on the shape and orientation of the fissure, the location of the fluid, and the completeness of the fissure (Raasch et al., 1982b). Some manifestations of interlobar fluid, such as the pseudotumor and middle lobe step sign, have often been illustrated. Pleural fluid collections less readily recognized are those occurring in patients with incomplete pleural fissures (Dandy, 1978). That most pleural fissures are incomplete is well accepted; patterns of fusion are described in detailed anatomic studies by Yamashita (1978) and, more recently, by Raasch and colleagues (1982b). Fluid may enter the plane of the fissure to the point of fissural fusion medially, resulting in a sharp perihilar lucency (Fig. 8–23). In cases of volume loss, a

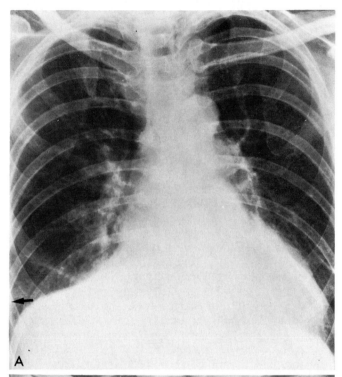

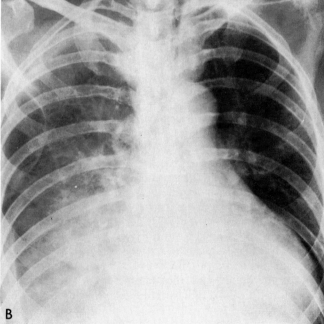

Figure 8–20. Pleural effusion. *A,* The anteroposterior (AP) upright radiograph demonstrates a density adjacent to the right border of the heart, representing either a right middle lobe collapse or medial fluid. In addition, the right hemidiaphragm is elevated, and minimal thickening of the lateral pleural space *(arrow)* is evident. *B,* Supine film taken several hours later demonstrates the fluid forming a layer over the entire right hemithorax, along the lateral lung and into the apex. In addition, an infiltrate is present at the right base medially, as demonstrated by the increased density and the air bronchogram.

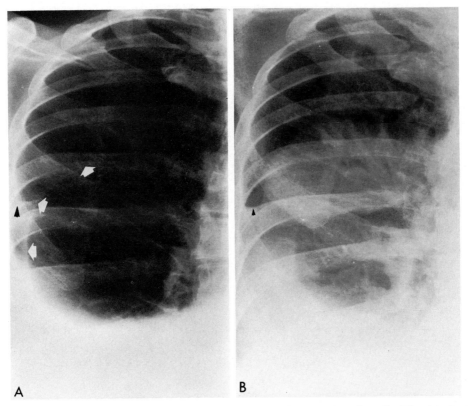

Figure 8–21. Pleural effusion. *A,* Upright portable radiograph demonstrates a large meniscus laterally. The right hemidiaphragm is not shown. Both the major *(white arrowhead)* and minor *(black arrowhead)* fissures are thickened. *B,* Supine radiograph demonstrates fluid trapped in both the major and minor fissures *(arrowhead).* The fluid delineates the upper extent of the major fissure. Note that the pulmonary vessels can be seen through the effusion.

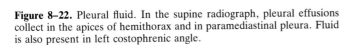

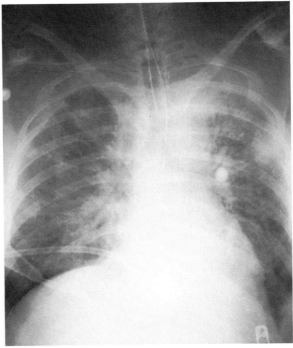

Figure 8–22. Pleural fluid. In the supine radiograph, pleural effusions collect in the apices of hemithorax and in paramediastinal pleura. Fluid is also present in left costophrenic angle.

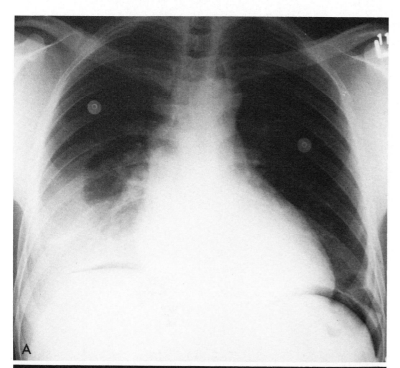

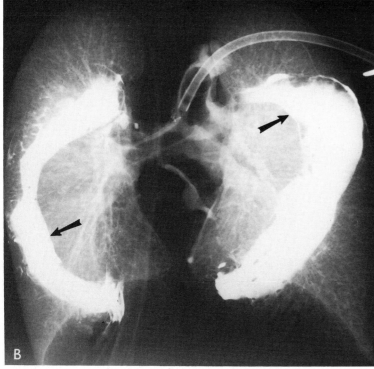

Figure 8–23. Incomplete fissure sign. *A,* Pneumoperitoneum and right hydrothorax after peritoneal dialysis. Fluid fills the lateral half of the major fissure, leaving a lucency medially. This radiographic appearance should not be confused with that of a bulla or cavity. (Courtesy of Dr. W.E. Dandy, Jr., Baltimore, MD.) *B,* Specimen radiograph of a different patient, with barium applied to the major fissures. The clear perihilar areas are due to an incomplete major fissure *(arrows).* (From Dandy, W.E.: Incomplete pulmonary interlobar fissure sign. Radiology 128:21–25, 1978, with permission.)

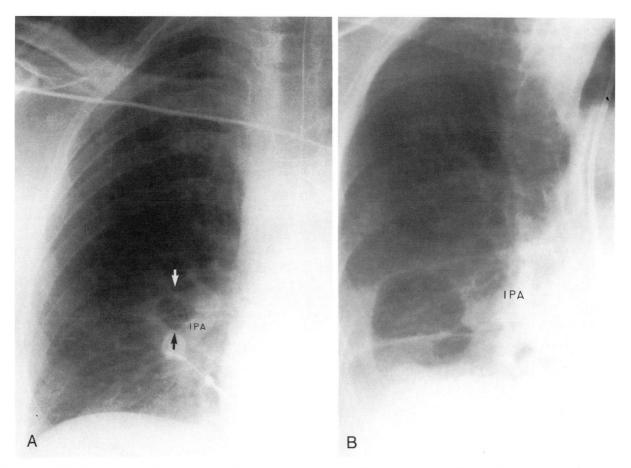

Figure 8–24. Fluid in incomplete fissures. *A,* Small lucency close to the right hilum represents fused lobes of lung surrounded by fluid in the incomplete fissures *(arrows). B,* In a different patient, a lucency simulating a lung lesion disappeared in a repeat radiograph in the sitting position. IPA, interlobar pulmonary artery.

common finding in ICU radiographs is the reorientation (Gross et al., 1988) of the fluid-filled incomplete fissures, which may result in an image simulating a lung cavity or pneumatocele. This "pseudocavity" is analogous to the pseudotumor. A repeated chest radiograph in the sitting or lateral decubitus position clarifies the nature of the finding, when the pseudocavity disappears and the pleural fluid becomes apparent (Fig. 8–24).

Several bedside maneuvers are available to confirm or rule out the presence of effusion. Decubitus radiographs in which the patient lies on a wooden board to prevent sagging can usually be obtained. Whenever possible, bilateral decubitus radiographs are obtained to rule out an unsuspected effusion on the opposite side. If the patient's condition or obesity precludes a decubitus position with the suspected side down, a radiograph obtained with the suspected side up may help differentiate pleural fluid from pleural thickening or lateral lower lobe infiltrate. If decubitus radiographs cannot be obtained, supine and erect radiographs may be obtained, demonstrating a generalized increased density on the supine film that disappears when the patient sits erect (see Figs. 8–20 and 8–21). A supine oblique radiograph may also demonstrate fluid between the lung and the lateral chest wall.

The totally immobilized patient and the individual with small effusions, massive effusions, and loculated collections may present diagnostic difficulties (Landay and Harless, 1977). Ultrasonography can readily detect free effusions and can locate loculated collections. Ultrasonographically guided thoracentesis greatly increases the chances of a successful tap of a local pleural pocket (Fig. 8–25); however, attempts to predict the likelihood of a successful tap based on the echogenicity of the focal collection have not been reliable. (Some echo-free collections do not yield fluid, whereas many complex collections do.) Thoracentesis under ultrasound guidance has one sixth of the pneumothorax rate of nonguided aspirations (Raptopoulos et al., 1991).

Computed tomography also graphically demonstrates the extent of the fluid, its loculations, and its relationship to other intrathoracic structures (Fig. 8–26) (see Figs. 5–11 and 5–12). Computed tomography has repeatedly demonstrated that portable radiographs grossly underestimate the amount of effusion. Ultrasonography is superior to computed tomography for demonstrating internal loculations.

Hydropneumothorax accounts for the dense appearance of certain pneumothoraces on supine radiographs. The pleural line is obliterated where only

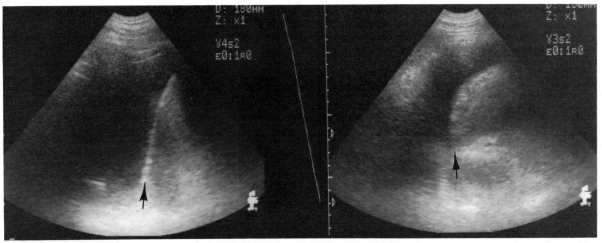

Figure 8–25. Pleural effusion. Fluid is seen above the diaphragm *(arrow)* on the longitudinal and transverse ultrasound images.

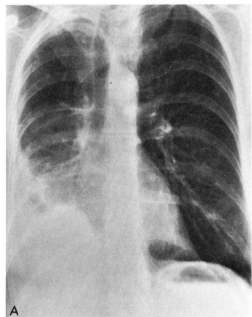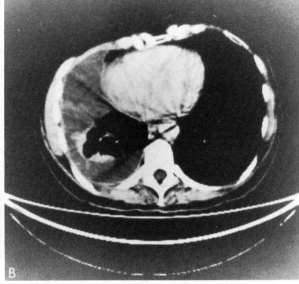

Figure 8–26. Loculated effusion. This patient with ovarian carcinoma developed an unexplained fever. Pneumonia was suspected clinically. *A,* Chest radiograph shows a definite right-sided effusion. A parenchymal process could not be excluded. Decubitus film did not demonstrate clearing of the right lower lobe. *B,* The CT scan demonstrates a loculated effusion at the base. Except for some minimal peripheral atelectasis, no parenchymal abnormality was demonstrated. The effusion was tapped and proved to be a sterile transudate. The fever eventually diminished without additional therapy.

fluid exists, becoming apparent at a point where the air and fluid separate, higher in the hemithorax. If the pleural effusion is sufficiently large, the pleural line may never become sufficiently visible, making the diagnosis of pneumothorax difficult. The absence of lung markings and visualization of the collapsed lung should be valuable clues. Decubitus and oblique radiographs are especially helpful when hydropneumothorax is suspected.

References

Andrew, T.A., and Milne, D.D.: Pneumoperitoneum associated with pneumothorax or pneumopericardium: A surgical dilemma in the injured patient. Injury 11:65, 1980.

Avery, M.E.: The Lung and Its Disorders in the Newborn Infant. Philadelphia, W.B. Saunders, 1968, p. 187.

Bernard, R.W., Stahl, W.M., and Chase, R.M.: Subclavian vein catheterizations: A prospective study. II. Infectious complications. Ann. Surg. 173:191, 1971.

Bone, R.C.: Complication of mechanical ventilation and positive end-expiratory pressure. Resp. Care 27:402, 1982.

Bone, R.C., Francis, P.B., and Pierce, A.K.: Pulmonary barotrauma complicating positive end-expiratory pressure. Am. Rev. Respir. Dis. 113:921, 1976.

Broadbent, J.C., Callahan, J.A., Kincaid, O.W., et al.: Congenital deficiency of the pericardium. Dis. Chest 50:237, 1966.

Campbell, R.E.: Intrapulmonary interstitial emphysema: A complication of hyaline membrane disease. AJR 110:449, 1970.

Cimmino, C.V.: Some radio-diagnostic notes on pneumomediastinum, pneumothorax, and pneumopericardium. Va. Med. Mon. 94:205, 1967.

Cyrlak, D., Milne, E.N.C., and Imray, T.J.: Pneumomediastinum: A diagnostic problem. Crit. Rev. Diagn. Imaging 23:75, 1984.

Dandy, W.E.: Incomplete pulmonary fissure sign. Radiology 128:21, 1978.

Elyaderani, M., and Gabriele, O.F.: Traumatic paramediastinal air cyst. Br. J. Radiol. 52:458, 1979.

Fleischner, F.G.: Atypical arrangement of free pleural effusion. Radiol. Clin. North Am. 1:347, 1963.

Gattinoni, L., Pesenti, A., Mascheroni, D., et al.: Low-frequency positive-pressure ventilation with extracorporeal CO_2 removal in severe acute respiratory failure. JAMA 256:881, 1986.

Gobien, R.P., Reines, H.D., and Schabel, S.J.: Localized tension pneumothorax: Unrecognized form of barotrauma in adult respiratory distress syndrome. Radiology 142:15, 1982.

Goodman, L.R., Foley, W.D., Wilson, C.R., et al.: Pneumothorax and other lung diseases: Effect of altered resolution and edge enhancement on diagnosis with digitized radiographs. Radiology 167:83, 1988.

Gordon, R.: The deep sulcus sign. Radiology 136:25, 1980.

Greene, R., McLoud, T.C., and Stark, P.: Pneumothorax. Semin. Roentgenol. 12:313, 1977.

Grosfeld, J.L., Kilman, J.W., and Frye, T.R.: Spontaneous pneumopericardium in the newborn infant. J. Pediatr. 76:614, 1970.

Gross, B.H., Spizarny, D.L., and Granke, D.S.: Sagittal orientation of the anterior minor fissure. Radiography and CT Radiology 166:1988.

Hammond, D.I.: The "ring-around-the-artery" sign in pneumomediastinum. Can. Assoc. Radiol. J. 35:88, 1984.

Heitzman, E.R.: The Lung: Radiologic-Pathologic Correlations. St. Louis, C.V. Mosby, 1984, p. 50.

Hoffer, F.A., and Ablow, R.C.: The cross-table lateral view in neonatal pneumothorax. AJR 142:1283, 1984.

Johnson, T.H., and Altman, A.R.: Pulmonary interstitial gas: First sign of barotrauma due to PEEP therapy. Crit. Care Med. 7:532, 1979.

Kassner, E.G., Baumstark, A., Balsam, D., and Haller, J.O.: Passage of feeding catheters into the pleural space: A radiographic sign of trauma to the pharynx and esophagus in the newborn. AJR 128:19, 1977.

Kurlander, G.J., and Helmen, C.H.: Subpulmonary pneumothorax. AJR 96:1019, 1966.

Lain, D.C., Dibenedetto, R., Morris, S.L., et al.: Pressure control inverse ratio ventilation as a method to reduce peak inspiratory pressure and provide adequate ventilation and oxygenation. Chest 95:1081, 1989.

Lams, P.M., and Jolles, H.: The effect of lobar collapse on the distribution of free intrapleural air. Radiology 142:309, 1982.

Landay, M., and Harless, W.: Ultrasonic differentiation of right pleural effusion from subphrenic fluid on longitudinal scans of the right upper quadrant: Importance of recognizing the diaphragm. Radiology 123:155, 1977.

Lane, E.F., Proto, A.V., and Phillips, T.W.: Mach bands and density perception. Radiology 121:9, 1976.

Latorre, F.J., Tomasa, A., Klamburg, J., et al.: Incidence of pneumothorax and pneumomediastinum in patients with aspiration pneumonia requiring ventilatory support. Chest 72:141, 1977.

Leeming, B.W.A.: Radiological aspects of pulmonary complications resulting from intermittent positive pressure ventilation (IPPV). Australas. Radiol. 12:361, 1968.

Levin, B.: The continuous diaphragm sign. Clin. Radiol. 24:337, 1973.

Levine, M.S., Scheiner, J.D., Rubesin, S.E., et al.: Diagnosis of pneumoperitoneum on supine abdominal radiographs. AJR 156:731, 1991.

Lewandowski, B.J., and Winsberg, F.: Sonographic demonstration of the right paramediastinal pleural space. Radiology 145:127, 1982.

Light, R.W., and George, R.B.: Incidence and significance of pleural effusions after abdominal surgery. Chest 69:621, 1976.

Macklin, M.I., and Macklin, C.C.: Malignant interstitial emphysema of the lungs and mediastinum as important occult complication in many respiratory diseases and other conditions: Interpretation of clinical literature in light of laboratory experiment. Medicine 23:281, 1944.

Markowitz, R.I.: The anterior junction line: A radiographic sign of bilateral pneumothorax in neonates. Radiology 167:717, 1988.

McLoud, T.C., Barash, P.G., and Ravin, C.E.: PEEP: Radiographic features and associated complications. AJR 129:209, 1977.

Moskowitz, P.S., and Griscom, N.T.: The medial pneumothorax. Radiology 120:143, 1976.

Naclerio, E.A.: The "V-sign" in the diagnosis of spontaneous rupture of the esophagus (an early Roentgen clue). Am. J. Surg. 93:291, 1957.

Nash, G., Blennerhassett, J.B., and Pontoppidan, H.: Pulmonary lesions associated with oxygen therapy and artificial ventilation. N. Engl. J. Med. 276:368, 1967.

Nightingale, R.C., and Flower, D.R.: Encysted pneumothorax: A complication of asthma. Br. J. Dis. Chest 78:98, 1984.

Ovenfors, C.: Pulmonary interstitial emphysema. Acta Radiol. Suppl. (Stockh.) 224:1, 1964.

Ovenfors, C., and Hedgcock, M.W.: Intensive care unit radiology problems of interpretation. Radiol. Clin. North Am. 16:407, 1979.

Pasternak, G.S., and O'Cain, C.F.: Thoracic complications of respiratory intensive care. In Herman, P.G. (ed.): Iatrogenic Thoracic Complications. New York, Springer-Verlag, 1983, p. 66.

Pratt, P.C.: Pathology of adult respiratory distress syndrome: Implications regarding therapy. Semin. Respir. Med. 4:79, 1982.

Proto, A.V., and Tocino, I.: Radiographic manifestations of lobar collapse. Semin. Roentgenol. 15:117, 1980.

Raasch, B.N., Carsky, E.W., Lane, E.J., et al.: Pleural effusion: Explanation of some typical appearances. AJR 139:899, 1982a.

Raasch, B.N., Carsky, E.W., Lane, E.J., et al.: Radiographic anatomy of the interlobar fissures: A study of 100 specimens. AJR 138:1043, 1982b.

Raptopoulos, V., Davis, L.M., Lee, G., et al.: Factors affecting the development of pneumothorax associated with thoracentesis. AJR 156:917, 1991.

Reid, L.: The connective tissue septa in the adult human lung. Thorax 14:138, 1959.

Rhea, J.T., Van Sonnemberg, E., and McLoud, T.C.: Basilar pneumothorax in the supine adult. Radiology 133:593, 1979.

Rohlfing, B., Webb, W., and Schlobohm, R.: Ventilator-related extra-alveolar air in adults. Radiology 121:25, 1976.

Ruskin, J.A., Gurney, J.W., Thorsen, M.K., and Goodman, L.R.: Detection of pleural effusions on supine chest radiographs. AJR 148:681, 1987.

Sagel, S.S., Wimbush, P., and Goldberg, D.: Tension pneumopericardium following assisted ventilation in hyaline membrane disease. Radiology 107:175, 1973.

Shapiro, M.P., and Gerzof, S.G.: Oxygen reservoir rebreathing mask simulating pneumothorax. Radiology 164:743, 1987.

Sherman, M., Levin, D., and Breidbart, D.: *Pneumocystis carinii* pneumonia with spontaneous pneumothorax: A report of three cases. Chest 90:609, 1986.

Spizarny, D.L., and Goodman, L.R.: Air in the minor fissure: A sign of right-sided pneumothorax. Radiology 160:329, 1986.

Steier, M., Ching, N., Roberts, E.B., and Nealon, T.F.: Pneumothorax complicating continuous ventilatory support. J. Thorac. Cardiovasc. Surg. 67:17, 1974.

Switzer, P., Pitman, R.G., and Fleming, J.P.: Pneumomediastinum associated with zypornetico-maxillary fracture. J. Can. Assoc. Radiol. 25:316, 1976.

Tocino, I.M.: Pneumothorax in the supine patient: Radiographic anatomy. Radiographics 5:557, 1985.

Tocino, I., and Armstrong, J.D.: Trauma to the lung. In Taveras, J.M., and Ferrocci, J.T. (eds.): Radiology Diagnosis-Imaging-Intervention. Philadelphia, J.B. Lippincott, 1988.

Tocino, I., and Miller, M.H.: Computed tomography in blunt chest trauma. J. Thorac. Imaging 2:45, 1987.

Tocino, I.M., and Watanabe, A.: Impending catheter perforation of superior vena cava: Radiographic recognition. AJR 146:487, 1986.

Tocino, I.M., Miller, M.H., and Fairfax, W.R.: Distribution of pneumothorax in the supine and semirecumbent critically ill adult. AJR 144:901, 1985.

Tocino, I.M., Miller, M.H., Frederick, P.R., et al.: CT detection of occult pneumothorax in head trauma. AJR 143:987, 1984.

Toomey, F.B., and Chinnock, R.F.: Subcutaneous emphysema, pneumomediastinum and pneumothorax in diabetic ketoacidosis. Radiology 116:543, 1975.

Volberg, F.M., Everett, C.J., and Brill, P.: Radiologic features of inferior pulmonary ligament air collections in neonates with respiratory distress. Radiology 130:357, 1979.

Wall, S.D., Federle, M.P., Jeffrey, R.B., and Brett, C.M.: CT diagnosis of unsuspected pneumothorax after blunt abdominal trauma. AJR 141:919, 1983.

Westcott, J.L., and Cole, S.R.: Interstitial pulmonary emphysema in children and adults: Roentgenographic features. Radiology 111:367, 1974.

Westcott, J.L., and Cole, S.: Barotrauma. In Herman, P.G. (ed.): Iatrogenic Thoracic Complications. New York, Springer-Verlag, 1983, p. 79.

Wiener-Kronish, J.P., and Matthay, M.A.: Pleural effusions associated with hydrostatic and increased permeability pulmonary edema. Chest 94:852, 1988.

Woodall, B.H., Winfield, D.F., and Bisset, G.S.: Inadvertent tracheobronchial placement of feeding tubes. Radiology 165:727, 1987.

Woodring, J.H.: Recognition of pleural effusion on supine radiographs: How much fluid is required? AJR 142:59, 1984.

Woodring, J.H.: Pulmonary interstitial emphysema in the adult respiratory distress syndrome. Crit. Care Med. 13:199, 1985.

Yamashita, H.: Roentgenologic Anatomy of the Lung. Tokyo, Igaku-Shoin, 1978, p. 49.

Ziter, F.M.H., Jr., and Westcott, J.L.: Supine subpulmonary pneumothorax. AJR 137:699, 1981.

Zwilich, C.W., Pierson, D.J., Creagh, C.E., et al.: Complications of assisted ventilation: A prospective study of 354 consecutive episodes. Am. J. Med. 57:161, 1974.

9

Pulmonary Embolism

■

Jud W. Gurney

*"This unsatisfactory state of affairs in a disease where
proper treatment offers a fair chance should prompt us to
improve our diagnostic acumen, and in particular, we
radiologists should take stock of how much we may
contribute to the correct diagnosis."*

(FLEISCHNER, 1962)

The topic of pulmonary embolism has stirred considerable confusion and controversy (Robin, 1977; Seckler-Walker, 1983). This circumstance is unfortunate, as pulmonary embolism is a common, serious, and potentially fatal condition that both clinicians and radiologists have a great deal of difficulty in diagnosing. *Pulmonary embolism has no telltale clinical signs, symptoms, or laboratory findings that strongly suggest its diagnosis* (Alderson and Martin, 1987; Sostman et al., 1986). Thus, the radiologist has a central role in the evaluation of patients suspected of having venous thromboemboli. Although the medical literature concerning pulmonary emboli is enormous, the evolution of medical and technologic progress in the diagnosis of pulmonary thromboembolism can be traced by a few landmark articles (Alderson et al., 1976; Biello et al., 1979a; Hampton and Castelman, 1940; Hull et al., 1983; Hull et al., 1985; McNeil et al., 1974; McNeil, 1980; PIOPED, 1990; Robin, 1977; UPET, 1970; Virchow, 1860; Wagner et al., 1964; Wagner et al., 1968; Westermark, 1938; Williams et al., 1963) (Fig. 9–1). Clearly, this important topic will continue to evolve in the 1990s.

One of the most important conceptual advances in the topic of pulmonary embolism is the recognition that pulmonary embolism itself is not a disease; rather, embolism is the end result of venous thrombosis (Hull et el., 1983; Hull et al., 1985; Moser, 1990). Although emboli may arise from nearly any vein, the overwhelming majority of thrombi arise in deep veins of the lower extremities (Havig, 1977; Hull et al., 1983; Sevitt and Gallagher, 1961).

SCOPE OF THE PROBLEM

Pulmonary embolism is the third most common cause of death (Rosenow et al., 1981). According to an alarming estimate, 90% of patients survive an initial embolic event but are undiagnosed two thirds of the time (Bell et al., 1977; Dalen and Alpert, 1975; Rosenow et al., 1981). These undiagnosed patients have a high rate of recurrent emboli and may die. Barker (1958) observed that untreated pulmonary emboli in postoperative patients were associated with a 33% chance of recurrence and an 18% chance of a fatal outcome. Anticoagulation is effective in decreasing the morbidity and mortality associated with thromboembolism but is not innocuous. Hemorrhagic complications of long-term anticoagulation range from 2% to 15% (Cheely et al., 1981).

PATHOPHYSIOLOGY

Deep Vein Thrombosis

The origin of a pulmonary embolus is a thrombus, usually from the deep veins of the leg or pelvis. In 1860, Virchow identified three factors responsible for thrombosis: stasis of blood, intimal injury, and a hypercoagulable state (Virchow, 1860). The most important factor is venous stasis, particularly that resulting from immobilization. The risk of embolization depends on the location and character of the thrombus. Distal thrombi are less likely to embolize than are thrombi more proximally located. Moreno-Cabral and colleagues (1976) reported lung scan evidence of pulmonary embolus in 30% of patients with calf vein thrombosis, 50% of those with popliteal vein thrombosis, and 66% of those with superficial femoral vein thrombosis. The character of the thrombus also determines the risk of embolization. Norris and as-

LANDMARK INVESTIGATIONS OF PULMONARY EMBOLISM

Virchow	1860	Pathogenesis of venous thromboemboli
Westermark	1938	Roentgen diagnosis of pulmonary embolus
Hampton and Castelman	1940	Pathology of pulmonary infarct
Williams et al.	1963	Angiography of pulmonary embolus
Wagner et al.	1964	Radioisotope scanning in pulmonary embolus
Wagner et al.	1968	Xenon scanning in pulmonary embolus
	1970	UPET
McNeil et al.	1974	Scintigraphic definition of pulmonary embolus
Alderson et al.	1976	Role of ventilation studies
Robin	1977	Overdiagnosis and overtreatment of pulmonary embolism
Biello et al.	1979–1980	Probability classification
Hull et al.	1983–1985	Prospective study of ventilation–perfusion scans
	1990	PIOPED
????		????

Figure 9–1. Landmark articles tracing chronologically the important developments in thromboembolic disease. UPET, Urokinase Pulmonary Embolism Trial; PIOPED, Prospective Investigation of Pulmonary Embolism Diagnosis.

sociates (1985) found that patients with free-floating (nonadherent) iliofemoral thrombi are much more prone to develop symptomatic pulmonary emboli than are patients with occlusive (adherent) thrombi. Embolization occurred in 60% (3/5) of the patients with free-floating thrombi, but in only 5.5% (4/73) of the patients with adherent thrombi.

Pulmonary Embolus

The pathophysiologic consequences of blockage of a pulmonary artery by an embolus are of two types: respiratory and hemodynamic (Moser, 1977). Major respiratory consequences include (1) persistent ventilation of nonperfused lung (alveolar dead space), (2) a transient, reflex volume reduction in the zone of embolized lung, and (3) loss of alveolar surfactant (Moser, 1977). The hemodynamic consequences of an embolus are related to the reduction in pulmonary vascular cross-sectional area (Moser, 1977). When more than 50% of the pulmonary vascular bed is occluded, pulmonary hypertension and right heart failure occur.

Commonly, the embolized lung maintains normal ventilation, but local ventilatory changes in the lung may occur. They complicate the interpretation of ventilation-perfusion studies. The acute blockage of a pulmonary artery may produce a decrease in ventilation by three mechanisms: (1) alveolar hypocapnic constriction of airways in the affected lung, (2) embolic induced release of bronchoconstrictor substances such as serotonin; and (3) reduction in surfactant. Acute ventilatory defects accompanying emboli have been demonstrated experimentally but are considered rare in clinical practice (Alderson et al., 1978; Kessler and McNeil, 1975). The reasons for their uncommon observation are unknown. Because the acute ventilatory response is transient, ventilation may have returned to a normal rate by the time the patient is scanned, or perhaps the hypoventilation is not detected, owing to the poor resolution of older xenon agents used to study the distribution of ventilation (Arborelius et al., 1985; Seckler-Walker, 1983).

CLINICAL MANIFESTATIONS

The clinical signs and symptoms of pulmonary embolism are neither sensitive nor specific. Patients with emboli may die suddenly or be completely asymptomatic. Silent embolization, in fact, may be a normal protective mechanism (Dorfman et al., 1987; Moreno-Cabral et al., 1976). Because the lungs are interposed between the venous and arterial circuits, they filter out small particulate materials from the blood that would embolize to the brain, kidneys, or heart if allowed into the arterial system. Of those patients having symptoms, dyspnea and pleuritic chest pain are most common, occurring in 81% and 72% respectively, of all individuals in the Urokinase Pulmonary Embolism Trial (UPET) study (1970). The most frequent sign of pulmonary emboli is tachypnea, which occurs in 81% of patients.

Multiple factors predispose a patient to the development of deep vein thrombosis and pulmonary embolism (Bell and Simon, 1982). These factors include a wide diversity of surgical and medical conditions, such as congestive heart failure, recent myocardial infarction, malignant disease, shock, obesity, pregnancy, and recent surgery, especially after major abdominal, thoracic, pelvic, or orthopedic procedures. Patients sustaining major trauma are also at high risk. In addition, thromboembolism is a common complication of polycythemia vera, the dysproteinemias, antithrombin-III deficiency, and the use of birth control pills. Ninety-four percent of the patients with documented emboli in the UPET study had one or more recognized predisposing conditions (Bell et al., 1977). The single most important risk factor, however, is a prior pulmonary embolus.

Seventy percent of patients with angiographically proven pulmonary emboli have proximal deep vein thrombosis (Hull et al., 1983). Unfortunately, the clinical diagnosis of deep vein thrombosis is also unreliable. Bounameaux and associates (1982) found that only half of the patients with clinically suspected thrombosis had the diagnosis confirmed by venography. Cranley and colleagues (1976) tabulated the clinical symptoms and signs of deep vein thrombosis in a group of 124 patients with 133 lower extremities suspected of harboring deep vein thrombosis. Clinical symptoms and signs of muscle pain, swelling, and tenderness, and Homan's sign were found to occur with approximately equal frequency in those limbs with and without deep vein thrombosis (see Chapter 16).

DIAGNOSIS

The goal of any imaging evaluation is direct visualization of the clot, whether it is in the deep venous system of the leg, or in the branches of the pulmonary arteries. This goal is obtained only at some cost of invasive testing. Until our diagnostic tools improve, we are left with a situation in which many of our noninvasive imaging techniques are able to visualize only the secondary effects of the clot, such as decreased perfusion in the lung, or absence of flow in deep veins of the leg.

IMAGING OF PULMONARY EMBOLISM

Chest Radiography

"In lung embolism without infarction the embolic lung area appeared anemic and pale besides being aerated. It is wedge-shaped, the apex being directed towards the hilum and the base towards the pleura."

(WESTERMARK, 1938)

The chest radiograph is the first level of investigation, although its sensitivity and specificity are low. Chest radiographs are, however, useful to screen out conditions that may clinically mimic pulmonary emboli, such as pneumothorax or pneumonia, and they are crucial to the proper interpretation of the ventilation-perfusion study. In fact, lung scans must be interpreted with current high-quality chest radiographs.

The majority of patients with pulmonary emboli have an abnormal chest radiograph. Moses and co-workers found that over 90% of patients with angiographically documented acute pulmonary emboli had some abnormality appearing on chest radiographs (Table 9–1). Unfortunately, these signs are nonspecific and are found in a wide variety of disorders. Curiously, a normal chest radiograph is more apt to be found in patients who have had a massive central embolus than in those with a small embolus.

Greenspan and colleagues (1982) studied the accuracy of chest radiographs for the diagnosis of pulmonary embolism. Single radiographs were reviewed independently by nine readers, who were asked, "Does this patient have pulmonary embolism?" A large number of radiographic signs were evaluated, including consolidation, atelectasis, Hampton's hump, a long-line shadow, pleural effusion, elevation of a hemidiaphragm, plump hilar vessels, focal oligemia, pulmonary hypertension, right ventricular or

Table 9–1. CHEST RADIOGRAPHIC FINDINGS IN PULMONARY EMBOLISM

Findings	Moses et al., 1974 (41 patients)	Bynum and Wilson, 1976 (155 patients)
Normal radiograph	7%	12%
Consolidation	54%	13%
Pleural effusion	51%	18%
Atelectasis	27%	6%
Elevated hemidiaphragm	17%	16%
Focal oligemia	2%	
Cardiomegaly/congestive heart failure	17%	<6%
Pulmonary arterial hypertension	5%	<6%
Two or more signs	44%	35%
Other		16%

left ventricular enlargement, and left atrial or right atrial enlargement. The sensitivity (true positive ratio) of the chest radiograph was poor, only 33%, while the specificity (true negative ratio) was 59%. The predictive index, which indicated the accuracy of the diagnosis was 40%, which is less than what would be expected by chance. The study did not include old radiographs for comparison, which are particularly important in evaluating such signs as enlargement of a hilar vessel or the detection of focal oligemia.

Vascular Alterations

One would expect vascular alterations in the lung to be common because emboli lodge in the pulmonary arteries. Unfortunately, they are uncommon. A central clot may enlarge and distort the normal contour of the pulmonary artery. This distortion is easier to recognize on the right side than on the left side. This sign is due not to pulmonary hypertension, but rather to the physical presence of the clot. On the right, the enlarged interlobar pulmonary artery often resembles a "knuckle" (Fig. 9–2). Palla and associates (1983) found that one quarter of their patients with acute embolism had this sausage-shaped appearance on the radiograph. Blood flow is markedly diminished in the peripheral arteries if the more proximal vessels are obstructed by a clot. This focal oligemia was first recognized by Westermark in 1938. This sign is infrequently identified, and detection requires previous high-quality films for comparison (Fig. 9–3).

Pleural Effusion

Pleural effusions are common in patients with pulmonary emboli. In one study, pleural effusions were seen in 51% of patients with pulmonary embolism and were thought to be directly related to embolic episodes in 40% (Bynum and Wilson, 1978). Pleural effusions were distributed equally between the right and left sides, and 5% of these patients had bilateral effusions. Those patients having pulmonary infarcts had larger and more persistent effusions than those

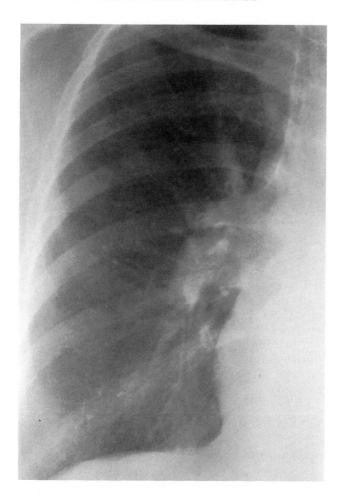

Figure 9–2. Knuckle sign. Enlarged sausage-shaped right pulmonary artery causes suspicion of an embolic episode.

without infarcts. Typically, effusions were maximal on the initial chest radiograph or within the first 3 days after the embolus was found. Only two patients (3%) had effusions that enlarged beyond the third day after admission. One of these patients had recurrent pulmonary emboli, and the other developed suppurative infection with empyema. In an additional two patients (3%) whose effusions were originally unilateral, a new contralateral pleural effusion appeared within 1 week after admission. Both patients had recurrent pulmonary emboli indicated by recurrence of symptoms and new lung scan defects. Although patients with infarcts are commonly expected to have pleural effusions, one third of patients with infarcts had no demonstrable pleural effusion (Bynum and Wilson, 1978).

Pulmonary Infarct

"The pulmonary infarct is a signal of a past embolic event. Treatment is directed to preventing further embolic episodes."

(FLEISCHNER, 1962)

In 1940, Hampton and Castleman initiated an ambitious project correlating postmortem radiographs with pathologic specimens. Fresh cadavers were suspended by a harness in the upright position to inflate the lungs, which were then fixed and correlated with the radiographic abnormalities. The authors clearly noted that infarcts come in a wide variety of shapes and appearances; however, the classic infarct has been repeatedly described in the literature as a wedge-shaped homogeneous opacity abutting the pleural edge with a hump-shaped apex pointing back toward the hilum (Fig. 9–4A). Unfortunately, an infarct having this appearance of Hampton's hump is unusual, and if one thought of infarcts only in these terms, the majority of lesions would be missed. In fact, Heitzman and associates (1972) have shown that infarcts have no predictable configuration, and that their differentiation from pneumonia or pulmonary edema is often impossible.

Approximately 10% of pulmonary thromboembolic episodes result in infarction (McCartney, 1981). Infarcts are uncommon because the lung has three routes of oxygen supply: (1) through the pulmonary artery, (2) through the bronchial arteries, and (3) through the airways. Also, infarcts are uncommon in the absence of underlying impairment—for instance, that due to chronic obstructive lung disease or heart disease. The location of an embolus within the pulmonary artery also determines the likelihood of infarction. Infarcts are more likely to occur with peripheral emboli than with emboli that are more centrally located. McNeil and colleagues (1974) found that only four of 120 patients with lobar or whole

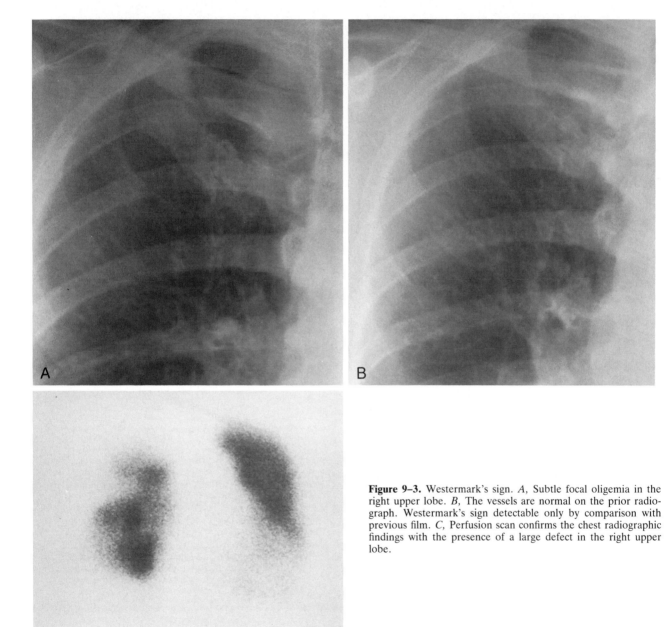

Figure 9–3. Westermark's sign. *A,* Subtle focal oligemia in the right upper lobe. *B,* The vessels are normal on the prior radiograph. Westermark's sign detectable only by comparison with previous film. *C,* Perfusion scan confirms the chest radiographic findings with the presence of a large defect in the right upper lobe.

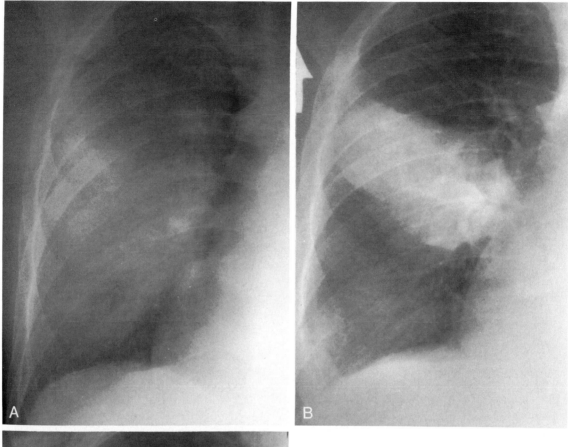

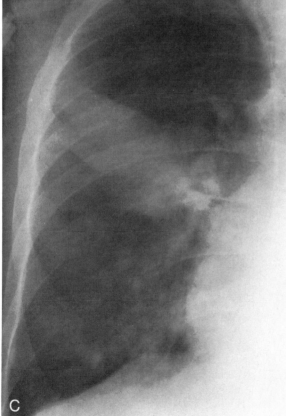

Figure 9–4. Pulmonary infarct. *A,* Sudden appearance of a homogeneous opacity in the middle of right lung. The edge is indistinct. Whether this abnormality is peripheral or central is not evident. The opacity is neither wedge-shaped nor humped. *B,* Six days later, the infarct is much more sharply defined, and the overall shape remains the same. *C,* Resolving infarct 21 days later. The infarct is melting. Note that the overall shape remains the same, as the infarct resolves from the outside in.

lung perfusion defects had associated roentgeno-graphic findings in the region of the perfusion defect, while 20 of 37 patients with segmental, subsegmental, or nonsegmental defects had associated abnormalities. This paradoxical observation is explained by the bronchial artery circulation, which provides collateral flow centrally but not peripherally (Dalen et al., 1977).

Some confusion exists regarding the use of the word infarct. Some use the word to describe any pulmonary opacity on a radiograph due to an embolus, while others use a stricter definition that reflects pathologic death of tissue (Fraser et al., 1990). The developing infarct represents both edema and hemorrhage (incomplete infarct) in aggregates of secondary pulmonary lobules. The incomplete infarct cannot be differentiated radiographically from actual tissue necrosis. Rarely does an infarct undergo liquification necrosis and cavitation. Infarcts vary in size from being barely visible to covering an entire lobe (Jacoby and Mindell, 1976). After embolization, a time lag of 12 to 24 hours often occurs before an opacity develops on the roentgenogram (Fleischner, 1962). At this point, the opacity is an ill-defined area of consolidation in the periphery of the lung, which over 2 to 4 days progresses to a more complete well-demarcated consolidated infarct (see Fig. 9–4B). This timing is only general, however, and there may be no time lag between embolization and infarction; conversely, an infarct may not develop for 1 week. Infarcts are more common in the lower lobes because of the greater perfusion to the lower lobes in the erect position. Infarcts are more common on the right side than on the left side, which reflects the greater volume in the right lower lobe and is perhaps also due to partial obscuration of the basilar segments of the left lower lobe by the opacity of the heart.

The resolution of roentgenographic pulmonary infarcts is variable. McGoldrick and co-workers (1979) studied 58 infarcts mostly drawn from patients in the UPET study. Infarcts cleared completely in 29 patients (50%), while 14 patients developed linear scars, nine formed pleural diaphragmatic adhesions, and six developed localized pleural thickening. Woesner and colleagues (1971) found that infarcts generally resolve from the outside in, in a manner analogous to that of a melting ice cube, which is in contrast to other pulmonary conditions, such as pneumonia or edema, which fade or resolve in a random manner throughout (see Fig. 9–3C). In pulmonary infarcts, the dead tissue lacks blood supply, and therefore the reparative process must begin at the periphery and work toward the center (melt), whereas in other acute inflammatory processes, such as pneumonia, which have a preserved blood supply, the entire involved area resolves at the same time (fades). The melting pattern is not specific for pulmonary infarction; the same pattern is found in the fibrotic organization of some pneumonias (Hendin, 1975).

Serial chest radiographs may be useful for evaluating patients suspected of having a pulmonary embolus. Vix (1983) found that 1 to 3 days after the onset of acute symptoms the appearance of a new radiographic opacity in a region of a perfusion scan defect was strongly associated with the presence of pulmonary embolus. This new opacity was found in 10 of 38 patients after an average interval of nearly 2 days (range: 4 hours to 5 days). Confirmation by angiography was available for five patients, and all five had pulmonary embolus. Certainly, the usefulness of this sign needs to be expanded to a larger patient population. Obtaining follow-up chest radiographs is not a common practice, however—nearly half of the patients in Vix's study did not receive follow-up studies. In two (9%) of the 23 patients with negative pulmonary angiograms, the appearance of a parenchymal opacity on the chest radiograph prompted a review of the pulmonary arteriogram, which revealed that pulmonary emboli had been missed—that is, pulmonary angiography yielded false-negative results (Vix, 1983).

The fact that a patient with a pulmonary embolus may have a normal chest radiograph cannot be overemphasized (Fig. 9–5). Some make the mistake of discounting the likelihood of emboli when the chest radiograph is normal. Davis and associates (1986) found that clinicians were more likely to wait until the chest radiograph became abnormal before requesting a ventilation-perfusion study. This strategy is counterproductive because not only does it delay the ultimate diagnosis, but the delay complicates the interpretation of the ventilation-perfusion scan and may turn a potential high probability scan into an indeterminate one.

Ventilation-Perfusion Scanning

Perfusion

The most sensitive examination for the detection of pulmonary emboli is perfusion scanning. In fact, a normal perfusion scan eliminates the diagnosis of pulmonary emboli. No case has been reported of a patient with a normal perfusion scan subsequently having a documented pulmonary embolus (Royal, 1989). Unfortunately, an embolus is only one of many disorders that can cause perfusion defects in the lung (Table 9–2). Differentiating an embolus from these other disorders is a tremendous challenge.

Table 9–2. NONEMBOLIC CAUSES OF
VENTILATION-PERFUSION DEFECTS

Emphysema
Congestive heart failure
Lung cancer
Pneumonia
Atelectasis
Pneumothorax
Elevated diaphragm
Asthma
Radiation therapy
Cardiomegaly
Pleural effusion
Bronchiectasis

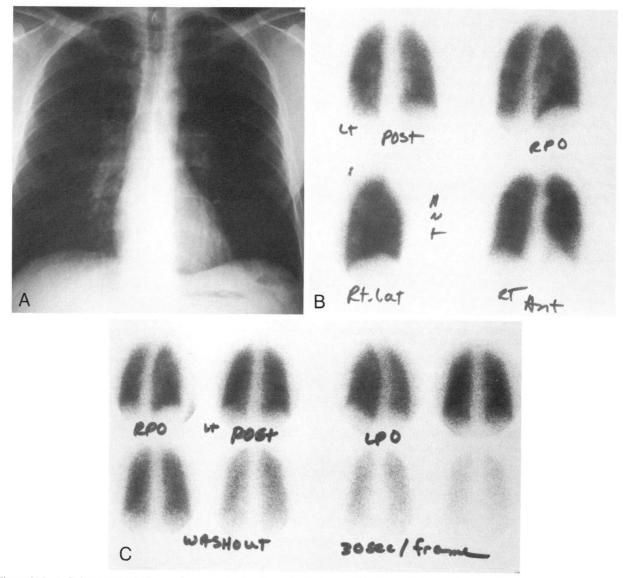

Figure 9–5. *A,* Pulmonary embolism and normal chest radiograph. Perhaps nothing in medicine can be so vexing as a patient in such dire straits with a normal radiograph. In general, the larger the embolus, the more likely it is that the result of the chest x-ray study is normal. *B,* The perfusion scan demonstrates multiple segmental defects. *C,* The ventilation scan appears normal.

Much of the confusion and controversy concerning the diagnosis of pulmonary embolism resolves around the role of ventilation-perfusion scanning (Robin, 1977). The confusion is due to the inherent limitations of a test that visualizes only the secondary effects of the clot rather than the clot itself. Nevertheless, ventilation-perfusion scanning has had a tremendous impact on patient management (Dismuke and Wagner, 1986; Mercandetti et al., 1985; Patton, 1985; Saenger et al., 1985).

When a clot breaks off from the deep veins of the leg and travels to the lung, it fragments in the right side of the heart, showering the lung with emboli that vary in size. An average of greater than eight vessels were embolized in the UPET data. Multiple (more than two) segmental or larger defects in perfusion should theoretically indicate pulmonary embolism; however, this observation does not carry even an

80% chance of being correct because perfusion defects are commonly found in a wide variety of other nonembolic disorders (Alderson et al., 1976; Poulose et al., 1968). Major perfusion defects may even be normal. Tetalman and colleagues (1973) found major perfusion defects in 5% of asymptomatic volunteers with normal chest radiographs. Although the specificity of perfusion scanning is poor, the clinical sensitivity for the detection of pulmonary embolism is 100%. Interestingly, the sensitivity of perfusion scans is actually less than that found experimentally. In dogs, the sensitivity of perfusion scans was 83% for detecting emboli that completely occlude pulmonary vessels, and 26% for partially occluding emboli (Alderson et al., 1978). Similarly, in humans, Arborelius and co-workers (1985) found that angiography demonstrated emboli in 10% of normally perfused lobes. Thus, in the majority of patients, the high sensitivity of perfusion scanning is due to the occurrence of multiple emboli, at least one of which gives rise to a perfusion defect.

Somewhat paradoxically, the detection of pulmonary emboli by perfusion scanning requires the embolization of small particles that temporarily occlude the pulmonary vascular bed (Neumann et al., 1980; Sostman et al., 1986). Technetium macroaggregated albumin (^{99m}Tc MAA) is the standard radiopharmaceutical used to study lung perfusion. Injected particles (200,000 to 500,000 particles per study) range in diameter from 20 to 40 μm. At this dose, approximately 0.1% of pulmonary arterioles (normal 200 to 300 million) are occluded, and these usually do not result in significant physiologic effects. Although the safety margin (greater than 1000×) is large, two deaths have been reported in patients with severely diminished pulmonary vascular beds (Dworkin et al., 1966; Vincent et al., 1968).

Ventilation

Major attempts have been made over the last 20 years to increase the specificity of the perfusion scan for the diagnosis of pulmonary embolus. Wagner and associates (1968) and DeNardo and colleagues (1970) suggested that ventilation imaging, when combined with perfusion imaging, would improve the specificity of diagnosis of pulmonary embolus because ventilation is maintained in nonperfused segments of lung. Alderson and co-workers (1976) evaluated the added role of xenon ventilation studies and found that ventilation-perfusion imaging was more discriminant than perfusion studies alone.

Whereas perfusion scanning is an established procedure, the proper agent and the proper method for performing a ventilation study remains controversial. The ideal ventilation agent is readily available and inexpensive, and is transportable to the intensive care unit for portable studies without contaminating the surrounding environment. The ideal study would be performed after perfusion scanning. If results of the perfusion scan are normal, then the ventilation scan need not be performed, which spares the patient the extra radiation exposure and expense. The physical characteristics of the ideal ventilatory agent should be such that its detection should not be degraded by technetium-99m (^{99m}Tc) used for the perfusion study. All phases of ventilation—inhalation, equilibrium, and exhalation—should be studied. Given the aforementioned preconditions, all currently available agents appear to have positive and negative features (Table 9–3).

Retrospective Studies

In the 1970s, investigators retrospectively evaluated the ventilation-perfusion scan patterns in patients who were proved to have pulmonary emboli by angiography. From this evaluation arose the concept of classifying scan patterns as high-probability, indeterminate, low-probability, or negative (normal) for pulmonary embolus.

Initially, the categorization of scan patterns was quite simple. For a segmental or greater perfusion defect with normal ventilation (mismatch), a high probability for pulmonary embolus was noted. For defects less than a segment, the probability for pulmonary embolus was either indeterminate or low, depending on the ventilation scan pattern (McNeil et al., 1974, 1976). Subsequent studies refined the scan categories by (1) using segmental equivalents, that is, adding the total area of subsegmental defects (Neumann et al., 1980), (2) comparing the perfusion defects with the size of any accompanying radiographic abnormality (Biello et al., 1979b), (3) evaluating scan patterns in patients with severe or significant obstructive airway disease (Alderson et al., 1981), and (4) qualitatively evaluating the scan defects such as the "stripe sign" (Sostman and Gottschalk, 1982). The various schemes used are listed in Table 9–4 (Biello et al., 1979a; McNeil, 1980; PIOPED, 1990). Previous areas of contention regarding the various schemes include the classification of ventilation-perfusion results and the proper sequence in performing ventilation-perfusion scanning (Blumhardt, 1986; Woods et al., 1989). Is one scheme better than another? Several large studies have found no significant difference between the criteria of Biello and colleagues (1979), McNeil (1980) and PIOPED (1990) (Sullivan et al., 1983; Webber et al., 1990; Woods et al., 1989).

Patient selection bias clouds the usefulness of data in any retrospective study (Sostman et al., 1982). The standard procedure used in all retrospective evaluations is pulmonary angiography, which is technically demanding and carries a definite risk for the patient. In all retrospective series, only a minority of the patients had pulmonary angiography, and the present diagnostic schemes have been derived from this select group of patients. More recent reports by nonradiologists have questioned the value of probability classifications and highlighted the importance of selection bias in any retrospective study. Selection bias decreases the probability of emboli in a high-probability classification, that is, results of high-probability scans are more likely to be false-positive because the only patients subjected to angiography are those with low

Table 9–3. VENTILATION IMAGING: IDEAL CHARACTERISTICS

Agent	Postperfusion Study	All Phases of Ventilation	Portable Studies
Xenon-133	N*	Y	N
Xenon-127	Y	Y	N
Krypton-81	Y	N	Y
Technetium-99m aerosols	Y	N	Y

*Controversial post-perfusion studies have been performed (McNeil, 1974; McNeil, et al., 1976; McNeil, 1980; Kipper and Alazraki, 1982).

Table 9–4. DIAGNOSTIC SCHEMES FOR PULMONARY EMBOLISM

Classification	Criteria		
	McNeil, 1980	*Biello et al., 1979a*	*PIOPED, 1990*
Normal	Normal perfusion	Normal perfusion	Normal perfusion or perfusion defects from extrinsic sources
Very low probability	–	–	<3 Small perfusion defects, normal chest radiograph
Low probability	Single subsegmental ventilation-perfusion mismatch Multiple subsegmental ventilation-perfusion match	Small ventilation-perfusion mismatches Ventilated-perfusion match(es), normal chest radiograph Perfusion defects substantially smaller than chest radiograph abnormality	Nonsegmental perfusion defects from extrinsic defect Single moderate segmental perfusion defect, normal chest radiograph, ventilation irrelevant Any perfusion defect substantially smaller than chest radiograph abnormality, ventilation irrelevant Ventilation-perfusion match <50% of lung including <75% of one lung zone with normal chest radiograph (or smaller than perfusion defects) >3 small perfusion defects, normal chest radiograph <3 small perfusion/chest radiograph matches
Indeterminate or intermediate	Mixed ventilation-perfusion match and mismatch Single segment ventilation-perfusion mismatch Perfusion defect matched to chest radiograph abormality	Severe COPD with perfusion defects Perfusion defect of same size as chest radiograph abnormality Single medium ventilation-perfusion V/P mismatch, normal chest radiograph	Abnormality not defined by "high" or "low" Borderline "high" or "low"
High probability	Single ventilation-perfusion mismatch, lobe or larger Multiple ventilation-perfusion mismatches, segmental or larger	Single large ventilation-perfusion mismatch, normal chest radiograph Perfusion defect substantially larger than chest radiograph abnormality Multiple medium or large ventilation-perfusion mismatches without matched chest radiograph abnormality	>2 large perfusion defects Normal ventilation and chest radiograph >2 large perfusion defects in which defect is substantially larger than either matching ventilation or chest radiograph abnormality >2 or more moderate perfusion defects and one large perfusion defect, normal ventilation and chest radiograph >4 moderate perfusion defects, normal ventilation and chest radiograph

COPD, chronic obstructive pulmonary disease; PIOPED, Prospective Investigation of Pulmonary Embolism Diagnosis. Definitions: small, <25% of an anatomic segment; nonsegmental: very small effusion, cardiomegaly, hilar impression, etc.; moderate: >25% and <75% of an anatomic segment; medium: 25%–90% of an anatomic segment; large: >75% of an anatomic segment.

clinical likelihood of disease (Frankel et al., 1986). Conversely, selection bias increases the probability of true embolus in a patient with a low-probability scan (i.e., low-probability scans are more likely to have false-negative results because the only patients subjected to angiography are those with a high clinical likelihood of having had a pulmonary embolus (Frankel et al., 1986). Not surprisingly, current assessments of the usefulness of pulmonary scintigraphy have shown a deterioration in the high- and low-probability scan classifications. For example, Caracci and associates (1988) found that only 65% of patients with a high-probability scan classification had pulmonary emboli, whereas 28% of patients with low to inter-

mediate probability for pulmonary embolus had pulmonary emboli.

Clinical care appears to be overly influenced by the ventilation-perfusion scan results without consideration of the clinical likelihood of pulmonary emboli. That is, too much reliance is given to the scan findings (Frankel et al., 1986). Sostman and co-workers (1982) reviewed the influence of scintigraphic diagnosis in patient care. Of 332 patients with a low-probability scan classification, only seven had angiography (one had pulmonary embolus). Of 101 patients who had an indeterminate result, over half were managed clinically without having had pulmonary angiography. The authors concluded that clinicians often incorrectly interpret low-probability results as normal results and fail to consider the clinical likelihood of having had an embolus. Because low-probability diagnostic categories include an estimated likelihood of pulmonary embolism of up to 20%, angiography probably should have been performed in more than 2% of patients with this scan classification. One cannot arrive at a clinical diagnosis of pulmonary embolus without considering the pretest clinical suspicion or likelihood of disease. Perhaps this matter would be less confusing if the scans results were reported in terms of likelihood ratios rather than probabilities (Table 9–5).

Are clinicians accurate in estimating the clinical likelihood of pulmonary embolus? Hull and colleagues (1983) found that in patients with prior estimates of "highly likely," "possible," and "unlikely," 79%, 38%, and 15%, respectively, were found to have pulmonary emboli on objective testing. In the PIOPED study (1990), clinicians were more often correct in excluding pulmonary embolus (correct: high probability in 68%, low probability in 9%, and intermediate probability in 30%). In postmortem studies, the accuracy is poor. In one such study, the frequency of a false-negative clinical diagnosis was 67%, and the frequency of a false-positive clinical diagnosis was 62% (Modan et al., 1972). Attempts have been made to improve the clinician's ability to diagnose pulmonary embolus by using discriminant analysis and standard questionnaires (Celi et al., 1989; Hoellerich and Wigton, 1986). Noninvasive testing for deep venous thrombosis, as was performed in the studies by Hull and co-workers (1983, 1985),

may aid in decision making. Further emphasis should be placed on developing simple, noninvasive tests that detect thrombi in general, both within the peripheral venous system and within the lung.

Prospective Studies

Two recent prospective studies have been performed to clarify the usefulness of ventilation-perfusion scanning. The Hamilton District Thromboembolism Programme headed by Hull and colleagues examined ventilation-perfusion scans, pulmonary angiography, and objective testing for the diagnosis of deep vein thrombosis (Hull et al., 1983; 1985). Of 305 patients who had abnormal ventilation-perfusion scans, the authors confirmed that patients with large perfusion defects, segmental or greater, and a ventilation mismatch had a high probability of having a pulmonary embolus. Unexpectedly, they found a false-negative rate of 25% to 30% in patients with low-probability scan results (Hull et al., 1983, 1985).

The unexpected finding of pulmonary emboli in 25% to 30% of patients with low-probability results has prompted much criticism of the methodology and possible biases in the series by Hull and colleagues (Alderson and Martin, 1987; Blumhardt, 1986; Royal, 1989; Seckler-Walker, 1983; Smith et al., 1987; Sostman et al., 1986; Spies et al., 1986; Wellman, 1986). No study, even prospective, can be nonbiased. A plausible explanation is that clinicians, knowing their patients would be subjected to the risks of pulmonary angiography, would have been hesitant to investigate

Table 9–5. LIKELIHOOD RATIOS FOR PULMONARY EMBOLI

Scan Results	Pulmonary Embolism Present	Pulmonary Embolism Absent	Likelihood Ratio*
Biello et al., 1979			
High probability	0.698	0.041	16.9
Low probability	0.037	0.548	0.07
Indeterminate	0.264	0.408	0.65
Alderson and Martin, 1987			
High probability	0.575	0.036	16.1
Low probability	0.025	0.048	0.05
Indeterminate	0.400	0.484	0.82
Hull et al., 1983 (Xenon-127)			
High probability	0.750	0.116	6.4
Low probability	0.200	0.651	0.31
Indeterminate	0.050	0.233	0.22†
Hull et al., 1985 (Aerosol)			
High probability	0.438	0.068	6.4
Low probability	0.500	0.727	0.69
Interminate	0.063	0.205	0.30†
PIOPED, 1990			
High probability	0.406	0.029	13.9
Indeterminate	0.418	0.452	0.93
Low probability	0.155	0.415	0.37
Near normal/normal	0.012	0.104	0.19

*The likelihood ratio (LR) is an intuitive method to determine the usefulness of a test. The larger the numerical value of the LR the more likely that the patient has embolic disease (post-test odds equals pretest odds × LR). As the LR approaches zero the more likely it is that pulmonary embolism is excluded. A test or result with a LR of 1 has no useful information, because pretest odds are not altered.

†Note that the LR for an indeterminate result is lower than for a low probability result, that is, a patient is less likely to have embolic disease with an indeterminate result than with a low probability result. This contradictory result suggests that selection bias is present.

PIOPED, Prospective Investigation of Pulmonary Embolism Diagnosis.

them for possible embolic disease. That this explanation is probably true is reflected in the clinicians' estimate that approximately 50% of the patients had a high likelihood for embolic disease prior to testing. Because clinical selection of patients has been shown to be notoriously inaccurate, the clinicians would have been aided in selecting patients if objective testing for deep vein thrombosis was performed prior to initiating an embolic work-up; indeed, the results of impedance plethysmography (IPG) were available prior to the clinical decision to investigate the patient for embolic disease. This selection bias would primarily skew the low-probability classification, for these patients (presumably at decreased risk for emboli) would have been most scrutinized by their referring clinician.

Other methodologic problems exist. Two different ventilation techniques, xenon-127 (^{127}Xe) and ^{99m}Tc aerosols were used. Whether these techniques are truly comparable to xenon-133 (^{133}Xe) is unknown. Studies using ^{127}Xe would be more sensitive than those using ^{133}Xe for ventilation abnormalities, and small defects not resolvable with ^{133}Xe (thus a mismatch) would have been detected with ^{127}Xe (thus a matched defect). Even with objective testing (IPG) for deep vein thrombosis in a select population, nearly half of the patients had normal perfusion scans, which suggests that a normal perfusion scan included a number of studies with small subsegmental defects that would have been classified as low-probability in other studies. Such scan interpretation would select a group of patients in the low-probability scan classification who were more likely to have embolic disease.

These authors emphasized the value of objective testing for deep vein thrombosis in identifing the precursors of pulmonary emboli. Interestingly, nearly one third of their patients with negative pulmonary angiograms had extensive deep vein thrombosis. If objective testing had not been performed in these patients, they would not have undergone anticoagulation and would have been at risk for pulmonary embolus. Substituting venograms, however, for pulmonary angiograms would not be prudent, because in patients with pulmonary emboli as documented by pulmonary angiography, the frequency of a negative venogram was nearly one third.

Outcomes

The usefulness of the low-probability classification was defended by Lee, Smith, Kahn, and their colleagues, who studied the clinical outcomes in a total of 372 patients with low-probability results. Only one patient had clinical evidence of pulmonary emboli (0.3%) over a follow-up period of 12 months (Kahn et al., 1989; Lee et al., 1985; Smith et al., 1987). These studies cast doubt on the high frequency of pulmonary embolus demonstrated in the studies by Hull and associates (1983; 1985). Two possibilities may explain this discrepancy. Either patients with

low-probability results have emboli that are of no clinical consequence, or the low-probability group of Hull and associates reflects the biases described earlier.

The PIOPED study (1990) has clarified some questions raised by the Hamilton group. This prospective study encompassed 931 patients from six participating institutions and confirmed the usefulness of the high-probability scan result (88% accuracy for pulmonary embolus; 96% accuracy when accompanied by a high clinical likelihood of disease). Likewise, patients with an intermediate scan classification were confirmed to be indeterminate for pulmonary embolus (33%). Patients with low-probability results (12%) and near normal scan results (4%) were less likely to have emboli demonstrated angiographically. Selection bias was also important in this prospective study. Patients with low and near normal scan results were less likely to undergo angiography than were those with other scan results. In this series, if the outcomes of the patients not undergoing angiography from the low-probability and near normal categories had not been analyzed, the rate of embolization would have increased to 16% in the low-probability group and increased to 9% in the near normal or normal group.

Although the results of this study confirm the usefulness of ventilation-perfusion scanning for both high- and low-probability classifications, particularly when combined with clinical estimates of disease, only a minority of the total patients fell into the high- or low-probability group. As a result, the majority of patients had an unknown status for embolic disease and generally required angiography for diagnosis. This sobering fact should be a stimulus for renewed efforts to develop other noninvasive tests that demonstrate the clot rather than the secondary effects of the clot.

DEEP VEIN THROMBOSIS

Although the clinical diagnosis of deep vein thrombosis is difficult, it is intimately related to the diagnosis of pulmonary embolism. Practically all pulmonary emboli arise from deep veins of the leg. Huisman and co-workers (1989) demonstrated a high prevalence of silent pulmonary embolism in outpatients with proven deep vein thrombosis. Fifty-one percent of their patients with symptomatic deep vein thrombosis had silent pulmonary emboli demonstrated by ventilation-perfusion scanning. This finding stresses the importance of objective testing for deep vein thrombosis, not only in patients clinically suspected of deep vein thrombosis, but also in patients at high risk for thromboembolic disease.

The ideal test for venous thrombosis should have high sensitivity, easy applicability, and no morbidity or mortality. Peripheral intravenous injection of iodine-125 (^{125}I) fibrinogen is highly sensitive for detection of deep vein thrombosis in calf veins, but is less sensitive for detection of the more significant thrombi in the deep veins of the thigh or pelvis (Kakkar et al., 1969). In addition, this radiopharmaceutical must be injected before clot formation so that fibrinogen may be incorporated into the clot. This test has been widely used in the past as an epidemiologic tool to identify the frequency of deep vein thrombosis in specific clinical populations. Venography has long been the standard procedure for detection of deep vein thrombosis (Holden et al., 1981). It has a high sensitivity for thrombi both in the calf and in the thigh; however, the procedure is invasive, painful, and costly and may itself induce venous thromboembolism (Albrechtsson and Olsson, 1976). Thus, it is not a useful screening examination. Impedance plethysmography has also been used to detect deep vein thrombosis. This test, when administered properly, has high sensitivity for the presence of thrombosis in the deep veins of the thigh, but much lower sensitivity for calf vein thrombosis (Moser and LeMoine, 1981). Finally, ultrasound assessment using vein compression can demonstrate deep vein thrombosis within the thigh with a high degree of sensitivity (Cronan et al., 1987). As compared with physiologic techniques, it has an increased sensitivity (90% to 98%) and specificity (85% to 95%) but is less useful for assessment of the deep veins of the calf, although its value may increase with further technical refinements and operator experience (Polak et al., 1989) (see Chapter 16).

PULMONARY ANGIOGRAPHY

The standard procedure for the diagnosis of pulmonary embolism is pulmonary angiography (Bookstein et al., 1980). Its ability to detect emboli is not perfect, however. In animal studies, the false-negative rate may be as high as 25% for small peripheral emboli. In clinical practice, the rate of false-negative examinations has been variably estimated from 1% to 9% (Wellman, 1986). This finding is not surprising, considering that injection of a pulmonary or lobar artery opacifies the vessels of several overlapping segments. The result is a profusion of crisscrossing and overlapping vessels, which make detection of small embolic defects difficult (Fig. 9–6). Like most radiologic techniques, pulmonary angiography is subject to observer variation. Greenspan measured interobserver disagreement between three angiographers and found that it exceeded 10% (Greenspan, 1983; UPET, 1970). The greatest disagreement occurred with emboli classified as subsegmental, that is, the smaller the emboli, the greater the chance of disagreement between observers or lack of recognition of emboli.

This less-than-perfect test becomes even worse if the technical performance of the examination is poor. What constitutes an adequate exam? Usually, the ventilation-perfusion scan should be used as a guide to determine the expected location of emboli. In this way, the projection that best profiles the perfusion defect can be chosen. Only two diagnostic signs suffice

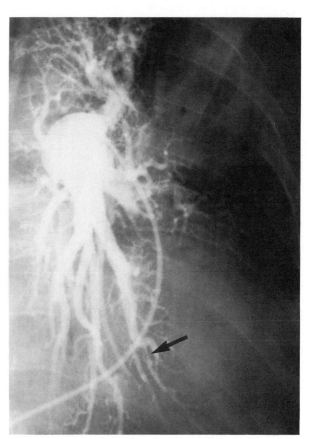

Figure 9–6. Infarct and embolic size. Note the small embolus *(arrow)* in a subsegmental branch of the left lower lobe. Patients with infarcts are more likely to have small emboli.

for the diagnosis of pulmonary embolism: either an intraluminal filling defect or vessel cutoff (Dalen et al., 1971) (Fig. 9–7). Secondary angiographic findings, such as decreased parenchymal staining, decreased perfusion, crowded vessels, delayed venous return, and shunting, are observed in other conditions as well. Such findings, however, should be viewed with suspicion, and in general, these areas should be further scrutinized with subselective angiograms (Johnsrude, 1982). Only when the primary angiographic criteria are clearly excluded can angiography be terminated. What role is there for digital subtraction angiography (DSA) (Ferris et al., 1984; Goodman and Brant, 1982; Pond et al., 1983)? Digital subtraction angiography is not equal to standard angiography except in cooperative patients. Artifacts from respiratory motion, cardiac motion, and patient motion all contribute to nondiagnostic angiograms. Under ideal circumstances, DSA is equivalent to pulmonary angiography (Pond, 1985).

What is the outcome of patients with negative pulmonary angiograms, particularly if the false-negative rate is high? Novelline and associates (1978) reviewed 180 consecutive patients with suspected pulmonary emboli and negative pulmonary arteriograms. Patients were followed clinically for at least 6 months.

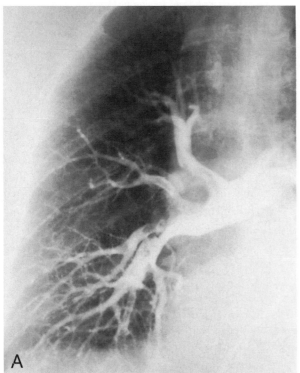

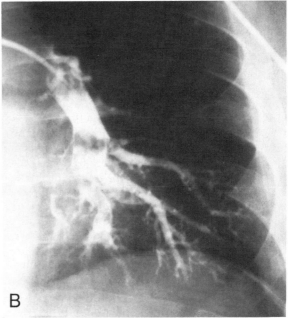

Figure 9–7. Angiographic study of pulmonary emboli. *A*, Right pulmonary angiogram. *B*, Left pulmonary angiogram. Both clearly show emboli in the central pulmonary arteries.

Of the 180 patients, 167 patients were untreated, 147 were alive at 6 months without evidence of recurrent thromboembolism and 20 had died prior to the 6-month follow-up examination. Ten of these last 20 patients had autopsy examinations. Pulmonary emboli were absent in seven patients, and small pulmonary emboli were present in three patients. Of the 13 patients treated with anticoagulation, all 13 were alive at 6 months without evidence of emboli. Thus, even though small pulmonary emboli may be missed, they are perhaps of no clinical consequence. Similar results were obtained in the PIOPED study (false-negative rate was 0.5%) (PIOPED, 1990). If one assumes a 1% false-negative rate for angiography, however, and a 30% mortality rate for untreated pulmonary emboli, then even in a series of 1000 patients, only three deaths are expected, a number that may not be observed by chance (Blinder and Coleman, 1985).

Indications

Pulmonary angiography is indicated in any patient with an indeterminate result of a ventilation-perfusion study or in patients with a high- or low-probability scan diagnosis and a strongly discordant clinical suspicion of embolic disease, usually a low-probability scan finding in a patient with high clinical likelihood of pulmonary emboli. In addition, pulmonary angiography is indicated prior to surgical embolectomy or placement of inferior vena cava (IVC) filters because of the morbidity and mortality associated with these treatments.

Angiography is an invasive procedure with potential complications, including a 2% death rate. Complications can be divided into those related to catheter manipulation through the heart and those related to contrast-medium reactions (Mills et al., 1980) (Table 9–6). Contrast injection increases the intravascular pressures, and in a patient with already elevated pulmonary artery pressures, the contrast load may induce acute cor pulmonale. The three deaths in the series by Mills and colleagues occurred in patients with right ventricular end-diastolic pressure that exceeded 20 mm Hg. Pulmonary artery pressures should be measured prior to the performance of angiography, and if the pressures are elevated, a limited study with subselective injection should be performed in these patients. Nonionic contrast does not appear to lessen this problem (Saeed et al., 1987).

Major arrythmias may occur during catheter manipulation through the heart—ventricular tachycardia, fibrillation, right bundle branch block, complete heart block, and bradycardia. Such complications

Table 9–6. COMPLICATIONS OF PULMONARY ANGIOGRAPHY (n = 1350)

Complication	No. of Patients
Death	3
Cardiac perforation	14
Cardiac injury	6
Major arrhythmia	11
Cardiac arrest	5
Contrast reactions	11
Miscellaneous	11

require that the examiner be prepared to pace the heart temporarily and treat major arrythmias if they occur. Contrast reactions, an infrequent but potentially serious problem, appear to be less frequent with nonionic agents (Saeed et al., 1987).

OTHER IMAGING TECHNIQUES

Computed Tomography

Godwin and colleagues (1980) reported three cases of pulmonary emboli detected by computed tomography (CT). In all cases, the clot appeared as a negative defect in the contrast-enhanced central pulmonary arteries. Clintapalli and associates (1988) reviewed the CT findings in 18 patients with pulmonary thromboembolism and infarction. Thrombus in the pulmonary arteries was identified in seven of 18 cases. The remainder of patients had parenchymal lesions consistent with pulmonary infarct. This series reflects clinical practice in which CT is, by chance, the first method of detecting pulmonary emboli in the pulmonary arteries, or in which CT is used to evaluate a nonspecific pulmonary abnormality that turns out to be an unsuspected pulmonary infarct (Fig. 9–8).

Experience with magnetic resonance imaging (MRI) is limited. This method, however, may detect pulmonary blood clots in the pulmonary arteries (Fisher and Higgins, 1986; Ovenfors and Batra, 1988; Stein et al., 1986). This technique has not been formally evaluated in a large series of patients.

TREATMENT

Anticoagulation and Fibrinolysis

Treatment of emboli is directed either at preventing the recurrence of emboli by using the anticoagulants heparin and coumadin, or at dissolving the clot using such agents as streptokinase. All of these drugs are hazardous and associated with significant bleeding and even death. Monitoring guidelines and treatment regimens are listed elsewhere (Heim and Des Prez, 1986).

Inferior Vena Cava Filter

Inferior vena cava (IVC) filters or ligation has been used in the past as a method of treating patients in whom anticoagulation therapy has failed, who have a contraindication to anticoagulation because of intercurrent disease, or who experience major bleeding as a result of anticoagulant therapy. The surgical mortality (15%) and morbidity for IVC interruption are high (Bomalaski et al., 1982). In a surgical series, the morbidity of postoperative leg swelling averaged 30%, and the rate of recurrent pulmonary embolism averaged 6%. More recently, percutaneous filters

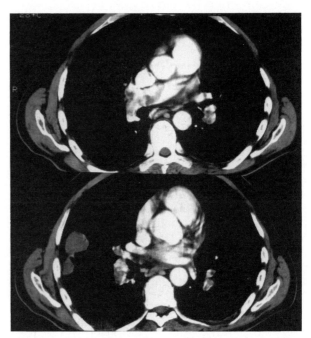

Figure 9–8. A CT scan performed to investigate a large mass in the right lung. Dynamic enhanced CT clearly demonstrates a large, unsuspected saddle embolus in the right and left pulmonary artery. The "mass" was a pulmonary infarct.

have been used to gain the same benefit without surgery. The most frequently used filter is the Greenfield filter (Wingerd et al., 1978). It has a low operative mortality and a morbidity of venous stasis of 5% to 15%. The incidence of recurring emboli averages 2% (see Chapter 16).

RESOLUTION

Considerable variability has been documented in the resolution of pulmonary emboli—ranging from several days to several weeks or months (Fred et al., 1966; Mathur et al., 1967; Sautter et al., 1967). As determined by perfusion scans, about 40% of individuals with less than 15% of lung involvement recovered completely in 28 days. When the scan defect was more extensive, with 15% to 30% of lung involvement, less than 40% of the patients had complete recovery at 28 days. When 31% to 58% of the lung was involved, less than 20% of the group had complete recovery at 28 days (Tow and Wagner, 1967). Paraskos and co-workers (1973) found incomplete resolution of perfusion defects in 35% of their patients, and approximately one third showed no resolution of their defects over an average follow-up interval of 29 months.

Resolution of pulmonary emboli occurs predominately through progressive fibrinolysis (Bell and Simon, 1982). The thrombolytic mechanism can result in resolution in as little as 30 hours, even in massive emboli. Of seven patients in a series by Fred and colleagues (1966), spontaneous resolution was complete in six patients within 7 to 19 days and was nearly complete in one patient within 16 days. In general, resolution depends on the size and maturity of the clot, the underlying health of the patient, and the timing and appropriateness of the treatment instituted (Bell and Simon, 1982).

Serial Lung Scintigraphy

If the diagnosis of pulmonary emboli is uncertain, serial lung scintigraphy may be useful. Alderson and colleagues (1983) found a high frequency of pulmonary emboli in patients with a changing perfusion pattern. They found that the sensitivity of a changing perfusion pattern for emboli was 74% (20 of 27), with a specificity of 75% (9 of 12). A changing perfusion pattern is not always due to additional pulmonary emboli; it may be due to resolution. Moser and colleagues (1973) reviewed the scintigraphic changes thought to indicate embolic recurrence. Emboli may migrate distally, resulting in new smaller peripheral defects with breakup of larger central emboli, or new

perfusion defects may arise because of a decrease in pulmonary vascular resistance in partially occluded arteries, which would turn a previously perfused zone into one that is not perfused. A changing perfusion pattern has been used as a tool to diagnose pulmonary embolism after major orthopedic procedures. Foley and associates (1989) compared preoperative with postoperative perfusion scans in 403 patients undergoing hip or knee repair. Twenty-two (5.5%) patients showed significant change in the postoperative studies. Silent emboli, in which patients are asymptomatic, were demonstrated by angiography in 13 patients. The overall frequency of emboli for both symptomatic and asymptomatic patients was 4% (16 of 403).

Serial scans are also useful in establishing a new baseline for lung perfusion after a known embolic episode. Optimal timing for follow-up perfusion scans is 1 week for confirmation of diagnosis, and 3 months following embolism, when the resolution should be nearly complete. Defects present at 3 months can be considered permanent (McCartney, 1981).

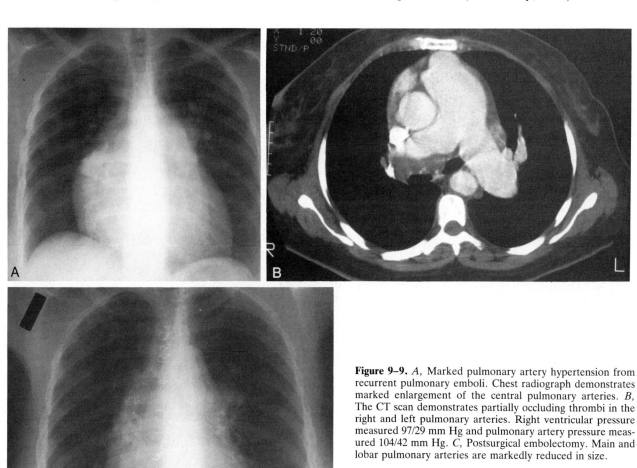

Figure 9–9. *A,* Marked pulmonary artery hypertension from recurrent pulmonary emboli. Chest radiograph demonstrates marked enlargement of the central pulmonary arteries. *B,* The CT scan demonstrates partially occluding thrombi in the right and left pulmonary arteries. Right ventricular pressure measured 97/29 mm Hg and pulmonary artery pressure measured 104/42 mm Hg. *C,* Postsurgical embolectomy. Main and lobar pulmonary arteries are markedly reduced in size.

CHRONIC EMBOLISM

The occurrence of pulmonary artery hypertension that is secondary to unresolved pulmonary emboli is uncommon and is generally reported in less than 1% of patients after an acute embolic event (Dalen and Alpert, 1975) (Fig. 9–9). Woodruff and co-workers (1985) reviewed the chest radiograph findings of chronic embolism in 22 patients. Cardiomegaly was the most frequent finding (86.4%). Other findings included an enlarged right pulmonary artery (54.5%), a small right pulmonary artery (9.1%), diminished vascularity in the lung (68.2%), chronic volume loss (27.3%), effusion or air-space disease (22.7%), and chronic pleural thickening (13.6%).

Perfusion scanning is an important diagnostic method in patients suspected of having chronic thromboembolic pulmonary hypertension and is particularly important in differentiating primary pulmonary hypertension from chronic thromboembolic disease (Lisbona et al., 1985). In primary pulmonary hypertension, the lung scan demonstrates peripheral nonsegmental defects in perfusion, whereas in thromboembolic hypertension, the scan is characterized by segmental or lobar defects in perfusion with or without subsegmental defects (Lisbona et al., 1985). Perfusion scanning, however, underestimates the severity of angiographic disease in patients with chronic thromboembolic pulmonary hypertension, as has been emphasized by Ryan and colleagues (1988).

SUMMARY

Radiologists must remain diligent in the search for embolic disease. Pulmonary emboli are common and are often undiagnosed. We have numerous tools at our disposal for this elusive diagnosis, but none are perfect, and work should be directed at developing noninvasive tests that directly image the clot, rather than the secondary effects of the clot.

References

Albrechtsson, U., and Olsson, C.: Thrombotic side effects of lower-limb phlebography. Lancet 1:723, 1976.

Alderson, P.O., and Martin, E.C.: Pulmonary embolism: Diagnosis with multiple imaging modalities. Radiology 164:297, 1987.

Alderson, P.O., Biello, D.R., Sacariah, K.G., and Siegel, B.A.: Scintigraphic detection of pulmonary embolism in patients with obstructive pulmonary disease. Radiology 138:661, 1981.

Alderson, P.O., Rujanavech, N., Sicker, W.R., and McKnight, R.C.: The role of ¹³³Xe ventilation studies in the scintigraphic detection of pulmonary embolism. Radiology 120:633, 1976.

Alderson, P.O., Doppman, J.L., Diamond, S.S., et al.: Ventilation-perfusion lung imaging and selective pulmonary angiography in dogs with experimental pulmonary embolism. J. Nucl. Med. 19:164, 1978.

Alderson, P.O., Dzebelo, N.N., Biello, D.R., et al.: Serial lung scintigraphy: Utility in diagnosis of pulmonary embolism. Radiology 149:797, 1983.

Arborelius, M.J., Fredin, H., Nyman, U., and Hellekant, C.: Angiographic evaluation of scintigraphic abnormalities in screening for pulmonary embolism after total hip replacement. Acta Radiol. 26:511, 1985.

Barker, N.W.: The diagnosis and treatment of pulmonary embolism. Med. Clin. North Am. 42:1053, 1958.

Bell, W.R., and Simon, T.L.: Current status of pulmonary thromboembolic disease: Pathophysiology, diagnosis, prevention, and treatment. Am. Heart J. 103:239, 1982.

Bell, W.R., Simon, T.L., and DeMets, D.L.: The clinical features of submassive and massive pulmonary emboli. Am. J. Med. 62:355, 1977.

Biello, D.R., Mattar, A.G., McKnight, R.C., and Siegel, B.A.: Ventilation-perfusion studies in suspected pulmonary embolism. AJR 133:1033, 1979a.

Biello, D.R., Mattar, A.G., Osei, W.A., et al.: Interpretation of indeterminate lung scintigrams. Radiology 133:189, 1979b.

Blinder, R.A., and Coleman, R.E.: Evaluation of pulmonary embolism. Radiol. Clin. North Am. 23:391, 1985.

Blumhardt, R.: Pulmonary angiography, ventilation lung scanning, and venography for clinically suspected pulmonary embolism with abnormal perfusion lung scan. Invest. Radiol. 21:940, 1986.

Bomalaski, J.S., Martin, G.J., Hughes, R.L., et al.: Inferior vena cava interruption in the management of pulmonary embolism. Chest 82:767, 1982.

Bookstein, J.J., Feigin, D.S., Seo, K.W., and Alazraki, N.P.: Diagnosis of pulmonary embolism: Experimental evaluation of the accuracy of scintigraphically guided pulmonary arteriography. Radiology 136:15, 1980.

Bounameaux, H., Krähenbühl, B., and Vukanovic, S.: Diagnosis of deep vein thrombosis by combination of Doppler ultrasound flow examination and strain gauge plethysmography: An alternative to venography only in particular conditions despite improved accuracy of the Doppler method. Thromb. Haemost. 47:141, 1982.

Bynum, L.J., and Wilson, J.E.: Characteristics of pleural effusions associated with pulmonary embolism. Arch. Intern. Med. 136:159, 1976.

Bynum, L.J., and Wilson, J.E.: Radiographic features of pleural effusions in pulmonary embolism. Am. Rev. Respir. Dis. 117:829, 1978.

Caracci, B.F., Rumbolo, P.M., Mainini, S., et al.: How accurate are ventilation-perfusion scans for pulmonary embolism? Am. J. Surg. 156:477, 1988.

Celi, A., Palla, A., Petruzzelli, S., et al.: Prospective study of a standardized questionnaire to improve clinical estimate of pulmonary embolism. Chest 95:332, 1989.

Cheely, R., McCartney, W.H., Perry, J.R., et al.: The role of noninvasive tests versus pulmonary angiography in the diagnosis of pulmonary embolism. Am. J. Med. 70:17, 1981.

Chintapalli, K., Thorsen, M.K., Olson, D.L., et al.: Computed tomography of pulmonary thromboembolism and infarction. J. Comput. Assist. Tomogr. 12:553, 1988.

Cranley, J.J., Canos, A.J., and Sull, W.J.: The diagnosis of deep vein thrombosis: Fallibility of clinical symptoms and signs. Arch. Surg. 111:34, 1976.

Cronan, J.J., Dorfman, G.S., Scola, F.H., et al.: Deep venous thrombosis: US assessment using vein compression. Radiology 162:191, 1987.

Dalen, J.E., and Alpert, J.S.: Natural history of pulmonary embolism. Prog. Cardiovasc. Dis. 17:259, 1975.

Dalen, J.E., Brooks, H.L., Johnson, L.W., et al.: Pulmonary angiography in acute pulmonary embolism: Indications, techniques, and results in 367 patients. Am. Heart J. 81:175, 1971.

Dalen, J.E., Haffajee, C.I., Alpert, J.E., et al.: Pulmonary embolism, pulmonary hemorrhage and pulmonary infarction. N. Engl. J. Med. 296:1431, 1977.

Davis, R.B., Schauwecker, D.S., Siddiqui, A.S., et al.: Indeterminate lung imaging: Can the number be reduced? Clin. Nucl. Med. 11:577, 1986.

DeNardo, G.L., Goodwin, D.A., Ravasini, R., et al.: The ventilatory lung scan in the diagnosis of pulmonary embolism. N. Engl. J. Med. 282:1334, 1970.

Dismuke, S., and Wagner, E.: Pulmonary embolism as a cause of death: The changing mortality in hospitalized patients. JAMA 255:2039, 1986.

Dorfman, G.S., Cronan, J.J., Tupper, T.B., et al.: Occult pulmonary embolism: A common occurrence in deep venous thrombosis. AJR 148:263, 1987.

Dworkin, H.J., Smith, J.R., and Bull, F.E.: A reaction following administration of macroaggregated albumin (MAA) for a lung scan. AJR 98:427, 1966.

Ferris, E.J., Holder, J.C., Lim, W.N., et al.: Angiography of pulmonary emboli: Digital studies and balloon-occlusion cineangiography. AJR 142:369, 1984.

Fisher, M., and Higgins, C.: Central thrombi in pulmonary artery hypertension detected by MR imaging. Radiology 158:223, 1986.

Fleischner, F.G.: Pulmonary embolism. Clin. Radiol. 13:169, 1962.

Foley, M., Maslack, M.M., Rothman, R.H., et al.: Pulmonary embolism after hip or knee replacement: Postoperative changes on pulmonary scintigrams in asymptomatic patients. Radiology 172:481, 1989.

Frankel, N., Coleman, R.E., Pryor, D.B., et al.: Utilization of lung scans by clinicians. J. Nucl. Med. 27:366, 1986.

Fraser, R.G., Paré, J.A.P., Paré, P.D., et al.: Diagnosis of Diseases of the Chest. Philadelphia, W.B. Saunders, 1990.

Fred, H.L., Axelrad, M.A., Lewis, J.M., and Alexander, J.K.: Rapid resolution of pulmonary thromboemboli in man. JAMA 196:1137, 1966.

Godwin, J.D., Webb, W.R., Gamsu, G., and Ovenfors, C.O.: Computed tomography of pulmonary embolism. AJR 135:691, 1980.

Goodman, P.C., and Brant, Z.M.: Digital subtraction pulmonary angiography. AJR 139:305, 1982.

Greenspan, R.H.: Angiography of pulmonary embolism. In Abrams, H.L. (ed.): Abrams Angiography: Vascular and Interventional Radiology, ed. 3. Boston, Little, Brown, 1983.

Greenspan, R.H., Ravin, C.E., Polansky, S.M., and McLoud, T.C.: Accuracy of the chest radiograph in diagnosis of pulmonary embolism. Invest. Radiol. 17:539, 1982.

Hampton, A.O., and Castleman, B.: Correlation of postmortem chest teleroentgenograms with autopsy findings, with special reference to pulmonary embolism and infarction. AJR 43:305, 1940.

Havig, O.: Source of pulmonary emboli. Acta Chir. Scand. 478:42, 1977.

Heim, C.R., and Des Prez, R.M.: Pulmonary embolism: A review. Adv. Intern. Med. 31:187, 1986.

Heitzman, E.R., Markarian, B., and Dailey, E.T.: Pulmonary thromboembolic disease: A lobular concept. Radiology 103:529, 1972.

Hendin, A.S.: Clearing patterns of pulmonary infarction and slowly resolving pneumonia. Radiology 114:557, 1975.

Hoellerich, V.L., and Wigton, R.S.: Diagnosing pulmonary embolism using clinical findings. Arch. Intern. Med. 146:1699, 1986.

Holden, R.W., Klatte, E.C., Park, H.M., et al.: Efficacy of noninvasive modalities for diagnosis of thrombophlebitis. Radiology 141:63, 1981.

Huisman, M.V., Buller, H.R., ten Cate, J.W., et al.: Unexpected high prevalence of silent pulmonary embolism in patients with deep venous thrombosis. Chest 95:498, 1989.

Hull, R.D., Hirsh, J., Carter, C.J., et al.: Pulmonary angiography, ventilation lung scanning, and venography for clinically suspected pulmonary embolism with abnormal perfusion lung scan. Ann. Intern. Med. 98:891, 1983.

Hull, R.D., Hirsh, J., Carter, C.J., et al.: Diagnostic value of ventilation-perfusion lung scanning in patients with suspected pulmonary embolism. Chest 88:819, 1985.

Jacoby, C.G., and Mindell, H.J.: Lobar consolidation in pulmonary embolism. Radiology 118:287, 1976.

Johnsrude, I.S.: Pulmonary embolism. Curr. Probl. Diagn. Radiol. 11:4, 1982.

Kahn, D., Bushnell, D.L., Dean, R., and Perlman, S.B.: Clinical outcome of patients with a "low probability" of pulmonary embolism on ventilation-perfusion lung scan. Arch. Intern. Med. 149:377, 1989.

Kakkar, V.V., Howe, C.T., Flanc, C., and Clarke, M.B.: Natural history of postoperative deep-vein thrombosis. Lancet 2:230, 1969.

Kessler, R.M., and McNeil, B.J.: Impaired ventilation in a patient with angiographically demonstrated pulmonary emboli. Radiology 114:111, 1975.

Kipper, M.S., and Alazraki, N.: The feasibility of performing Xe-133 ventilation imaging following the perfusion study. Radiology 144:581, 1982.

Lee, M.E., Biello, D.R., Kumar, B., and Siegel, B.A.: "Low-probability" ventilation-perfusion scintigrams: Clinical outcomes in 99 patients. Radiology 156:497, 1985.

Lisbona, R., Kreisman, H., Novales-Diaz, J., and Derbekyan, V.: Perfusion lung scanning: Differentiation of primary from thromboembolic pulmonary hypertension. AJR 144:27, 1985.

Mathur, V.S., Dalen, J.E., Evans, H., et al.: Pulmonary angiography one to seven days after experimental pulmonary embolism. Invest. Radiol. 2:304, 1967.

McCartney, W.H.: Ventilation-perfusion lung scanning in pulmonary embolus. Clin. Nucl. Med. 6:27, 1981.

McGoldrick, P.J., Rudd, T.G., Figley, M.M., and Wilhelm, J.P.: What becomes of pulmonary infarcts? AJR 133:1039, 1979.

McNeil, B.J.: Ventilation-perfusion studies and the diagnosis of pulmonary embolism: Concise communication. J. Nucl. Med. 21:319, 1980.

McNeil, B., Holman, L., and Adelstein, J.: The scintigraphic definition of pulmonary embolism. JAMA 227:753, 1974.

McNeil, B.J., Hessel, S.J., Branch, W.T., et al.: Measures of clinical efficacy. III. The value of the lung scan in the evaluation of young patients with pleuritic chest pain. J. Nucl. Med. 17:163, 1976.

Mercandetti, A., Kipper, M., and Moser, K.: Influence of perfusion and ventilation scans on therapeutic decision making and outcome in cases of possible embolism. West. J. Med. 142:208, 1985.

Mills, S.R., Jackson, D.C., Older, R.A., et al.: The incidence, etiologies, and avoidance of complications of pulmonary angiography in a large series. Radiology 136:295, 1980.

Modan, B., Sharon, E., and Jelin, N.: Factors contributing to the incorrect diagnosis of pulmonary embolic disease. Chest 62:388, 1972.

Moreno-Cabral, R., Kistner, R., and Nordyke, R.: Importance of calf vein thrombophlebitis. Surgery 80:735, 1976.

Moser, K.M.: Pulmonary embolism. Am. Rev. Respir. Dis. 115:829, 1977.

Moser, K.M.: Venous thromboembolism. Am. Rev. Respir. Dis. 141:235, 1990.

Moser, K.M., and LeMoine, J.R.: Is embolic risk conditioned by location of deep venous thrombosis? Ann. Intern. Med. 94:439, 1981.

Moscr, K.M., Longo, A.M., Ashburn, W.L., and Guisan, M.: Spurious scintiphotographic recurrence of pulmonary emboli. Am. J. Med. 55:434, 1973.

Moses, D.C., Silver, T.M., and Bookstein, J.J.: The complementary roles of chest radiography, lung scanning, and selective pulmonary angiography in the diagnosis of pulmonary embolism. Circulation 49:179, 1974.

Neumann, R.D., Sostman, H.D., and Gottschalk, A.: Current status of ventilation-perfusion imaging. Semin. Nucl. Med. 10:198, 1980.

Norris, C.S., Greenfield, L.J., and Herrmann, J.B.: Free-floating iliofemoral thrombus: A risk of pulmonary embolism. Arch. Surg. 120:806, 1985.

Noveline, R.A., Baltarowich, O.H., Athanasoulis, C.A., et al.: The clinical course of patients with suspected pulmonary embolism and a negative pulmonary arteriogram. Radiology 126:561, 1978.

Ovenfors, C.O., and Batra, P.: Diagnosis of peripheral pulmonary emboli by MR imaging: An experimental study in dogs. Magn. Reson. Imaging. 6:487, 1988.

Palla, A., Donnamaria, V., Petruzzelli, S., et al.: Enlargement of the right descending pulmonary artery in pulmonary embolism. AJR 141:513, 1983.

Paraskos, J.A., Adelstein, S.J., Smith, R.E., et al.: Late prognosis of acute pulmonary embolism. N. Engl. J. Med. 289:55, 1973.

Patton, D.: The efficacy of lung scans: The emperor had clothes all along. J. Nucl. Med. 26:812, 1985.

PIOPED I.: Value of ventilation/perfusion scan in acute pulmonary embolism: Results of the prospective investigation of pulmonary embolism diagnosis (PIOPED). JAMA 263:2753, 1990.

Polak, J.F., Culter, S.S., and O'Leary, D.H.: Deep veins of the calf: Assessment with color Doppler flow imaging. Radiology 171:481, 1989.

Pond, G.D.: Pulmonary digital subtraction angiography. Radiol. Clin. North Am. 23:243, 1985.

Pond, G.D., Ovitt, T.W., and Capp, M.P.: Comparison of conventional pulmonary angiography with intravenous digital subtraction angiography for pulmonary embolic disease. Radiology 147:345, 1983.

Poulose, K., Reba, R.C., and Wagner, H.N.: Characterization of the shape and location of perfusion defects in certain pulmonary disorders. N. Engl. J. Med. 279:1020, 1968.

Robin, E.D.: Overdiagnosis and overtreatment of pulmonary embolism: The emperor may have no clothes. Ann. Intern. Med. 87:775, 1977.

Rosenow, E.C., Osmundson, P.J., and Brown, M.L.: Pulmonary embolism. Mayo Clin. Proc. 56:161, 1981.

Royal, H.D.: Radionuclide imaging of the lung. Current Opinion Radiology 1:446, 1989.

Ryan, K.L., Fedullo, P.F., Davis, G.B., et al.: Perfusion scan findings understate the severity of angiographic and hemodynamic compromise in chronic thromboembolic pulmonary hypertension. Chest 93:1180, 1988.

Saeed, M., Braun, S.D., Cohan, R.H., et al.: Pulmonary angiography with iopamidol: Patient comfort, image quality, and hemodynamics. Radiology 165:345, 1987.

Saenger, E., Buncher, C., Specker, B., et al.: Determination of clinical efficacy: Nuclear medicine as applied to lung scanning. J. Nucl. Med. 26:793, 1985.

Sautter, R.D., Fletcher, F.W., Ousley, J.L., and Wenzel, F.J.: Extremely rapid resolution of a pulmonary embolus: Report of a case. Dis. Chest 52:825, 1967.

Seckler-Walker, R.H.: On purple emperors, pulmonary embolism, and venous thrombosis. Ann. Intern. Med. 98:1006, 1983.

Sevitt, S., Gallagher, N.G.: Venous thrombosis and pulmonary embolism: A clinicopathologic study in injured and burned patients. Br. J. Surg. 48:475, 1961.

Smith, R., Maher, J.M., Miller, R.I., and Alderson, P.O.: Clinical outcomes of patients with suspected pulmonary embolism and low-probability aerosol-perfusion scintigrams. Radiology 164:731, 1987.

Sostman, H.D., and Gottschalk, A.: The stripe sign: A new sign for diagnosis of nonembolic defects on pulmonary perfusion scintigraphy. Radiology 142:737, 1982.

Sostman, H.D., Rapoport, S., Gottschalk, A., and Greenspan, R.H.: Imaging of pulmonary embolism. Invest. Radiol. 21:443, 1986.

Sostman, H.D., Ravin, C.E., Sullivan, D.C., et al.: Use of pulmonary angiography for suspected pulmonary embolism: Influence of scintigraphic diagnosis. AJR 139:673, 1982.

Spies, W.G., Burstein, S.P., Dillehay, G.L., et al.: Ventilation-perfusion scintigraphy in suspected pulmonary embolism: Correlation with pulmonary angiograpy and refinement of criteria for interpretation. Radiology 159:383, 1986.

Stein, M.G., Crues, J.E., Bradley, W.J., et al.: MR imaging of pulmonary emboli: An experimental study in dogs. AJR 147:1133, 1986.

Sullivan, D.C., Coleman, R.E., Mills, S.R., et al.: Lung scan interpretation: Effect of different observers and different criteria. Radiology 149:803, 1983.

Tetalman, M.R., Hoffer, P.B., Heck, L.L., et al.: Perfusion scans in normal volunteers. Radiology 106:595, 1973.

Tow, D.E., and Wagner, H.J.: Recovery of pulmonary arterial blood flow in patients with pulmonary embolism. N. Engl. J. Med. 276:1053, 1967.

UPET: Urokinase pulmonary embolism trial. Phase 1 results: A cooperative study. JAMA 214:2163, 1970.

Vincent, W.R., Goldberg, S.J., and Desilets, D.: Fatality immediately following rapid infusion of macroaggregates of ^{99m}Tc albumin (MAA) for lung scan. Radiology 91:1181, 1968.

Virchow, R.: "Cellular Pathology." New York, Dewitt, 1860.

Vix, V.A.: The usefulness of chest radiographs obtained after a demonstrated perfusion scan defect in the diagnosis of pulmonary emboli. Clin. Nucl. Med. 8:497, 1983.

Wagner, H.N., Jr., Lopez-Majano, V., Langan, J.K., et al.: Radioactive xenon in the differential diagnosis of pulmonary embolism. Radiology 91:1168, 1968.

Wagner, H.N., Jr., Sabiston, D.J., Jr., McAfee, J.G., et al.: Diagnosis of massive pulmonary embolism in man by radioisotope scanning. N. Engl. J. Med. 271:377, 1964.

Webber, M.M., Gomes, A.S., Roe, D., et al.: Comparison of Biello, McNeil, and PIOPED criteria for the diagnosis of pulmonary emboli on lung scans. AJR 154:975, 1990.

Wellman, H.N.: Pulmonary thromboembolism: Current status report on the role of nuclear medicine. Semin. Nucl. Med. 16:236, 1986.

Westermark, N.: On the roentgen diagnosis of lung embolism. Acta Radiol. 19:357, 1938.

Williams, J., Wilcox, W., Andrews, G., et al.: Angiography in pulmonary embolism. JAMA 184:473, 1963.

Wingerd, M., Bernhard, V.M., Maddison, F., and Towne, J.B.: Comparison of caval filters in the management of venous thromboembolism. Arch. Surg. 113:1264, 1978.

Woesner, M.E., Sanders, I., and White, G.W.: The melting sign in resolving transient pulmonary infarction. AJR 111:782, 1971.

Woodruff, W.E., Hoeck, B.E., Chitwood, W.J., et al.: Radiographic findings in pulmonary hypertension from unresolved embolism. AJR 144:681, 1985.

Woods, E.R., Iles, S., and Jackson, S.: Comparison of scintigraphic diagnostic criteria in suspected pulmonary embolism. Can. Assoc. Radiol. J. 40:194, 1989.

10

The Immunocompromised Patient

■

Dewey J. Conces, Jr.

One of the greatest challenges that a clinician can face is the evaluation and treatment of an immunocompromised patient with suspected pulmonary infection. Various factors contribute to the difficulty of these cases. Immunocompromised patients are susceptible to a large number of different bacteria, fungi, viruses, and protozoa, many of which do not normally cause infection in the immunocompetent individual. The manifestations of infection in an immunocompromised patient tend to be more variable than in the normal host. A further source of confusion in the clinical picture is that these patients may develop a variety of noninfectious conditions that mimic infection clinically. In addition, these infections can progress rapidly. If not treated adequately and early, they often have a fatal outcome. These factors produce a sense of both urgency and frustration in the evaluation of a patient with a suspected pulmonary infection.

The chest radiograph, which can help in identifying the presence of a pulmonary process, is unable to provide a diagnosis, because the radiographic findings are never specific for a given organism or pathologic process (Williams et al., 1976). This lack of specificity, however, does not mean that the radiologic findings are not useful. On the contrary, when information provided by the chest radiograph is combined with a number of clinical clues, it can significantly decrease the number of possible diagnoses. Through the narrowing of the range of diagnostic possibilities, a logical selection of diagnostic tests can be made, possibly leading to a specific diagnosis. When empiric therapy is deemed necessary, the narrowed list of diagnostic possibilities allows a rational selection of therapeutic agents.

This chapter discusses important clinical clues that are useful in the evaluation of the immunocompromised patient with suspected pulmonary infection. These clues are found in the patient's history, physical examination, and initial laboratory studies. This information is best obtained by close communication with the clinical services responsible for the care of the compromised patient. This information allows a more meaningful interpretation of the chest radiograph.

Several general concepts need to be kept in mind while one evaluates infiltrates in immunocompromised patients. First, the possibility that the infiltrates are due to a noninfectious etiologic mechanism must always be considered. Also, when infection is present, it may be caused by more than one organism. In addition, the patient may develop sequential infections caused by different organisms (Fig. 10–1). Thus, a patient who worsens while receiving therapy for a specific infection may represent not a failure to respond, but actually a new infection by a different organism or the development of a new noninfectious process (Fig. 10–2).

HISTORICAL INFORMATION

Of the clinical clues available for the evaluation of chest radiographs, the most useful are historical. Information is sought regarding the history of the current illness as well as the history of past illnesses and therapy. Epidemiologic factors are evaluated to identify possible infectious exposures. The information that is obtained needs to be constantly updated to determine how changes in the chest radiograph correlate with a changing clinical situation.

Nature of Immune Defect

The pulmonary defense mechanisms can be divided into three main categories: mechanical, phagocytic,

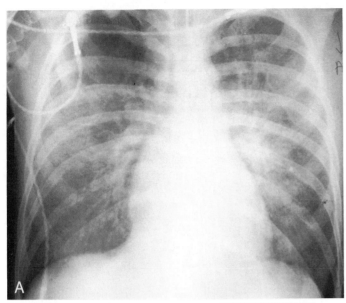

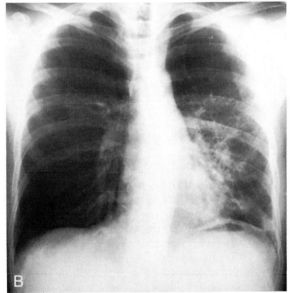

Figure 10–1. Patient with acquired immunodeficiency syndrome (AIDS) and non-Hodgkin's lymphoma who developed *Pneumocystis carinii* pneumonia during a period of granulocytopenia following chemotherapy. *A,* Chest radiograph demonstrates diffuse bilateral interstitial infiltrates. Following antiprotozoal therapy, the patient developed recurrent fever, which persisted for several weeks. *B,* Chest radiograph eventually showed a lingular infiltrate. Bronchoscopy revealed *Histoplasma capsulatum.*

Figure 10–2. Three months following a cadaveric renal transplant, the patient developed cytomegalovirus pneumonia. Chest radiograph demonstrates diffuse bilateral interstitial infiltrates. While recovering from the viral pneumonia, the patient developed increasing dyspnea. A pulmonary angiogram demonstrated a left lower lobe pulmonary embolus *(not shown).*

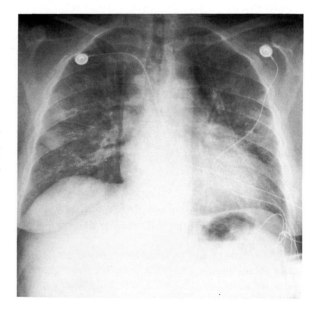

and specific immune defenses (Kaltreider, 1988; Reynolds, 1988). The mechanical defenses consist of the filtration and impaction of inhaled particles, the epithelial barriers, and the clearance debris from the airways. Phagocytic defenses are provided by the pulmonary macrophages and polymorphonuclear leukocytes. Specific defense against microbiologic agents is provided by the antibody-producing B-lymphocytes and the cellular immune response of the T-lymphocytes.

The function of the various components of the pulmonary defenses can be affected both by the underlying disease of the patient and by the therapeutic methods employed in the treatment of the disorder. Specific defects in the immune defense system predispose the patient to infections by particular groups of organisms (Table 10–1). Thus, knowledge of the type of defect present provides clues regarding the specific organisms to which the patient has increased susceptibility. When considering the nature of the immune defects in an individual patient, one must remember that disease processes and therapeutic interventions may disable more than one branch of the immune system. An example of this phenomenon is cyclophosphamide, a potent lymphocytotoxic drug. Its effects on the B-lymphocytes result in altered primary and secondary responses to microbial antigens (Gershwin et al., 1974). By acting on the T-lymphocytes, the drug inhibits cell-mediated immunity (Balow et al., 1975).

One must also consider the net immune state of the patient. Adequate nutrition is required for optimal function of the immune system (Chandra, 1983). The presence of a metabolic disorder such as diabetes mellitus, renal failure, or liver failure can result in a diminished immune response (van der Meer, 1988). The elderly exhibit decline in both humeral and cell-mediated responses (Roberts-Thomson et al., 1974). Infections by immune-modulating viruses such as cytomegalovirus (CMV), Epstein-Barr virus, and human immunodeficiency virus (HIV) can result in depressed immunity (Beck and Shellito, 1989; Junker et al., 1986; Rubin et al., 1977).

The rate at which the immune defect occurs affects the susceptibility to infection. Acute development of immune defects is typically associated with more frequent and severe infections than is a chronic change. The rapid decrease in circulating granulocytes that occurs following the administration of chemotherapy is associated with severe infection by the gram-negative bacteria or fungi such as those of *Candida* and *Aspergillus* (Winston et al., 1979a, 1979b). In contrast, patients suffering from the rare disorder of chronic neutropenia experience little problem with infections (Dale et al., 1979; Kyle and Linman, 1968). The severity of the defect should be considered when evaluating the patient. The absolute granulocyte count is a guide to the functioning of the phagocytic defenses. When the absolute granulocyte count falls below 500/mm^3 (0.5×10^9/liter), a marked increase occurs in the frequency and severity of infections (Bodey et al., 1966) (Fig. 10–3).

Table 10–1. IMMUNOLOGIC DEFECTS AND ASSOCIATED MICROORGANISM

Immune Defect	Underlying Disease	Associated Organism
Immunoglobulin abnormalities (B-lymphocyte)	Hypogammaglobulinemia Corticosteroids Immunosuppressive agents Lymphoma Lymphocytic leukemia Multiple myeloma Splenectomy	*Streptococcus pneumoniae* *Hemophilus influenzae* *Neisseria meningitidis* *Staphylococcus aureus* Gram-negative bacteria

Cell-mediated immune dysfunction (T-lymphocyte)	Lymphoma
	Corticosteroids
	Immunosuppressive agents
	Radiation therapy
	Viral infection (Acquired immunodeficiency syndrome)
	Uremia
		Viruses
		  Cytomegalovirus
		  Herpes simplex
		  Varicella-zoster
		Parasites
		  Pneumocystis carinii
		  Toxoplasma gondii
		  Strongyloides stercoralis
		Fungi
		  Cryptococcus neoformans
		  Candida
		  Histoplasma capsulatum
		  Coccidioides immitis
		Bacteria
		  Legionella
		  Nocardia
		  Listeria
		  Mycobacterium

Phagocytic defense disorders (polymorphonuclear leukocyte)	Granulocytopenia Corticosteroids Acute myelocytic leukemia	*Staphylococcus aureus* Gram-negative bacteria *Aspergillus* *Candida* Zygomycetes

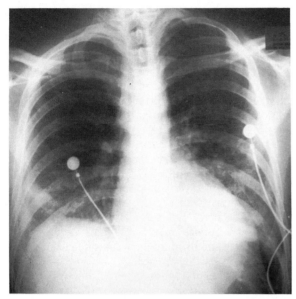

Figure 10–3. Patient who developed a fever while receiving chemotherapy for acute lymphocytic leukemia. Absolute granulocyte count was 0/mm³ (0.0 × 10⁹/liter). Chest radiograph shows bilateral basilar alveolar infiltrates and a right pleural effusion. Blood cultures were positive for *Staphylococcus aureus, Escherichia coli, Klebsiella* organisms and two strains of *Streptococcus* organisms.

Temporal Relationship to Transplantation

Infections following transplantation tend to occur in a certain temporal relationship that is related to the time interval since transplantation. One pattern is seen following solid organ transplantation (Anderson and Jordan, 1990; Austin et al., 1989; Dummer, 1990; Kusne et al., 1988; Mermel and Maki, 1990; Ramsey et al., 1980; Rubin et al., 1981; Wilson et al., 1989) (Table 10–2). A second pattern occurs following bone marrow transplantation (Meyers and Thomas, 1988; Young, 1984) (Table 10–3). These temporal patterns of infection are related to the changing status of the immune defenses.

Following solid organ transplantation, patients are placed on high doses of immunosuppressive agents to prevent organ rejection. The full effects of this immune suppression, however, is not realized until several weeks later. Because of this delay in the effect

Table 10–2. TEMPORAL OCCURRENCE OF INFECTIONS FOLLOWING SOLID ORGAN TRANSPLANTATION

< 1 Month	1–4 Months	> 4 Months
Bacterial	*Pneumocystis*	*Cryptococcus*
Wound infection	*Aspergillus*	*Pneumocystis*
Catheter sepsis	Zygomycetes	
Aspiration	*Nocardia*	
	Mycobacterium	
	Cytomegalovirus	
	Other viruses	

Table 10–3. TEMPORAL OCCURRENCE OF INFILTRATES FOLLOWING BONE MARROW TRANSPLANTATION

0–30 Days	30–100 Days	> 100 Days
Aspiration	*Pneumocystis*	*Streptococcus*
Gram-negative	Cytomegalovirus	*pneumoniae*
	Other viruses	*Staphylococcus*
	Idiopathic	Varicella-zoster
	Hemorrhage	Graft-vs.-host

on the immune system, the pulmonary infections encountered in the immediate post-transplant period are due to bacterial organisms that typically cause infection in the immunocompetent patient (Rubin, 1988). Immune suppression is greatest 1 to 4 months following transplantation with T-lymphocyte–mediated immunity at its lowest functional level. During this period, infections by herpesviruses, especially CMV, are most common (Anderson and Jordan, 1990) (see Fig. 10–2). Cytomegalovirus is itself an immune system–modulating virus that further suppresses immune function by infecting T-lymphocytes and producing neutropenia (Gentry and Zeluff, 1988). These changes result in superinfection by opportunistic organisms such as *Pneumocystis carinii* (Wilson et al., 1985) (Fig. 10–4).

Organ transplant patients in the late period, greater than 120 days, can be divided into two groups: (1) those who show no evidence of rejection and are receiving minimal immunosuppressive agents and (2) those patients who experience continued transplant organ rejection and require high doses of immunosuppressive therapy (Rubin, 1988). In those individuals who are on low-maintenance doses of immunosuppressive agents, most pneumonias are

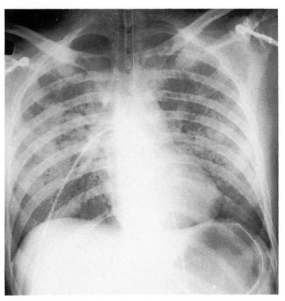

Figure 10–4. Renal transplant patient who developed *Pneumocystis carinii* pneumonia. Chest radiograph demonstrates diffuse bilateral infiltrates.

caused by the usual infections present in the general population. The continued administration of immunosuppressive drugs, however, does result in a persistent mild suppression of T-lymphocyte function. As a result, occasional opportunistic infections are encountered, with *Cryptococcus neoformans* infection being the most common. Those patients who require high doses of immunosuppressive agents to prevent organ rejection continue to be predisposed to infections typically seen during the period of severe immunosuppression, 1 to 4 months following transplantation.

The nature and severity of the immune defect following bone marrow transplantation differ from those seen with solid organ transplantation. A different spectrum of infections results (Meyers and Thomas, 1988; Young, 1984). Prior to transplanta-

tion, the recipient's bone marrow is conditioned, which results in a severe depletion of all cell lines in the bone marrow. As a result, circulating granulocytes are virtually absent at the time of transplantation, which predisposes the patient to severe bacterial infections, especially gram-positive cocci and gram-negative rods (Winston et al., 1979a; Young, 1984).

Granulocyte recovery typically occurs around 30 days following transplantation. Following marrow engraftment and until 100 days after transplantation, the most common pneumonias are interstitial in nature (Crawford et al., 1989; Neiman et al., 1977; Wingard et al., 1988). Idiopathic interstitial pneumonitis accounts for 40% of these cases. Cytomegalovirus is the most common infectious etiologic agent, with *Pneumocystis carinii* infection and other viruses accounting for the remainder (Fig. 10–5). After 100

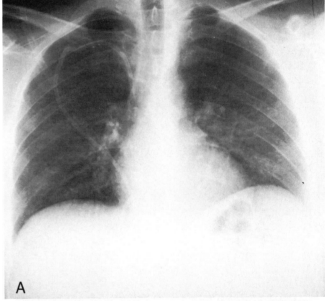

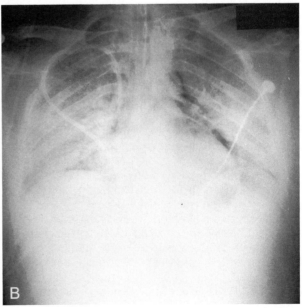

Figure 10–5. Fever developed in a patient 56 days following bone marrow transplant for leukemia. *A,* Initial chest radiograph demonstrates an early infiltrate in the left lower lobe. Cytomegalovirus pneumonia diagnosed by bronchoscopy. *B,* Pneumonia progressed to bilateral consolidation over the next 6 days. Air outlines the aortic knob and left heart border as a result of respirator-induced barotrauma. Other radiographs showed air in the neck. A pneumothorax never developed.

days, the incidence of infection decreases. In the late period, an increased risk of infection continues, owing to residual immune dysfunction that is present in all patients. In those with allogenic transplants who develop graft-versus-host disease (GVHD), additional immunosuppression is present because of the effects of GVHD on the immune system as well the immunosuppressive therapy used to treat GVHD (Meyers and Thomas, 1988). During the late period, incidence of *Streptococcus pneumoniae* infections is increased, presumably owing to the patient's inability to produce opsonizing antibodies (Winston et al., 1979b).

Therapy

In addition to the alterations in immune function produced by chemotherapeutic and immunosuppressive agents, a number of other therapeutic interventions can increase the chance of infection. Mechanical defenses can be bypassed with the placement of intravenous lines, endotracheal tubes, and chest tubes. Endotracheal tubes, which bypass the filtration of the upper airways, predispose the patient to the development of pneumonia. The incidence of pneumonia is related to the duration of ventilatory support, increasing from 5% in patients receiving 1 day of support to 68% in those receiving more than 30 days of support (Langer et al., 1989). The epithelial barrier of the skin is bypassed with vascular catheters. These lines may become infected and produce hematogenous spread of the infection to the lung. Catheter-related hematogenous pneumonia is most frequently due to *Staphylococcus* or *Candida* organisms (Clarke and Raffin, 1990; Press et al., 1984) (Fig. 10–6). Triple-lumen catheters have a higher incidence of infection than do single-lumen catheters (Hilton et al., 1988; Yeung et al., 1988).

Blood transfusions as well as organ transplants can result in transmission of an organism from an infected donor to the recipient. Viral infections, such as hepatitis, CMV, and HIV, are the infections most commonly transmitted by transfusion of blood products (Barbara and Tedder, 1984). Viral infections are also the most frequent type of infection transmitted by the transplanted organ itself (Gottesdiener, 1989). Transmission of CMV from a seropositive donor to a seronegative recipient is a major risk factor for the development of severe, and sometimes fatal, CMV pneumonia following transplantation (Hutter et al., 1989). Transmission of bacterial infection is usually related to contamination during harvesting and preparation of the organ for transplantation, and fungal and mycobacterial transmission is rare.

Broad-spectrum antibiotics, which are often administered for the empiric treatment of febrile patients with suspected infection, predispose patients to the development of infections by fungal organisms (Harvey and Myers, 1987; Komshian et al., 1989; Wey et al., 1989). The administration of prophylactic

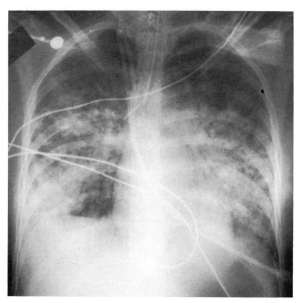

Figure 10–6. Patient became febrile 2 weeks after bone marrow transplant for acute lymphocytic leukemia. Chest radiograph demonstrates bilateral patchy alveolar infiltrates. Hickman catheter, blood, and skin lesion cultures grew *Candida* organisms.

trimethoprim-sulfamethoxazole results in a marked reduction of infections by *Pneumocystis* organisms (Young, 1986). Inhaled pentamidine administered for prophylaxis against *Pneumocystis* organisms has been shown to alter the appearance of *Pneumocystis* pneumonia, with the infiltrates being confined to the apices of the lungs (Chaffey et al., 1990; Conces et al., 1989). Radiation therapy also alters the pattern of infiltrates in *Pneumocystis* infection, with the irradiated lung being spared (Panicek et al., 1987). Splenectomy such as that performed during a staging laparotomy for Hodgkin's disease increases the patient's susceptibility to infections by *Streptococcus pneumoniae*. Conversely, pneumococcal vaccination decreases susceptibility to pneumococcal infection.

Epidemiologic Risk Factors

Information from the patient's epidemiologic history may be important. Exposure to an organism known to cause dormant infections, or previous history of such exposure, may provide a clue to the current illness. A number of organisms, including those of *Histoplasma, Coccidioides, Mycobacterium, Toxoplasma, Pneumocystis,* CMV, herpes simplex virus, and varicella virus, may remain in a dormant state following the initial infection (Anderson and Jordan, 1990; Dummer, 1990; McCabe and Remington, 1990; Sinnott and Emmanuel, 1990; Zeluff, 1990). With decreasing immune status, these organisms may reactivate, producing a recurrent infection. Patients with asymptomatic *Strongyloides stercoralis* infection may develop disseminated disease when given corticosteroids or immunosuppressive agents (Stone and Schaffner, 1990).

Infections that are community-acquired frequently are due to organisms that cause pneumonia in normal individuals. Hospitalization of the patient, however, is associated with a change in the flora of the upper airways (Woods, 1988). The normal gram-positive, low-virulence organisms are replaced by gram-negative bacilli, which when aspirated can result in a serious gram-negative pneumonia (Pennington, 1986) (see Chapter 5). When nosocomial infections do occur, knowledge of current hospital epidemiology may provide clues to the etiologic agent. The occurrence of two or more cases of gram-negative or fungal infection that are related by either time or location should raise the possibility of a point-source outbreak. Point-source outbreaks have also been associated with infection by *Legionella* and *Mycobacterium* organisms (Arnow et al., 1982; Di Perri et al., 1989). Epidemics occurring in the community, such as with infection by *Histoplasma* organisms, frequently involve individuals with compromised immune function (Wheat et al., 1982). Travel to, or previous residence in, regions with endemic infections may result in infection by organisms of such genera as *Histoplasma*, *Coccidioides*, and *Strongyloides* (Stone and Schaffner, 1990; Zeluff, 1990) (see Fig. 10–1*B*).

Rate of Progression

A useful clue in the evaluation of the compromised patient with suspected pneumonia is the rate at which the disease process developed. The pulmonary process can be classified as acute, subacute, or chronic. This information is useful because organisms have characteristic rates of progression (Table 10–4). Acute processes, those that develop in less than 24 hours, are typically bacterial infections or due to such noninfectious processes as edema or hemorrhage (Fig. 10–7). Subacute processes occur over 1 to 7 days and are seen with infections due to organisms of *Aspergillus*, *Nocardia*, *Legionella*, and *Pneumocystis*, and to viruses (see Fig. 10–5). Chronic development is said to occur when the progression is gradual and lasts for a period longer than 1 week. Mycobacterial and fungal infections frequently are responsible for these slowly developing infiltrates (see Fig. 10–1*B*). Some organisms may have a variable rate of progression. An example is *Pneumocystis*

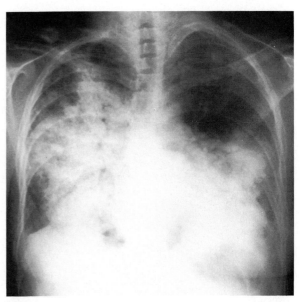

Figure 10–7. Patient receiving steroids for systemic lupus erythematosus and serum sickness developed dyspnea accompanied by mild hemoptysis over a period of several hours. Chest radiograph demonstrates widespread alveolar infiltrates, which on bronchoscopy were found to represent blood. Pulmonary hemorrhage was felt to be secondary to the patient's vasculitis.

organisms, which have a much more insidious course in patients with acquired immunodeficiency syndrome (AIDS). In one series, the median duration of symptoms at the time of diagnosis was 28 days in AIDS patients as compared with 5 days in non-AIDS patients (Kovacs et al., 1984).

Extrapulmonary Findings

Extrapulmonary physical findings and clinical factors can provide clues to the nature of a suspected pneumonia. Dissemination of organisms from a lung infection may result in the development of skin and soft-tissue infections (Wolfson et al., 1985). Ecthyma gangrenosum is a cutaneous lesion that may develop in granulocytopenic patients with *Pseudomonas aeruginosa* pneumonia. Bacteremia during pneumonia from *Staphylococcus* or *Nocardia* organisms may result in the development of subcutaneous abscesses. Skin lesions may also be observed with infections by *Cryptococcus*, *Candida*, and *Mycobacterium avium* organisms (see Fig. 10–6).

Meningoencephalitis and brain abscess may occur with infections by *Cryptococcus*, *Nocardia*, *Toxoplasma*, and *Mycobacterium* organisms (Armstrong and Polsky, 1988) (Fig. 10–8). In granulocytopenic patients, dissemination of the central nervous system by bacteria, such as *Pseudomonas* and *Staphylococcus* organisms, as well as by *Aspergillus* fungi, may occur. The sinuses and upper respiratory tract may be infected by Zygomycetes organisms and respiratory syncytial virus (Englund et al., 1988; Zeluff, 1990). In addition to causing pneumonitis, CMV may also

Table 10–4. RATE OF DEVELOPMENT OF PULMONARY INFECTIONS

Acute (< 24 hr)	Subacute (1–7 days)	Chronic (> 7 days)
Streptococcus pneumoniae	*Pneumocystis*	*Mycobacterium*
Staphylococcus	*Aspergillus*	*Cryptococcus*
Gram-negative	Zygomycetes	*Nocardia*
Legionella	*Cryptococcus*	
	Nocardia	
	Mycobacterium	
	Cytomegalovirus	
	Other viruses	

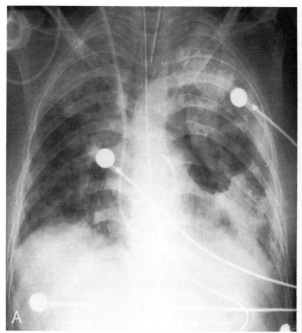

Figure 10–8. Patient who developed cough, fever, and mental status changes while receiving prednisone for pulmonary fibrosis. *A,* Chest radiograph demonstrates a cavitary infiltrate superimposed on the underlying changes of pulmonary fibrosis. *Nocardia* organisms identified by bronchoscopy. *B,* Computed tomographic (CT) scan of the head demonstrates enhanced choroid plexitis with dilated ventricles. Ventricular tap yielded pus with *Nocardia* organisms.

cause hepatitis, ulcerative gastroenteritis, and retinitis (Anderson and Jordan, 1990). Gastrointestinal symptoms sometimes occur with pneumonia due to *Legionella* organisms (Fairbank et al., 1983; Moore et al., 1984). Dissemination of *Nocardia* organisms may result in septic arthritis (Wilson et al., 1989).

LABORATORY STUDIES

A definitive diagnosis of pneumonia requires that the organism be identified either by microscopic examination or by culture. As a rule, this information is not available at the time of the initial evaluation. Certain laboratory studies that may provide insight into the pulmonary process are initially available. The partial pressure of oxygen is typically lowered with infections by bacteria, viruses, and *Pneumocystis carinii*. Hypoxia associated with a normal chest radiograph in a febrile immunocompromised patient should raise the question of infection by *Pneumocystis* organisms or a virus (Young, 1986). In contrast, hypoxia is not typically seen with early involvement by *Nocardia* or *Mycobacterium* organisms, or by fungi. The preservation of oxygenation in these patients is probably due to shunting of blood flow away from the infected lung (Rubin, 1988). Hepatitis,

which sometimes occurs with CMV pneumonia, produces elevation of the hepatic enzymes (Anderson and Jordan, 1990).

CHEST RADIOGRAPHY

The chest radiograph is the primary tool used in screening the febrile immunocompromised patient for a suspected pulmonary infection. Although the chest radiograph is excellent for identifying abnormalities in the thorax, it does not allow a specific diagnosis (Williams et al., 1976). In spite of this limitation, the

Table 10–5. RADIOGRAPHIC APPEARANCE OF INFILTRATES

Consolidation	Nodular/Cavitary	Diffuse
Bacteria	*Cryptococcus*	*Pneumocystis*
Nocardia	*Aspergillus*	Virus
Legionella	*Legionella*	Pulmonary edema
Cryptococcus	*Nocardia*	Hemorrhage
Aspergillus	Bacterial abscess	Radiation
Mycobacterium	Septic emboli	Drug
Hemorrhage	Neoplasm	Lymphangitic tumor
Pulmonary embolus		
Radiation		

information available on the chest radiograph can provide major insight into the pulmonary disease process. Both infectious and noninfectious disease processes tend to produce characteristic radiographic changes, which allows the list of potential differential diagnostic possibilities to be significantly narrowed (Table 10–5). The initial radiographic pattern can be divided into three main groups: consolidative, nodular, and diffuse.

Consolidative Patterns

Consolidation represents filling of the alveolar air spaces with material of fluid density. These infiltrates may be lobar, segmental, or subsegmental in distribution. Air bronchograms may be present. Bacterial infections, including those of the species of *Legionella* and *Nocardia*, typically produce alveolar consolidation (Feigin, 1986; Mermel and Maki, 1990; Modilevsky et al., 1989; Moore et al., 1984) (Fig. 10–9). A consolidative pattern may also be produced by infections due to fungal organisms, such as those of *Aspergillus, Cryptococcus, Histoplasma, Coccidioides,* and *Candida* (Ampel et al., 1989; Buff et al., 1982; Khoury et al., 1984; Pagani and Libshitz, 1981; Zeluff, 1990). A bronchopneumonic pattern, which is characterized by patchy areas of consolidation, may be present. This pattern may occur in infections due to species of *Staphylococcus, Legionella,* and *Candida* (Buff et al., 1982; Kaye et al., 1990; Moore et al., 1984; Pagani and Libshitz, 1981; Zeluff, 1990). Postobstructive pneumonia appears as an area of consolidation, frequently with associated volume loss, which involves lung distal to the bronchial obstruction.

Nodular Patterns

Nodular densities may develop when the pulmonary infection is focal in nature. This pattern is frequently seen with fungal infections by species of *Aspergillus, Cryptococcus, Coccidioides, Histoplasma,* and Zygomycetes (Ampel et al., 1989; Khoury et al., 1984; Pagani and Libshitz, 1981; Zeluff, 1990) (Fig. 10–10). The lesions may be single or multiple; often, multiple lesions are clustered in the same lobe. Rounded or nodular infiltrates may also be produced by infections due to *Legionella, Nocardia,* and anaerobic bacteria (Feigin, 1986; Moore et al., 1984).

Septic emboli in the immunocompromised patient are most commonly associated with an infected indwelling venous catheter, which seeds the lung with infected thrombi. Hematogenous pneumonia due to line sepsis is usually caused by either *Staphylococcus* or *Candida* infection (Clarke and Raffin, 1990; Press et al., 1984). The characteristic chest radiographic findings are multiple nodular densities whose margins are often indistinct (Fig. 10–11*A*). The nodular densities may show evidence of cavitation. In some patients, these findings are equivocal and not definitive for septic emboli. In these cases, computed tomography (CT) may suggest the diagnosis because septic emboli produce a number of characteristic findings (Huang et al., 1989; Kuhlman et al., 1990) (see Fig. 10–11*B*). The most frequent finding is multiple peripheral nodules, which may show evi-

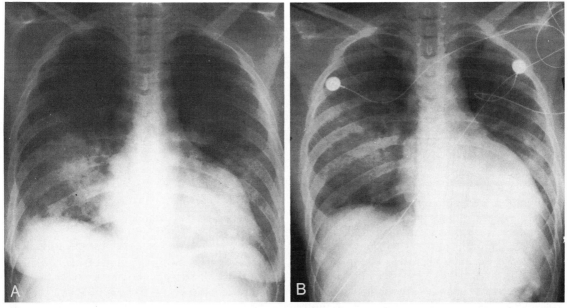

Figure 10–9. Patient with systemic lupus erythematosus who developed sudden onset of fever and a productive cough while receiving steroids. *Hemophilus influenzae* was identified in sputum. *A,* Initial radiograph demonstrating bilateral basilar alveolar infiltrates. *B,* Twelve hours later, significant progression of the left lower lobe infiltrate has occurred.

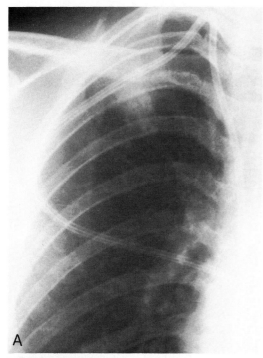

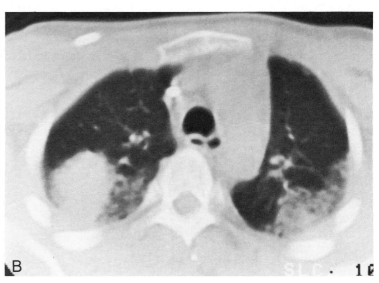

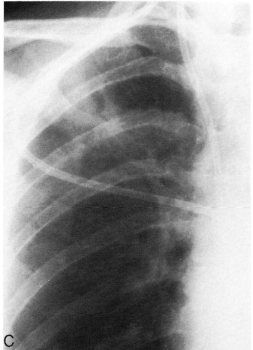

Figure 10–10. Patient developed fever 2 weeks following bone marrow transplant for testicular carcinoma. Patient was profoundly granulocytopenic. *A,* Initial chest radiograph shows a nodular infiltrate in the right upper lobe. Needle biopsy identified *Aspergillus* organisms. *B,* Chest CT scan demonstrates a right upper lobe mass and left upper lobe infiltrate. A narrow zone of low attenuation, representing the halo sign, surrounds the mass. *C,* Following bone marrow recovery, air crescent sign develops within the infiltrate.

dence of cavitation. A feeding vessel can frequently be identified. Air bronchograms may be present within the nodule. Wedge-shaped subpleural lesions are also common, and pleural effusions may occur.

Some infections result in necrosis of lung parenchyma. When necrosis occurs, the necrotic material may drain, resulting in the development of an air-filled cavity. Organisms that may produce cavitation include those of *Aspergillus,* Zygomycetes, *Legionella, Nocardia, Mycobacterium, Staphylococcus,* anaerobic bacteria, and gram-negative bacilli (Feigin,

1986; Kaye et al., 1990; Modilevsky et al., 1989; Moore et al., 1984; Pagani and Libshitz, 1981; Zeluff, 1990) (see Figs. 10–8 and 10–10).

The finding of the air-crescent sign strongly suggests invasive aspergillosis (Gefter et al., 1985; Gross et al., 1982). This sign is characterized by a nodular infiltrate that contains a crescent-shaped air collection surrounding a central density (see Fig. 10–10C). These changes are the result of vascular invasion by *Aspergillus* mycelia resulting in vascular occlusion and subsequent infarction and necrosis of the involved lung. The central density seen within the cavity is composed of necrotic debris and mycelia. This disease process must not be confused with an aspergilloma, which represents mycelia that have colonized a preexisting cavity. The development of the air-crescent sign corresponds with granulocytic recovery (Gefter et al., 1985). Its appearance is associated with improved survival and is usually accompanied by improvement in the infiltrate within 2 to 3 days. It typically appears late in the infection, an average of 15 days after onset.

A number of CT findings have been described for invasive aspergillosis (Hruban et al., 1987; Kuhlman et al., 1985, 1988) (see Fig. 10–10B). Early in the infection, single or multiple nodules or nodular infiltrates develop. When multiple nodules are seen, a dominant mass may be present. A halo of low attenuation surrounding the nodule may develop. These nodules subsequently undergo cavitation and may develop a mural nodule within the cavity, producing an air-crescent sign. Magnetic resonance imaging (MRI) of invasive aspergillosis demonstrates target lesions. The low-density center is due to coagulation necrosis, and the higher signal rim is due to subacute hemorrhage or hemorrhagic infarction (Herold et al., 1989).

Diffuse Patterns

Small opacities may develop in the peribronchial and perivascular regions, producing an interstitial infiltrate. This pattern is typical of viral infections by such agents as CMV, respiratory syncytial virus, herpes simplex virus, and varicella (Anderson and Jordan, 1990). Cytomegalovirus is the most common cause of viral pneumonia in the immunocompromised host (Crawford et al., 1989; Ramsey et al., 1980;

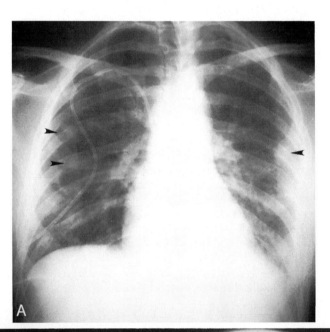

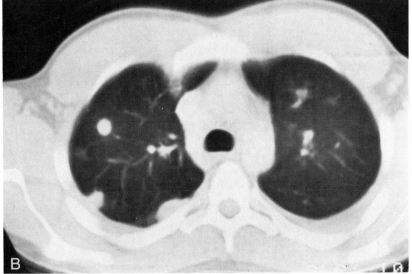

Figure 10–11. Patient receiving high-dose steroids developed *Staphylococcus aureus* septic emboli. *A,* Chest radiograph demonstrates scattered ill-defined nodular infiltrates *(arrowheads). B,* The CT scan shows nodules with feeding vessels, pleural-based lesion, and bilateral pleural effusions.

Wingard et al., 1988). These infections represent either reactivation of a pre-existing dormant virus or transmission of the virus via transfused blood or transplanted organs. The onset of the infection may be acute but is typically subacute in nature. Radiographically, the infection may appear as areas of consolidation, as interstitial infiltrates, or as a combination of the two patterns (Olliff and Williams, 1989) (see Figs. 10–2 and 10–5). Nodules and lobar consolidation have been reported with this infection, but these appearances are uncommon (Ravin et al., 1977; Schulman, 1987). The infiltrates usually are bilateral when first seen, but they may be unilateral. Initially, the infiltrates develop in the middle and lower portions of the lung, but as the infection progresses, they become diffuse (see Fig. 10–5). Incidence of pneumothoraces is increased in patients with CMV pneumonia.

Pneumocystis carinii infection may also produce diffuse infiltrates. In its early stages, the infection appears as a reticular nodular infiltrate that is typically perihilar or basilar in location (Forrest, 1972). As the infection progresses, the infiltrates become diffuse in distribution and alveolar in appearance. *Pneumocystis* infection in patients with AIDS has a much more varied appearance, with focal, nodular, and apical infiltrates being reported (Klein et al., 1989; Milligan et al., 1985) (see Fig. 10–4). In AIDS patients, however, the presence of lobar consolidation, nodules, infiltrates with effusions, and isolated pleural effusions should suggest bacterial infection rather than *Pneumocystis* infection (Amorosa et al., 1990). Patients with AIDS may develop pneumatoceles following *Pneumocystis* pneumonia (Sandhu and Goodman, 1989). These cysts may be present on the initial radiograph or may develop during therapy. The pneumatoceles are often multiple and thin-walled and do not contain intracystic material (Fig. 10–12). Rupture of these cysts may be responsible for the increased incidence of pneumothoraces observed in AIDS pa-

tients with *Pneumocystis* infection (Goodman et al., 1986; Sandhu and Goodman, 1989).

Patients may have an active *Pneumocystis* infection yet have a normal chest radiograph at initial presentation. An abnormally low arterial partial pressure of oxygen (Pa_{O_2}) is frequently noted in this situation. Gallium scintigraphy, which is highly sensitive in detecting *Pneumocystis* infection (94% to 100%), is useful in these cases although not specific. The results are usually abnormal when the chest radiograph is normal (Barron et al., 1985; Kramer et al., 1989; Woolfenden et al., 1987).

Another diffuse pattern occurs with dissemination of fungal and tuberculous infections. This miliary pattern is made up of multiple diffuse nodules, which measure less than 3 mm. Cryptococcal pneumonia in AIDS patients most commonly appears on radiographs as adenopathy and interstitial infiltrates, which may be nodular (Miller et al., 1990). This pattern differs from that seen in immunocompetent and non-AIDS immunocompromised patients, which typically contains nodules and alveolar infiltrates.

Pleural Effusion

Pleural effusions occur with bacterial infections and infections due to organisms of *Legionella*, *Nocardia*, *Mycobacterium*, *Coccidioides*, and *Cryptococcus* (Ampel et al., 1989; Fairbank et al., 1983; Feigin, 1986; Modilevsky et al., 1989; Moore et al., 1984). Infections due to viruses and to *Pneumocystis* and *Aspergillus* organisms rarely cause pleural effusions. When they do occur, they are usually small. Immunocompromised patients who have unexplained pleural effusions should be thoroughly investigated for infections by *Mycobacterium* and *Cryptococcus* organisms, because these infections may be difficult to diagnose and pleural effusion may be their sole radiographic manifestation (Conces et al., 1990; Woodring et al., 1986).

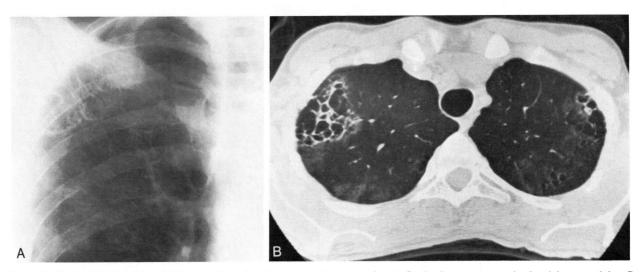

Figure 10–12. An AIDS patient with history of previous *Pneumocystis* pneumonia. *A,* Cystic changes present in the right upper lobe. *B,* The CT scan demonstrates multiple bilateral pneumatoceles, which are thin-walled and do not contain any intracystic material.

Lymphadenopathy

Adenopathy may develop in infections due to species of *Coccidioides, Histoplasma,* and *Mycobacterium* (Ampel et al., 1989; Modilevsky et al., 1989). In AIDS patients, infections due to *Mycobacterium avium* complex and *Cryptococcus* organisms are the most common causes of hilar and mediastinal adenopathy (Suster et al., 1986). Adenopathy occurs infrequently with *Nocardia* infection and rarely occurs with bacterial, viral, *Pneumocystis,* or *Aspergillus* infection (Feigin, 1986; Pagani and Libshitz, 1981). Neoplasm, either primary or recurrent, and lymphoma must always be considered as a possible cause of lymph node enlargement.

NONINFECTIOUS ETIOLOGIC FACTORS

Pulmonary abnormalities that develop in the immunocompromised host are not always due to infection; noninfectious processes may be responsible for many of the infiltrates that develop in the patient. These abnormalities may represent progression or a complication of the underlying disease. Therapy for the underlying disease may, at times, produce complications resulting in the development of infiltrates. Seriously ill patients are also prone to development of unrelated disease processes that involve the lung. Noninfectious causes must be identified to spare the patient unnecessary diagnostic tests and potentially harmful therapeutic procedures.

Pulmonary Edema

Fluid overload or congestive heart failure may produce infiltrates that may simulate infection in the compromised host. This effect may be due to unrelated coronary artery disease or may result from treatment for the underlying disease. Chemotherapeutic agents (e.g., doxorubicin hydrochloride [Adriamycin]) may damage the myocardium (Perry, 1986), and radiation therapy may produce myocarditis or constrictive pericarditis (Niewtzow and Reynolds, 1986).

Noncardiac pulmonary edema may develop from a variety of causes, including bacteremia and drug reactions. Acute pulmonary edema due to a leukoagglutinin reaction may develop following a blood transfusion (Ward, 1970). It results from a reaction between transfused antibodies and the recipient's white blood cells. This reaction, which usually occurs within 4 hours of the transfusion, is associated with dyspnea, fever, urticaria, and hypotension. A progressive fatal congestive cardiomyopathy has been reported in AIDS patients (Corboy et al., 1987).

Neoplasm

Neoplasm, representing either recurrent or new malignancy, may develop in the immunocompromised host. Patients maintained on prolonged immunosuppressive therapy have an increased incidence of neoplasms, including lung cancer, breast cancer, non-Hodgkin's lymphoma, and leukemia (Rosenow et al., 1985). Patients with AIDS may develop Kaposi's sarcoma and lymphoma (Sider et al., 1989; Sivit et al., 1987).

Metastatic lesions may appear as nodules, adenopathy, pleural effusions, or lymphangitic spread. Lymphangitic spread produces diffuse interstitial infiltrates, which over time become coarser in appearance and may be associated with nodular densities. In AIDS patients, Kaposi's sarcoma tends to involve the lung diffusely, producing either linear or nodular densities (Sivit et al., 1987).

Patients with recurrent Hodgkin's disease frequently present with adenopathy but may demonstrate infiltrates, nodules, and pleural effusions (Rosenow et al., 1985) (Fig. 10–13). The majority of lymphomas developing in patients with AIDS or organ transplants are non-Hodgkin's lymphomas (Penn, 1989; Sider et al., 1989). A relation between post-transplant lymphomas and Epstein-Barr viral infection has been hypothesized. Reduction in immunosuppression may be associated with regression of these tumors. These lymphomas may demonstrate adenopathy but are more frequently found to be extranodal, with pleural effusions, nodules, and interstitial and alveolar disease developing.

Leukemia may directly involve the lung with the development of infiltrates (Rosenow et al., 1985). The high white blood cell counts observed with acute leukemias may produce pulmonary leukostasis (van Buchem et al., 1987). This process results in leukemic cell thrombi of the vasculature with resulting cerebral, cardiac, and pulmonary dysfunction. The chest radio-

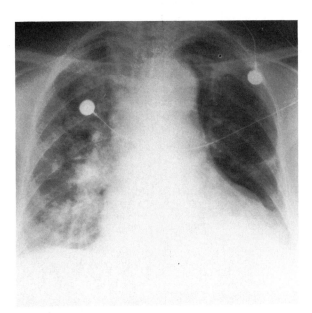

Figure 10–13. Heart transplant patient who developed shortness of breath 19 months following transplantation. Bilateral alveolar infiltrates were present, which on open lung biopsy proved to be non-Hodgkin's lymphoma.

graph may appear normal or show changes of pulmonary edema. Leukemic cell-lysis pneumonopathy is a disorder observed following the treatment of acute leukemia, and it results in the development of noncardiac pulmonary edema (Tryka et al., 1982a).

Drug Reactions

Chemotherapeutic agents not only suppress the immune system, making the patient susceptible to infection, but also may have direct toxic effects on the lung. Drug-induced pulmonary disease can be divided into two categories: cytotoxic and noncytotoxic reactions (Snyder and Hertz, 1988) (Table 10–6). Drug reactions frequently produce infiltrates, and the patient often has fever, which clinically mimics infection.

Cytotoxic reactions are the most common type encountered, with the symptoms usually beginning 2 to 6 months after initiation of therapy. Clinically, they are characterized by the insidious development of cough, dyspnea, and fever. The symptoms slowly progress and often do not resolve with discontinuation of the drug. Radiographically, development of diffuse infiltrates appears; it may consist of either alveolar opacities or interstitial changes (Fig. 10–14). Small pleural effusions develop in 10% of patients. These patients are hypoxic, and their pulmonary function tests reveal a restrictive pattern. The reaction may be accelerated by administration of oxygen or irradiation of the lungs (Tryka et al., 1982b).

The two types of noncytotoxic drug-induced pulmonary disease are hypersensitivity lung disease and noncardiac pulmonary edema (Snyder and Hertz, 1988). The hypersensitivity reaction develops relatively acutely, with symptoms appearing within hours to days of the initiation of drug therapy. Clinically, the patient develops cough, dyspnea, and fever. The patient may have peripheral eosinophilia. The chest radiographic changes tend to involve interstitial infiltrates. Usually, the result of discontinuation of the drug, of administration of glucocorticoids, or of both is resolution of the clinical and radiographic findings. Noncardiac pulmonary edema is an uncommon drug reaction that may occur with administration of cytosine arabinoside, methotrexate, interleukin-2, or cy-

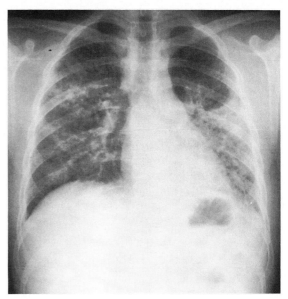

Figure 10–14. Patient with recurrent Hodgkin's disease who was treated with a regimen of chemotherapy that included bleomycin. Chest radiograph demonstrated development of bilateral perihilar infiltrates, which on open lung biopsy were consistent with bleomycin toxicity.

clophosphamide (Snyder and Hertz, 1988; Conant et al., 1989).

Radiation Pneumonitis

Irradiation of the lung may damage the lung parenchyma, producing radiation pneumonitis (Gross, 1977; Libshitz and Southard, 1974). Radiation pneumonitis is most frequently seen in patients treated for breast cancer, lung cancer, and Hodgkin's disease. The radiation injury produces a biphasic clinical pattern: acute radiation pneumonitis and radiation fibrosis, which develops later.

Radiation pneumonitis usually becomes clinically evident between 2 to 3 months following completion of radiation therapy. Cough is the most prominent symptom, with dyspnea and fever occurring in severe cases. The initial radiographic findings are characterized by the development of a ground-glass appearance within the radiation fields, which may progress to an area of alveolar consolidation. The infiltrates have sharp edges that cross anatomic boundaries and correspond to the radiation field. Air bronchograms are frequently present, and pleural or pericardial effusion may develop.

Most patients become asymptomatic with resolution of the radiation pneumonitis but develop some degree of radiation fibrosis. These changes gradually develop 12 to 24 months following completion of therapy. Radiographically, radiating streaklike densities develop in the original area of pneumonitis. Contraction of the involved lung may occur, with

Table 10–6. CHEMOTHERAPEUTIC AGENTS THAT CAUSE PULMONARY DISEASE

Cytotoxic Reaction	Noncytotoxic Reaction
Azathioprine	Bleomycin
Bleomycin	Cytosine arabinoside
Busulfan	Methotrexate
Chlorambucil	Procarbazine
Cyclophosphamide	
Melphalan	
Mitomycin C	
Nitrosourea agents	
Procarbazine	

resultant displacement of hilar structures and compensatory hyperinflation of adjacent lung. Pleural reaction may also be observed.

Interstitial Pneumonia

Interstitial pneumonia develops in 55% of bone marrow transplant patients who survive more than 30 days after transplantation (Bortin et al., 1989; Neiman et al., 1977; Wingard et al., 1988). This disorder typically develops between 30 and 90 days following transplantation. Most of these infiltrates are due to infection, with CMV being the most common organism recovered from these patients. In 40% of the patients, however, the interstitial pneumonitis is idiopathic. These disorders are indistinguishable clinically and radiographically. The exact cause of the idiopathic pneumonitis is not known, but it appears to be related to radiation and chemotherapy toxicity.

Patients with AIDS frequently develop interstitial infiltrates. The most common cause is infection by *Pneumocystis carinii*. These patients, however, are prone to development of noninfectious interstitial infiltrates. Lymphocytic interstitial pneumonia develops in AIDS patients and is characterized by a diffuse infiltration of the interstitium by lymphocytes, histiocytes, and plasma cells (Guillon et al., 1988; Oldham et al., 1989). Radiographically, this disorder may appear as a fine or coarse reticular nodular infiltrate, which may have superimposed areas of alveolar infiltrate. This disorder may appear as isolated pneumonitis or as part of a diffuse infiltrative lymphocytosis syndrome with involvement of multiple organs (Itescu et al., 1990). Another form of interstitial pneumonitis has been reported in conjunction with HIV infection and is characterized histologically by nonspecific interstitial pneumonitis (Simmons et al., 1987). Both of these disorders produce diagnostic dilemmas because they can not be distinguished radiographically from *Pneumocystis carinii* infection.

Other Noninfectious Disease Processes

Pulmonary hemorrhage may occur spontaneously during development of severe thrombocytopenia, which usually involves a platelet count of less than 15,000/mm³ (15 × 10⁹/liter) of blood. Hemorrhage may also follow such procedures as transbronchial biopsy and percutaneous needle biopsy of the lung. Hemoptysis may not be present. Radiographically, the hemorrhage may appear as either focal or diffuse areas of consolidation (see Fig. 10–7 and Chapter 5). Infiltrates may develop following a pulmonary embolus if infarction occurs. The infiltrates are typically pleural-based and wedge-shaped. A pleural effusion may be associated with the infiltrate (see Chapter 9). Bronchoalveolar lavage, which is frequently used to evaluate infiltrates in the immunocompromised pa-

tient, may produce areas of consolidation that correspond with the regions of the lung that underwent lavage (Gurney et al., 1987). These infiltrates tend to clear within 24 hours following the procedure.

References

Amorosa, J.K., Nahass, R.G., Nosher, J.L., and Gocke, D.J.: Radiologic distinction of pyogenic pulmonary infection from *Pneumocystis carinii* pneumonia in AIDS patients. Radiology 175:721, 1990.

Ampel, N.M., Wieden, M.A., and Galgiani, J.N.: Coccidioidomycosis: Clinical update. Rev. Infect. Dis. 11:897, 1989.

Anderson, D.J., and Jordan, M.C.: Viral pneumonia in recipients of solid organ transplants. Semin. Respir. Infect. 5:38, 1990.

Armstrong, D., and Polsky, B.: Central nervous system infections in the compromised host. *In* Rubin, R.H., and Young, L.S. (eds.): Clinical Approach to Infection in the Compromised Host, ed. 2. New York, Plenum, 1988, p. 165.

Arnow, P.M., Chou, T., Weil, D., et al.: Nosocomial Legionnaires' disease caused by aerosolized tap water from respiratory devices. J. Infect. Dis. 146:460, 1982.

Austin, J.H.M., Schulman, L.L., and Mastrobattista, J.D.: Pulmonary infection after cardiac transplantation: Clinical and radiologic correlations. Radiology 172:259, 1989.

Balow, J.E., Hurley, D.L., and Fauci, A.S.: Cyclophosphamide suppression of established cell-mediated immunity. J. Clin. Invest. 56:65, 1975.

Barbara, J.A.J., and Tedder, R.S.: Viral infections transmitted by blood and its products. Clin. Haematol. 13:693, 1984.

Barron, T.F., Birnbaum, N.S., Shane, L.B., et al.: *Pneumocystis carinii* pneumonia studied by gallium-67 scanning. Radiology 154:791, 1985.

Beck, J.M., and Shellito, J.: Effects of human immunodeficiency virus on pulmonary host defenses. Semin. Respir. Infect. 4:75, 1989.

Bodey, G.P., Buckley, M., Sathe, Y.S., and Freireich, E.J.: Quantitative relationships between circulating leukocytes and infection in patients with acute leukemia. Ann. Intern. Med. 64:328, 1966.

Bortin, M.M., Ringden, O., Horowitz, M.M., et al.: Temporal relationships between the major complications of bone marrow transplantation for leukemia. Bone Marrow Transplant. 4:339, 1989.

Buff, S.J., McLelland, R., Gallis, H.A., et al.: *Candida albicans* pneumonia: Radiographic appearance. AJR 138:645, 1982.

Chaffey, M.H., Klein, J.S., Gamsu, G., et al.: Radiographic distribution of *Pneumocystis carinii* pneumonia in patients with AIDS treated with prophylactic inhaled pentamidine. Radiology 175:715, 1990.

Chandra, R.K.: Nutrition, immunity, and infection: Present knowledge and future directions. Lancet 1:688, 1983.

Clarke, D.E., and Raffin, T.A.: Infectious complications of indwelling long-term central venous catheters. Chest 97:966, 1990.

Conant, E.F., Fox, K.R., and Miller, W.T.: Pulmonary edema as a complication of interleukin-2 therapy. AJR 152:749, 1989.

Conces, D.J., Vix, V.A., and Tarver, R.D.: Pleural cryptococcosis. J. Thorac. Imaging 5:84, 1990.

Conces, D.J., Kraft, J.L., Vix, V.A., and Tarver, R.D.: Apical *Pneumocystis carinii* pneumonia after inhaled pentamidine prophylaxis. AJR 152:1192, 1989.

Corboy, J.R., Fink, L., and Miller, W.T.: Congestive cardiomyopathy in association with AIDS. Radiology 165:139, 1987.

Crawford, S.W., Hackman, R.C., and Clark, J.G.: Biopsy diagnosis and clinical outcome of persistent focal pulmonary lesions after marrow transplantation. Transplantation 48:266, 1989.

Dale, D.C., Guerry, D., Wewerka, J.R., et al.: Chronic neutropenia. Medicine 58:128, 1979.

Di Perri, G., Cruciani, M., Danzi, M.C., et al.: Nosocomial epidemic of active tuberculosis among HIV-infected patients. Lancet 2:1502, 1989.

Dummer, J.S.: *Pneumocystis carinii* infections in transplant recipients. Semin. Respir. Infect. 5:50, 1990.

Englund, J.A., Sullivan, C.J., Jordan, M.C., et al.: Respiratory syncytial virus infection in immunocompromised adults. Ann. Intern. Med. 109:203, 1988.

Fairbank, J.T., Mamourian, A.C., Dietrich, P.A., and Girod, J.C.: The chest radiograph in Legionnaires' disease. Radiology 147:33, 1983.

Feigin, D.S.: Nocardiosis of the lung: Chest radiographic findings in 21 cases. Radiology 159:9, 1986.

Forrest, J.V.: Radiographic findings in *Pneumocystis carinii* pneumonia. Radiology 103:539, 1972.

Gefter, W.B., Albelda, S.M., Talbot, G.H., et al.: Invasive pulmonary aspergillosis and acute leukemia: Limitations in the diagnostic utility of the air crescent sign. Radiology 157:605, 1985.

Gentry, L.O., and Zeluff, B.: Infection in the cardiac transplant patient. *In* Rubin, R.H., and Young, L.S. (eds.): Clinical Approach to Infection in the Compromised Host, ed. 2. New York, Plenum, 1988, p. 623.

Gershwin, M.E., Goetzl, E.J., and Steinberg, A.D.: Cyclophosphamide: Use in practice. Ann. Intern. Med. 80:531, 1974.

Goodman, P.C., Daley, C., and Minagi, H.: Spontaneous pneumothorax in AIDS patients with *Pneumocystis carinii* pneumonia. AJR 147:29, 1986.

Gottesdiener, K.M.: Transplanted infections: Donor-to-host transmission with the allograft. Ann. Intern. Med. 110:1001, 1989.

Gross, B.H., Spitz, H.B., and Felson, B.: The mural nodule in cavitary opportunistic pulmonary aspergillus. Radiology 143:619, 1982.

Gross, N.J.: Pulmonary effects of radiation therapy. Ann. Intern. Med. 86:81, 1977.

Guillon, J.M., Autran, B., Denis, M., et al.: Human immunodeficiency virus–related lymphocytic alveolitis. Chest 94:1264, 1988.

Gurney, J.W., Harrison, W.C., Sears, K., et al.: Bronchoalveolar lavage: Radiographic manifestations. Radiology 163:71, 1987.

Harvey, R.L., and Myers, J.P.: Nosocomial fungemia in a large community teaching hospital. Arch. Intern. Med. 147:2117, 1987.

Herold, C.J., Kramer, J., Sertl, K., et al.: Invasive pulmonary aspergillosis: Evaluation with MR imaging. Radiology 173:717, 1989.

Hilton, E., Haslett, T.M., Borenstein, M.T., et al.: Central catheter infections: Single- versus triple-lumen catheters. Am. J. Med. 84:667, 1988.

Hruban, R.H., Meziane, M.A., Zerhouni, E.A., et al.: Radiologic-pathologic correlation of the CT halo sign in invasive pulmonary aspergillosis. J. Comput. Assist. Tomogr. 11:534, 1987.

Huang, R.M., Naidich, D.P., Lubat, E., et al.: Septic pulmonary emboli: CT-radiographic correlation. AJR 153:41, 1989.

Hutter, J.A., Scott, J., Wreghitt, T., et al.: The importance of cytomegalovirus in heart-lung transplant recipients. Chest 95:627, 1989.

Itescu, S., Brancato, L.J., Buxbaum, J., et al.: A diffuse infiltrative CD8 lymphocytosis syndrome in human immunodeficiency virus (HIV) infection: A host immune response associated with HLA-DR5. Ann. Intern. Med. 112:3, 1990.

Junker, A.K., Ochs, H.D., Clark, E.A., et al.: Transient immune deficiency in patients with acute Epstein-Barr virus infection. Clin. Immunol. Immunopathol. 40:436, 1986.

Kaltreider, H.B.: Phagocytic, antibody and cell-mediated immune mechanisms. *In* Murray, J.F., and Nadel, J.A. (eds.): Textbook of Respiratory Medicine, vol. 1. Philadelphia, W.B. Saunders, 1988, p. 332.

Kaye, M.G., Fox, M.J., Bartlett, J.G., et al.: The clinical spectrum of *Staphylococcus aureus* pulmonary infection. Chest 97:788, 1990.

Khoury, M.B., Godwin, J.D., Ravin, C.E., et al.: Thoracic cryptococcosis: Immunologic competence and radiologic appearance. AJR 141:893, 1984.

Klein, J.S., Warnock, M., Webb, W.R., and Gamsu, G.: Cavitating and noncavitating granulomas in AIDS patients with *Pneumocystis* pneumonitis. AJR 152:753, 1989.

Komshian, S.V., Uwaydah, A.K., Sobel, J.D., and Crane, L.R.: Fungemia caused by *Candida* species and *Torulopsis glabrata* in the hospitalized patient: Frequency, characteristics, and evaluation of factors influencing outcome. Rev. Infect. Dis. 11:379, 1989.

Kovacs, J.A., Hiemenz, J.W., Macher, A.M., et al.: *Pneumocystis carinii* pneumonia: A comparison between patients with the acquired immunodeficiency syndrome and patients with other immunodeficiencies. Ann. Intern. Med. 100:663, 1984.

Kramer, E.L., Sanger, J.H., Garay, S.M., et al.: Diagnostic implications of Ga-67 chest-scan patterns in human immunodeficiency virus–seropositive patients. Radiology 170:671, 1989.

Kuhlman, J.E., Fishman, E.K., and Siegelman, S.S.: Invasive pulmonary aspergillosis in acute leukemia: Characteristic findings on CT, the CT halo sign, and the role of CT in early diagnosis. Radiology 157:611, 1985.

Kuhlman, J.E., Fishman, E.K., and Teigen, C.: Pulmonary septic emboli: Diagnosis with CT. Radiology 174:2112, 1990.

Kuhlman, J.E., Fishman, E.K., Burch, P.A., et al.: CT of invasive pulmonary aspergillosis. AJR 150:1015, 1988.

Kusne, S., Dummer, J.S., Singh, N., et al.: Infections after liver transplantation: An analysis of 101 consecutive cases. Medicine 67:132, 1988.

Kyle, R.A., and Linman, J.W.: Chronic idiopathic neutropenia. N. Engl. J. Med. 279:1015, 1968.

Langer, M., Mosconi, P., Cigada, M., and Mandelli, M.: Long-term respiratory support and risk of pneumonia in critically ill patients. Am. Rev. Respir. Dis. 140:302, 1989.

Libshitz, H.I., and Southard, M.E.: Complications of radiation therapy: The thorax. Semin. Roentgenol. 9:41, 1974.

McCabe, R.E., and Remington, J.S.: *Toxoplasma gondii. In* Mandell, G.L., et al. (eds.): Principles and Practice of Infectious Diseases, ed 3. New York, Churchill Livingstone, 1990, p. 2090.

Mermel, L.A., and Maki, D.G.: Bacterial pneumonia in solid organ transplantation. Semin. Respir. Infect. 5:10, 1990.

Meyers, J.D., and Thomas, E.D.: Infection complicating bone marrow transplantation. *In* Rubin, R.H., and Young, L.S. (eds.): Clinical Approach to Infection in the Compromised Host, ed. 2. New York, Plenum, 1988, p. 525.

Miller, W.T., Edelman, J.M., and Miller, W.T.: Cryptococcal pulmonary infection in patients with AIDS: Radiologic appearance. Radiology 175:735, 1990.

Milligan, S.A., Stulbarg, M.S., Gamsu, G., and Golden, J.A.: *Pneumocytis carinii* pneumonia radiographically simulating tuberculosis. Am. Rev. Respir. Dis. 132:1124, 1985.

Modilevsky, T., Sattler, F.R., and Barnes, P.F.: Mycobacterial disease in patients with human immunodeficiency virus infection. Arch. Intern. Med. 49:2201, 1989.

Moore, E.H., Webb, W.R., Gamsu, G., and Golden, J.A.: Legionnaires' disease in the renal transplant patient: Clinical presentation and radiographic progression. Radiology 153:589, 1984.

Neiman, P.E., Reeves, W., Ray, G., et al.: A prospective analysis of interstitial pneumonia and opportunistic viral infection among recipients of allogenic bone marrow grafts. J. Infect. Dis. 136:754, 1977.

Niewtzow, R.C., Reynolds, R.D.: Radiation therapy and the heart. *In* Kapoor, A.S., and Reynolds, R.D. (eds.): Cancer and the Heart. New York, Springer-Verlag, 1986, p. 232.

Oldham, S.A.A., Castillo, M., Jacobson, F.L., et al.: HIV-related lymphocytic interstitial pneumonia: Radiologic manifestations and pathologic correlation. Radiology 170:83, 1989.

Olliff, J.F.C., and Williams, M.P.: Radiological appearances of cytomegalovirus infections. Clin. Radiol. 40:463, 1989.

Pagani, J.J., and Libshitz, H.I.: Opportunistic fungal pneumonias in cancer patients. AJR 137:1033, 1981.

Panicek, D.M., Groskin, S.A., Chung, C.T., et al.: Atypical distribution of *Pneumocystis carinii* infiltrates during radiation therapy. Radiology 163:689, 1987.

Penn, I.: Risk of cancer in the transplant patient. *In* Flye, M.W. (ed.): Principles of Organ Transplantation. Philadelphia, W.B. Saunders, 1989, p. 634.

Pennington, J.E.: Gram-negative bacterial pneumonia in the immunocompromised host. Semin. Respir. Infect. 1:145, 1986.

Perry, M.C.: Effects of chemotherapy on the heart. *In* Kapoor,

A.S., and Reynolds, R.D. (eds.): Cancer and the Heart. New York, Springer-Verlag, 1986, p. 223.

Press, O.W., Ramsey, P.G., Larson, E.B., et al.: Hickman catheter infections in patients with malignancies. Medicine 63:189, 1984.

Ramsey, P.G., Rubin, R.H., Tolkoff-Rubin, N.E., et al.: The renal transplant patient with fever and pulmonary infiltrates: Etiology, clinical manifestations, and management. Medicine 59:206, 1980.

Ravin, C.E., Smith, G.W., Ahern, M.J., et al.: Cytomegaloviral infection presenting as a solitary pulmonary nodule. Chest 71:220, 1977.

Reynolds, H.Y.: Normal and defective respiratory host defenses. In Pennington, J.E. (ed.): Respiratory Infections: Diagnosis and Management, ed. 2. New York, Raven Press, 1988, p. 1.

Roberts-Thomson, I.C., Whittingham, S., Youngchaiyud, U., et al.: Ageing, immune response, and mortality. Lancet 2:368, 1974.

Rosenow, E.C., Wilson, W.R., and Cockerill, F.R.: Pulmonary disease in the immunocompromised host (first of two parts). Mayo Clin. Proc. 60:473, 1985.

Rubin, R.H.: Infection in the renal and liver transplant patient. In Rubin, R.H., and Young, L.S. (eds.): Clinical Approach to Infection in the Compromised Host, ed. 2. New York, Plenum, 1988, p. 557.

Rubin, R.H., Wolfson, J.S., Cosimi, A.B., and Tolkoff-Rubin, N.E.: Infection in the renal transplant recipient. Am. J. Med. 70:405, 1981.

Rubin, R.H., Cosimi, A.B., Tolkoff-Rubin, N.E., et al.: Infectious disease syndromes attributable to cytomegalovirus and their significance among renal transplant recipients. Transplantation 24:458, 1977.

Sandhu, J.S., and Goodman, P.C.: Pulmonary cysts associated with Pneumocystis carinii pneumonia in patients with AIDS. Radiology 173:33, 1989.

Schulman, L.L.: Cytomegalovirus pneumonitis and lobar consolidation. Chest 91:558, 1987.

Sider, L., Weiss, A.J., Smith, M.D., et al.: Varied appearance of AIDS-related lymphoma in the chest. Radiology 171:629, 1989.

Simmons, J.T., Suffredini, A.F., Lack, E.E., et al.: Nonspecific interstitial pneumonitis in patients with AIDS: Radiologic features. AJR 149:265, 1987.

Sinnott, J.T., and Emmanuel, P.J.: Mycobacterial infections in the transplant patient. Semin. Respir. Infect. 5:65, 1990.

Sivit, C.J., Schwartz, A.M., and Rockoff, S.D.: Kaposi's sarcoma of the lung in AIDS: Radiologic-pathologic analysis. AJR 148:25, 1987.

Snyder, L.S., and Hertz, M.I.: Cytotoxic drug-induced lung injury. Semin. Respir. Infect. 3:217, 1988.

Stone, W.J., and Schaffner, W.: Strongyloides infections in transplant recipients. Semin. Respir. Infect. 5:58, 1990.

Suster, B., Akerman, M., Orenstein, M., and Wax, M.R.: Pulmonary manifestations of AIDS: Review of 106 episodes. Radiology 161:87, 1986.

Tryka, A.F., Godleski, J.J., and Fanta, C.H.: Leukemic cell lysis pneumonopathy: A complication of treated myeloblastic leukemia. Cancer 50:2763, 1982a.

Tryka, A.F., Skornik, W.A., Godleski, J.J., and Brain, J.D.: Potentiation of bleomycin-induced lung injury by exposure to 70% oxygen: Morphologic assessment. Am. Rev. Respir. Dis. 126:1074, 1982b.

van Buchem, M.A., Wondergem, J.H., Kool, L.J.S., et al.: Pulmonary leukostasis: Radiologic-pathologic study. Radiology 165:739, 1987.

van der Meer, J.W.M.: Defects in host-defense mechanisms. In Rubin, R.H., and Young, L.S. (eds.): Clinical Approach to Infection in the Compromised Host, ed. 2. New York, Plenum, 1988, p. 131.

Ward, H.N.: Pulmonary infiltrates associated with leukoagglutinin transfusion reactions. Ann. Intern. Med. 73:689, 1970.

Wey, S.B., Mori, M., Pfaller, M.A., et al.: Risk factors for hospital-acquired candidemia. Arch. Intern. Med. 149:2349, 1989.

Wheat, L.J., Slama, T.G., Norton, J.A., et al.: Risk factors for disseminated or fatal histoplasmosis: Analysis of a large urban outbreak. Ann. Intern. Med. 96:159, 1982.

Williams, D.M., Krick, J.A., and Remington, J.S.: Pulmonary infection in the compromised host. Part 1. Am. Rev. Respir. Dis. 114:359, 1976.

Wilson, J.P., Turner, H.R., Kirchner, K.A., and Chapman, S.W.: Nocardial infections in renal transplant recipients. Medicine 68:38, 1989.

Wilson, W.R., Cockerill, F.R., and Rosenow, E.C.: Pulmonary disease in the immunocompromised host (second of two parts). Mayo Clin. Proc. 60:630, 1985.

Wingard, J.R., Mellits, E.D., Sostrin, M.B., et al.: Interstitial pneumonitis after allogenic bone marrow transplantation. Medicine 67:175, 1988.

Winston, D.J., Gale, R.P., Meyer, D.V., and Young, L.S.: Infectious complications of human bone marrow transplantation. Medicine 58:1, 1979a.

Winston, D.J., Schiffman, G., Wang, D.C., et al.: Pneumococcal infections after human bone-marrow transplantation. Ann. Intern. Med. 91:835, 1979b.

Wolfson, J.S., Sober, A.J., and Rubin, R.H.: Dermatologic manifestations of infections in immunocompromised patients. Medicine 64:115, 1985.

Woodring, J.H., Vandiviere, H.M., Fried, A.M., et al.: Update: The radiologic features of pulmonary tuberculosis. AJR 146:497, 1986.

Woods, D.E.: Bacterial colonization of the respiratory tract: Clinical significance. In Pennington, J.E. (ed.): Respiratory Infections: Diagnosis and Management, ed. 2. New York, Raven Press, 1988, p. 34.

Woolfenden, J.M., Carrasquillo, J.A., Larson, S.M., et al.: Acquired immunodeficiency syndrome: Ga-67 citrate imaging. Radiology 162:383, 1987.

Yeung, C., May, J., and Hughes, R.: Infection rate for single lumen v. triple lumen subclavian catheters. Infect. Control Hosp. Epidemiol. 9:154, 1988.

Young, L.S.: An overview of infection in bone marrow transplant recipients. Clin. Haematol. 13:661, 1984.

Young, L.S.: Protozoal infections in the lungs of immunocompromised patients. Semin. Respir. Infect. 1:186, 1986.

Zeluff, B.J.: Fungal pneumonia in transplant recipients. Semin. Respir. Infect. 5:80, 1990.

11

Acute Thoracic Trauma

■

Caroline Chiles
Charles E. Putman

Trauma is the most common cause of death in people between 15 and 45 years of age. Twenty-five percent of these deaths result from chest trauma.

To reduce the morbidity and mortality related to trauma, the American College of Surgeons established trauma center criteria (American Medical Association, 1981). The criteria for a dedicated Level I or II trauma center include the in-hospital presence of an emergency room physician, an anesthesiologist, and a trauma surgeon 24 hours a day. A board-certified radiologist or senior radiology resident must be on call and promptly available. The emergency room must contain radiographic equipment, and a radiology technologist qualified in general radiography, angiography, and computed tomography (CT) must be in the hospital 24 hours a day. Equipment for CT, ultrasonography, nuclear scanning, and angiography must be immediately available for emergency studies.

Appropriate triage of the trauma victim is an important factor in reducing mortality. Because 84% of patients with chest trauma also have extrathoracic injuries which usually involve the head and extremities (Schorr et al., 1987), the evaluation and management of these patients are often complicated.

Conventional radiography remains the mainstay of imaging for trauma victims. The presence of radiographic units within the emergency room allows radiographs to be obtained promptly and with minimal interruption of life-support measures. Angiography is performed in a selected population of trauma victims, based on clinical or radiographic evidence of vascular injury. Computed tomography does not allow optimal patient monitoring and should be reserved for patients who are hemodynamically stable. Magnetic resonance imaging (MRI), owing to the large magnetic field involved, interferes with monitoring equipment to such a degree that it is rarely used in the acute trauma setting.

Chest trauma may be the result of either penetrating injury (e.g., gunshot or stab wound) or blunt trauma (e.g., motor vehicle accident). The radiologist with knowledge of the clinical history is more likely to interpret correctly any imaging studies obtained. For example, a patient with a history of deceleration injury is at risk for aortic transection. The patient with stab wounds over the thorax is likely to have a pneumothorax. The mechanism of injury may help to explain some of the nonspecific abnormalities seen on conventional radiographs, CT scans, ultrasound scans, or nuclear medicine examinations.

PULMONARY PARENCHYMAL INJURY

Pulmonary Contusion

Pulmonary contusion occurs as a result of either blunt or penetrating trauma to the chest. The diagnosis is established by obtaining the history of thoracic trauma and recognizing the characteristic opacities on the chest radiograph. Pulmonary contusion is usually present on the admission chest radiograph but may be delayed in onset for up to 6 hours (Goodman and Putman, 1981). The areas of contusion are frequently adjacent to solid structures, such as ribs, sternum, and vertebral bodies. The opacities may appear as either areas of homogeneous air-space consolidation or an interstitial form of irregular coarse infiltration (Fig. 11–1 A).

Homogeneous consolidation represents intra-alveolar hemorrhage and can be distinguished from atelectasis or pneumonia by its failure to conform to segmental or lobar boundaries. The coarse infiltrate represents hemorrhage into peribronchial and perivascular spaces (Stevens and Templeton, 1965; Williams and Bonte, 1963).

Pulmonary contusion begins to resolve in 24 to 48

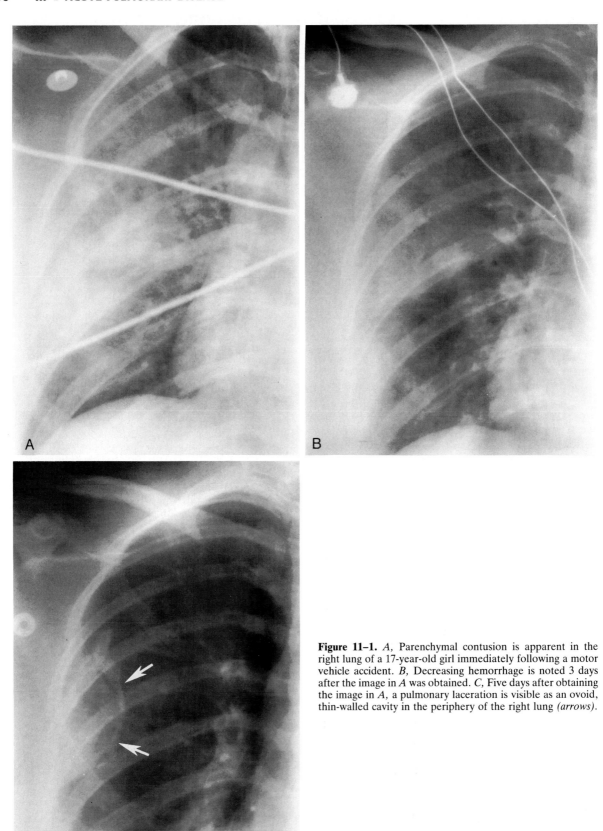

Figure 11–1. *A*, Parenchymal contusion is apparent in the right lung of a 17-year-old girl immediately following a motor vehicle accident. *B*, Decreasing hemorrhage is noted 3 days after the image in *A* was obtained. *C*, Five days after obtaining the image in *A*, a pulmonary laceration is visible as an ovoid, thin-walled cavity in the periphery of the right lung *(arrows)*.

hours and is often completely resolved at 1 week (see Fig. 11–1B). Progression of abnormality after 48 hours should prompt consideration of a superimposed process such as infection or adult respiratory distress syndrome (ARDS). Patients with pulmonary contusion may complain of dyspnea and chest pain. Hemoptysis may or may not be present. Hypoxemia that is out of proportion to the radiographic abnormality may be present (Hankins et al., 1973). Although pulmonary contusion usually resolves without sequelae, ARDS may occur after severe pulmonary contusion.

Pulmonary Laceration

Thoracic trauma may also produce pulmonary laceration. Computed tomography shows that pulmonary laceration occurs more frequently than previously suspected. Using CT, Wagner and colleagues (1988) found 99 pulmonary lacerations in 85 patients, whereas chest radiographs demonstrated lacerations in only five of these patients.

Pulmonary lacerations may be divided into four categories based on the mechanism of injury. Type 1 lacerations, the most common form, occur as a result of sudden compression of a pliable chest wall, causing rupture of the air-containing lung. Type 1 laceration appears as an air-filled linear structure or as an intraparenchymal cavity, with or without an air–fluid level. If the laceration extends to the visceral pleura, the parenchymal cavity is accompanied by a pneumothorax. Type 2 lacerations occur as a result of sudden compression of the pliable lower chest wall, which causes the lower lobe to shift suddenly across

the vertebral body, producing a shear injury. Type 2 laceration, like Type 1 laceration, appears as an air-filled cavity, but occurs in the paravertebral areas of the lower lobes.

Type 3 lacerations are due to penetration of the lung by a fractured rib. Such injury is usually associated with pneumothorax and appears as a small peripheral cavity or linear radiolucency. Type 4 lacerations occur in patients with pre-existing pleural adhesions, which cause the lung to tear when the chest wall is violently moved inward or is fractured. These lacerations can be diagnosed only surgically or at autopsy (Wagner et al., 1988).

Pulmonary lacerations may be obscured initially by intra-alveolar hemorrhage produced by torn vessels (Fig. 11–2; see Fig. 11–1C). Pulmonary lacerations due to compression of the chest wall may be multiple; those due to penetration by a fractured rib are usually single. Air-filled lacerations decrease in size at a rate of 1 to 2 cm per week; lacerations containing blood resolve more slowly. Pulmonary lacerations completely resolve in a period of several weeks to months after injury.

Fat Embolism

Fat embolism syndrome is a serious but relatively uncommon disorder characterized by pulmonary, cerebral, and cutaneous manifestations occurring 12 to 72 hours after trauma (Batra, 1987; Lahiri and ZuWallack, 1977). Fat droplets within small pulmonary vessels are a frequent pathologic finding in patients with multiple fractures and can be found in 96% of accident victims who survive for at least 6

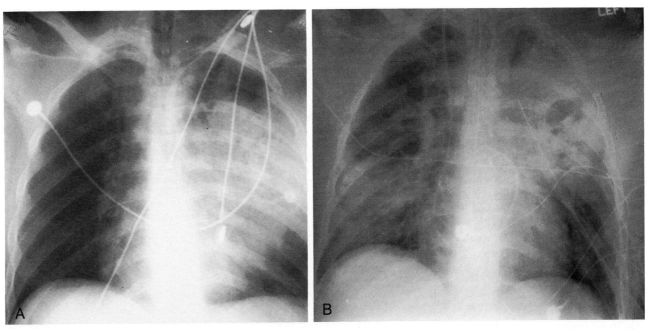

Figure 11–2. A, Parenchymal contusion in left lung after shotgun blast to left thorax. Note fractured left clavicle and metallic fragments in left shoulder. B, Subsequent pneumatocele formation due to pulmonary laceration at the time of injury.

hours after their injury (Palmovic and McCarroll, 1965). Less than 1% of patients with severe or multiple bone injuries, however, show clinical or radiographic evidence of the fat embolism syndrome (Maruyama and Little, 1962; Peltier et al., 1974).

The lipids cause mechanical occlusion of lung capillaries and chemical injury due to lipolysis and to release of free fatty acids. Aggravating conditions, such as shock, hypovolemia, sepsis, or disseminated intravascular coagulation, may be necessary factors in converting the presence of fat emboli into fat embolism syndrome (Gong, 1977).

The typical clinical setting involves a young adult with skeletal injury, often with multiple fractures involving the long bones and pelvis. Clinical signs include fever, tachypnea, tachycardia, and a characteristic pattern of petechiae on the base of the neck, in the axilla, and on the conjunctiva. The patient's symptoms are due to the decrease in perfusion to various organs. The patient develops dyspnea and cyanosis as a result of decreased pulmonary perfusion, disorientation and delirium due to loss of cerebral perfusion, and oliguria due to decreased renal perfusion (Evarts, 1970). The patient is hypoxemic, often with an arterial oxygen pressure (P_{O_2}) of less than 50 mm Hg.

The appearance of the chest radiograph does not correlate with the low P_{O_2} (Peltier, 1971). The chest radiograph initially appears normal but develops patchy opacities and then widespread diffuse opacity within 72 hours of injury (Feldman et al., 1975). Air bronchograms are often visible. The pulmonary opacity resembles alveolar pulmonary edema, with perihilar and basilar predominance, and sparing of the lung apices. A peripheral predominance in some patients may help in distinguishing this entity from cardiogenic edema (Fig. 11–3). The chest radiograph

in fat embolism syndrome may also be distinguished from cardiogenic edema by the normal heart size, normal pulmonary vasculature, normal vascular pedicle, and absence of pleural effusions. In addition, the pulmonary opacity does not clear after diuresis. The distinction on the chest radiograph between fat embolism and other causes of noncardiogenic edema or pulmonary contusion may be more difficult. Whereas pulmonary contusion is radiographically apparent immediately after injury, the appearance of fat embolism is delayed for up to 72 hours after trauma. Contusion clears rapidly (24 to 48 hours). Fat embolism may be recognized in some cases only by the slower rate of clearing (7 to 10 days) on serial chest radiographs.

Pulmonary Edema

Pulmonary edema may occur as a result of cardiac disease, overhydration, or increased capillary permeability. Determination of the cause of the edema facilitates appropriate management of the patient. The chest radiograph is valuable in detecting edema and in distinguishing the three categories of pulmonary edema (Milne et al., 1985). Cardiac edema can be recognized by cardiomegaly, pleural effusions, and a homogeneous pattern of edema. Septal lines and enlargement of the vascular pedicle may be present as well. Overhydration edema shares these features of cardiac edema but may demonstrate a more central edematous pattern.

The patient who appears in the emergency room as a result of trauma is likely to demonstrate capillary permeability edema. Permeability edema may occur as a result of injury to the gas-exchanging membrane, either from the alveolar side (smoke inhalation or

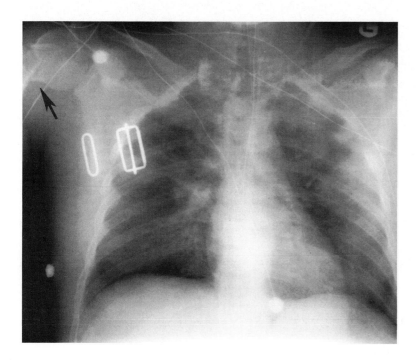

Figure 11–3. Patchy edema due to fat emboli is present bilaterally in 27-year-old man who was struck by an automobile while riding his bicycle. Note the fractures of the proximal right humerus *(arrow)* and of the right seventh and eighth ribs. The patient was febrile, tachypneic, and hypoxemic (P_{O_2} = 54 on 40% oxygen).

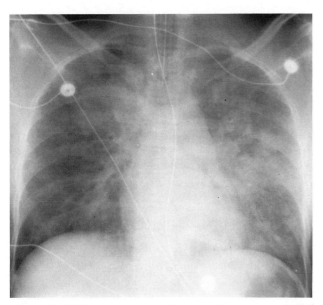

Figure 11–4. Near drowning. A 21-year-old woman was pulled from a freshwater pond after a 10-minute submersion. Her chest radiograph shows pulmonary edema and a normal heart size.

near drowning) or from the capillary side (sepsis or fat embolism) (Greene, 1987; Marini, 1989) (Fig. 11–4). Several radiographic features help to distinguish permeability edema from cardiac edema. In permeability edema, the heart size is normal, the width of the vascular pedicle is normal, and the edema pattern is often patchy and peripheral. Septal lines and pleural effusions are absent, although air bronchograms are commonly seen. The pulmonary capillary wedge pressure in patients with permeability edema remains normal, and the edema does not respond to diuresis. The reader is referred to Chapters 6 and 7 for further discussion of ARDS.

Atelectasis

The patient in distress in the emergency room is unlikely to provide an optimal inspiration for chest radiographs. Atelectasis is a common finding in this situation, but it is usually symmetric and confined to subsegmental areas of the lower lobes. Asymmetric opacity should raise suspicion of pulmonary injury, such as contusion. Atelectasis of an entire lobe or lung may be due to foreign body aspiration, mucous plugging, or ruptured bronchus (see Chapter 5).

Aspiration

The patient who has lost consciousness may have aspirated gastric contents. The chest radiograph is often normal initially but within several hours of the aspiration shows increasing air-space opacity in the posterior segments of the upper lobes or in the superior segments of the lower lobes (see Chapter 5).

Lobar Torsion

Torsion of a lobe or of a complete lung is an uncommon event but can occur after blunt trauma to the chest, after thoracic surgery, or in association with pneumonia or bronchogenic carcinoma (Felson, 1987). Traumatic compression of the lower thorax may cause upward displacement of a lower lobe, severing the inferior pulmonary ligament and allowing torsion to occur (Moser and Proto, 1987). Lobar torsion is more likely to occur in the setting of pneumothorax or pleural effusion (Berkmen et al., 1989).

On chest radiographs, the diagnosis of lobar torsion may be suspected when a collapsed or consolidated lobe is noted in an unusual position. The hilum may be displaced in a direction inappropriate for the atelectatic lobe (Felson, 1987). The lobe may opacify rapidly after trauma, or the opacified lobe may change position on sequential radiographs.

ABNORMALITIES OF THE PLEURAL SPACE

Pneumothorax and hemopneumothorax are common occurrences in the trauma patient. Recognition of pneumothorax, particularly in supine patients, is important and has been emphasized in Chapter 8. A pneumothorax sufficiently large to cause respiratory symptoms requires chest tube placement. Chest tubes may also be indicated when penetrating injury to the chest has occurred and positive-pressure ventilation is contemplated (Millikan et al., 1980), despite failure to identify a pneumothorax radiographically. A pneumothorax that is not visible radiographically is present in 2% to 4% of patients undergoing abdominal CT after trauma (Rhea et al., 1989; Wall et al., 1983). An occult pneumothorax is present in an even higher percentage (44%) of patients undergoing brain CT for trauma (Tocino et al., 1984). One should be aware of the potential for even a small pneumothorax to develop into a tension pneumothorax in a patient who is intubated and is receiving mechanical ventilation in the operating room or critical care unit.

The presence of subcutaneous emphysema over the chest wall in a patient with a history of trauma to the chest should alert the radiologist to the possibility of an occult pneumothorax as a source of the air in the soft tissues. Subcutaneous emphysema may also be focal and related to a soft-tissue laceration or penetrating injury (e.g., stab wound). More widespread subcutaneous emphysema is a frequent development following barotrauma caused by mechanical ventilation (see Chapter 8).

Fluid in the pleural space in the patient following acute trauma to the thorax most likely represents blood. Hemothorax may be due to disruption of a systemic vessel in the chest wall, mediastinum, or diaphragm, or disruption of a pulmonary vessel. Because of the tendency for hemothorax to produce pleural fibrosis, chest tube drainage is often indicated.

Rupture of the thoracic duct is uncommon but produces a characteristic chylothorax, with milky fluid recovered through thoracentesis. Rupture of the thoracic duct in the lower thorax produces right-sided chylothorax. The thoracic duct crosses the midline in the midthorax, so that injury above this level produces a left-sided chylothorax.

CARDIOVASCULAR TRAUMA

Aortic Transection

Transection of the aorta is the cause of death in 10% to 15% of all traffic fatalities. The majority (80% to 90%) of these individuals die instantly; only 10% to 20% survive long enough to reach an emergency room. Diagnosis and repair are essential. Without surgical repair, 90% of those who survive the initial event die within the following 4 months (Bennett and Cherry, 1967; Parmley et al., 1958). Surgical repair results in an 83% survival rate (Symbas et al., 1973).

The injury to the aorta occurs at the level of the aortic isthmus in 70% to 95% of patients receiving medical attention, and just above the aortic valve in only 5% to 30% of patients. The aortic isthmus is the primary site of injury because of several mechanical factors. The major force operating on the aortic isthmus during deceleration is a shear stress produced by differing deceleration rates of the mobile aortic arch and the descending thoracic aorta (Greendyke, 1966). The diagnosis of aortic trauma should be considered after any deceleration injury. The most common event is a motor vehicle accident. Other causes include falls from a height, an airplane crash, and elevator accidents.

The patient may complain of retrosternal or subscapular chest pain, hoarseness, dyspnea, or dysphagia. After a motor vehicle accident or other serious accident, however, trauma to other parts of the body may dominate the clinical situation. The physical examination may be noncontributory to the diagnosis. A systolic murmur is heard in 17% to 39% of patients with aortic transection. An acute coarctation syndrome, characterized by hypertension in the upper extremities and hypotension in the lower extremities, is produced by compression of the distal aorta by mediastinal hematoma or an obstructing intimal flap.

The chest radiograph plays a major role in the diagnosis of aortic transection. The presence of mediastinal hemorrhage on the chest radiograph identifies the patient who has sustained a significant deceleration injury. The diagnosis of aortic transection is then confirmed by aortography. The mediastinal hemorrhage may not be directly related to the aortic injury, because the adventitia of the aorta remains intact in 60% of aortic ruptures. Instead, the mediastinal hemorrhage arises from smaller mediastinal arteries and veins that have torn at the time of impact.

The many radiographic features of mediastinal hemorrhage are related to the resultant displacement of mediastinal structures (Mirvis et al., 1987a; Woodring et al., 1984) (Table 11–1). A widened mediastinum is the most frequently recognized abnormality, and this finding should prompt a search for other radiographic indicators of mediastinal hemorrhage (Marnocha et al, 1984; Seltzer et al., 1981). Shift of the trachea to the right (so that the left wall of the trachea is to the right of the spinous process of the fourth thoracic vertebral body) and shift of a nasogastric tube within the esophagus (to the right of the T4 spinous process) are the most reliable, although infrequent, indicators of mediastinal hemorrhage and aortic injury (Gerlock et al., 1980; Marnocha and Maglinte, 1985; Tisnado et al., 1977). Additional signs include obscuration of the aortic knob or of the lateral wall of the descending thoracic aorta, left apical cap (Simeone et al., 1975, 1981), displacement of the left and right paraspinal interfaces (Peters and Gamsu, 1980), depression of the left main bronchus, thickening of the right paratracheal stripe (Woodring et al., 1982a), left hemothorax, and rib fractures (Fig. 11–5). Isolated fractures of the first and second ribs, once thought to indicate severe mediastinal trauma, do not correlate with aortic rupture and are not by themselves an indication for aortography (see "Fractures of the Thoracic Skeleton," later in this chapter).

Some authors recommend that aortography be performed in any patient with the appropriate mechanism of injury (e.g., deceleration), regardless of the normal appearance of the mediastinum (Fisher et al., 1981; Kirsh et al., 1976a). Others have suggested that certain signs can be used to exclude the diagnosis of aortic rupture in patients with blunt chest trauma. Marnocha and Maglinte (1985) reviewed the chest radiographs of 86 consecutive patients with blunt chest trauma and suspected aortic rupture. When the aortic knob and contour appeared normal, and no deviation of the trachea and nasogastric tube was present, no case of aortic rupture was found.

This study was followed by a review of chest radiographs of 205 patients who underwent thoracic aortography to exclude aortic rupture (Mirvis et al., 1987b). The most discriminating signs were loss of the aorticopulmonary window, abnormality of the

---

Table 11–1. RADIOGRAPHIC SIGNS OF MEDIASTINAL HEMORRHAGE

Lateral displacement of the trachea
Lateral displacement of the nasogastric tube
Obscured top of the aortic arch
Obscured lateral margin of the descending aorta
Apical cap
Widened right paratracheal stripe
Displaced right paraspinal interface
Displaced left paraspinal interface
Wide mediastinum
Inferior displacement of left main bronchus

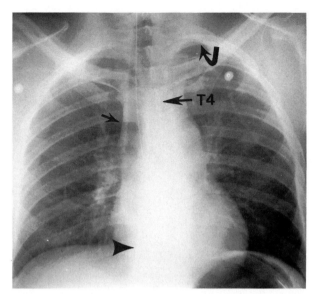

Figure 11–5. Frontal radiograph of a 20-year-old motorcyclist involved in an automobile–motorcycle collision. The trachea and the nasogastric tube are displaced to the right of the spinous process of the fourth thoracic vertebral body (T4). The top of the aortic arch is obscured. A left apical cap *(curved arrow)*, a thick right paratracheal stripe *(arrow)*, and a displaced right paraspinous interface *(arrowhead)* support the diagnosis of mediastinal hematoma. Aortography revealed aortic transection at the level of the aortic isthmus.

aortic arch, rightward tracheal shift, and displacement of the left paraspinal interface. In this patient population, no single radiographic sign or combination of signs was sufficient for diagnosis of all cases of aortic transection without the performance of a large number of negative aortograms. The absence of any radiographic sign (i.e., a normal chest radiograph) had a 96% negative predictive value, based on radiographs obtained with patients in a supine position, and a 98% negative predictive value, based on radiographs obtained with patients in an erect position (Mirvis et al., 1987b). In a review of 32 cases of acute traumatic rupture of the brachiocephalic arteries and aortic isthmus, Woodring and King (1989) also found that in two patients, the chest radiographs showed no specific signs of mediastinal hemorrhage (Woodring and King, 1989). Based on these two studies, one can conclude that 2% to 6% of patients with traumatic rupture of the aorta have an essentially normal chest radiograph.

Computed tomography may show direct signs of aortic injury, including (1) pseudoaneurysm, (2) linear lucency within the aortic lumen produced by the torn edge of the aortic wall, (3) irregularity of the aortic wall, and (4) aortic dissection, or indirect signs of aortic injury, including periaortic or intramural hematoma (Heiberg et al., 1983). The sensitivity and specificity of these signs have not been fully determined. They are likely to be helpful when present, but they are of limited negative predictive value. Although mediastinal hematoma and hemothorax are limited as positive predictors of aortic injury, some

authors have suggested that the absence of mediastinal hematoma on CT may be used to eliminate the need for thoracic aortography in selected cases (Mirvis et al., 1987c). In patients undergoing CT for trauma to the head or abdomen, scanning of the mediastinum to exclude the possibility of aortic injury may be reasonable.

Mirvis and associates (1987c) and Madayag and associates (1991) recommend aortography as the procedure of choice in the patient with unequivocal radiographic evidence of mediastinal hematoma. In the patient with equivocal mediastinal abnormalities or severe blunt trauma and a normal radiograph, thoracic CT may be performed, using 1-cm contiguous scans from the top of the manubrium to the level of the carina. The scans should be performed in a dynamic fashion following a bolus injection of intravenous contrast material. Evidence of aortic injury or mediastinal hematoma as revealed by CT is an indication for aortography. The use of CT in this manner, particularly in patients being evaluated by CT for other injuries, reduces the need for aortography in trauma patients (see Chapter 16).

Either fractures or dislocations of the lower cervical, thoracic, or upper lumbar spine, or both, are the source of mediastinal bleeding in 9% to 18% of patients with mediastinal hemorrhage (Sandor, 1967; Woodring et al., 1988) (Fig. 11–6). In patients with evidence of mediastinal hematoma, the radiologist should closely examine the radiographs for evidence of spinal fracture (Dennis and Rogers, 1989).

Cardiac Contusion

Myocardial injury can occur as a consequence of blunt trauma to the chest, including a direct blow to the chest from a steering wheel, a sports injury, or a fall from a high elevation. Myocardial injury may also result from closed chest massage during cardio-

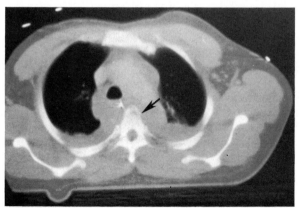

Figure 11–6. Chest computed tomography (CT) in a patient following a motor vehicle accident. Chest radiograph had revealed evidence of mediastinal hematoma, but aortography revealed no evidence of aortic transection. A fracture of the fourth thoracic vertebra *(arrow)* is visible on CT scan and is probably responsible for the hematoma.

pulmonary resuscitation, because of compression of the heart between the sternum and the thoracic spine (Tenzer, 1985). Myocardial trauma causes a spectrum of injuries, ranging from cardiac concussion to cardiac contusion and myocardial rupture. Cardiac concussion describes an injury to the heart that can produce arrhythmias but does not cause myocardial cellular damage, and therefore causes no release of creatine phosphokinase (CPK) from the myocardium. A myocardial contusion describes extravasation of red blood cells into and between myocardial muscle fibers and necrosis of myocardial muscle fibers (Tenzer, 1985). Myocardial contusion is associated with a rise in the circulating MB isoenzyme of CPK (CPK-MB), which peaks within 24 hours of injury. Myocardial rupture is the most serious injury, typically involving the right ventricle in its vulnerable position behind the sternum.

Recognition of myocardial injury is important because of the serious arrhythmias that can occur. Myocardial injury is difficult to diagnose, however, but should be suspected in the patient with the appropriate mechanism of injury. Electrocardiography and serial CPK isoenzyme detection remain the most commonly used screening tests (Waxman et al., 1986). Additional tests have been recommended to identify patients with myocardial injury. Frazee and associates (1986) have used serum CPK-MB screening followed by two-dimensional echocardiography in victims of blunt trauma. An elevated CPK-MB level was present in 20% (58/291) of patients. Two-dimensional echocardiography was performed in those 58 patients and revealed wall-motion abnormalities, chamber dilatation, or wall thinning in 40% (23/58) of patients.

Nuclear medicine examinations, including thallium-201 (^{201}Tl) single-photon emission computed tomography (SPECT), have also been recommended to detect patients at risk of developing serious arrhythmias after blunt trauma (Waxman et al., 1986). In 25 of 48 patients, ^{201}Tl SPECT scans were abnormal. Serious arrhythmias requiring therapy developed in five of those 25 patients (20%) and in none of the patients with normal ^{201}Tl SPECT scans.

Echocardiography is also useful in detecting hemopericardium, with or without tamponade, and serous or serosanguinous pericardial effusions that can occur after cardiac injury.

The chest radiograph plays only a minor role in the evaluation of myocardial injury. Its greatest value lies in detecting associated injuries (rib fractures, sternum fractures, and pulmonary contusion), which can increase clinical suspicion of myocardial injury.

Pneumopericardium

Pneumopericardium, a rare problem, can occur as a result of either blunt or penetrating trauma to the chest (Fig. 11–7). It is more commonly seen in patients who are intubated and receiving mechanical

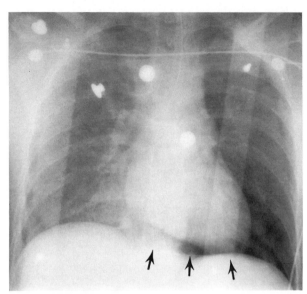

Figure 11–7. A 16-year-old boy involved in a head-on collision developed severe hypotension. An anteroposterior supine radiograph reveals bilateral pneumothoraces, and pneumopericardium, which outlines the inferior aspect of the heart *(arrows)*.

ventilation and is often accompanied by other signs of barotrauma, including pneumothorax, pneumomediastinum, and subcutaneous emphysema.

Tension pneumopericardium can produce cardiac tamponade, recognizable clinically by a deterioration in the patient's hemodynamic status despite adequate intravascular volume. Serial measurements of the cardiothoracic ratio may facilitate the diagnosis of impending tamponade in patients with pneumopericardium (Mirvis et al., 1986). In four cases of post-traumatic tension pneumopericardium, Mirvis described a sudden substantial (10% to 20%) decrease in the cardiothoracic ratio. The transverse cardiac diameter decreased by at least 2 cm. A 2-cm change in cardiac diameter cannot be attributed to systolic-diastolic variation, which produces a difference of no more than 0.9 cm in 93% of normal individuals. In a study of 359 patients reported by Gammill and co-workers (1970), no patient had a change of more than 1.7 cm that was based on systolic and diastolic variation alone.

Intravascular Missiles

Determination of the type of firearm projectile seen on a radiograph may be important for forensic purposes (Dodd and Budzik, 1990). The caliber of a bullet may be calculated from the following equation:

True bullet size (caliber) =
$$\frac{\text{(focal spot-to-bullet distance) (bullet image size)}}{\text{(focal spot-to-film distance)}}$$

The number of bullets can be easily counted unless

extensive fragmentation has occurred. Handguns fire a solitary, relatively low-velocity projectile, but they are also capable of firing multiple, small metal pellets (birdshot or ratshot). Shotguns fire multiple metal pellets, which may vary in size from larger buckshot to smaller birdshot. Rifles fire high-velocity solitary bullets.

Two views of the chest are usually sufficient to localize a bullet or missile fragment within the chest wall or lung. Bullets that have entered the cardiovascular system, however, may require additional evaluation, usually with fluoroscopy. Missiles superimposed on the cardiac silhouette may be present within the pericardial space, may be free within a cardiac chamber, or may be partially or completely embedded within myocardium. Bullets free in the left atrium or ventricle quickly embolize into a systemic artery (Symbas et al., 1989). Although bullets in the right atrium or ventricle may embolize into the pulmonary vascular bed, these may instead become trapped in the coarse trabeculae of the right ventricle. Bullets occasionally reach the right side of the heart by migration via a systemic vein after a peripheral injury. A number of factors affect the tendency of a missile to migrate, including missile size, body position, the force of blood flow, and the vascular anatomy.

Blurring of a missile on a radiograph due to motion suggests an intravascular or intracardiac position (Wallace and Slovis, 1987). If surgery is being performed for an intracardiac bullet, a portable radiograph should be obtained after general anesthesia induction to assure that the bullet has not embolized during transport to the operating room.

TRACHEOBRONCHIAL FRACTURE

Injury to the tracheobronchial tree may occur as a result of a penetrating wound or blunt trauma. Penetrating wounds are usually the result of gunshot or knife wounds and usually involve the cervical trachea. The presence of cervical subcutaneous emphysema in a patient with a penetrating neck wound should alert the radiologist to the possibility of tracheal injury. Patients with penetrating injuries of the trachea may have accompanying esophageal or arterial injuries.

Blunt trauma may involve a direct blow to the trachea, which primarily affects the cervical trachea (Fig. 11–8), or blunt trauma to the chest, which produces injury to the thoracic trachea and central bronchi. During a motor vehicle accident, the passenger may strike the windshield, causing extension of the neck and impact of the larynx or trachea against the dashboard (Butler and Moser, 1968).

Tracheal laceration due to blunt trauma produces an injury within 2.5 cm of the carina in 80% of cases (Kirsh et al., 1976b). The right and left main bronchi are involved more often than the intrathoracic trachea.

Fracture of the intrathoracic tracheobronchial tree is a difficult injury to recognize. Tracheobronchial injury almost invariably produces subcutaneous emphysema. Subcutaneous emphysema is, however, a common finding in the acute care setting and is more often related to pulmonary trauma or mechanical ventilation. Other indirect findings of tracheobronchial rupture are pneumomediastinum and pneumothorax. Tracheobronchial rupture may produce a ten-

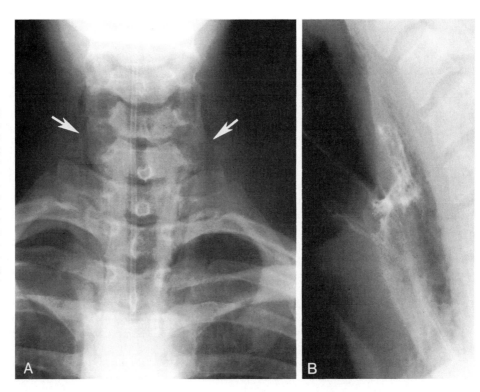

Figure 11–8. *A,* A 21-year-old man received blunt trauma to the head, neck, and chest when he was thrown against the steering wheel and windshield of his automobile. He complained of hoarseness, and subcutaneous emphysema was noted in the soft tissues of his neck *(arrows). B,* A meglumine diatrizoate swallow showed extravasation of contrast material from a posterior hypopharyngeal leak. Direct laryngoscopy confirmed a 2.5-cm-long midline laceration in the hypopharynx.

sion pneumothorax, or continued air leak even after chest tube placement. The failure of a lung to re-expand after chest tube placement should evoke suspicion of tracheobronchial injury.

A direct, but uncommon, sign of bronchial rupture is the "fallen lung" sign. Originally described by Oh and associates (1969), this sign refers to the collapsed lung falling away from the hilum. In patients with tension pneumothorax and lung collapse without bronchial rupture, the lung is tethered by the hilar structures and inferior pulmonary ligament and therefore collapses medially and inferiorly. In the patient with bronchial rupture, tension pneumothorax and lung collapse also occur, but the lung may fall away from the hilum if the laceration is complete (Petterson et al., 1989). On supine radiographs, the collapsed lung lies posteriorly and laterally. On upright radiographs, the superior aspect of the collapsed lung is caudal to the level of the upper lobe bronchus (Kumpe et al., 1970).

Fracture of one of the first three ribs may be associated with tracheobronchial injury, occurring in 58% (52/90) of patients with bronchial rupture (Burke, 1962). A study of 50 patients with fractures of the first and second ribs as a result of blunt chest trauma showed that only 2% of patients had a ruptured bronchus (Woodring et al., 1982b). The patient with a ruptured bronchus is likely to have fractured ribs as well; the patient with first and second rib fractures rarely has a ruptured bronchus (Albers et al., 1982). An additional sign of bronchial rupture is the presence of a sleeve of air surrounding the bronchus. Abnormalities of the endotracheal tube may also allow recognition of tracheal injury. The endotracheal tube or the inflated balloon cuff may lie outside the trachea, suggesting tracheal rupture (Unger et al., 1989). Bronchial rupture has also been recognized on CT, when the mediastinal structures were displaced toward the compromised lung, but the trachea was retracted in the opposite direction, indicating discontinuity (Weir et al., 1988). The diagnosis of tracheobronchial rupture is confirmed by bronchoscopy (Grover et al., 1979).

ESOPHAGEAL RUPTURE

Injury to the esophagus in blunt chest trauma is extremely uncommon. Spontaneous rupture of the esophagus (Boerhaave's syndrome) is more likely to occur in patients who have been vomiting or retching. The perforation is usually found on the left posterolateral wall of the distal esophagus (Han et al., 1985). The severe chest pain may cause confusion with other diagnoses, including myocardial infarction, aortic dissection, and perforated ulcer. The chest radiograph typically demonstrates pneumomediastinum, pleural effusion or hydropneumothorax, and subcutaneous emphysema (Fig. 11–9). Rupture of the distal esophagus produces pleural effusion on the left, whereas rupture of the midesophagus produces pleural effu-

sion on the right. The diagnosis is confirmed at fluoroscopy using water-soluble contrast material or with endoscopy.

FRACTURES OF THE THORACIC SKELETON

Fractures of the thoracic skeleton often alert the radiologist to the history of severe chest trauma and to the large amount of energy that has been imparted to the chest wall and thoracic viscera (Schorr et al., 1987). Fractures of the ribs, scapulae, sternum, and clavicles, either alone or in combination, occur in 75% of patients admitted to the emergency room with blunt chest trauma. Rib fractures predominate and are often multiple. When multiple adjacent ribs are fractured, a segment of chest wall that is discontinuous with the remainder of the thorax is created. This condition constitutes a flail chest and is associated with paradoxical respirations and often significant underlying pulmonary injury.

In the past, some authors have recommended arteriography to rule out aortic laceration for all patients with fractures of the first and second ribs (Richardson et al., 1975). More recent analysis of patients with fractures of the first and second ribs, however, suggests that the presence of such a fracture does not in itself constitute an indication for arteriography. Fisher and colleagues (1982) reviewed arteriograms performed in patients with blunt trauma. The incidence of aortic or brachiocephalic trauma was similar (20%) for patients with and without inlet rib fractures.

A second study by Woodring and colleagues (1982b) divided patients into two groups: (1) those with fractures of the first rib, second rib, or both that are associated with other radiographic abnormalities suggestive of mediastinal hematoma, and (2) those with fractures of the first rib, second rib, or both that are associated with no more than apical extrapleural capping. Injury to the thoracic aorta or brachiocephalic vessels was present in 13.8% of those with rib fractures and associated mediastinal abnormalities and in none of those with isolated fractures. Therefore, arteriography should be based on clinical history and radiographic evidence of mediastinal hematoma. The isolated presence of a first or second rib fracture should not prompt arteriography.

DIAPHRAGMATIC RUPTURE

Diaphragmatic rupture may occur because of either blunt trauma or a penetrating injury and can also occur as a complication of surgery. An early diagnosis avoids the higher morbidity and mortality rates associated with bowel strangulation and obstruction due to a delay in repair.

The diagnosis of traumatic diaphragmatic rupture with herniation of abdominal contents into the thorax

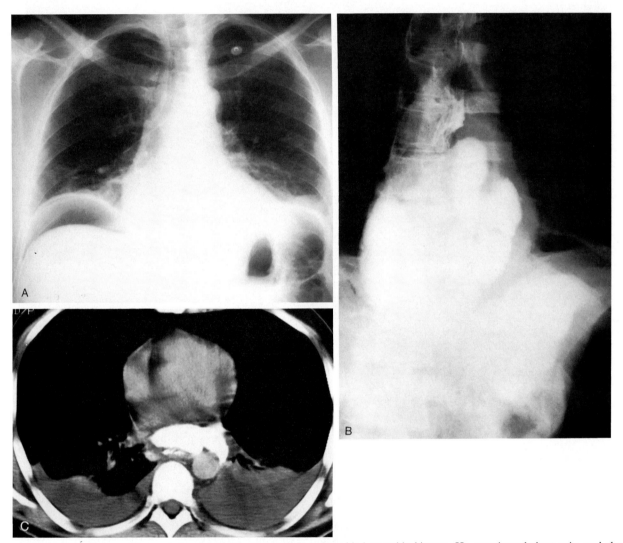

Figure 11–9. *A,* Á 50-year-old man induced vomiting in an effort to stop his intractable hiccups. He experienced chest pain, and chest radiograph reveals pneumoperitoneum and bibasilar atelectasis. *B,* Meglumine diatrizoate swallow shows extravasation of contrast material due to esophageal rupture (Boerhaave's syndrome). *C,* Axial chest CT shows bilateral pleural effusions and extravasation of esophageal contrast material.

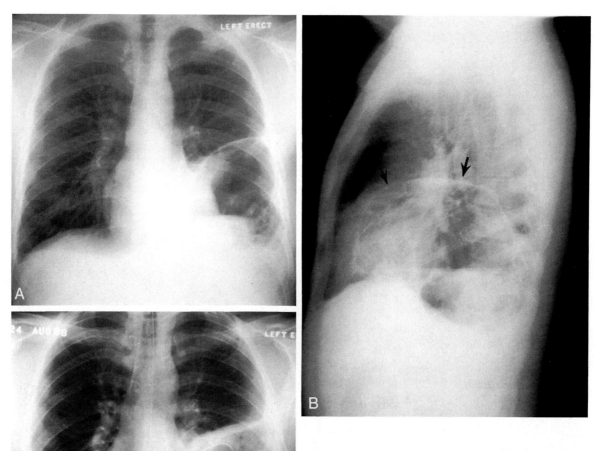

Figure 11–10. *A,* Frontal chest radiograph of a 22-year-old man with a history of trauma reveals gas-filled structures above the expected position of the left hemidiaphragm. *B,* Lateral view shows a thin-walled viscus *(arrows)* in the thorax and bilateral pleural effusions. *C,* Placement of a nasogastric tube *(arrows)* helps to distinguish rupture of the diaphragm from eventration. In this patient with diaphragmatic rupture, the nasogastric tube descends through the gastroesophageal junction in a normal position, and then curves upward into the stomach, which has herniated into the thorax through a central defect in the left hemidiaphragm.

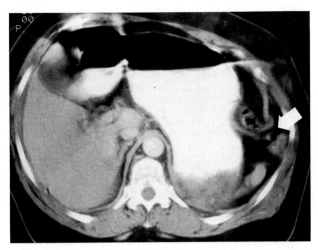

Figure 11–11. In a 65-year-old woman injured in a motor vehicle accident, CT reveals discontinuity of the diaphragm *(arrow)* and herniation of omental fat and of the small bowel through a lateral tear.

is more readily made if the injury is recent, if the tear is large and involves the left hemidiaphragm, and if strong suspicion of the diagnosis is maintained (Ball et al., 1982). If the trauma was remote, if the history of trauma is not obtained, or if the tear involves the right hemidiaphragm, the diagnosis is less likely to be made. An early diagnosis of diaphragmatic rupture is established in less than 50% of cases.

The chest radiograph is often helpful in suggesting the correct diagnosis. Radiographic signs of diaphragmatic rupture include apparent elevation of the diaphragm and an intrathoracic air bubble (Fig. 11–10 A and B). Diaphragmatic rupture is difficult to distinguish from eventration or paralysis of the diaphragm. Placement of a nasogastric tube may help in suspected left hemidiaphragm rupture (Perlman et al., 1984). Because most diaphragmatic tears are centrally located, sparing the esophageal hiatus, the esophagogastric junction and cardia of the stomach lie in a normal position. The fundus and greater curvature of the stomach are more likely to herniate through the central tear. A nasogastric tube in this case extends inferiorly below the normal esophagogastric junction and then forms an upward curve into the herniated stomach within the left hemithorax (see Fig. 11–10C).

An upper gastrointestinal study or barium enema is helpful in demonstrating bowel herniation. The bowel loops are pinched together as they pass through the defect in the diaphragm, creating the "lovebird" sign described by Felson (1986). For tears involving the right hemidiaphragm, a liver–spleen scan may show a characteristic linear deformity around the herniated portion of liver, created by the constrictive effect of the diaphragm. Ultrasonography, CT, and MRI have all been used to document diaphragmatic rupture. On CT scans, herniation of bowel or omental fat may be visible through an abrupt discontinuity in the diaphragm (Heiberg et al., 1980) (Fig. 11–11). On ultrasound scans, the thoracic and abdominal cavities are normally clearly separated by the curvi-

linear echo of the diaphragm. Real-time ultrasonography may allow visualization of not only a mass above the diaphragm, but also bowel peristalsis (Ammann et al., 1983). Ultrasonography may simply show a discontinuity of the diaphragm. Ultrasonography may be limited either by the acoustic barrier created by the presence of gas in the splenic flexure and stomach, or by subcutaneous emphysema accompanying chest trauma. Magnetic resonance imaging allows direct imaging in sagittal and coronal planes, which provides easy recognition of the diaphragm and visceral herniation (Mirvis et al., 1988).

References

Albers, J.E., Rath, R.K., Glaser, R.S., and Poddar, P.K.: Severity of intrathoracic injuries associated with first rib fractures. Ann. Thorac. Surg. 33:614, 1982.

American Medical Association: Provisional Guidelines for the Optimal Categorization of Hospital Emergency Capabilities. Chicago, American Medical Association, 1981.

Ammann, A.M., Brewer, W.H., Maull, K.I., and Walsh, J.W.: Traumatic rupture of the diaphragm: Real-time sonographic diagnosis. AJR 140:915, 1983.

Ball, T., McCrory, R., Smith, J.O., and Clements, J.L., Jr.: Traumatic diaphragmatic hernia: Errors in diagnosis. AJR 138:633, 1982.

Batra, P.: The fat embolism syndrome. J. Thorac. Imag. 2:12, 1987.

Bennett, D.E., and Cherry, J.K.: Natural history of traumatic aneurysms of the aorta. Surgery 61:516, 1967.

Berkmen, Y.M., Yankelevitz, D., Davis, S.D., and Zanzonico, P.: Torsion of the upper lobe in pneumothorax. Radiology 173:447, 1989.

Burke, J.F.: Early diagnosis of traumatic rupture of the bronchus. JAMA 181:682, 1962.

Butler, R.M., and Moser, F.H.: The padded dash syndrome: Blunt trauma to the larynx and trachea. Laryngoscope 78:1172, 1968.

Dennis, L.N., and Rogers, L.F.: Superior mediastinal widening from spine fractures mimicking aortic rupture on chest radiographs. AJR 152:27, 1989.

Dodd III, G.D., and Budzik, R.F., Jr.: Identification of retained firearm projectiles on plain radiographs. AJR 154:471, 1990.

Evarts, C.M.: The fat embolism syndrome: A review. Surg. Clin. North Am. 50:493, 1970.

Feldman, F., Ellis, K., and Green, W.M.: The fat embolism syndrome. Radiology 114:535, 1975.

Felson, B.: Armchair research and the practicing radiologist. AJR 147:881, 1986.

Felson, B.: Lung torsion: Radiographic findings in nine cases. Radiology 162:631, 1987.

Fisher, R.G., Ward, R.E., Ben-Manachem, Y., et al.: Laceration of the thoracic aorta and brachiocephalic arteries by blunt trauma: Report of 54 cases and review of the literature. Radiol. Clin. North Am. 19:91, 1981.

Fisher, R.G., Ward, R.E., Ben-Menachem, Y., et al.: Arteriography and the fractured first rib: Too much for too little? AJR 138:1959, 1982.

Frazee, R.C., Mucha, P., Jr., Farnell, M.B., and Miller, F.A., Jr.: Objective evaluation of blunt cardiac trauma. J. Trauma 26:510, 1986.

Gammill, S.L., Krebs, C., Meyers, P., et al.: Cardiac measurements in systole and diastole. Radiology 94:115, 1970.

Gerlock, A.J., Jr., Muhletaler, C.A., Coulam, C.M., and Hayes, P.T.: Traumatic aortic aneurysm: Validity of esophageal tube displacement sign. AJR 135:713, 1980.

Gong, H.: Fat embolism syndrome: A puzzling phenomenon. Postgrad. Med. 62:40, 1977.

Goodman, L.R., and Putman, C.E.: The S.I.C.U. chest radiograph after massive blunt trauma. Radiol. Clin. North Am. 19:111, 1981.

Greendyke, R.M.: Traumatic rupture of aorta: Special reference to automobile accidents. JAMA 195:119, 1966.

Greene, R.: Adult respiratory distress syndrome: Acute alveolar damage. Radiology 163:57, 1987.

Grover, F.L., Ellestad, C., Arom, K.V., et al.: Diagnosis and management of major tracheobronchial injuries. Ann. Thorac. Surg. 28:384, 1979.

Han, S.Y., McElvein, R.B., Aldrete, J.S., and Trishler, J.M.: Perforation of the esophagus: Correlation of site and cause with plain film findings. AJR 145:537, 1985.

Hankins, J.R., Attar, S., Turney, S.Z., et al.: Differential diagnosis of pulmonary parenchymal changes in thoracic trauma. Am. Surg. 39:309, 1973.

Heiberg, E., Wolverson, M.K., Sundaram, M., and Shields, J.B.: CT in aortic trauma. AJR 140:1119, 1983.

Heiberg, E., Wolverson, M.K., Hurd, R.N., et al.: CT recognition of traumatic rupture of the diaphragm. AJR 135:369, 1980.

Kirsh, M.M., Behrendt, D.M., and Orringer, M.B.: The treatment of acute traumatic rupture of the aorta: A 10-year experience. Ann. Surg. 184:308, 1976a.

Kirsh, M.M., Orringer, M.B., Behrendt, D.M., and Sloan, H.: Management of tracheobronchial disruption secondary to neopenetrating trauma. Ann. Thorac. Surg. 22:93, 1976b.

Kumpe, D.A., Oh, K.S., and Wyman, S.M.: A characteristic pulmonary finding in unilateral complete bronchial transection. AJR 110:704, 1970.

Lahiri, B., and ZuWallack, R.: The early diagnosis and treatment of fat embolism syndrome: A preliminary report. J. Trauma 17:956, 1977.

Madayag, M.A., Kirshenbaum, K.J., Nadimpalli, S.R., et al.: Thoracic aortic trauma: Role of dynamic CT. Radiology 179:853, 1991.

Marini, J.J.: Adult Respiratory Distress Syndrome: Current Therapy of Respiratory Disease 3. Toronto, B.C. Decker, 1989, p. 330.

Marnocha, K.E., and Maglinte, D.D.T.: Plain-film criteria for excluding aortic rupture in blunt chest trauma. AJR 144:19, 1985.

Marnocha, K.E., Maglinte, D.D.T., Woods, J., et al.: Mediastinal-width/chest-width ratio in blunt chest trauma: A reappraisal. AJR 142:275, 1984.

Maruyama, Y., and Little, J.B.: Roentgen manifestations of traumatic pulmonary fat embolism. Radiology 79:945, 1962.

Millikan, J.S., Moore, E.E., Steiner, E., et al.: Complications of tube thoracostomy for acute trauma. Am. J. Surg. 140:738, 1980.

Milne, E.N.C., Pistolesi, M., Miniati, M., and Giuntini, C.: The radiologic distinction of cardiogenic and noncardiogenic edema. AJR 144:879, 1985.

Mirvis, S.E., Indeck, M., Schorr, R.M., and Diaconis, J.N.: Posttraumatic tension pneumopericardium: The "small heart" sign. Radiology 158:663, 1986.

Mirvis, S.E., Keramati, B., Buckman, R., and Rodriguez, A.: MR imaging of traumatic diaphragmatic rupture. J. Comput. Assist. Tomogr. 12:147, 1988.

Mirvis, S.E., Bidwell, J.K., Buddemeyer, E.U., et al.: Imaging diagnosis of traumatic aortic rupture: A review and experience at a major trauma center. Invest. Radiol. 22:187, 1987a.

Mirvis, S.E., Bidwell, J.K., Buddemeyer, E.U., et al.: Value of chest radiography in excluding traumatic aortic rupture. Radiology 163:487, 1987b.

Mirvis, S.E., Kostrubiak, I., Whitley, N.O., et al.: Role of CT in excluding major arterial injury after blunt thoracic trauma. AJR 149:601, 1987c.

Moser, E.S., and Proto, A.V.: Lung torsion: Case report and literature review. Radiology 162:639, 1987.

Oh, K.S., Fleishner, F.G., and Wyman, S.M.: Characteristic pulmonary finding in traumatic complete transection of a mainstem bronchus. Radiology 92:371, 1969.

Palmovic, V., and McCarroll, J.R.: Fat embolism in trauma. Arch. Pathol. 80:630, 1965.

Parmley, L.F., Mattingley, T.W., Manion, W.C., and Jahnke, E.J., Jr.: Nonpenetrating traumatic injury of the aorta. Circulation 17:1086, 1958.

Peltier, L.F.: The diagnosis and treatment of fat embolism. J. Trauma 11:661, 1971.

Peltier, L.F., Collins, J.A., Evarts, C.M., and Sevitt, S.: Fat embolism. Arch. Surg. 109:12, 1974.

Perlman, S.J., Rogers, L.F., Mintzer, R.A., and Mueller, C.F.: Abnormal course of nasogastric tube in traumatic rupture of left hemidiaphragm. AJR 142:85, 1984.

Peters, D.R., and Gamsu, G.: Displacement of the right paraspinous interface: A radiographic sign of acute traumatic rupture of the thoracic aorta. Radiology 134:599, 1980.

Petterson, C., Deslauries, J., and McClish, A.: A classic image of complete right main bronchus avulsion. Chest 96:1415, 1989.

Rhea, J.T., Novelline, R.A., Lawrason, J., et al.: The frequency and significance of thoracic injuries detected on abdominal CT scans of multiple trauma patients. J. Trauma 29:502, 1989.

Richardson, J.D., McElvein, R.B., and Trinkle, J.K.: First rib fracture: A hallmark of severe trauma. Ann. Surg. 181:251, 1975.

Sandor, F.: Incidence and significance of traumatic mediastinal haematoma. Thorax 22:43, 1967.

Schorr, R.M., Crittenden, M., Indeck, M., et al.: Blunt thoracic trauma: Analysis of 515 patients. Ann. Surg. 206:200, 1987.

Seltzer, S.E., D'Orsi, C., Kirshner, R., and DeWeese, J.A.: Traumatic aortic rupture: Plain radiographic findings. AJR 137:1011, 1981.

Simeone, J.F., Deren, M.M., and Cagle, F.: The value of the left apical cap in the diagnosis of aortic rupture: A prospective and retrospective study. Radiology 139:35, 1981.

Simeone, J.F., Minagi, H., and Putman, C.E.: Traumatic disruption of the thoracic aorta: Significance of the left apical extrapleural cap. Radiology 117:265, 1975.

Stevens, E., and Templeton, A.W.: Traumatic nonpenetrating lung contusion. Radiology 85:247, 1965.

Symbas, P.N., Tyras, D.H., Ware, R.E., and Hatcher, C.R.: Rupture of the aorta. Ann. Thorac. Surg. 15:405, 1973.

Symbas, P.N., Vlasis-Hale, S.E., Picone, A.L., and Hatcher, C.R.: Missiles in the heart. Ann. Thorac. Surg. 48:192, 1989.

Tenzer, M.L.: The spectrum of myocardial contusion: A review. J. Trauma 25:620, 1985.

Tisnado, J., Tsai, F.Y., Als, A., and Roach, J.F.: A new radiographic sign of acute traumatic rupture of the thoracic aorta: Displacement of the nasogastric tube to the right. Radiology 125:603, 1977.

Tocino, I.M., Miller, M.H., Federick, P.R., et al.: CT detection of occult pneumothorax in head trauma. AJR 143:987, 1984.

Unger, J.M., Schuchmann, G.G., Grossman, J.E., and Pellett, J.R.: Tears of the trachea and main bronchi caused by blunt trauma: Radiologic findings. AJR 153:1175, 1989.

Wagner, R.B., Crawford, W.O., Jr., and Schimpf, P.P.: Classification of parenchymal injuries of the lung. Radiology 167:77, 1988.

Wall, S.D., Federle, M.P., Jeffrey, R.B., and Brett, C.M.: CT diagnosis of unsuspected pneumothorax after blunt abdominal trauma. AJR 141:919, 1983.

Wallace, K.L., and Slovis, C.M.: Hepatic vein bullet embolus as a complication of left thoracic gunshot injury. Ann. Emerg. Med. 16:102, 1987.

Waxman, K., Soliman, M.H., and Braunstein, P.: Diagnosis of traumatic contusion. Arch. Surg. 12:689, 1986.

Weir, I.H., Muller, N.L., and Connell, D.G.: CT diagnosis of bronchial rupture. J. Comput. Assist. Tomogr. 12:1035, 1988.

Williams, J.R., and Bonte, F.J.: Pulmonary damage in nonpenetrating chest injuries. Radiol. Clin. North Am. 1:439, 1963.

Woodring, J.H., and King, J.G.: The potential effects of radiographic criteria to exclude aortography in patients with blunt chest trauma. J. Thorac. Cardiovasc. Surg. 97:456, 1989.

Woodring, J.H., Lee, C., and Jenkins, K.: Spinal fractures in blunt chest trauma. J. Trauma 28:789, 1988.

Woodring, J.H., Loh, F.K., and Kryscio, R.J.: Mediastinal hemorrhage: An evaluation of radiographic manifestations. Radiology 151:15, 1984.

Woodring, J.H., Pulmano, C.M., and Stevens, R.K.: The right paratracheal stripe in blunt chest trauma. Radiology 143:605, 1982.

Woodring, J.H., Fried, A.M., Hatfield, D.R., et al.: Fractures of first and second ribs: Predictive value for arterial and bronchial injury. AJR 138:211, 1982b.

12

Imaging After Thoracotomy
∎
Lawrence R. Goodman

NORMAL RADIOGRAPHIC APPEARANCE FOLLOWING LUNG SURGERY

Following lung surgery, numerous changes in the postoperative chest radiograph merely reflect the procedure performed and are of little clinical significance, whereas other alterations may herald major clinical problems. After recuperation, certain residual radiographic changes are frequently seen and are not important, but others suggest a delayed surgical complication. To evaluate the postoperative radiograph properly, one must be familiar with the expected radiographic changes and those that indicate a potential complication (Brooks, 1984; Goodman, 1980; Spirn et al., 1988).

Pneumonectomy

After removal of a lung, great care is taken to expand the remaining lung maximally and to assure that the mediastinum has returned to the midline. In the operating room, air may be added or withdrawn from the pneumonectomy space to ensure that no significant mediastinal shift has occurred. Further adjustments may be required during the following days. The immediate postpneumonectomy radiograph should show a fully expanded contralateral lung, an approximately midline trachea, and a vacant hemithorax with little or no fluid. A clamped chest tube may be inserted for use in the case of complications (Adkins and Slovin, 1975; Malamed et al., 1977) (Fig. 12–1).

During the first several days, the mediastinum should remain stationary or *gradually* shift *toward* the operated side. A *gradual* shift *away from* the surgical side indicates atelectasis of the remaining lung or the rapid accumulation of fluid on the operative side at a rate faster than that at which the air can be resorbed.

A rapid mediastinal shift toward the remaining lung usually indicates massive atelectasis or increased tension in the surgical space from a bronchopleural fistula or bleeding (Adkins and Slovin, 1975; Malamed et al., 1977). The vacant hemithorax fills with fluid from chest wall bleeding, transudation from the pleural surface, or lymphatic leakage. The rate of accumulation of fluid is extremely variable, and standards are difficult to set. Within the first 4 to 7 days, the lower one half to two thirds of the hemithorax usually fills with fluid (see Fig. 12–1*B*). Total obliteration of the pleural space usually takes several weeks (see Fig. 12–1*C*).

Fluid accumulation is more rapid following an extrapleural pneumonectomy or the lysis of multiple adhesions. Under these circumstances, total opacification of the hemithorax may occur over several days, suggesting serious bleeding. When fluid accumulates more rapidly than air can be resorbed, the mediastinum may shift to the contralateral side, and air may be forced through the thoracotomy incision, stimulating a bronchopleural fistula.

As the vacant hemithorax fills with fluid, the mediastinum and heart gradually shift *toward* that side. Following a right pneumonectomy, the heart moves to the right and posteriorly. The left lung herniates across the midline, anteriorly in relation to the rotated heart. Following left pneumonectomy, the heart merely shifts, and the right lung herniates anteriorly in relation to the heart. In approximately one half of the patients, the right lung also crosses behind the heart (Biondetti et al., 1982). Once the mediastinum has started to shift, any movement *away from* the side of the operation suggests excess pressure on that side (empyema, bronchopleural fistula, or hemorrhage) (Barker et al., 1966; Christiansen et al., 1965).

The ultimate fate of the pleural space after pneumonectomy is variable. Using computed tomography (CT), Biondetti and associates (1982) demonstrated that in approximately one third of patients, all of the pleural fluid eventually resorbs. This resorption is

213

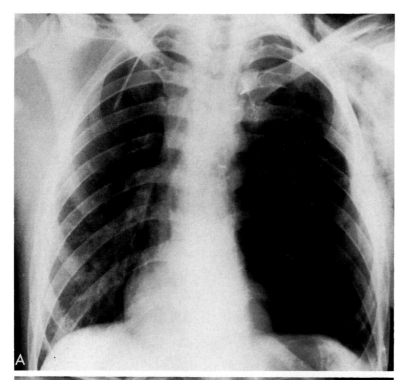

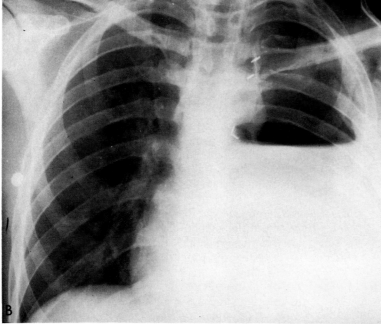

Figure 12–1. Radiographs following left pneumonectomy for carcinoid tumor. *A,* Postoperative 18-hour radiograph. Left pneumothorax, minimal mediastinal shift to the right, and minimal right lower lobe atelectasis are present. No chest tube is present. Posterior fourth rib is resected, and air appears in the soft tissues on the left. *B,* Postoperative day 6. Fluid appears in lower half of left hemithorax; trachea is shifted to the midline. Right lower lobe atelectasis is cleared; subcutaneous emphysema is resolving. *C,* Postoperative day 12. Hemithorax is opaque, left hemidiaphragm is elevated, and heart and mediastinum are shifted further to the left. (From Goodman, L.R.: Postoperative chest radiograph: II. Alterations after major intrathoracic surgery. AJR 134:803–813, 1980, with permission. © 1980, American Roentgen Ray Society.)
Illustration continued on following page

associated with a marked shift of mediastinal structures, overinflation of the contralateral lung, a variable elevation of the diaphragm, and contraction of the rib interspaces. In the other two thirds of patients, a variable amount of fluid remains in the hemithorax for years, and the shifts are less dramatic. In an autopsy series of 37 patients, Suarez and colleagues (1969) found that 27 had residual fluid in the thorax. Seven of the 27 patients were studied at least 2 years following pneumonectomy, the longest postoperative period being 8 years. The remaining 10 patients demonstrated total resorption of fluid. Fibrothorax

due to organization of fluid in the hemithorax was not seen in any of the 57 patients studied in these two series. Most likely, empyemas occurring several years after the surgical procedure occur in patients with residual fluid.

Lobectomy

Following lobectomy, the radiograph shows modest mediastinal shift and diaphragmatic elevation. Usually, an anterosuperior chest tube for draining air and a posteroinferior chest tube for draining fluid are

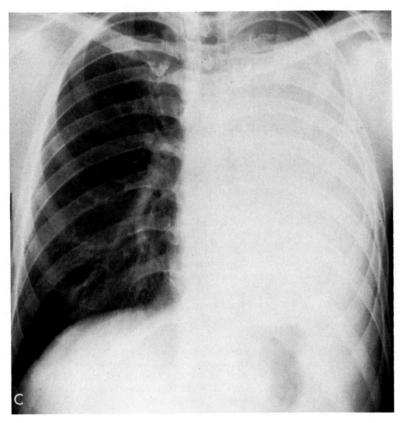

Figure 12–1. *Continued.*

present. A row of staples closing the bronchus is frequently noted. In the majority of patients, fissures are not complete, and lung tissue must be crossed and stapled to complete the lobectomy. Therefore, air leaks are common, but they usually seal within several days (Brooks, 1984). Within the first few days, the residual lung hyperinflates to fill the hemithorax. The lung may fail to hyperinflate, owing to underlying fibrosis, pleural adhesions, scarring of the mediastinum, or postoperative atelectasis on either side. Ipsilateral atelectasis requires prompt re-expansion to prevent the development of pneumonia or an exudative pleural effusion that may form a "peel" and prevent further lung expansion.

After lobectomy, a predictable pattern of reorientation of the remaining lobes occurs. After right upper or lower lobectomy, the middle lobe rotates and hyperinflates to occupy the majority of the residual space. When the middle lobe or lingula is removed, both upper and lower lobes expand and rotate slightly to fill the void (Holbert et al., 1987; Malamed et al., 1977). The reorientation is visible on both chest radiographs and CT scans (Fig. 12–2). After right upper lobectomy, the hilum moves superiorly and laterally, and fewer markings are visible than on the normal side. A "neofissure" forms between the superior segment of the lower lobe and the reoriented middle lobe. On the lateral chest radiographs of approximately one third of the patients, this neofissure is visible and continuous with the major fissure. On the CT scans of two thirds of the patients, the neofissure is parallel to the major fissure; in the

remaining third, the lower fissure swings forward into a sagittal plane (Mahoney and Shipley, 1988). After lower lobectomy, a similar reorientation of the minor fissure occurs, and the hilum is considerably smaller, owing to the absence of the large truncus inferior.

After lobectomy, the radiograph may simulate collapse of the resected lobe. For example, the "upper triangle sign" of right lower lobe collapse and the "aortic knob sign" of left lower lobe collapse may appear after lower lobectomy. A "juxtaphrenic peak," which is often seen with upper lobe collapse, may be visible after upper lobectomy (Spirn et al., 1988). Conversely, right middle lobe collapse following right upper lobectomy may be difficult to diagnose. The neofissure swings into the sagittal plane and allows the middle lobe to collapse against the mediastinum, simulating mediastinal widening. Shift of the mediastinum to the right, elevation of the hilum, and superomedial shift of the staples securing the middle to the lower lobe help confirm the diagnosis (Shiply and Mahoney, 1988). Shifting mediastinal structures or residual loculated fluxed collections may simulate recurrent tumor (Fig. 12–3).

A continuous row of staples across the bronchus is the surest indication of bronchial resection. The staple lines tend to have a constant appearance from film to film, and any spreading or angulation of the staples suggests adjacent problems (recurrent tumor, infection, or bronchopleural fistula) (Fig. 12–4). Evaluation of the stability of the staples should be part of serial radiographic examinations (S. Reich, M.D., verbal communication, 1989).

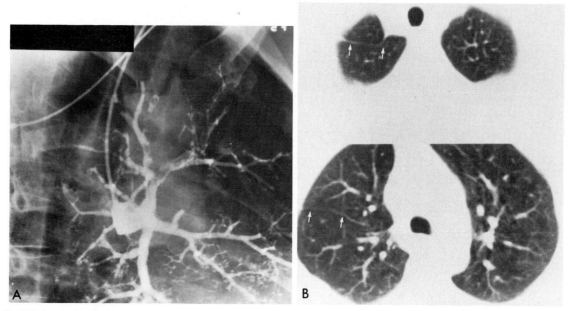

Figure 12–2. Lobar realignment after lobectomy (two patients). *A,* Oblique radiograph of a left bronchogram after a left lower lobectomy. The apical posterior bronchus supplies the upper third of the lung. The anterior upper lobe bronchus supplies the middle third of the lung, and the lingula bronchus supplies the lower third of the lung. *B,* CT scan of a patient after right upper lobectomy. The "neofissure" *(arrows)* is visible on cuts through the middle and lower lung fields. The middle lobe occupies the anterior portion of the chest, and the lower lobe is elevated, occupying the posterior portion.

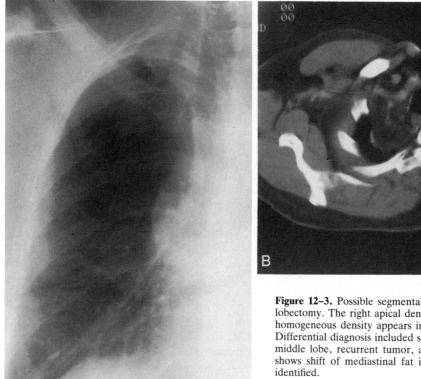

Figure 12–3. Possible segmental collapse or recurrent tumor after right upper lobectomy. The right apical density occurred many months after surgery. *A,* A homogeneous density appears in the right apex with a concave lateral margin. Differential diagnosis included segmental collapse of the medial segment of the middle lobe, recurrent tumor, and an apical fluid collection. *B,* The CT scan shows shift of mediastinal fat into the apex. No pathologic abnormality was identified.

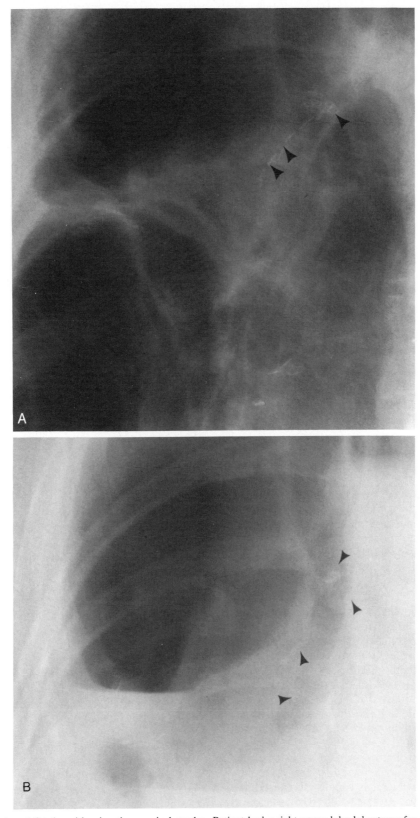

Figure 12–4. Bronchopleural fistula, with migrating surgical staples. Patient had a right upper lobe lobectomy for atypical tuberculosis. *A,* Chest radiograph, several weeks after surgery, shows a persistent air collection in the right hemithorax. The residual lung was not capable of expanding to fill the void. Bronchial staples of the right upper lobe appears in a straight line *(arrowheads). B,* A follow-up chest radiograph obtained 2 months later shows a fluid level at the base of the air collection. The surgical staples are in a random distribution *(arrowheads).* The spreading of the staples indicates a disruption of the bronchial closure (confirmed at surgery).

The residual bronchial stump should also be assessed on each radiograph. The total length of the stump should be less than 1 cm, producing a visible air column within the stump of only several millimeters. Long stumps are associated with retained secretions, infection, and occasional purulent tracheal bronchitis, hemoptysis, and bronchopleural fistula. Rarely, re-amputation of the stump is required (Brooks, 1984).

Segmental or Lesser Resections

The radiograph following segmental or lesser resections is similar to that seen after lobectomy, with several important differences. These resections involve cutting across pulmonary parenchyma and require repleuralization or stapling to minimize air leakage. Therefore, postoperative air leaks from the surface are quite common, and a persistent pneumothorax requiring prolonged tube drainage is not uncommon. Postoperative consolidation in the involved lobe is frequent and represents a combination of hemorrhage, contusion, and atelectasis. Although the consolidation usually resolves over a period of several days to weeks, a parenchymal scar or pseudotumor may persist (Malamed et al., 1977). Any postoperative shift of the mediastinum or diaphragm indicates atelectasis because there should be little parenchymal rearrangement due to the resection itself.

Bronchoscopy and Mediastinoscopy

Complications of diagnostic bronchoscopy are uncommon and are usually due to trauma to the upper airway, trachea, or bronchi (Ferguson, 1979). Upper airway trauma includes broken teeth, which may be aspirated, or lacerations of the pharynx or larynx, in which the patient may present with deep cervical emphysema or a mass from bleeding or infection. Injury to the tracheobronchial tree is most often due to the biopsy forceps or brush. This injury may result in pneumothorax or pneumomediastinum. Increasing opacification of the lung after bronchoscopy is most often due to endobronchial bleeding. Progressive opacification may also be due to the endobronchial spread of infection from entering an area of postobstructive pneumonia or an obstructed cavity. Diagnostic bronchopulmonary lavage uses a relatively small amount of liquid and therefore results in no, or transient, focal opacification of the lung (Gurney et al., 1987).

Mediastinoscopy, when performed by experienced hands, involves a 2% complication rate. Bleeding, the most frequent problem, is usually diagnosed and treated at the time of surgery. Other complications include pneumothorax, mediastinitis, esophageal perforation, and injury to the phrenic or recurrent pharyngeal nerve (Ferguson, 1979). The immediate post-procedure radiograph often demonstrates slight mediastinal widening and localized mediastinal air. Large or progressive collections suggest one of the foregoing complications (Fig. 12–5).

COMPLICATIONS OF LUNG SURGERY

Rigorous preoperative evaluation, improved surgical techniques, improved anesthesia, and sophisticated postoperative care have dramatically reduced the mortality and morbidity associated with lung resection. Several recent series report a postoperative mortality rate of approximately 2% for lobectomy and 6% for pneumonectomy. The postoperative morbidity rate, however, remains high with complication rates of 17% to 40% reported for lobectomy and rates as high as 60% reported for pneumonectomy. The vast majority of fatal and nonfatal complications are cardiorespiratory in origin. The leading causes of postoperative morbidity include intractable atelectasis, pneumonia, acute respiratory failure, cardiac problems (e.g., myocardial infarctions, acute arrythmia), and complications directly related to surgery (e.g., bleeding, air leaks) (Keagy et al., 1985; Motta and Ratto, 1989; Nagasaki et al., 1982). Major risk factors include limited cardiopulmonary reserve, old age (greater than 70 years old), the presence of preoperative infection—especially tuberculosis—and right pneumonectomy. Most of the complications discussed in the following sections occur after pneumonectomy, lobectomy, or lesser resections. A few are unique to one procedure.

Postoperative Spaces

Persistent pleural air collections are noted in 10% to 20% of patients who have undergone lobectomy and in a higher percentage of patients who have had smaller resections. This condition is usually due to atelectasis, fibrosis, or adhesions that prevent the residual lung from hyperinflating or to a persistent bronchial leak. In the vast majority of patients, no fever or leukocytosis occurs, and the radiograph shows little pleural thickening or effusion. Most of these spaces have a benign, self-limited course (Fig. 12–6); the lung eventually expands to fill the void, or the space fills with fluid. On occasion, a small apical air collection may persist for several weeks or months without apparent ill effects (Adkins and Slovin, 1975; Brooks, 1984; Christiansen et al., 1965; Kirsh et al., 1975; Malamed et al., 1977) (see Fig. 12–4A). A small percentage of postoperative air spaces follow a more serious clinical course. They are associated with fever, leukocytosis, and a persistent or expanding space with effusions and thickened, irregular pleura. This is most often due to a low-grade infection or a small bronchopleural fistula. Most postoperative air spaces can be treated with prolonged chest tube drainage and antibiotics, rather than surgical intervention.

Empyema

Significant infection of the pleural space occurs in less than 5% of pneumonectomies and in a smaller

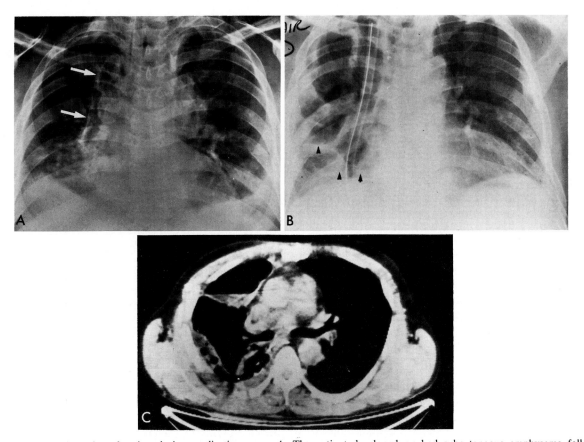

Figure 12–5. Esophageal perforation during mediastinoscopy. *A,* The patient developed marked subcutaneous emphysema following mediastinoscopy for evaluation of adenopathy. The radiograph demonstrates marked subcutaneous emphysema and pneumomediastinum on the right *(arrows).* The air along the left cardiac border probably represents pneumomediastinum as well; however, pneumopericardium cannot be excluded. The patient was explored, and a rent in the esophagus was repaired. *B,* After several weeks of tube drainage and antibiotic therapy, fever reappeared. The radiograph shows multiple air–fluid levels *(arrowheads)* and multiple densities throughout the lung. One could not determine from the radiographs alone whether lung abscesses, as well as pleural loculations, were present. *C,* The CT scan below the carina shows two pleural collections, one anterior and one posterior. No significant parenchymal disease was noted. Based on the CT findings, percutaneous drainage of both collections was instituted. The fever resolved.

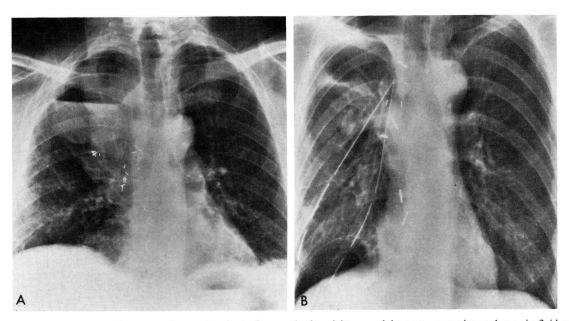

Figure 12–6. Benign postoperative spaces (two patients). *A,* One week after right upper lobectomy, a persistent, large air–fluid collection appeared at the right apex. The patient was asymptomatic. Over the next few weeks, slight further re-expansion of the lung occurred. The remainder of the space filled with fluid. *B,* Following removal of the right upper lobe and the superior segment of the right lower lobe for tuberculosis, the remaining lung never expanded into the apex. This radiograph, obtained approximately 8 days after surgery, shows a persistent air collection at the right apex as well as a subpulmonic air collection. The patient was asymptomatic, and the chest tubes were removed 2 days later without incident.

percentage of lesser resections. Empyema may occur alone, may follow a bronchopleural fistula, or may cause a bronchopleural fistula by disrupting the stump closure. Most infections occur in the immediate post-operative period because of soilage at the time of surgery or via a bronchial leak. *Staphyloncus, Pseudomonas, Streptococcus,* and *Aerobacter* organisms are most frequently involved (Brooks, 1984; Spirn et al., 1988; Young and Perryman, 1979). Empyemas may also occur months to years after pneumonectomy, presumably in patients with persistent pleural fluid. These late infections are usually not due to a bronchopleural fistula and are assumed to be secondary to hematogenous spread.

Considerable variation occurs in both the clinical and radiographic appearance of the empyema. Patients presenting with infection shortly after the surgical procedure tend to have both local and constitutional signs and symptoms, whereas those with delayed infections often have relatively mild constitutional symptoms that do not necessarily suggest their source.

Following pneumonectomy, the varied radiographic appearance depends on the state of the hemithorax at the onset of the infection. If the hemithorax is partially filled, the air–fluid level may rise rapidly. If the hemithorax is already full, the mediastinum may shift toward the contralateral lung (Fig. 12–7). Mediastinal shift, however, was present in only one of the nine of Kerr's patients with late onset empyemas (Kerr, 1977). Examination by CT of a delayed empyema may show the mediastinal pleura as concave *toward* the mediastinum rather than the normal convexity toward the thorax (Heater et al., 1985). The pleura may be thick and enhance with intravenous contrast. If a fistulous connection is present, the air–fluid level drops or air reappears in a previously opaque hemithorax (Fig. 12–8). Rarely, a gas-forming organism causes air to reappear in the hemithorax (Kerr, 1977; Lams, 1980).

After lobectomy or a lesser resection, empyema is usually suggested by the combination of fever, leukocytosis, pleural thickening, and fluid accumulation. Multiple loculated pockets are common. Differentiation between pleural and parenchymal disease is often difficult in the postoperative thorax. Computed tomography clearly delineates the pleural collections, their relationship to the chest tubes, and the presence of parenchymal disease (see Fig. 12–5; see Chapter 5). Small collections of air may be visible in the pleural space, indicating an empyema or a bronchopleural fistula if a chest tube has not been recently placed. Aspiration with CT or ultrasound guidance may be necessary to obtain cultures. Guided drainage of local collections often obviates the need for more aggressive therapy.

The term "technical empyema" refers to a prolonged external drainage procedure via a tube or surgical flap to vent a persistent air leak, an infected pleural space, or a space created by failure of the remaining lung to re-expand. The tube or flap drains the pleural space to the skin surface until the lung re-expands or the space granulates in. Although not frankly infected, it is assumed to be contaminated. The radiograph usually demonstrates a partially obliterated pleural space with a thickened pleura and a tube in the residual air pocket, or a track in the chest wall. Air–fluid levels may come and go if this space is being irrigated with saline or other solutions (Dorman et al., 1973; Kirsh et al., 1975).

Bronchopleural Fistula

Small air leaks from the cut lung surface or bronchial stump are common in the immediate postoperative period and usually close spontaneously with conservative management. Large or persistent air collections are usually due to bronchopleural fistula. In the immediate postsurgical period, bronchial leaks are rare and usually due to faulty closure of the bronchus. After the first week, bronchopleural fistula is much more common and usually due to infection or residual tumor of the stump (Young and Perryman, 1979); it may even appear years after the surgery (O'Meara and Slade, 1974; Spirn et al., 1988). Spreading of the staples closing the bronchus may provide a clue to the state of the bronchus.

Again, the radiographic changes depend on the state of the hemithorax at the time of the leak (Adkins and Slovin, 1975; Kerr, 1977; Kirsh et al., 1975; Malamed et al., 1977).

Following pneumonectomy, one or more of the following signs may be visible when a bronchopleural fistula is present:

1. Persistent or progressive pneumothorax despite tube drainage.
2. Failure of the hemithorax to fill with fluid at the expected rate.
3. Shift of the mediastinum to the contralateral side due to increased intrathoracic pressure (see Fig. 12–7). Expiratory radiographs may produce a false-positive shift because the mediastinum often shifts to the nonsurgical side in expiration (Wechsler and Goodman, 1985) (Fig. 12–9).
4. A drop of 2 cm or more in a pre-existing air–fluid level or the reappearance of air in an opaque hemithorax.
5. Air in the soft tissue, possibly indicating a bronchopleural cutaneous fistula (empyema necessitatis).

A bronchopleural fistula occurring after lobectomy is usually indicated by a localized increase of fluid or the reappearance or persistence of air in the pleural space.

Bleeding

Postoperative hemorrhage is usually due to bleeding that involves the systemic circulation and intercostal vessels or mediastinal vessels. Hemorrhage

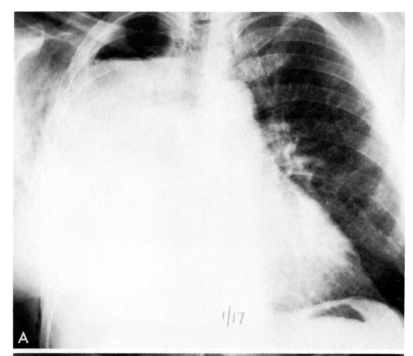

Figure 12–7. Empyema and bronchopleural fistula after pneumonectomy. *A,* Postoperative day 6. The patient is asymptomatic. Fluid occupies most of the right hemithorax, more than is usually found at this stage. The mediastinum is shifted slightly to the right, however, and a small amount of subcutaneous air is still present. *B,* Postoperative day 13. The patient developed a mild fever. The entire hemithorax is opaque, and the trachea is shifted slightly to the left. The significance of the tracheal shift was not appreciated. During the next 10 days, the patient's fever persisted without apparent explanation.

Illustration continued on following page

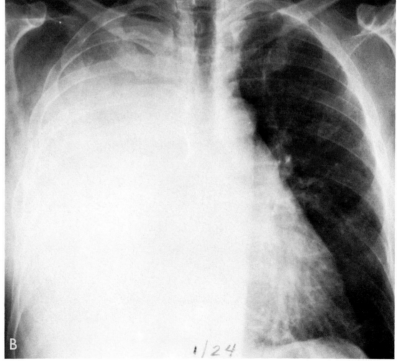

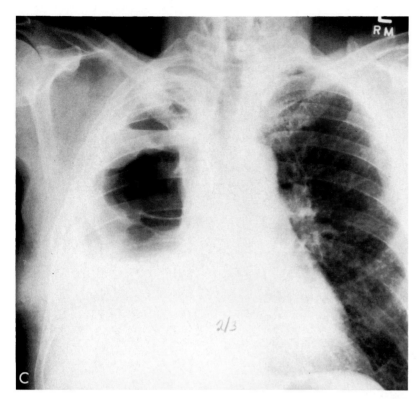

Figure 12–7. *Continued. C,* Postoperative day 23. A large quantity of pus drained spontaneously through the original surgical incision. A radiograph shows multiple air–fluid levels in the right hemithorax, and the mediastinum is again shifted to the right. The patient was treated with prolonged drainage and antibiotics. Eventually, the entire hemithorax was re-opacified with fluid. (From Goodman, L.R.: Postoperative chest radiograph: II. Alterations after major intrathoracic surgery. AJR 134:803–813, 1980, with permission. © 1980, American Roentgen Ray Society.)

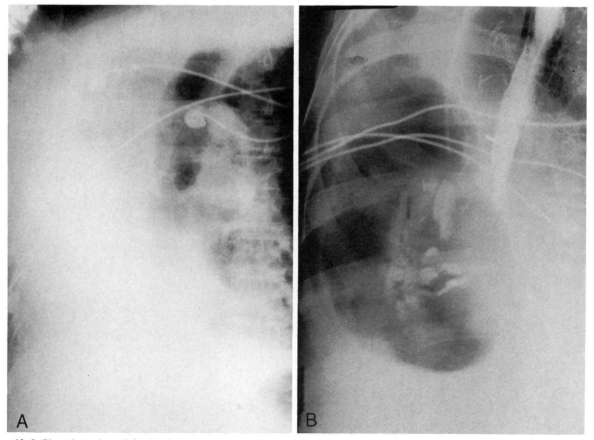

Figure 12–8. Pleural esophageal fistula after pneumonectomy. *A,* The right hemithorax is opaque; the mediastinum and heart are shifted to the right. *B,* Two days later, the fluid in the right hemithorax has been replaced by air. A water-soluble contrast study of the esophagus demonstrates a fistula between the lower esophagus and the pleural space.

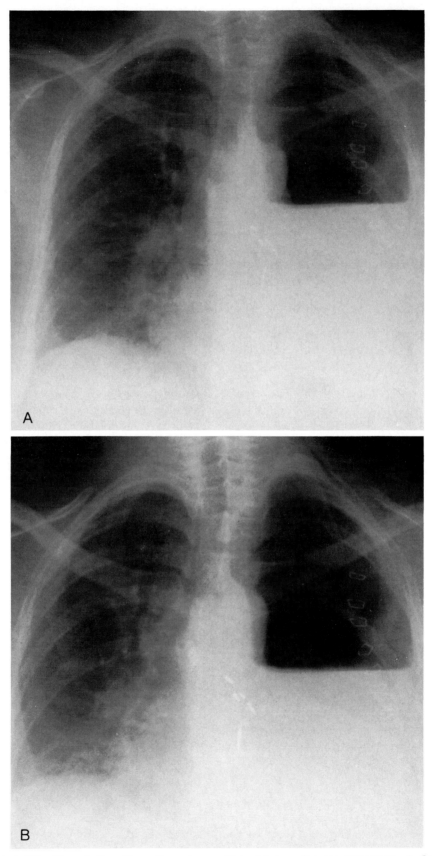

Figure 12–9. Mediastinal shift with expiration. The radiograph was obtained 3 days after pneumonectomy. *A,* On inspiration, the right heart border is 37 mm from the spine. *B,* On expiration, the right heart border is 47 mm from the spine. This type of shift on expiration is a normal physiologic phenomenon and does not indicate a problem.

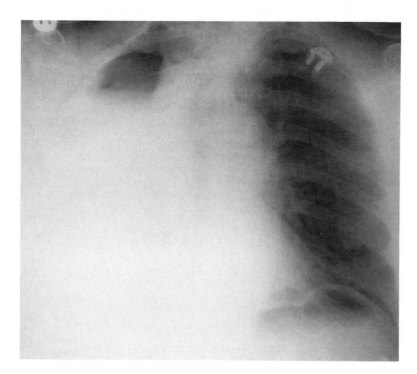

Figure 12–10. Severe postoperative hemorrhage after right pneumonectomy. The patient developed hypotension and tachycardia 1 day after surgery. The radiograph shows opacification of three fourths of the right hemithorax. (Courtesy of the Royal Brompton Hospital, London, England.)

from the pulmonary vessels is unusual. In the majority of cases, the combination of bleeding from the chest tube and the rapid opacification of the hemithorax provide the diagnosis. On occasion, however, a large amount of blood may accumulate in the thorax if the chest tube is obstructed by clot or isolated in a pleural loculation (Fig. 12–10). After lobectomy, the blood accumulating in the pleural space compresses the residual lung, and a "peel" traps the lung in an atelectatic condition. Surgical intervention is often required to control bleeding and remove the peel (Brooks, 1984; McLaughlin and Hankins, 1979).

The differential diagnosis of rapid fluid accumulation may also include chylothorax due to thoracic duct injury or the infusion of "intravenous" fluid into the thorax via an improperly positioned catheter (Adkins and Slovin, 1975; Brooks, 1984; Malamed et al., 1977). The severity of the dyspnea in these two

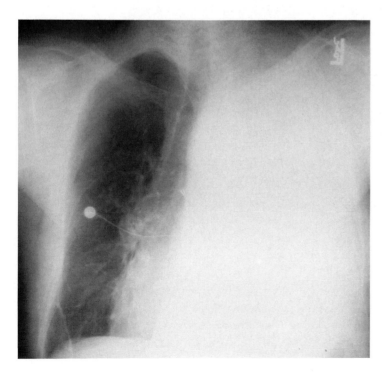

Figure 12–11. Chylothorax. The patient had had a pneumonectomy many years previously. Since then, the patient returned to the hospital several times for gradually increasing shortness of breath. On each occasion, the mediastinum was found shifted to the right side by a huge pleural effusion. Thoracentesis always yielded chyle without evidence of malignancy or infection. The patient's symptoms were relieved following thoracentesis.

conditions is usually proportional to the volume and speed of fluid accumulation (Fig. 12–11).

Cardiac Herniation

Herniation of the heart through a pericardial defect following intrapericardial pneumonectomy is a rare but often lethal complication. Herniation usually occurs in the immediate postoperative period and is manifested by signs of obstruction of venous return when herniation is to the right, and of hypotension and tachycardia when the heart projects to the left.

When the heart herniates to the right, the apex may move laterally or rotate posteriorly. Air may outline the empty pericardial sac. When the heart herniates to the left, a notch may be present along the upper left border of the heart, where the heart protrudes through the pericardium. A rapid diagnosis is imperative if surgical reduction is to be successful (Atkins and Slovin, 1975; Arndt et al., 1978; Kirsh et al., 1975).

Less frequently, herniation occurs more gradually, over a period of several hours or days after surgery. Prior to complete herniation, a portion of the heart may be visible radiographically as it protrudes through the defect. Gurney and colleagues (1986) likened the radiographic appearance of the partially herniated heart to that of a "snow cone" (Fig. 12–12). Although this appearance has only been demonstrated in a few cases, it appears to be specific and to indicate the need for surgical intervention to prevent complete herniation.

Esophagopleural Fistula

Esophagopleural fistula is a rare complication that usually occurs following right pneumonectomy for tuberculosis or cancer. The vast majority of cases arise within 6 weeks of surgery. During the first 2 weeks, the fistula is usually secondary to direct esophageal injury or compromise of the blood supply to the lower esophagus at the time of surgery. Late rupture is usually due to adjacent empyema or lymphadenitis, a bronchopleural fistula, or recurrent cancer. The diagnosis is frequently delayed because clinically and radiographically the picture resembles bronchopleural fistula, empyema, or recurrent tumor. Any patient who develops postoperative dysphagia, or clinical or radiographic evidence of bronchopleural fistula without demonstrable bronchial leak, should have an esophagogram to rule out an esophageal fistula (Adkins and Slovin, 1975; Kirsh et al., 1975; Sethi and Takaro, 1978) (see Fig. 12–8).

Lobar Torsion and Gangrene

After lobectomy, an ipsilateral lobe may rotate on its bronchovascular pedicle, compromising its circulation. Initially, venous flow is impeded, causing severe venous engorgement and parenchymal congestion. This process rapidly progresses to ischemia and lobar gangrene. This rare complication occurs most often after right upper lobectomy with torsion of the middle lobe. Initially, the middle lobe appears large and dense. The vascular pedicle may appear inverted

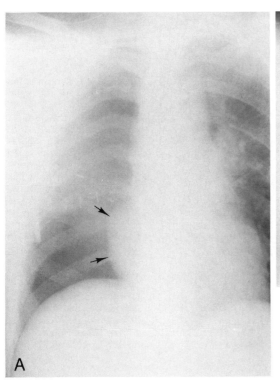

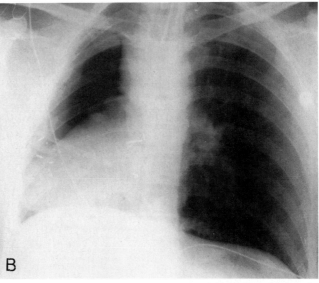

Figure 12–12. Cardiac herniation following a right intrapericardial pneumonectomy for a stab wound. *A,* Initial postoperative radiograph in the recovery room demonstrates a hemispheric bulge along the right border of the heart *(arrows).* This bulge resembles a "snow cone." The patient was clinically stable. *B,* Ninety minutes later, the patient became acutely hypotensive. The portable radiograph shows complete cardiac herniation with volvulus into the right hemithorax. The pericardium is full of air. (From Gurney, J.W., et al.: Impending cardiac herniation: The snow cone sign. Radiology 161:653–655, 1986, with permission.)

(Moser and Proto, 1987), and the surgical clips or staples may appear to be displaced. These signs are followed by volume loss, complete opacification of the lobe, and pleural effusion. The patient is usually gravely ill, and the chest tube may drain foul-smelling material (Fig. 12–13). Rapid confirmation by angiography or bronchoscopy may be required before surgical re-exploration. Even with prompt diagnosis, the prognosis is poor (Adkins and Slovin, 1975; Brooks, 1984; Kirsh et al., 1975; Pinstein et al., 1985). Pulmonary gangrene due to obstruction of the pulmonary veins may simulate lobar torsion.

Thoracic Dehiscence

Separation of the posterolateral thoracotomy incision may be complete or may occur with the skin intact. It is seen most often in debilitated patients or in the presence of chest wall infection, seroma, or hematoma (Brooks, 1984; McLaughlin and Hankins, 1979). When the skin is intact, subcutaneous air or herniated lung is visible radiographically. These changes are accentuated by expiration. The radiograph or CT scan may also show progressive separation of the involved ribs (Fig. 12–14).

THORACOPLASTY

Prior to the development of specific chemotherapy, thoracoplasty was developed to treat severe cavitary tuberculosis, with or without empyema. Thoracoplasty and other space-altering procedures are still used occasionally for treatment of severe cavitary tuberculosis, persistent empyemas, and empyemas and bronchopleural fistulas associated with pulmonary resection (Hopkins et al., 1985).

Thoracoplasty involves the extraperiosteal removal of multiple ribs and transverse processes, with or without the removal of intrathoracic muscles. It is usually limited to the removal of three or four posterior ribs and adjacent transverse processes to allow the chest wall to obliterate the pleural space. More extensive chest wall resections are often staged to allow chest wall stabilization between procedures and thus to minimize the effects of the surgically created flailed chest (Fig. 12–15).

Following thoracoplasty, the radiograph usually demonstrates the absence of the ribs, diminished volume of the hemithorax, marked "pleural thickening," and a variable amount of mediastinal shift and scoliosis. The underlying lung is often fibrotic as a result of the primary disease. Examination by CT shows pleural thickening, chest wall deformity, and rotary scoliosis (Moore et al., 1988). Bronchiectasis and bullae are frequently present, especially in patients treated for tuberculosis. If successful, the collapsed chest wall should obliterate the space, and little or no fluid should remain. Fluid collections that persist or enlarge beyond the immediate postoperative period strongly suggest persistent or recurrent infection or the presence of an underlying bronchopleural fistula. The significance of asymptomatic fluid

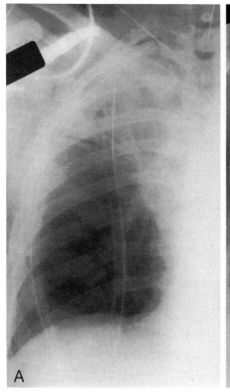

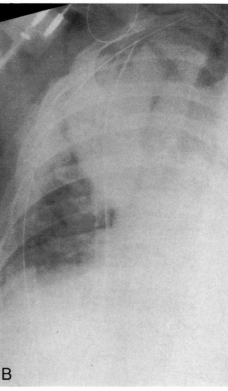

Figure 12–13. Torsion of the right middle lobe. *A,* The immediate postoperative radiograph after a right upper lobectomy for a penetrating injury shows increased density in the upper thorax corresponding to the re-oriented right middle lobe. *B,* Twenty-four hours later, the right middle lobe is totally consolidated and enlarged. The patient was asymptomatic at this point, and bronchoscopy showed no endobronchial lesion. Over the next 24 hours, the patient developed increasing pleural effusion and signs of systemic toxicity. A thoracotomy was performed, and the right middle lobe was found to be rotated on its pedicle and engorged with blood. (Courtesy of Dr. Robert Goren, Philadelphia, Pennsylvania.)

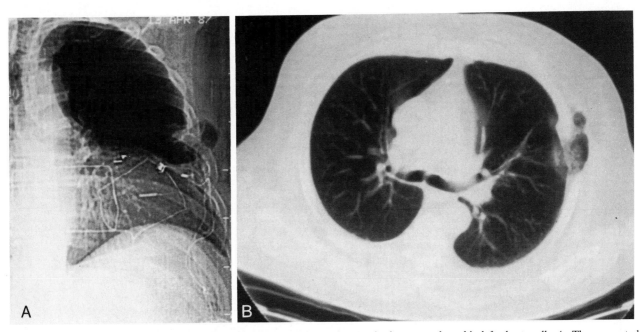

Figure 12–14. Lung herniation. Several weeks after thoracotomy, patient noticed a mass along his left chest wall. *A,* The computed radiograph scan shows a collection of air continuous with the lung in the sixth anterior lateral interspace. *B,* An axial scan through this level shows a defect in the chest wall with the lung herniating through the defect.

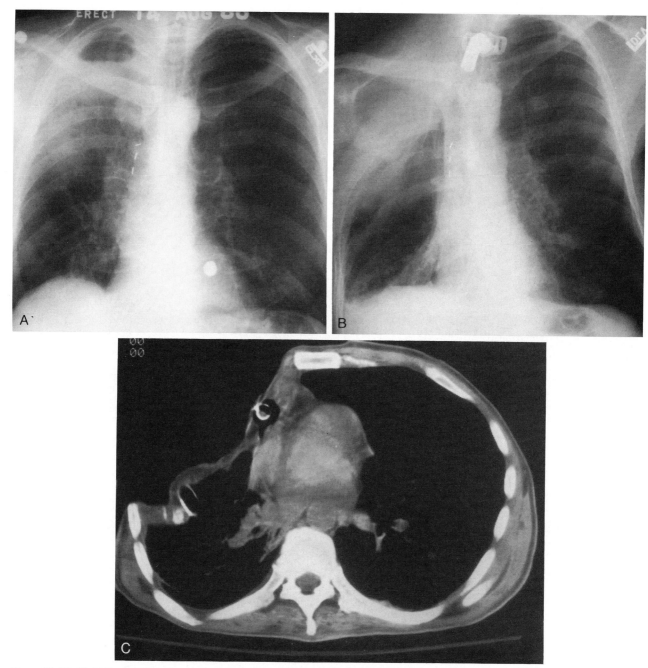

Figure 12–15. Right thoracoplasty for persistent empyema. *A,* A persistent air–fluid level appears in the right apex, several weeks after a right upper lobectomy. The infection failed to respond to conservative management. *B,* The first through fifth ribs have been removed to close a right apical empyema space. *C,* Approximately 2 weeks later a CT scan through the midthorax shows that the chest wall has collapsed to meet the lung. No residual space is present. Two thoracostomy tubes appear in the pleural space.

collection persisting for several years after surgery is less certain. Moore and associates (1988) found three persistent fluid collections in 33 patients who were studied for an average of 36 years after thoracoplasty for tuberculosis. They suggest that these collections contain active tuberculous organisms that may cause clinical disease at a later time.

The pleural-tent procedure (apicolysis) involves an extrathoracic dissection of the parietal pleura with application of the parietal pleura to the residual lung surface. This procedure obliterates the intrapleural space but creates an extrapleural space (Goodman et al., 1977). In recent years, muscle flaps and omentum have been turned into the thorax to reinforce bronchopleural fistula repairs, to bring additional blood supply to the thorax, and to occupy space (Fig. 12–16). This procedure often produces bizarre chest radiographs and CT scans, which can only be interpreted with a precise knowledge of the surgical procedure.

HEART–LUNG AND LUNG TRANSPLANTATION

Heart–Lung Transplantation

Heart–lung transplantation has been performed primarily in patients with cardiopulmonary failure due to severe pulmonary artery hypertension or Eisenmenger's syndrome. The 2-year actuarial survival rate is 62% with most deaths occurring within 2 months of surgery. The surgical implantation involves an end-to-end anastomosis of the distal trachea, an end-to-end anastomosis of the proximal aorta, and suturing of a cuff of the host's right atrium (containing the superior vena cava and inferior vena cava) to the donor's right atrium. The recipient's phrenic, vagus, and recurrent laryngeal nerves are preserved, but cardiopulmonary innervation, lymphatic circulation, and bronchial arterial circulation are sacrificed (Bonser et al., 1989).

Numerous problems of radiographic interest occur in the postoperative period. Posterior mediastinal bleeding from difficult-to-ligate, bronchopulmonary collateral vessels as well as from coagulopathy, is frequent and may necessitate reoperation. Disruption of the nerve supply to the lungs obliterates the cough reflex, and retained secretions and atelectasis are frequent. Similarly, injury to the vagus nerve is often associated with gastric outlet obstruction and reflux.

Pulmonary edema universally occurs several days to 1 week after surgery. The radiograph usually demonstrates mid- and lower-zone interstitial edema, peribronchial cuffing, and septal lines. This edema peaks within several days and gradually resolves. This phenomenon has been termed "the implant response," and it is probably due to a combination of

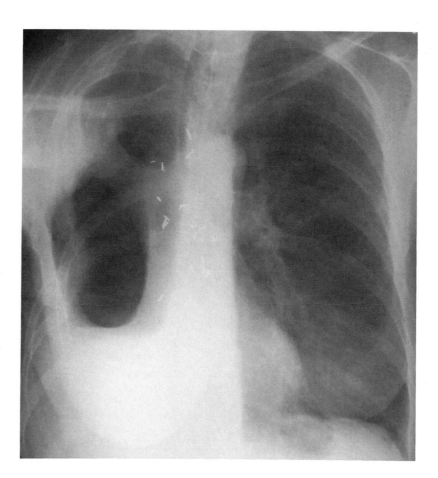

Figure 12–16. Latissimus dorsi flap for a bronchopleural fistula. The patient underwent pneumonectomy for atypical tuberculosis that resulted in a persistent bronchopleural fistula. Closure was finally obtained when the latissimus dorsi muscle was wrapped around the bronchial stump. Chest radiograph shows an opaque band running supralaterally to intramedially. This band represents the muscle crossing the thorax.

surgically related factors, including ischemia, trauma, and interruption of the pulmonary lymphatics and of pulmonary innervation (Bonser et al., 1989; Chiles et al., 1985). Pleural effusions are also frequent, probably owing to the interruption of lymphatic circulation. Pneumothorax is frequent and usually self-limited.

Acute rejection of the lung is also common in the postoperative period. It may occur synchronously or asynchronously with or without evidence of cardiac rejection. Distinguishing acute rejection from infection is extremely difficult, both clinically and radiographically. Millet and co-workers (1989) studied 23 patients with acute rejection within the first month and 22 patients with acute rejection beyond the first month. Of the former group, 75% had abnormal chest radiographs, whereas in the latter group, only 23% had abnormal radiographs. The abnormal radiographic appearances were similar for both groups. The majority of patients presented with lower- and mid-zone nodules that often became confluent or progressed to focal consolidation. The vast majority also had pleural effusions, and septal lines were present in half. With the exception of septal lines, the radiographic appearance was similar to cytomegalovirus (CMV) infection frequently seen during the first month and *Pneumocystis* infection frequently seen beyond the first month.

Bergin and colleagues (1990) found that the combination of septal lines and new or enlarging effusions without evidence of further cardiac enlargement, fur-

ther enlargement of the vascular pedicle, or vascular redistribution was a good indication of rejection. They found a sensitivity of 68%, specificity of 90%, and accuracy of 83% (Fig. 12–17). Transbronchial biopsy was the most effective tool for distinguishing infection from rejection.

Long-term survivors face the additional risk of bronchiolitis obliterans. This condition results in airflow obstruction and restrictive lung disease in 10% to 50% of patients (Millet et al., 1989; Skeens et al., 1989). Pathologically, there is evidence of inflammatory bronchiolitis and small airway plugging that leads to fibrosis. There are also muscular changes in the pulmonary arteries. The cause is unknown but is most likely chronic rejection. The radiographic pattern runs the entire gamut from normal to reticular nodular changes, to multiple discrete or confluent nodules, to pulmonary consolidation. The parenchymal changes are indistinguishable from infection. A possible unique feature, however, is central airway dilatation with bronchial wall thickening, which was found in nine out of 11 patients in the study by Skeens and colleagues (1989).

Unilateral and Bilateral Lung Transplantation

Unilateral or bilateral lung transplantation is a recent alternative for patients with severe end-stage lung disease without concomitant cardiac disease.

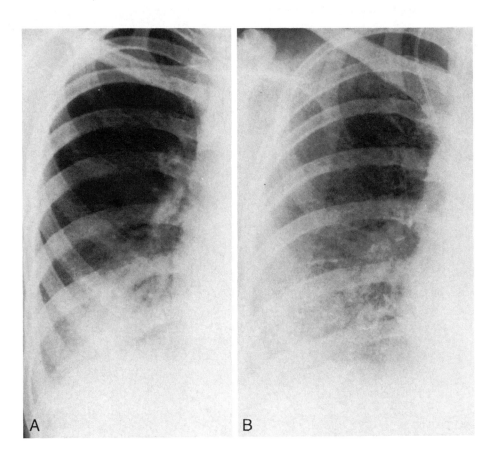

Figure 12–17. Acute lung rejection. *A,* Ill-defined nodular densities appear in the right midlung field, progressing to coalescence consolidation in the lower lung zone. A small effusion appears on the right as well. Similar, but less severe changes were visualized on the left. *B,* Kerley's lines and diffuse interstitial thickening are noted throughout the lung. Pleural effusion is also present at the right base. Similar changes were present on the left side. (From Millet, B., et al.: The radiographic appearances of injection and acute rejection of the lung after heart-lung transplantation. Am. Rev. Respir. Dis. 140:62, 1989, with permission.)

A   B

Bilateral lung transplantation involves end-to-end anastomosis of the distal trachea or of both bronchi, the main pulmonary artery, and a cuff of the recipient's left atrium and pulmonary veins to the donor's left atrium. For a single-lung transplant, the pulmonary artery and proximal main stem bronchus are anastomosed end to end or in a telescope fashion, with the donor's bronchus inside the host bronchus. The donor's and the recipient's left atria are joined.

Necrosis of the tracheal anastomosis due to loss of bronchial circulation has been a major cause of morbidity and mortality following lung transplantation. To reinforce the tracheal anastomosis and to bring additional blood supply to the area, the omentum is brought up through the diaphragm, is tunneled beneath the sternum, and is wrapped around the bronchus. This structure is usually visible as a paratracheal mass on the chest radiograph. The fatty nature of the mass is clear on the CT scan (Herman et al., 1989a, 1989b; The Toronto Lung Transplant Group, 1988). The omental wrap may not be necessary with the telescoping anastomosis.

The parenchymal problems of "reimplantation syndrome," acute rejection, and infection are similar to those of heart–lung transplant patients. In addition, necrosis and stricture at the site of tracheal anastomosis remain a serious problem. In four cases of tracheal necrosis reported by Herman and associates (1989b), mediastinal gas was present in three chest radiographs and CT scans. Delayed bronchial strictures were more difficult to visualize on radiographs and required CT or bronchoscopy for evaluation.

Lymphomas related to immunosuppressive therapy occur in a small percentage of heart–lung and lung transplant patients. The average duration from transplant to onset of lymphoma is approximately 8 months (see Fig. 10–13). The typical radiographic appearance includes pulmonary nodules and lymphadenopathy. These changes are often considerably more rapid than those associated with conventional lymphomas. In the majority of patients, lowering of the cyclosporine dose is associated with regression or resolution (Harris et al., 1987).

References

Adkins, P.C., and Slovin, A.J.: Complications of pulmonary resection. In Artz, C.P., and Hardy, J.D. (eds.): Management of Surgical Complications, ed 3. Philadelphia, W.B. Saunders, 1975, p. 309.

Arndt, R.D., Frank, C.G., Schmitz, A.L., and Haveson, S.B.: Cardiac herniation with volvulus after pneumonectomy. AJR 130:155, 1978.

Barker, W.L., Langston, H.T., and Neffah, P.: Postresectional thoracic spaces. Ann. Thorac. Surg. 2:299, 1966.

Bergin, C.J., Castellino, R.A., Blank, N., et al.: Acute lung rejection after heart-lung transplantation: Correlation of findings on chest radiographs with lung biopsy results. AJR 155:23, 1990.

Biondetti, P.R., Fiore, D., Sartori, F., et al.: Evaluation of the postpneumonectomy space by computed tomography. Comput. Assist. Tomogr. 6:238, 1982.

Bonser, R.S., Fragomeni, L.S., and Jamieson, S.W.: Heart–lung transplantation. Invest. Radiol. 24:310, 1989.

Brooks, J.W.: Complications of pulmonary and chest wall resection. In Greenfield, L.J. (ed.): Complications in Surgery and Trauma. Philadelphia, J.B. Lippincott, 1984, p. 285.

Chiles, C., Guthaner, D.F., Jamieson, S.W., et al.: Heart–lung transplantation: The postoperative radiograph. Radiology 54:299, 1985.

Christiansen, K.H., Morgan, S.W., Karich, A.F., and Takaro, T.: The pleural space following pneumonectomy. Ann. Thorac. Surg. 1:298, 1965.

Dorman, J.P., Campbell, D., Grover, F.L., et al.: Open thoracostomy drainage of post-pneumonectomy empyema with bronchopleural fistula. J. Thorac. Cardiovasc. Surg. 66:979, 1973.

Ferguson, T.B.: Complications of bronchoscopy and mediastinoscopy. In Cordell, A.R., and Ellison, R.G. (eds.): Complications of Intrathoracic Surgery. Boston, Little, Brown, 1979, p. 289.

Goodman, L.R.: Postoperative chest radiograph: II. Alterations after major intrathoracic surgery. AJR 134:803, 1980.

Goodman, P.C., Minagi, H., and Thomas, A.N.: Radiographic appearance of the chest after pleural space reduction procedures: Construction of a pleural tent and phrenoplasty. AJR 129:229, 1977.

Gurney, J.W., Arnold, S., and Goodman, L.R.: Impending cardiac herniation: The snow cone sign. Radiology 161:653, 1986.

Gurney, J.W., Harrison, W.L., Sears, K., et al.: Bronchoalveolar lavage: Radiographic manifestations. Radiology 163:71, 1987.

Harris, K.M., Schwartz, M.L., Slasky, B.S., et al.: Posttransplantation cyclosporine-induced lymphoproliferative disorders: Clinical and radiologic manifestations. Radiology 162:697, 1987.

Heater, K., Revzani, L., and Rubin, J.M.: CT evaluation of empyema in the postpneumonectomy space. AJR 145:39, 1985.

Herman, S.J., Rappaport, D.C., Weisbrod, G.L., et al.: Single lung transplantation: Imaging features. Radiology 170:89, 1989a.

Herman, S.J., Weisbrod, G.L., Weisbrod, L., et al.: Chest radiographic findings after bilateral lung transplantation. AJR 153:1181, 1989b.

Holbert, J.M., Chasen, M.H., Libshitz, H.I., and Mountain, C.F.: The postlobectomy chest: Anatomic considerations. Radiographics 7:889, 1987.

Hopkins, R.A., Ungerleider, R.M., Staub, E.W., et al.: The modern use of thoracoplasty. Ann. Thorac. Surg. 40:181, 1985.

Keagy, B.A., Loros, M.E., Starek, P.J., et al.: Elective pulmonary lobectomy: Factors associated with morbidity and operative mortality. Ann. Thorac. Surg. 40:349, 1985.

Kerr, W.F.: Late-onset post-pneumonectomy empyema. Thorax 32:149, 1977.

Kirsh, M.M., Rotman, H., Behrendt, D.M., et al.: Complications of pulmonary resection. Ann. Thorac. Surg. 20:215, 1975.

Lams, P.: Radiographic signs in postpneumonectomy bronchopleural fistula. Can. Assoc. Radiol. J. 31:178, 1980.

Mahoney, M.C., and Shipley, R.T.: Neofissure after right upper lobectomy: Radiographic evaluation. Radiology 166:721, 1988.

Malamed, M., Hipona, F.A., Reynes, C.J., et al.: The adult postoperative chest. Springfield, IL, Charles C Thomas, 1977.

McLaughlin, J.S., and Hankins, J.R.: Wound complications following chest wall surgery. In Cordell, A.R., and Ellison, R.G. (eds.): Complications of Intrathoracic Surgery. Boston, Little, Brown, 1979, p. 333.

Millet, B., Higenbottam, T.W., Flower, C.D., et al.: The radiographic appearances of infection and acute rejection of the lung after heart–lung transplantation. Am. Rev. Respir. Dis. 140:62, 1989.

Moore, N.R., Phillips, M.S., Shneerson, J.M., et al.: Appearances of computed tomography following thoracoplasty for pulmonary tuberculosis. Br. J. Radiol. 61:573, 1988.

Moser, E.G., and Proto, A.V.: Lung torsion: Case report and literature review. Radiology 162:639, 1987.

Motta, G., and Ratto, G.B.: Complications of surgery in the treatment of lung cancer: Their relationship with the extent of resection and preoperative respiratory function tests. Acta Chir. Belg. 89:161, 1989.

Nagasaki, F., Flehinger, B.J., and Martini, N.: Complications of surgery in the treatment of carcinoma of the lung. Chest 82:25, 1982.

O'Meara, J.B., and Slade, P.R.: Disappearance of fluid from the postpneumonectomy space. J. Thorac. Cardiovasc. Surg. 67:621, 1974.

Pinstein, M.L., Winer-Maram, H., Eastridge, C., et al.: Middle lobe torsion following right upper lobectomy. Radiology 155:580, 1985.

Sethi, G.K., and Takaro, T.: Esophagopleural fistula following pulmonary resection. Ann. Thorac. Surg. 25:74, 1978.

Shipley, R.T., and Mahoney, M.C.: Right middle lobe collapse following right upper lobectomy. Radiology 166:725, 1988.

Skeens, J.L., Fuhrman, C.R., and Yousem, S.A.: Bronchiolitis obliterans in heart–lung transplantation patients: Radiologic findings in 11 patients. AJR 153:253, 1989.

Spirn, P.W., Gross, G.W., Wechsler, R.J., and Steiner, R.M.: Radiology of the chest after thoracic surgery. Semin. Roentgenol. 23:9, 1988.

Suarez, J., Clagett, O.T., and Brown, A.L., Jr.: The postpneumonectomy space: Factors influencing its obliteration. J. Thorac. Cardiovasc. Surg. 57:539, 1969.

The Toronto Lung Transplant Group: Experience with single lung transplantation for pulmonary fibrosis. JAMA 259:2258, 1988.

Wechsler, R.J., and Goodman, L.R.: Mediastinal position and air-fluid height after pneumonectomy: The effect of the respiratory cycle. AJR 145:1173, 1985.

Young, W.G., and Perryman, R.A.: Complications of pneumonectomy. *In* Cordell, A.R., and Ellison, R.G. (eds.): Complications of Intrathoracic Surgery. Boston, Little Brown, 1979, p. 257.

ACUTE CARDIOVASCULAR DISEASE

PART IV

13

Acute Myocardial Infarction

Glenn E. Newman

This chapter reviews the current therapeutic management of acute myocardial infarction (AMI) and the relative roles of myocardial imaging techniques in AMI. The details of the myocardial imaging methods in AMI are beyond the scope of this chapter, but the principles of these imaging methods as well as the controversial issues in the management of AMI are reviewed.

Coronary artery disease (CAD) remains the most common cause of death in the United States annually, even though the incidence of coronary artery disease and the mortality rate associated with AMI in patients with CAD have decreased in the past 20 years (American Heart Association, 1987).

Numerous noninvasive myocardial imaging techniques have been developed in the past 20 years, and these techniques complement cardiac catheterization with coronary angiography in the management of patients suffering from AMI.

The conservative approach of general supportive care with hemodynamic and electrophysiologic monitoring of patients with a documented AMI in acute coronary care units has been replaced by a more aggressive and interventional approach (Alpert and Francis, 1987; Becker and Alpert, 1989; Wasserman and Ross, 1989). New strategies in the management of AMI continue to be developed, but the central principle in the more aggressive approach in the management of these patients is related to limitation of infarct size and preservation of ventricular function by salvaging viable myocardium (Becker and Alpert, 1989). These evolving strategies have primarily involved the recently developed pharmacologic therapy with thrombolysis, and mechanical therapy using balloon angioplasty.

HISTORY AND DEVELOPMENT

The history of cardiac catheterization and subsequent developments is brief compared with the orig-

inal clinical description of angina in 1768 by Heberden, and with that of AMI in 1912 by Herrick.

In 1929, Forssmann used fluoroscopy to catheterize his own right atrium from the left antecubital vein, but Judkins did not describe what came to be the most widely applied method of coronary angiography in the world until 1967 (Judkins, 1968; Steckelberg et al., 1979). In the interim, many significant developments occurred.

Cournand and Ranyes (1941) and Richards (1945) rediscovered the technique of right heart catheterization. Seldinger did not report his technique of vascular access until 1953, and selective coronary angiography was first reported in 1959 by Sones (Amplatz, 1983; Sones, 1970). Coronary angiography with preformed catheters was not reported until 1962 by Rickets and Abrams. Abrams had described image-amplified cineangiography only 4 years earlier, in 1958.

The first contrast agent that was relatively satisfactory in terms of toxicity and radiodensity—meglumine diatrizoate (Renografin) in Germany and cysto-meglumine diatrizoate (Hypaque) in the United States—was not available until the middle 1950s (Newman, 1989). The first organic iodide had been described in 1929, and iodopyrocet (Diodrast) was the safest contrast agent used throughout the 1940s (Newman, 1989).

Heparin was discovered by McClean in 1916, but the first therapeutic use of heparin was reported in 1941 for venous thrombosis and pulmonary embolism (Clason, 1941; Crafoord, 1941; McClean, 1959). Streptokinase, a thrombolytic agent, was not described until 1933, and urokinase was not described until 1957 (Ploug and Kjeldgaard, 1957; Tillet and Garner, 1933). Several thrombolytic trials were initiated from the late 1950s through the 1970s, but thrombolytic therapy was not approved for intracoronary use in patients with AMI until 1982, and it was approved for intravenous use in this same patient population in 1987 (Becker and Alpert, 1989; Ellis,

1990; Wasserman and Ross, 1989). Human tissue–type plasminogen activator (t-PA) was first identified in 1947, but it was not isolated until the late 1960s and was not purified in sufficient quantity for investigation until 1982 (Astrup and Permin, 1947; Collen et al., 1982).

The concept of percutaneous transluminal angioplasty (PTCA) was not documented until 1964, when Dotter and Judkins used a coaxial catheter system to improve flow in patients with peripheral vascular disease (Dotter and Judkins, 1964). Thirteen years later, in 1977, Gruntzig and colleagues (1979) performed the first coronary balloon angioplasty in man.

Thus, not until the late 1970s and early 1980s did cardiologists have at their disposal the capability to challenge the conventional, supportive approach in the management of patients with AMI with the more aggressive approach of pharmacologic and mechanical therapy (Becker and Alpert, 1989; Wasserman and Ross, 1989).

APPROACH TO PATIENT

Patients complaining of symptoms consistent with an acute myocardial infarction must undergo efficient clinical evaluation (Becker and Alpert, 1989; Wasserman and Ross, 1989). The clinician must determine by history, physical examination, and electrocardiogram (ECG) whether the patient's symptoms are likely to be a manifestation of myocardial ischemia, and if so, whether an AMI is probable (Alpert and Francis, 1987; Becker and Alpert, 1989; Wasserman and Ross, 1989). Frequently, these patients complain of crushing substernal chest pain, which may or may not radiate to the neck, jaw, left arm, or infrequently the right arm. Unfortunately, as many as 25% of the patients may have no or minimal chest pain but may have weakness, cold perspiration, and a general sense of not feeling well (Alpert and Francis, 1987). On physical examination, these patients frequently appear anxious with cool, clammy skin. The cardiovascular and respiratory examinations may reflect the impending AMI, the sequela of previous myocardial events, or both. On the ECG, the development of Q waves or loss of R waves is the electrocardiographic hallmark of Q-wave or transmural infarction. A non-Q wave infarction—nontransmural infarction—may be accompanied by persistent minor or major ST-segment or T-wave changes on the ECG.

The diagnosis of an acute myocardial infarction should not be excluded, however, by a normal ECG alone. The chest radiograph not only allows assessment of relative cardiac size, chamber enlargement, interstitial or alveolar edema, and pulmonary vascular redistribution, but also excludes other diagnostic possibilities. Blood samples for serum enzyme determinations should also be initially and serially obtained. Although most samples reach a peak after the infarction, they may serve to establish a diagnosis or rule out the diagnosis of AMI. The serum levels of MB isoenzyme of creative phosphokinase (CPK-MB) generally rise within 6 to 8 hours of onset of infarction and peak at 24 hours. The serum glutamic-oxaloacetic transaminase (SGOT) levels generally rise within 8 to 12 hours of onset of infarction and peak at 18 to 36 hours. The serum lactate dehydrogenase (LDH) levels generally rise within 24 to 48 hours of onset of infarction and peak at 3 to 6 days (Alpert and Francis, 1987).

DIFFERENTIAL DIAGNOSIS

The differential diagnosis of AMI is well established, but the ability to differentiate patients who are suffering an AMI from those who are not is critical (Alpert and Francis, 1987; Alpert and Rippe, 1988). In general, the differential diagnosis may be categorized by anatomic or organ system. Anatomically, the possibilities are chest wall pain, pleuritic pain, pulmonary (lung) pain, esophageal pain, or myocardial pain. The differential diagnosis, however, is expanded and more complete when considered by organ system. These possibilities include musculoskeletal pain such as broken ribs, strained muscles, and degenerative disc disease. Differential possibilities of the pulmonary system include pulmonary embolism, pneumothorax, and pneumonia. The differential possibilities from the gastrointestinal system include esophagitis, esophageal spasm, esophageal reflux, esophageal perforation, peptic ulcer disease, hiatal hernia, and acute cholecystitis or acute cholelithiasis. Vascular possibilities include aortic dissection and thoracic aneurysm.

The astute clinician must establish a reasonable differential diagnosis by history, physical examination, and simple laboratory data and must be prepared to explore the most life-threatening possibility. In patients with an established history of angina pectoris, the clinical diagnosis may be obvious. On the other hand, the diagnosis in a patient with acute onset of chest pain and no history of angina may be more problematic. Silent ischemia may be even more challenging to the clinician.

PATHOLOGY

Independently, Levine in 1929 and Mallory and White in 1939 pioneered the pathology of AMI (Levine, 1929; Mallory et al., 1939). An understanding of the serial pathologic developments in the myocardium is critical to understanding the therapeutic regimens in the evolving AMI and in the post-infarct treatment of the patient (Mallory et al., 1939).

Because the histologic features of an evolving infarct are so dynamic and specific during the first 3 weeks, the age of infarct can be accurately determined pathologically. In less than 24 hours, myocardial necrosis is easily demonstrated pathologically, but definite histologic evidence of necrosis is difficult to establish before approximately 6 hours after the cessation of blood flow. In general, the necrosis is histologically uniform throughout the area of infarct. From the third day through the fourth day, a progressive increase occurs in infiltration of the infarcted area with polymorphonuclear leukocytes. During the fifth day, the initial signs of myocardial muscle fiber phagocytosis appear histologically. By the seventh day, phagocytosis of myocardial muscle fibers appears, beginning at the periphery of the infarcted area and proceeding centripetally. By the tenth day, the necrotic myocardial muscle fibers have been almost completely removed in small infarcts. In general, the removal of muscle fibers continues in moderate-sized infarcts beyond the fourteenth day.

The ingrowth of blood vessels and connective tissue cells is usually not demonstrated before the fifth day, but it can extend dramatically beyond 21 days, depending on the size of the infarct. The pattern of ingrowth of these blood vessels and connective tissue cells is similar to that pattern seen with the removal of the myocardial muscle cells from the infarct. In other words, as these myocardial muscle cells are being removed progressively from the periphery of the infarcted area, they are being replaced by the ingrowth of blood vessels and connective tissues. Thus, when myocardial rupture occurs, usually it occurs within 7 days but may even occur between 7 and 14 days, following the infarction. Myocardial rupture after 14 days is rare.

The speed of healing of a myocardial infarct depends on the size and the position of the infarct and is somewhat variable, depending on the state of the remaining myocardial circulation. In general, however, by histologic criteria, much of the necrotic myocardial muscle cells have been phagocytized and replaced by connective tissue cells between 14 days and 21 days following the infarction. Small infarcts are usually not completely healed, however, until after 5 weeks, and large infarcts may not be healed pathologically until 8 weeks, following the infarction.

By understanding the evolving pathologic and histologic changes of a myocardial infarct, one recognizes that the time from the onset of symptoms to the actual documented cellular death is approximately only 6 hours (Alpert and Francis, 1987; Becker and Alpert, 1989; Mallory et al., 1939; Reimer et al., 1977). Thus, the elapsed time to initiation of therapy designed to establish myocardial reperfusion is critical (Mallory et al., 1939; Reimer et al., 1977). Knowledge of the temporal changes in a healing myocardial infarction allows one clinical insight into the potential complications of a myocardial infarction. These complications include arrhythmias, scar formation, aneurysm formation, thrombus formation within the ventricle over the area of the infarct, and myocardial rupture. This information also provides insight into the management of these patients during the infarction and during the post-infarct recovery period.

Currently, this immediate post-infarct recovery period is used to determine those factors that may have an adverse prognosis for the patient, so that appropriate therapy can be established (Gibbons, 1990; Massel et al., 1990). These issues are independently reviewed in a later section, "Imaging During and After Acute Myocardial Infarction."

MANAGEMENT

General Medical Therapy

The current management of patients with AMI is dedicated to the concept of preserving viable myocardial tissue and thus ventricular function (Becker and Alpert, 1989; Gibbons, 1990; Massel et al., 1990; The Multicenter Postinfarction Research Group, 1983; Wasserman and Ross, 1989). During the past 10 to 12 years, the conventional, conservative approach of supportive therapy has been replaced by more aggressive approaches (Becker and Alpert, 1989; Wasserman and Ross, 1989). The fact that most myocardial infarctions develop in patients with an acute thrombosis at a critical coronary artery stenosis has led to a number of clinical investigations designed to elucidate the best aggressive management of AMI—that is, to restore ventricular function by salvaging viable myocardium (Becker and Alpert, 1989; DeWood et al., 1980; Falk, 1983; Wasserman and Ross, 1989) (Fig. 13–1). These aggressive investigations have involved pharmacologic therapy, specifically thrombolytic therapy, mechanical therapy with a balloon angioplasty catheter, or both, and have focused on the relative roles of each of these two techniques in the management of patients with AMI.

In general, patients with a documented AMI are admitted to an intensive coronary care unit when general treatment of the AMI is initiated (Alpert and Francis, 1987; Becker and Alpert, 1989; Wasserman and Ross, 1989). Bedrest and sedation reduce stress to the patient. This general treatment is therapeutic in itself in that myocardial oxygen demand and consumption may be reduced. In addition, supplemental oxygen is provided. Patients with a suspected, but not documented, AMI should be admitted to the intensive coronary care unit until a myocardial infarction is excluded.

During the time in which the general medical treatment of AMI is being established, each patient should be continuously monitored for impending hemodynamic complications (Becker and Alpert, 1989; Wasserman and Ross, 1989). Each patient should be monitored for blood pressure, heart rate, and cardiac rhythm. When indicated, patients should undergo central venous catheterization for pressure measurements, pulmonary arterial catheterization for determination of pulmonary wedge pressures and cardiac output, or both. Appropriate monitoring of these patients allows constant assessment of the hemodynamic and electrical activity of the heart.

Complications of AMI include significant cardiac

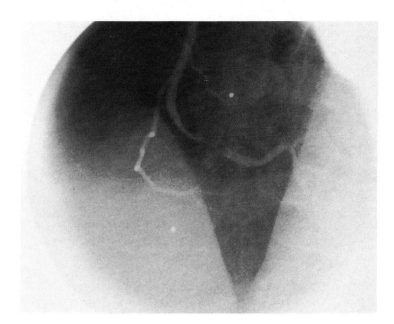

Figure 13–1. An angiographic image of a selected right coronary arteriogram in a patient with symptoms of an acute myocardial infarction (AMI). This image demonstrates the clot—the intraluminal filling defect—in the right coronary artery. The clot-associated stenosis is less apparent on this image.

arrhythmia. Bradycardia and tachycardia may occur, as may ventricular fibrillation.

Hemodynamic monitoring of patients is performed to assess the degree of right or left ventricular failure, which can be as profound as cardiogenic shock.

Acute ischemic left heart failure is a frequent complication of AMI and may occur transiently in 40% to 50% of patients (Becker and Alpert, 1989). Thus, while the acute infarct is developing, the systolic and diastolic functions of the heart may be markedly altered, depending on the extent of the acute infarction and previous infarctions. In general, the treatment strategy for heart failure induced by acute ischemic myocardial infarction depends on the assessment of the intravascular volume, cardiac rhythm, and right and left ventricular function. Ventricular performance is determined by the size of the evolving infarct, which is quite variable, and the size and severity of any previously completed myocardial infarcts.

Cardiogenic shock is manifested by systemic hypotension, tachycardia, pulmonary edema, oliguria, and peripheral hypoperfusion. Unfortunately, severe cardiogenic shock is associated with a mortality rate of 80% to 90% and implies myocardial necrosis involving approximately 40% of the left ventricular mass (Becker and Alpert, 1989; Page et al., 1971).

Other complications of AMI that severely affect patient mortality and involve the mechanical function of the ventricle are the development of acute mitral insufficiency from papillary necrosis, rupture, or both; rupture of the ventricular septum; and rupture of the free wall of the left ventricle. Rupture of the ventricular septum, the free wall of the left ventricle, or both is rare, but the occurrence and risk factors as well as physiologic features of these two complications have been outlined (Delborg et al., 1985; Randford et al., 1981; Tele and Edmonds, 1980).

Specific Medical Therapy

A correlation has been established between the degree of left ventricular dysfunction and the extent of myocardial necrosis (Alpert and Francis, 1987; Becker and Alpert, 1989; Wasserman and Ross, 1989). Additional publications have documented a relationship between the extent of necrosis from a single AMI and that from serial myocardial infarctions, which are additive and result in patient death. In other words, when approximately 40% of the left ventricular myocardium has undergone infarction, whether from a single infarction or from multiple infarctions, death is likely (Becker and Alpert, 1989; Page et al., 1971). Thus, the primary goal in the treatment of the myocardial infarction is limitation of myocardial necrosis, establishment of early myocardial reperfusion, or both, so that function may be preserved (Alpert and Francis, 1987; Becker and Alpert, 1989; Gibbons, 1990; Wasserman and Ross, 1989).

β-Adrenergic Blockers

The development of β-adrenergic blocking agents has had a significant impact on the management of AMI patients (Alpert and Francis, 1987; Becker and Alpert, 1989; Massel et al., 1990). By reducing heart rate, systemic blood pressure, and myocardial contractility, β-blockers reduce the myocardial oxygen demand. In addition, β-blockers have antiarrhythmic properties, which serve to protect against some of the tachyarrhythmias. β-blockers have contraindications, however, which include bronchial asthma, existing congestive heart failure, systemic hypotension, heart block, and bradycardia.

The benefits of the intravenous use of β-adrenergic blocking agents have been documented by multiple randomized trials (ISIS-1 Collaborative Group, 1986; Rossi et al., 1983; Yusuf et al., 1983, 1985). These benefits include reduction of infarct size, reduction in the incidence of complex ventricular arrhythmias, and reduction in early mortality and frequency of reinfarction and cardiac arrest.

Nitrates

Pharmacologically, the use of nitrates and related drugs reduces myocardial oxygen demand by reducing left ventricular filling pressure and myocardial wall stress (Becker and Alpert, 1989; Jugdutt, 1983, 1985; Yusuf and Collins, 1985). These agents have been investigated in several randomized trials, which support their use because of their beneficial reduction in early mortality from AMI. Additional studies have documented reduced early morbidity and mortality as well as a reduction in long-term mortality (Jugdutt, 1985).

The use of intravenous nitrates during AMI, however, may be counterproductive in those situations in which the reduction of afterload compromises coronary artery perfusion pressure. In such situations, myocardial ischemia may be enhanced (Becker and Alpert, 1989).

Calcium Channel Blockers

Calcium antagonists, or calcium channel blockers, have been documented to decrease myocardial oxygen demand by lowering the systemic blood pressure, heart rate, and myocardial contractility through pharmacologic properties similar to those of the β-blockers (Becker and Alpert, 1989; Massel et al., 1990; The Multicenter Postinfarction Research Group, 1983). In contrast to the β-blocker investigations to date, however, the calcium channel blockers have failed to demonstrate a favorable reduction in infarct size or in early morbidity or mortality during the AMI.

Thrombolysis

Immediate Thrombolytic Therapy

The development and subsequent availability of thrombolytic agents have had a tremendous impact on the management of patients with AMI for several pathophysiologic reasons (Becker and Alpert, 1989; Massel et al., 1990; The Multicenter Postinfarction Research Group, 1983; Wasserman and Ross, 1989). Experimental evidence documents that early (less than 6-hour) coronary reperfusion reduces myocardial infarct progression (Mallory et al., 1939; Reimer et al., 1977). In addition, clinical investigations have established that AMI is caused by an acute thrombus at the site of a significant coronary arterial lesion (DeWood et al., 1980; Falk, 1983). Thrombolytic agents, per se, are more effective in dissolving acute thrombus than are conventional anticoagulants such as heparin (Becker and Alpert, 1989) (Fig. 13–2).

In 1959, Fletcher and colleagues reported the use of thrombolytic agents in the treatment of patients with myocardial infarctions. Several subsequent reports substantiated this concept and investigated the benefit, risk, and efficacy of systemic (intravenous) thrombolytic therapy in patients with AMI. Chazov and colleagues (1976) and Rentrop and associates (1979) reported the use of selective intracoronary (intra-arterial) thrombolytic therapy in patients undergoing AMI. Subsequent investigations in which this selective intracoronary thrombolytic infusion technique was used demonstrated the therapeutic benefit of this form of thrombolytic therapy in achieving coronary artery patency and improved short- and long-term survival (Anderson et al., 1983; Kennedy

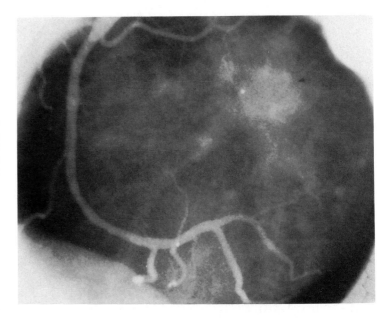

Figure 13–2. An image of a selective right coronary arteriogram after successful immediate thrombolytic therapy and balloon angioplasty of the lesion in the area of the previously defined clot. An excellent result is apparent. (This image is from the same patient as in Fig. 13–1.)

et al., 1983, 1985; Leiboff et al., 1984; Weinstein, 1982).

When the efficacy of the intravenous (systemic) form of thrombolytic therapy, however, was compared with that of the selective intracoronary technique, no demonstrable difference in infarct-related coronary patency rates was found (Alpert and Francis, 1987; Becker and Alpert, 1989). In addition, neither technique was superior in terms of preservation of left ventricular function or reduced mortality. Thus, the more invasive selective intracoronary approach was not proved superior, and the intravenous (systemic) approach was adopted, not only because of the reduced risk, but also because the intravenous approach has a significantly greater availability for a larger number of patients. Approximately 20% of hospitals in the United States have the capability of performing cardiac catheterization with selective coronary angiography (Becker and Alpert, 1989).

In 1986, the GISSI (*G*ruppo *I*taliano per lo *S*tudio Della *S*treptochinas, Nell' *I*nfarto Miocardico) trial was published. This study compared intravenous thrombolytic (streptokinase) therapy to standard therapy in patients suspected of having AMI who were seen within 12 hours of the onset of symptoms. Results demonstrated a reduced 21-day mortality rate and a survival benefit at 1 year. Since this investigation, a number of large prospective randomized trials have been designed to investigate not only the optimal thrombolytic agent or combination of agents, but also the optimal doses of the agent or agents (Becker and Alpert, 1989; Wasserman and Ross, 1989). In addition, adjunctive therapy—including aspirin, heparin, and β-adrenergic blockers—has been explored in some of these trials. Controversy persists, however, because the specified end points in the randomized prospective trials are inconsistent and therefore cannot necessarily be extrapolated from one study to another.

The AIMS Study Group trial (1988) reported a therapeutic benefit of an intravenous thrombolytic agent (anisoylated plasminogen–streptokinase activator complex) compared with a placebo in terms of reduction in mortality rates at 1 month and 1 year. This trial randomized patients suspected of having AMI to a therapeutic program of either a thrombolytic agent plus heparin or a placebo plus heparin. The patient receiving the thrombolytic agent plus heparin had an improved 1 month survival. The European Cooperative Study randomized patients to a thrombolytic agent (recombinant tissue plasminogen activator [rt-PA]), aspirin, heparin, and a β-blocker or to a placebo, aspirin, heparin, and β-blocker (Van de Werf et al., 1988). Those patients receiving the intravenous thrombolytic agent had a higher left ventricular ejection fraction and fewer cardiovascular complications of the initial infarct—such as ventricular fibrillation and cardiogenic shock—when compared with the placebo group. In addition, this group of patients had improved 2-week and 1-month survival. The Second International Study of Infarct Survival (ISIS-2) Collaborative Study Group (1988) considered patients with AMI who were seen within the first 24 hours after the onset of symptoms and randomized them into four therapeutic groups: (1) intravenous thrombolytic therapy (streptokinase), (2) aspirin, (3) both intravenous thrombolytic therapy and aspirin, and (4) neither agent. The mortality was significantly reduced in the group treated with the combination therapy compared with patients treated with either agent alone.

As a result of these randomized prospective clinical trials involving intravenous thrombolytic therapy, the best evidence suggests that patients seen within 6 hours after the onset of symptoms in relation to an AMI should receive a thrombolytic agent unless it is contraindicated (Becker and Alpert, 1989; Wasserman and Ross, 1989). In addition, adjunctive therapy that includes anticoagulant therapy, antiplatelet therapy, and β-adrenergic agents seems to be beneficial, if not synergistic, with myocardial infarction in terms of reduced mortality. The published trials and early evidence from the ongoing trials provide increasing evidence that patency of the infarct-related artery decreases infarct expansion and thus improves or, better, preserves left ventricular function and healing of the acute infarction (Becker and Alpert, 1989; Ohman and Califf, 1990; Wasserman and Ross, 1989). The optimum doses of these thrombolytic agents, antiplatelet agents, anticoagulant agents, and β-blockers, however, have yet to be determined (Becker and Alpert, 1989; Massel et al., 1990; Wasserman and Ross, 1989). Additional randomized prospective data are necessary to resolve some of these controversies (Becker and Alpert, 1989; Massel et al., 1990; Wasserman and Ross, 1989).

Late Thrombolytic Therapy

Prospective randomized trials have been performed to evaluate the efficacy of thrombolytic therapy in the temporal relationship with the onset of myocardial infarction (Becker and Alpert, 1989; Massel et al., 1990; Wasserman and Ross, 1989). In one study, therapy was initiated within 5 hours of symptom onset and demonstrated a significantly lower 1-year mortality rate in patients who achieved early patency of infarct-related vessels (Kennedy et al., 1983, 1985). One trial failed to demonstrate a benefit for patients when treatment was initiated 6 or more hours after the onset of symptoms (Dalen et al., 1988). Another more recent trial, however, the ISIS-2 (Second International Study of Infarct Survival), reported a significant reduction in mortality for patients treated up to 24 hours after the onset of symptoms (ISIS-2 Collaborative Study Group, 1988). Again, additional randomized studies are necessary.

Invasive Therapy—Percutaneous Transluminal Coronary Angioplasty

Since the development of the percutaneous balloon angioplasty catheter by Gruntzig, the role of percutaneous transluminal coronary angioplasty (PTCA) as an elective therapeutic technique in patients with angina has become well established (Becker and Alpert, 1989; Gruntzig et al., 1979). Controversy persists, however, regarding the use of PTCA in the emergency situation, that is, in the patient with AMI (Becker and Alpert, 1989; Ohman and Califf, 1990; Wasserman and Ross, 1989). Multiple prospective randomized trials designed to determine the optimum role of PTCA in patients with an evolving myocardial infarction have been performed. The question is, Should the angioplasty be performed during the initial thrombolytic therapy or immediately after clot lysis in patients without contraindications to thrombolytic therapy, directly in patients with contraindications to thrombolytic therapy, on a deferred (elective) basis in patients with successful thrombolytic therapy, or as a "rescue" procedure in patients who fail thrombolytic therapy (Becker and Alpert, 1989; Wasserman and Ross, 1989)?

Percutaneous Transluminal Coronary Angioplasty Immediately Following Thrombolysis

The role of immediate coronary angioplasty—that is, PTCA—after successful thrombolytic therapy has been evaluated in several clinical trials (Becker and Alpert, 1989; Ohman and Califf, 1990; Wasserman and Ross, 1989). The TIMI-IIA trial was designed to evaluate PTCA immediately after thrombolytic therapy as compared with PTCA deferred 18 to 48 hours after the onset of the symptoms of acute myocardial infarction (Passamani et al., 1987) (see Fig. 13–2). The left ventricular ejection fraction at discharge was the end point of the study and did not differ between the two groups. Also, no differences in death or reinfarction were found between the two groups. Those patients undergoing immediate PTCA, however, subsequently underwent emergency coronary artery bypass graft (CABG) more frequently. The TIMI-I trial was designed to compare immediate PTCA with that of deferred (elective) PTCA 7 to 10 days later in a group of patients treated with intravenous thrombolytic agent within 6 hours of symptoms and a patent infarct-related coronary artery (Topol et al., 1987). The left ventricular ejection fraction at discharge was comparable between the two groups. Those patients undergoing the immediate angioplasty, however, were associated with a higher mortality rate and required CABG more frequently.

The European Cooperative Study also assessed patients who were treated with immediate PTCA and were receiving thrombolytic therapy in comparison with a similar group undergoing a noninvasive therapeutic strategy (Verstraete et al., 1985). This trial was prematurely terminated because of a documented lack of benefit in those patients undergoing immediate PTCA. Lack of benefit was related to infarct size and left ventricular ejection fraction. In addition, the patients undergoing immediate PTCA had an increased mortality rate, greater incidence of recurrent ischemia, and a greater incidence of totally occluded infarct-related vessel at coronary artery angiography prior to discharge. Thus, the clinical trials performed to date have failed to document an increased global left ventricular function in the group undergoing immediate PTCA as assessed by left ventricular ejection fraction at discharge (Becker and Alpert, 1989; Ohman and Califf, 1990; Wasserman and Ross, 1989). In addition, these patients have a higher rate of morbidity than those patients not undergoing immediate PTCA.

Direct Percutaneous Transluminal Coronary Angioplasty

The concept of direct PTCA developed from analysis of data from the large prospective randomized trials investigating intravenous thrombolytic therapy in patients suffering an AMI (Becker and Alpert, 1989; Ohman and Califf, 1990; Wasserman and Ross, 1989). Analysis of this data demonstrated that thrombolytic therapy is contraindicated in as many as 30% to 40% of patients undergoing an AMI (Becker and Alpert, 1989; Wasserman and Ross, 1989; Wilcox et al., 1988). The efficacy of direct PTCA has been assessed in nonrandomized trials. The combined results of these nonrandomized trials reveal that PTCA is successful in establishing reperfusion in 83% to 95% of the patients, with an acute re-occlusion rate of 0% to 14% and an in-hospital mortality of 6.3% to 9.3% (Kimura et al., 1986; Marco et al., 1987; O'Neill et al., 1986; Rothbaum et al., 1987; Topol, 1988).

The number of patients who present with symptoms of an AMI and in whom thrombolytic therapy is contraindicated is significant (Becker and Alpert, 1989; Dalen et al., 1988; Wasserman and Ross, 1989). In other words, these patients are not candidates for the best first-line therapy—thrombolysis—and they may not have access to the number of hospitals capable of performing emergency PTCA in a timely fashion. In addition, the rate of complications in patients undergoing direct PTCA may be higher than that in patients undergoing thrombolysis with immediate PTCA.

Deferred or Elective Percutaneous Transluminal Coronary Angioplasty

Deferred, or elective, PTCA as defined by the clinical trials to date is PTCA performed between 1 day and 10 days after the onset of symptoms and successful thrombolytic therapy. Thus, with such a broad range, the optimal time for deferred PTCA remains controversial. In the Johns Hopkins study, patients were randomized to be treated with intravenous thrombolytic therapy (rt-PA) or placebo therapy, and they underwent immediate coronary angiography (Guerci et al., 1987). These patients were again randomized to either PTCA on the third day or to no PTCA during the subsequent 10 days. The patients in the group undergoing PTCA on day 3 had similar left ventricular ejection fractions at rest as compared with the noninvasive treatment group, and no difference was noted in the 10-day mortality between the groups. The patients in the invasive group, however, had greater left ventricular ejection fractions during submaximal exercise and a reduced incidence of post-infarction angina in the 10-day study compared with the other group.

A subset of patients in the TIMI-I trial were randomly assigned to a conservative strategy that included coronary angiography and PTCA only in those patients with spontaneous ischemia, exercise-induced ischemia, or both (The TIMI Study Group, 1989). In this group, only the left ventricular ejection fraction during exercise was significantly different at 6 weeks. This group also suffered adverse cumulative effects, however, including death, nonfatal infarction, intracranial hemorrhage, and a need for emergency bypass grafting after PTCA. The conservative group in this trial had a 10.5% incidence of coronary bypass grafting, a 6% incidence of recurrent infarction, a 13% incidence of ischemia on exercise testing, a 25% incidence of recurrent chest pain, and a 16% incidence of PTCA. Thus, these two trials involving deferred PTCA have failed to define the optimal time of PTCA following thrombolytic therapy for an AMI. Ventricular function with exercise was improved, however.

Rescue Percutaneous Transluminal Coronary Angioplasty

From experience with the clinical trials involving thrombolytic therapy, investigators have documented that initial thrombolytic therapy is unsuccessful in approximately 25% of patients with AMI (Becker and Alpert, 1989; Ellis, 1990; Wasserman and Ross, 1989). In the setting of failed thrombolytic therapy, PTCA is defined as rescue PTCA (Becker and Alpert, 1989; Ellis, 1990; Wasserman and Ross, 1989). In the TIMI-I trial, the subgroup of patients who did not undergo successful reperfusion after thrombolytic therapy underwent PTCA, which resulted in reperfusion with less than a 50% residual coronary artery stenosis in 73 of the 86 patients (Topol et al., 1987). Percutaneous transluminal coronary angioplasty failed to achieve any reperfusion in 11% of these patients. Mortality in these patients—that is, failed PTCA after failed thrombolytic therapy—was 44%. In addition, in those patients with failed thrombolytic therapy and successful PTCA, the re-occlusion rate was almost 30%. Conversely, the mortality was zero in the 10 patients who failed thrombolytic therapy but did not have PTCA. In the TIMI-IIA trial, the results also suggest that PTCA performed after failed thrombolytic therapy provided no benefit to the patient (The TIMI Research Group, 1988; The TIMI Study Group, 1985). The infarct-related arterial patency at discharge of the TIMI-II patients with com-

bination therapy was 96% in those patients undergoing rescue angioplasty for failed thrombolytic therapy (Topol et al., 1988). In the TIMI-V trial, rescue PTCA performed after failed thrombolytic therapy yielded a total infarct-related arterial patency of approximately 95% for single or combination thrombolytic therapy (Califf et al., 1991). Clearly, additional trials are necessary to establish the long-term benefit of rescue PTCA.

Coronary Artery Bypass Surgery

Coronary artery bypass grafting (CABG) is an established elective therapeutic procedure to restore blood flow in patients with CAD (Favaloro et al., 1970), and studies have demonstrated the efficacy of CABG in restoring blood flow in patients with an AMI (Berg et al., 1981; Goldman and Webel, 1986; Mock et al., 1982; Phillips et al., 1979). DeWood and colleagues (1983, 1989) have reported an in-hospital mortality of 3.1% for non–Q-wave infarction treated with CABG and a mortality of 5.2% for Q-wave infarction treated with CABG. In the same studies, they emphasize the importance of elapsed time for CABG in patients with AMI. In those patients undergoing CABG within 6 hours of the onset of symptoms, the in-hospital mortality was 3.8%, and the 10-year survival was 83%. In those patients undergoing CABG after 6 hours of symptoms, however, in-hospital mortality was 8%, and 10-year survival was 66%. In one randomized trial of emergency CABG for AMI, 3-month mortality was reported to be 2.9% in patients undergoing CABG but 20.6% in medically treated patients (Koshal et al., 1988).

The general indications for emergency CABG in patients with AMI have been established (Becker and Alpert, 1989). Emergency CABG may be performed in patients when thrombolytic therapy, PTCA, or both have been unsuccessful, provided that the symptoms of AMI are less than 6 hours in duration. Emergency CABG may be performed in patients with documented multivessel CAD who also have persistent pain, hemodynamic instability, or both. Emergency CABG may also be performed in patients with the combination of CAD not amendable by PTCA and angina that is resistant to maximal medical therapy. Furthermore, emergency CABG may be performed in hemodynamically unstable patients who have multivessel CAD requiring an intra-aortic balloon pump; a compromising complication of AMI, such as a ventricular septal defect or papillary muscle rupture; or both.

Unresolved Issues

Thrombolytic therapy has an established benefit in patients with a Q-wave myocardial infarction who are treated early (less than 6 hours following the infarction) (Becker and Alpert, 1989; Ellis, 1990; Ohman and Califf, 1990; Wasserman and Ross, 1989). For several patient groups, however, the efficacy of thrombolytic therapy remains controversial (Guerci, 1990). The relative risks and benefits of thrombolytic therapy in elderly patients with Q-wave infarctions, in patients with inferior infarctions, and in patients with non–Q-wave or non–ST-segment infarctions are not well established. Additional investigations are necessary to resolve questions regarding treatment of these problematic patients.

Additional investigations are required to establish the optimal management not only of patients in whom thrombolytic therapy is initially unsuccessful but also of patients in whom coronary artery re-occlusion develops (Muller and Topol, 1990). Moreover, the optimal management of patients with Q-wave infarctions presenting more than 6 hours after the onset of symptoms has been insufficiently addressed.

IMAGING DURING AND AFTER ACUTE MYOCARDIAL INFARCTION

A number of noninvasive imaging techniques are capable of assessing the heart's anatomic aspects, functional aspects, or both (Feigenbaum, 1986; Gibbons, 1990; Kiat and Berman, 1989a, 1989b; Kisslo et al., 1988; Reske, 1989). These noninvasive imaging techniques have an important role in the assessment of patients with stable or even progressive angina, and they are more important in the assessment of patients recovering from AMI than in the assessment of these patients during the early stages (hours) of the acute infarction itself. The details of each of these imaging methods is beyond the scope of this chapter, but the important capabilities of each are briefly reviewed.

These noninvasive imaging techniques are important for multiple reasons (Feigenbaum, 1986; Gibbons, 1990; Kiat and Berman, 1989a, 1989b; Kisslo et al., 1988; Reske, 1989). They are usually more available to patients, yet because of their noninvasive nature, they carry less risk to the patient in terms of complications than do invasive diagnostic procedures. Moreover, these imaging techniques, individually and collectively, allow specific diagnoses, which if established, represent complications related to the initial myocardial infarction. They are also capable, however, of stratifying patients in relation to yet another cardiac event, that is, to either re-infarction or death. This capability, to stratify patients according to future risk, clearly has therapeutic and prognostic implications.

Chest Radiography

Despite the development of such noninvasive techniques as echocardiography, radionuclide studies, computed tomography (CT), and magnetic resonant imaging (MRI), chest radiography continues to be a foundation of cardiopulmonary imaging because of its general availability and established value in most patients with acute cardiopulmonary disease (Chen, 1987). Moreover, chest radiography with fluoroscopy may be used as a screening procedure for CAD and may be used functionally in the management of patients suffering an AMI.

In patients with cardiac symptoms, coronary arterial calcifications detected by chest radiography, by fluoroscopy, or by both are highly predictive of major CAD (Chen, 1987). Unfortunately, a truly "normal" chest radiograph does not exclude significant CAD.

The chest radiograph is invaluable in the management of patients who have acute cardiopulmonary disease (Chen, 1987). It allows evaluation of the pulmonary vascularity, general size of the heart, and specific chamber enlargement, and it reflects the underlying cardiopulmonary function of the patient. The chest radiographic signs of AMI are usually nonspecific and must be correlated with the results of physical examination and further imaging procedures. In patients with AMI, the most common finding on the chest radiograph is pulmonary edema with a "normal" heart. Serial chest radiographs frequently document the resolution of pulmonary edema produced by therapy in patients with uncomplicated AMI. Persistent or severe pulmonary edema, however, may suggest the development of complications arising from the initial myocardial infarction. These complications include left ventricular aneurysm formation, mitral insufficiency after rupture of the papillary muscle, and perforation of the ventricular septum.

Assessment of the pulmonary vasculature in patients suffering an AMI is clinically important (Chen, 1987). Usually, during the acute phase of the myocardial infarction, left-sided heart failure occurs, which appears radiographically as a combination of alveolar pulmonary edema in a perihilar or hilar distribution, normal heart size, and lack of cephalization of the pulmonary vasculature. If cardiomegaly or specific chamber enlargement appears radiographically, then cardiopulmonary disease or the previous myocardial events is evident. Chronic left-sided heart failure is manifested radiographically as cephalization of the pulmonary vasculature, interstitial pulmonary edema, septal lines, and notable cardiomegaly. Extreme left-sided heart failure can also cause right-sided heart failure, which is manifested radiographically as reduced pulmonary blood flow, a reduced pattern of cephalization, right-sided heart chamber enlargement, and perhaps even less prominently, left-sided heart enlargement. In patients with CAD, severe left-sided heart failure is the most common cause of right-sided heart failure.

Echocardiography

Echocardiography has developed rapidly and is currently capable of providing both anatomic and relative functional information regarding the heart (Feigenbaum, 1986; Kisslo et al., 1988). Echocardiography is capable of assessing anatomic information, including cardiac chamber size, myocardial wall thickness, presence of mural thrombi, presence of ventricular aneurysm, and valve motion. Echocardiography is also capable of providing functional information such as that regarding segmental and global wall-motion abnormalities. When echocardiography is serially applied, it can assess changes in these potential anatomic and functional abnormalities.

In patients with ischemic heart disease, echocardiography is capable of providing both functional and anatomic information simultaneously (Feigenbaum, 1986; Kisslo et al., 1988). Assessment of left ventricular function is accomplished by comparison of diastolic and systolic echocardiographic images to detect global and regional wall-motion patterns and abnormalities, or by "real-time" assessment of the wall motion throughout the cycle (Kisslo et al., 1988). In general, during and following the infarction, the myocardium demonstrates wall-motion abnormalities whose severity is described as hypokinetic, akinetic, dyskinetic, or aneurysmal, depending on the size, extent, and age of the infarct. Associated findings include thinning and scarring of the infarcted myocardium.

Echocardiography may also provide specific anatomic diagnoses that represent complications as sequelae of myocardial infarctions (Feigenbaum, 1986; Kisslo et al., 1988). These sequelae include pericardial effusion (Dressler's syndrome), post-infarction ventricular septal defect, papillary muscle rupture, left ventricular aneurysm with or without a mural thrombus, pseudoaneurysm, and myocardial rupture (Fig. 13–3).

Nuclear Medicine Imaging

Functional Imaging

Functional imaging of the heart—assessment of left ventricular ejection fraction and regional wall motion—can be performed by two generally accepted radionuclide angiocardiographic techniques (Gibbons, 1990). One is the multiple-gated acquisition (MUGA) technique, which involves gated acquisition of images after an injection of technetium agent, which "tags" the red blood cells. The other technique is the "first-pass" technique, which averages images from two to four cardiac cycles as the radiopharmaceutical traverses the heart. Each technique can be performed in the resting and exercise states. The assessment of myocardial function at rest and during exercise provides information that allows diagnostic, therapeutic, and prognostic decisions to be made by clinicians caring for patients who have suffered a myocardial infarction (Gibbons, 1990).

Resting Ejection Fraction

The measurement of left ventricular ejection fraction at rest after a myocardial infarction permits an estimation of the size of the infarct and documents the residual function of the left ventricle (Kiat and Berman, 1989a, 1989b). In addition, the left ventricular ejection fraction at rest has prognostic value for the patient following an AMI (Defeyter et al., 1982; Sanz et al., 1982). A correlation exists between left ventricular ejection fraction at rest after an AMI and the survival at 12 months (The Multicenter Postinfarction Research Group, 1983). That is, the 1-year cardiac mortality is inversely related to the resting ejection fraction in a continuous fashion. The 1-year cardiac mortality steadily increases as the resting ejection fraction of the left ventricle decreases. In patients with an ejection fraction greater than 60%, the 1-year cardiac mortality is less than 5%. At the other extreme, in patients with a left ventricular ejection fraction at rest of less than 20%, 1-year cardiac mortality is almost 50%.

Exercise Radionuclide Angiography

Just as the resting left ventricular ejection fraction after myocardial infarction is related to the extent of myocardial damage, so are the presence and extent of exercise-induced ischemia also predictors of patient outcome following myocardial infarction (Gibbons, 1990). This finding is documented by the work of Corbett and associates (1983a, 1983b), who studied patients after uncomplicated acute myocardial infarctions. Of those patients who failed to increase their

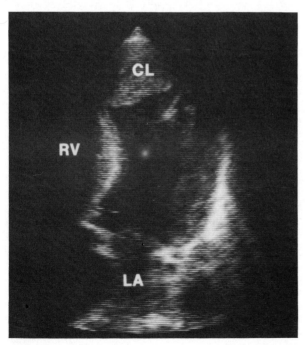

Figure 13–3. Isolated image from an echocardiogram. This two-dimensional apical four-chamber view demonstrates a left ventricular aneurysm, which is associated with an apical thrombus (clot [CL]). The right ventricle (RV) and left atrium (LA) are also labeled.

ejection fraction with exercise, 95% suffered a myocardial event within 6 months of the original infarction. In contrast, less than 10% of the patients who increased their ejection fraction with exercise had a subsequent myocardial event during the 6-month follow-up. These findings were substantiated by a second investigation by Dewhurst and Muir (1983). In yet another study by Morris and colleagues (1985), the left ventricular ejection fraction during exercise was found to be the single most important of 12 clinical parameters in predicting survival (Corbett et al., 1983a). The expected 2-year mortality was 56% in patients with an exercise ejection fraction of 15% and 29% in patients with an exercise ejection fraction of 30%, but it was only 11% in patients with an exercise ejection fraction of 50% (Lebowitz et al., 1975; Nielson et al., 1979).

Infarct Imaging

Myocardial infarct imaging is a well-developed imaging technique that utilizes technetium-99m (^{99m}Tc) pyrophosphate, which localizes in areas of myocardial necrosis (Wackers et al., 1976; Willerson et al., 1975). In transmural infarctions, the sensitivity of this technique is 95% to 100% and is probably only slightly less in nontransmural or subendocardial infarctions (Willerson et al., 1975). Despite the excellent sensitivity of this imaging technique, however, its clinical usefulness is variable because the temporal relationship between the onset of symptoms and the development of a positive scan is a major limitation (Willerson et al., 1975). That is, with the current technique of infarct imaging, the images do not become reliably positive until approximately 24 hours or more after infarction. This problem has thus limited the use of this imaging technique to patients with non–Q-wave infarcts and pre-existent abnormal ECGs (Willerson et al., 1975).

Perfusion (Myocardial) Imaging

The use of myocardial perfusion imaging at rest and during exercise in patients with angina is well established, and several studies have described the use of thallium-201 (^{201}Tl) imaging not only to detect, localize, and size AMI, but also to determine prognosis (Silverman et al., 1980; Smitherman et al., 1978; Wackers et al., 1976). In one study, the sensitivity was 100% when imaging was performed within 6 hours of the initial symptoms that suggested the acute infarction. Because a given perfusion defect is not specific for an acute myocardial event, however, the use of ^{201}Tl to diagnose AMI is limited in some situations. The perfusion defect of healed infarct could thus not be differentiated from the perfusion defect of acute infarction (Wackers et al., 1976). Serial perfusion imaging to detect infarct extension may be of greater value in patients with post-infarction pain.

The morbidity and mortality of AMI correlate with the extent of the necrosis and degree of left ventricular functional impairment (Silverman et al., 1980). The extent of the perfusion defects appearing on thallium imaging studies at rest can help estimate the extent of the myocardial damage. Investigators have documented differences in patient survival based on the extent of perfusion defects. Silverman and coworkers (1980) documented with both planar and tomographic imaging techniques that large defects in the images identified patients at risk of a cardiac event within 18 months. Patients with small perfusion defects had only a 7% incidence of a myocardial event (angina, myocardial infarct, sudden death), but patients with large perfusion defects had a 92% incidence of a myocardial event (Silverman et al., 1980).

Just as exercise radionuclide assessment of ventricular function has been found to correlate with patient outcome, so has post-exercise thallium imaging been employed to identify patients at risk for subsequent cardiac events due to exercised-induced ischemia (Gibson et al., 1983). Multiple investigations have been reported, and they suggest that patients may be stratified on the basis of thallium imaging studies according to risk of a subsequent myocardial event (Gibson, 1988). Gibson (1988) performed exercise thallium imaging, exercise treadmill testing, and coronary angiography on 140 conservatively treated patients after they underwent an uncomplicated myocardial infarction. The high-risk thallium group was identified by the presence of redistribution on 4-hour delayed images, increased lung uptake, or perfusion defects in more than a single coronary artery. The high-risk thallium group had a similar incidence of events (death, infarction, Class III and IV angina) as those groups identified by either high-risk exercise treadmill testing or high-risk coronary angiography. The low-risk thallium group, defined by one perfusion defect and no redistribution, had a significantly reduced probability of an event when compared with the low-risk subgroups undergoing coronary angiography and exercise treadmill testing. Thus, the low-risk thallium subgroup appeared to be "protected" from an event in this study.

Abraham and colleagues (1986) performed a similar study and reported that exercise thallium imaging had only a modest prognostic value. Hung and associates (1984), however, compared the prognostic value of exercise treadmill testing with exercise MUGA imaging in 117 men within 3 weeks of AMI. The single best prognostic indicator was the change in left ventricular ejection fraction from rest to exercise. When the ejection fraction with exercise decreased from that of rest by 0.05 or greater, 38% of the patients had an event (death or myocardial infarction) within 1 year. Yet, only 3% of patients without this decrease suffered an event within 1 year.

Thus, because of differences in patient populations, end points of investigation, and stratification schemes, the single best predictor of future myocardial events is difficult to know for sure, but exercise functional imaging and exercise thallium imaging are clearly among the best indicators (Gibbons, 1990).

Positron-Emission Tomography

Positron-emission tomography (PET) permits the noninvasive investigation of the metabolism of myocardial tissue (Schelbert, 1987; Storch-Becker et al., 1988). It can thus evaluate and quantify substrate fluxes, biochemical reaction rates, oxidative metabolism, and blood flow in the myocardium.

Research investigations with PET imaging have focused on stress-induced myocardial ischemia, chronic myocardial ischemia, and AMI (Schelbert, 1987; Storch-Becker et al., 1988). Moreover, PET metabolic imaging in AMI can detect metabolic activity and myocardial viability in areas of Q-wave infarction and areas of necrosis identified by ECG (Braunwald and Rutherford, 1986; Brunker et al., 1986; Chava, 1983) (Fig. 13–4). Thus, given the sensitive metabolic imaging capabilities of PET, intensive research may be of value in determining newer and more innovative methods of treating patients

with myocardial infarction so that viable myocardium is salvaged.

Positron-emission tomography is an expensive imaging system with limited availability to patients with AMI (Schelbert, 1987; Storch-Becker et al., 1988). Specific research interest, however, and developments in PET imaging in patients with AMI may provide information that will ultimately reach a larger patient population.

Magnetic Resonance Imaging

Magnetic resonance imaging (MRI) is a developing imaging procedure that has had a tremendous clinical impact in several areas, especially neuroradiology, but it has not yet had a significant clinical impact in patients with myocardial infarcts (Swenson et al., 1989). To some extent, the information currently obtainable by MRI can also be obtained by other noninvasive imaging techniques, such as echocardiography or nuclear medicine imaging (Swenson et al., 1989). Currently, MRI can detect and localize myocardial infarctions, wall-motion abnormalities, and myocardial thinning after an infarction (Fig.

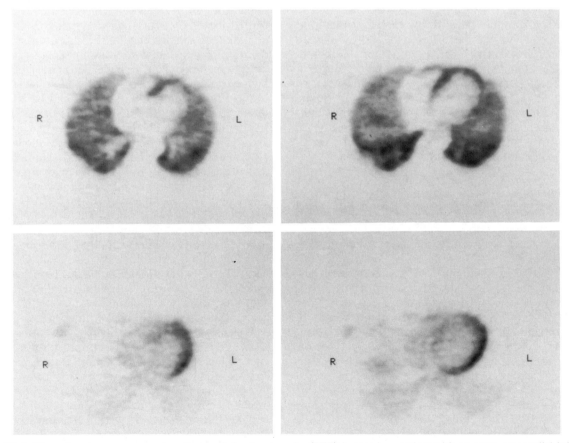

Figure 13–4. These four images represent positron-emission tomography (PET) images in a patient with an acute myocardial infarction. The top two images are perfusion images with nitrogen-13 (^{13}N) ammonia as a perfusion agent. In the lower two images, fluorodeoxyglucose was used as an imaging agent of glucose metabolism. The top two images demonstrate reduced perfusion to the lateral wall of the left ventricle and also increased lung activity secondary to congestive heart failure. The lower two images demonstrate increased glucose uptake in the lateral wall of the left ventricle, which represents ischemic but viable myocardium.

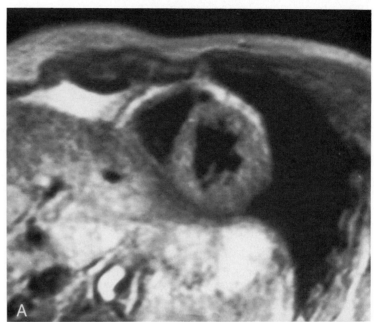

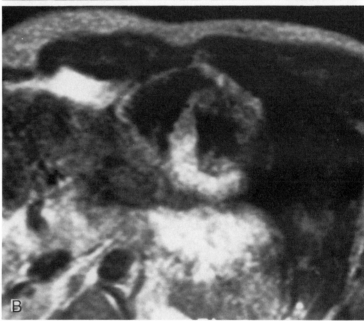

Figure 13–5. Cardiac gated oblique magnetic resonance imaging (MRI) examination (left ventricular short-axis projection). *A,* First echo (20-msec time to echo [TE]) image through the left ventricle demonstrates normal flow void in the left and right ventricular cavities, with no definite abnormal signal intensity in the left ventricular myocardium. *B,* Second echo (60-msec TE) image demonstrates abnormal high signal intensity in the inferior septum and inferior wall of the left ventricle. This finding is typical in acute myocardial infarction and represents edema and necrosis.

13–5). With additional research and development, however, MRI may have greater importance in the future for patients who suffer myocardial infarcts.

SUMMARY

Coronary artery disease is the most common cause of death in the United States. Myocardial infarctions generally occur when an acute thrombus forms at a coronary arterial stenosis. The therapeutic goal in the treatment of patients suffering an AMI is the timely re-establishment of myocardial perfusion (less than 6 hours following the onset of symptoms), to limit infarct size, and to preserve left ventricular function.

Prospective randomized trials have involved thrombolytic therapy primarily, and adjunctive administration of heparin, aspirin, or β-adrenergic blockers, to salvage the infarcting myocardium. In general, these trials have documented reduced mortality and improved residual ventricular function. The efficacy of PTCA has been investigated as well. These trials suggest that PTCA is indicated after successful thrombolytic therapy, but in the deferred (elective) states rather than immediately. Thrombolytic failures, and patients with contraindications to thrombolytic therapy, present challenges to clinicians. Controversy persists regarding thrombolytic therapy in the elderly, thrombolytic therapy in the inferior infarct, the treatment of non–Q-wave infarcts, and treatment of patients with re-occlusion of the infarct-related artery. Additional research is necessary to resolve these problems.

Several imaging techniques that are currently available permit assessment of the extent of the infarct and of complications related to the infarct. Most of these imaging procedures are noninvasive and can be applied serially. Functional data obtained via these techniques permit stratification of patients according to risk of a subsequent myocardial event and are therefore prognostically important. Continued research with PET imaging may advance the treatment of patients with AMI.

References

Abraham, R.D., Freedman, S.B., Dunn, R.F., et al.: Prediction of multivessel coronary artery disease and prognosis early after acute myocardial infarction by exercise electrocardiography and thallium-201 myocardial perfusion scanning. Am. J. Cardiol. 58:423, 1986.

Abrams, H.L.: An approach to biplane cineangiocardiography. Radiology 72:735, 741, 1958.

The AIMS Study Group: Effect of intravenous APSAC on mortality after acute myocardial infarction: Preliminary report of a placebo-controlled clinical trial. Lancet 1:545, 1988.

Alpert, J.S., and Francis, G.S.: Manual of Coronary Care, ed. 4. Boston, Little, Brown, 1987, p. 47.

Alpert, J.S., and Rippe, J.M.: Manual of Cardiovascular Diagnosis and Therapy, ed. 3. Boston, Little, Brown, 1988, p. 172.

American Heart Association: Heart Facts. Dallas, American Heart Association, National Center for Health Statistics: Monthly Vital Statistics Report. Sept. 1986, Vol. 34, no. 13.

Amplatz, K.: Rapid film changes. In Abrams, H.L. (ed.): Abrams Angiography: Vascular and Interventional Radiology, ed. 3. Boston, Little, Brown, 1983.

Anderson, J.L., Marshall, H.W., Bray, B.E., et al.: A randomized trial of intracoronary streptokinase in the treatment of acute myocardial infarction. N. Engl. J. Med. 308:1312, 1983.

Astrup, T., and Permin, P.W.: Fibrinolysis in animal organism. Nature 159:681, 1947.

Becker, R.C., and Alpert, J.S.: Current management of acute myocardial infarction. Curr. Probl. Cardiol. 14:505, 1989.

Berg, R., Jr., Selinger, S.L., and Leonard, J.J.: Immediate coronary artery bypass for acute evolving myocardial infarction. J. Thorac. Cardiovasc. Surg. 81:493, 1981.

Braunwald, E., and Rutherford, J.D.: Reversible ischemic left ventricular dysfunction: Evidence for the "hibernating myocardium." J. Am. Coll. Cardiol. 8:1467, 1986.

Brunken, R., Tillisch, J., Schwaiger, M., et al.: Regional perfusion, glucose metabolism and wall motion in chronic electrocardiographic Q-wave infarctions: Evidence for persistence of viable tissue in some infarct regions by positron emission tomography. Circulation 73:951, 1986.

Califf, R.M., Topol, E.J., George, B.S. et al.: Importance of Recurrent Ischemia as an Adverse Outcome After Thrombolytic Therapy. (Abstract.) Atlanta, American Heart Association, 1991.

Chava, N.R.: Transient QRS changes in variant angina simulating acute myocardial infarction. Am. Heart J. 105:695, 1983.

Chazov, E.L., Mateeva, L.S., Mazaev, A.V., et al.: Intracoronary administration of fibrinolysin in acute myocardial infarction. Ter. Arkh. 48:8, 1976.

Chen, J.T.T.: Essentials of Cardiac Roentgenology. Boston, Little, Brown, 1987, p. 167.

Clason, S.: Three cases of pulmonary embolism following confinement, treated with heparin. Acta Med. Scand. 107:131, 1941.

Collen, D., Rijken, D.C., Van Damme, J., and Billiau, A.: Purification of human tissue-type plasminogen activator in cen-

tigram quantities from human melanoma cell culture fluid and its conditioning for use in vivo. Thromb. Haemost. 48:294, 1982.

Corbett, J.R., Nicod, P.H., Huxley, R.L., et al.: Left ventricular functional alterations at rest and during submaximal exercise in patients with recent myocardial infarction. Am. J. Med. 74:577, 1983a.

Corbett, J.R., Nicod, P., Lewis, S.E., et al.: Prognostic value of submaximal exercise radionuclide ventriculography after myocardial infarction. (Abstract.) Am. J. Cardiol. 52:82, 1983b.

Cournand, A., and Ranyes, H.A.: Catheterization of the right auricle in man. Proc. Soc. Exp. Biol. Med. 46:462, 1941.

Crafoord, C.: Heparin as a prophylactic against thrombosis. JAMA 116:2831, 1941.

Dalen, J.E., Gore, J.M., Braunwald, E., et al.: Six- and twelve-month follow-up of the Phase I TIMI Trial. Am. J. Cardiol. 62:179, 1988.

Defeyter, P.J., Van Ecinige, M.J., Dighton, D.H., et al.: Prognostic value of exercise testing, coronary angiography, and left ventriculography six to eight weeks after myocardial infarction. Circulation 66:527, 1982.

Delborg, M., Held, P., and Swedberg, K.: Rupture of the myocardium: Occurrence and risk factors. Br. Heart J. 54:11, 1985.

Dewhurst, N.G., and Muir, A.L.: Comparative prognostic value of radionuclide ventriculography at rest and during exercise in 100 patients after first myocardial infarction. Br. Heart J. 49:111, 1983.

DeWood, M.A., Notske, R.N., Berg, R., Jr., et al.: Medical and surgical management of early Q wave myocardial infarction. I. Effects of surgical reperfusion on survival, recurrent myocardial infarction, sudden death and functional class at 10 or more years of follow-up. J. Am. Coll. Cardiol. 14:65, 1989.

DeWood, M.A., Spores, J., Berg, R., et al.: Acute myocardial infarction: A decade of experience with surgical reperfusion in 701 patients. Circulation 68(Suppl. II):II-8, 1983.

DeWood, M.A., Spores, J., Notske, R., et al.: Prevalence of total coronary occlusion during the early hours of transmural myocardial infarction. N. Engl. J. Med. 303:897, 1980.

Dotter, C.T., and Judkins, M.P.: Transluminal treatment of arteriosclerotic obstruction. Circulation 30:654, 1964.

Ellis, S.G.: Interventions in acute myocardial infarction. Circulation 81(Suppl. IV):IV-43, 1990.

Falk, E.: Plaque rupture with severe pre-existing stenosis precipitating coronary thrombosis: Characteristics of coronary artery plaque underlying fatal occlusive thrombus. Br. Heart J. 50:127, 1983.

Favaloro, R.G., Effler, D.B., Groves, L.K., et al.: Severe segmental obstruction of the left main coronary artery and its divisions: Surgical treatment by the saphenous vein graft technique. J. Thorac. Cardiovasc. Surg. 60:469, 1970.

Feigenbaum, H.: Echocardiography, ed. 4. Philadelphia, Lea & Febiger, 1986, p. 402.

Fletcher, A.P., Sherry, S., Alkjaersig, N., et al.: The maintenance of a sustained thrombolytic state in man. II. Clinical observations on patients with myocardial infarction and other thromboembolic disorders. J. Clin. Invest. 38:1111, 1959.

Gibbons, R.J.: The use of radionuclide techniques for identification of severe coronary disease. Curr. Probl. Cardiol. 15:305, 1990.

Gibson, R.S.: Non-Q-wave myocardial infarction: Diagnosis, prognosis, and management. Curr. Probl. Cardiol. 13:1, 1988.

Gibson, R.S., Watson, D.D., Craddock, G.B., et al.: Prediction of cardiac events after uncomplicated myocardial infarction: A prospective study comparing predischarge exercise thallium-201 scintigraphy and coronary angiography. Circulation 68:321, 1983.

Goldman, B.S., and Webel, R.D.: Surgical reperfusion of acute myocardial ischemia: A clinical review. Journal of Cardiac Surgery 1:167, 1986.

Gruntzig, A.R., Senning, A., and Siegenthaler, W.E.: Non-operative dilation of coronary artery stenosis: Percutaneous transluminal coronary angioplasty. N. Engl. J. Med. 301:61, 1979.

Gruppo Italiano per lo Studio Della Streptochinas, Nell' Infarto Miocardico (GISSI): Effectiveness of intravenous thrombolytic treatment in acute myocardial infarction. Lancet 1:397, 1986.

Guerci, A.D.: Unresolved issues: Treatment of elderly patients and patients with inferior infarction and non–ST-segment infarcts. Coronary Artery Disease 1:34, 1990.

Guerci, A.D., Gerstenblith, G., Brinker, J.A., et al.: A randomized trial of intravenous t-PA for acute myocardial infarction with subsequent randomization to elective coronary angioplasty. N. Engl. J. Med. 317:1613, 1987.

Herberden, W.: Commentaries on the history and cure of disease. Boston, Wells and Lilly, 1768, p. 292.

Herrick, J.B.: Clinical features of sudden obstruction of the coronary arteries. JAMA 59:2015, 1912.

Hung, J., Goris, M.L., Nash, E., et al.: Comparative value of maximal treadmill testing, exercise thallium myocardial perfusion scintigraphy and exercise radionuclide ventriculography for distinguishing high- and low-risk patients soon after acute myocardial infarction. Am. J. Cardiol. 53:1221, 1984.

ISIS-1 Collaborative Group: A randomized trial of intravenous atenolol among 16,027 cases of suspected acute myocardial infarction. Lancet 2:57, 1986.

ISIS-2 (Second International Study of Infarct Survival) Collaborative Study Group: Randomized trial of intravenous steptokinase, oral aspirin, both or neither among 17,187 cases of suspected acute myocardial infarction. Lancet 2:349, 1988.

Judkins, M.P.: Percutaneous transfemoral selective coronary arteriography. Radiol. Clin. North Am. 6:467, 1968.

Jugdutt, B.I.: Myocardial salvage by intravenous nitroglycerin in conscious dogs: Loss of beneficial effect with marked nitroglycerin-induced hypotension. Circulation 68:673, 1983.

Jugdutt, B.I.: Delayed effects of early infarct-limiting therapies on healing after myocardial infarction. Circulation 72:907, 1985.

Kennedy, J.W., Ritchie, J.L., Davis, K.B., et al.: Western Washington randomized trial of intracoronary streptokinase in acute myocardial infarction. N. Engl. J. Med. 301:1477, 1983.

Kennedy, J.W., Ritchie, J.L., Davis, K.B., et al.: Western Washington randomized trial of intracoronary streptokinase in acute myocardial infarction: A 12-month follow-up. N. Engl. J. Med. 312:1073, 1985.

Kiat, H., and Berman, D.S.: Clinical radionuclide imaging of myocardial perfusion. Current Opinion in Radiology 1:418, 1989.

Kiat, H., and Berman, D.S.: Clinical radionuclide imaging of myocardial viability. Current Opinion in Radiology 1:435, 1989.

Kimura, T., Nosaka, H., Ueno, K., and Nobuyoshi, M.: Role of coronary angioplasty in acute myocardial infarction. Circulation 74(Suppl. II):II-22, 1986.

Kisslo, J.A., Abrams, D.B., and Leech, G.J.: Essentials of Echocardiography: Heart Muscle Disease. New York, Medi Cine Prod, 1988, p. 1.

Koshal, A., Beanlands, D.S., Davies, R.A., et al.: Urgent surgical reperfusion in acute evolving myocardial infarction: A randomized controlled study. Circulation 78(Suppl. I):I-171, 1988.

Lebowitz, E., Greene, M.W., Fairchild, R., et al.: Thallium-201 for medical use. J. Nucl. Med. 16:1512, 1975.

Leiboff, R.H., Katz, R.J., Wasserman, A.G., et al.: A randomized angiography-controlled trial of intracoronary streptokinase in acute myocardial infarction. Am. J. Cardiol. 53:404, 1984.

Levine, S.: Coronary thrombosis: Its various clinical features. Medicine 8:245, 1929.

Mallory, G.K., White, P.D., and Salcedo-Salgar, J.: Speed of healing of myocardial infarction: Study of pathologic anatomy in 72 cases. Am. Heart J. 18:647, 1939.

Marco, J., Caster, L., Szatmary, L.J., et al.: Emergency percutaneous transluminal coronary angioplasty without thrombolysis as initial therapy in acute myocardial infarction. Int. J. Cardiol. 15:55, 1987.

Massel, D., Gill, J.B., and Cairus, J.A.: Management of the patient following coronary thrombolysis. Clin. Cardiol. 13:591, 1990.

McClean, J.: The discovery of heparin. Circulation 19:75, 1959.

Mock, M.B., Ringquist, I., Fisher, L.D., et al.: Survival of medically treated patients in the Coronary Artery Surgery Study (CASS) registry. Circulation 66:562, 1982.

Morris, K.G., Palmeri, S.T., Califf, R.M., et al.: Value of radionuclide angiography for predicting specific cardiac events after acute myocardial infarction. Am. J. Cardiol. 55:318, 1985.

Muller, D.W.M., and Topol, E.J.: Unresolved issues: Late reperfusion, lytic failure, and reocclusion. Coronary Artery Disease 1:39, 1990.

The Multicenter Postinfarction Research Group: Risk stratification

and survival after myocardial infarction. N. Engl. J. Med. 309:331, 1983.

Newman, G.E.: Pulmonary embolism: A historical perspective. J. Thorac. Imaging 4:1, 1989.

Neilson, A., Morris, K.G., Murdock, R.H., et al.: Linear relationship between distribution of Tl-201 and blood flow in ischemic and non-ischemic myocardium during exercise. Circulation 59-60:11, 1979.

Ohman, E.M., and Califf, R.M.: Thrombolytic therapy: Overview of clinical trials. Coronary Artery Disease 1:23, 1990.

O'Neill, W., Timmis, G.C., Bourdillon, P., et al.: A prospective randomized clinical trial of intracoronary streptokinase versus coronary angioplasty therapy of acute myocardial infarction. N. Engl. J. Med. 314:813, 1986.

Page, D.L., Caulfield, J.B., Kastor, J.A., et al.: Myocardial changes associated with cardiogenic shock. N. Engl. J. Med. 285:133, 1971.

Passamani, E., Hodges, M., Herman, M., et al.: The thrombolysis in myocardial infarction (TIMI) Phase II Pilot Study: Tissue plasminogen activator followed by percutaneous transluminal coronary angioplasty. J. Am. Coll. Cardiol. 10:5113, 1987.

Phillips, S.J., Kongtahworn, C., and Zeff, R.H.: Emergency coronary artery revascularization: A possible therapy for acute myocardial infarction. Circulation 60:241, 1979.

Ploug, J., and Kjeldgaard, N.O.: Urokinase: An activator of plasminogen from human urine. I. Isolation and properties. Biochim. Biophys. Acta 24:278, 1957.

Randford, M.J., Johnson, R.A., Daggett, W.M., et al.: Ventricular septal rupture: A review of clinical and physiologic features and an analysis of survival. Circulation 64:545, 1981.

Reimer, K.A., Lower, J.E., Rasmussen, M.M., et al.: The wavefront phenomenon of ischemic cell death. Circulation 56:786, 1977.

Rentrop, K.P., Blanke, H., Karsche, K.R., et al.: Initial experience with transluminal recanalization of the recently occluded infarct-related coronary artery in acute myocardial infarction. Clin. Cardiol. 2:92, 1979.

Reske, S.N.: Cardiac radionuclide imaging. Current Opinion in Radiology 1:147, 1989.

Richards, D.W., Jr.: Cardiac output by catheterization technique in various clinical conditions. Fed. Proc. 4:215, 1945.

Rickets, H.J., and Abrams, H.L.: Percutaneous selective coronary cine arteriography. JAMA 181:620, 1962.

Rossi, P.R.F., Yusuf, S., Ramsdale, O., et al.: Reduction of ventricular arrhythmias by early intravenous atenolol in suspected acute myocardial infarction. Br. Med. J. 286:506, 1983.

Rothbaum, D.A., Linnemeier, T.J., Landin, R.J., et al.: Emergency percutaneous transluminal coronary angioplasty in acute myocardial infarction: A 3-year experience. J. Am. Coll. Cardiol. 10:264, 1987.

Sanz, G., Costaner, A., Betrin, A., et al.: Determinants of prognosis in survivors of myocardial infarction. N. Engl. J. Med. 306:1065, 1982.

Schelbert, H.R.: Positron emission tomography: Diagnostic and therapeutic implications in human myocardial ischemia. Int. J. Card. Imaging 2:199, 1987.

Silverman, K.J., Becker, L.C., Bulkley, B.H., et al.: Value of early thallium-201 scintigraphy for predicting mortality in patients with acute myocardial infarction. Circulation 61:996, 1980.

Smitherman, T.C., Osborn, R.C., and Norahora, K.A.: Serial myocardial scintigraphy after a single dose of thallium-201 in men after acute myocardial infarction. Am. J. Cardiol. 42:177, 1978.

Sones, F.M., Jr.: Cine coronary arteriography. In Hurst, J.W., and Logue, R.B. (eds.): Heart, ed. 2. New York, McGraw-Hill, 1970, p. 377.

Steckelberg, J.M., Vliestra, R.E., Ludwig, J., et al.: Werner Forssmann (1904–1979) and his unusual success story. Mayo Clin. Proc. 54:746, 1979.

Storch-Becker, A., Kaiser, K.P., and Feinendegen, L.E.: Cardiac nuclear medicine: Positron emission tomography in clinical medicine. Eur. J. Nucl. Med. 13:648, 1988.

Swenson, S.J., Ehman, R.L., and Brown, L.R.: Magnetic resonance imaging of the thorax. J. Thorac. Imaging 4:19, 1989.

Tele, N.A., and Edmonds, L.H.: Operation for acute post-infarction mitral insufficiency and shock. J. Thorac. Cardiovasc. Surg. 89:525, 1980.

Tillet, W.S., and Garner, R.L.: The fibrinolytic activity of streptococci. J. Exp. Med. 58:485, 1933.

The TIMI Study Group: The Thrombolysis in Myocardial Infarction (TIMI) Trial: Phase I findings. N. Engl. J. Med. 312:932, 1985.

The TIMI Research Group: Immediate vs. delayed catheterization and angioplasty following thrombolytic therapy for acute myocardial infarction: TIMI-IIA results. JAMA 260:2849, 1988.

The TIMI Study Group: Comparison of invasive and conservative strategies after treatment with intravenous t-PA in acute myocardial infarction: Results of the TIMI Phase II Trial. N. Engl. J. Med. 320:618, 1989.

Topol, E.J.: Direct or sequential PTCA. *In* Topol, E.J. (ed.): Acute Coronary Intervention. New York, Alan R. Liss, 1988, p. 79.

Topol, E.J., Califf, E.M., George, B.S., et al.: A randomized trial of immediate versus delayed elective angioplasty after intravenous tissue plasminogen activator in acute myocardial infarction. N. Engl. J. Med. 317:581, 1987.

Topol, E.J., Califf, R.M., George, B.S., et al.: Coronary arterial thrombolysis with combined infusion of recombinant tissue-type plasminogen activator and urokinase in patients with acute myocardial infarction. Circulation 77:1100, 1988.

Van de Werf, F., Arnold, A.E.R., and the European Cooperative Study Group for Recombinant Tissue-Type Plasminogen Activator (rt-Pa): Intravenous rt-Pa and size of infarct, left-ventricular function and survival in acute myocardial infarction. Br. Med. J. 297:2374, 1988.

Verstraete, M., Bernard, R., Bory, M., et al.: Randomized trial of intravenous recombinant tissue-type plasminogen activator versus intravenous streptokinase in acute myocardial infarction: Report from the European Cooperative Study Group for Recombinant Tissue-Type Plasminogen Activator. Lancet 1:842, 1985.

Wackers, F.J., Sokole, E.B., Samson, G., et al.: Value and limitations of thallium-201 scintigraphy in the acute phase of myocardial infarction. N. Engl. J. Med. 295:1, 1976.

Wasserman, A.G., and Ross, A.M.: Coronary thrombolysis. Curr. Probl. Cardiol. 14:5, 1989.

Weinstein, J.: Treatment of myocardial infarction with intracoronary streptokinase: Efficacy and safety data from 209 United States cases in the Hoecst-Roussel Registry. Am. Heart J. 104:894, 1982.

Wilcox, R.G., Olsson, C.G., Skewe, A.M., et al.: The ASSET Study Group. Trial of tissue plasminogen activator for mortality reduction in acute myocardial infarction: Anglo-Scandinavian Study of Early Thrombolysis (ASSET). Lancet 1:525, 1988.

Willerson, J.T., Parkey, R.W., Bonte, F.J., et al.: Acute subendocardial myocardial infarction in patients: Its detection by technetium-99m stannous pyrophosphate myocardial scintigrams. Circulation 51:436, 1975.

Yusuf, S., and Collins, R.: Intravenous nitroglycerin and nitroprusside therapy in acute myocardial infarction reduces mortality: Evidence from randomized controlled trials. Circulation 72(Suppl. III):III-224, 1985.

Yusuf, S., Peto, R., Lewis, J., et al.: Beta-blockade during and after myocardial infarction: An overview of the randomized trials. Prog. Cardiovasc. Dis. 37:335, 1985.

Yusuf, S., Sleight, P., Rossi, P., et al.: Reduction in infarct size, arrhythmias and chest pain and morbidity by early intravenous beta blockade in suspected acute myocardial infarction. Circulation 67:I32, 1983.

14

Pericardial Disease

■

Barbara L. McComb
Robert M. Steiner

The increasing importance of manifestations of pericardial disease in the critically ill patient parallels the frequency of cardiac and noncardiac thoracic surgery, thoracic irradiation, and the use of an array of therapeutic agents that can affect the pericardium. In addition, the frequent diagnosis of acute and chronic pericarditis reflects increasingly sophisticated diagnostic imaging techniques, including echocardiography (ECHO), computed tomography (CT), and magnetic resonance imaging (MRI) as well as plain film radiography. In this chapter, the role of diagnostic imaging in diseases of the pericardium, including pathologic conditions found in the medical and surgical critical care patient, is discussed.

ANATOMY AND PHYSIOLOGY

The pericardium is a double-layered fibroserosal envelope that surrounds the heart, great vessels, and veins (Moncada et al., 1982). It aids in maintaining ventricular compliance when ventricular end-diastolic pressures are elevated and prevents sudden dilation of the cardiac chambers due to hypervolemia (Mangano et al., 1985). The pericardium assists atrial filling during ventricular systole as negative intrapericardial pressure develops during ventricular ejection. Aided by 20 to 25 ml of lymphoid fluid within the pericardial space, it reduces friction between the heart and contiguous structures (Holt, 1970; Mangano et al., 1985; McKiernan, 1988; Shabetai et al., 1979; Spodick, 1983). By virtue of its immunologic components, it retards the spread of inflammation from the lung and pleural space (Shabetai et al., 1979).

The pericardium consists of an outer fibrous layer formed by a dense collagen network and an inner serous layer. The serous layer is composed of visceral and parietal portions. The visceral portion, or epicardium, covers the heart and the proximal half of the

ascending aorta and extends to the bifurcation of the main pulmonary artery. The visceral pericardium is reflected on itself at the level of the sternal notch to form the serous layer of the parietal pericardium (Warwick and Williams, 1973). The fibrous layer extends superiorly over the aorta and the superior vena cava and blends with the vascular adventitia (Warwick and Williams, 1973).

The fibrous portion of the parietal pericardium adheres to the diaphragm at the central tendon and is attached anteriorly to the chest wall by the sternopericardial ligaments. Laterally, it is separated from the lungs by the mediastinal pleura. Posteriorly, the pericardium is contiguous with the main bronchi, the esophagus, the descending aorta, and the posterior mediastinal surface of each lung. The inferior vena cava enters the pericardium through the central tendon of the diaphragm and is not covered by the fibrous pericardial layer (Warwick and Williams, 1973) (Fig. 14–1).

The visceral pericardial layer adheres to the heart and great vessels, forming a complex network of communicating sinuses and recesses (Aronberg et al., 1984; Chiles et al., 1986; Choe et al., 1967; Im et al., 1988; Levy-Ravetch et al., 1985; Shin et al., 1986; Vesely and Cahill, 1986). Familiarity with this anatomy is essential when interpreting CT (Aronberg et al., 1984; Levy-Ravetch et al., 1985) and MRI (Im et al., 1988) images because fluid within recesses may simulate thymic masses (Levy-Ravetch et al., 1985; Shin et al., 1986), aortic dissection (Chiles et al., 1986), or lymphadenopathy (Shin et al., 1986). In addition, cysts or tumors may develop within pericardial sinuses or recesses (Moncada et al., 1982; Shin et al., 1986).

The sinuses and recesses of the pericardium have been inconsistently named in the literature leading Vesely and Cahill (1986) to propose a standard nomenclature. That portion of the pericardial cavity

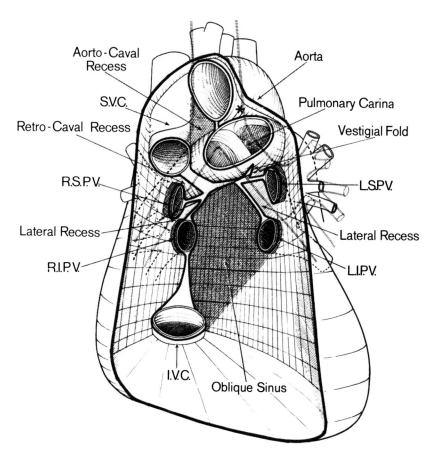

Figure 14–1. Diagrammatic representation of the normal pericardial reflections. In this anteroposterior projection, an anterior window is created in the fibrous pericardium. The *solid dark line* outlines the pericardium. LSPV, Left superior pulmonary vein, LIPV, left inferior pulmonary vein, IVC, inferior vena cava, RIPV, right inferior pulmonary vein, RSPV, right superior pulmonary vein, SVC, superior vena cava. Aortocaval recess and * represent the superior aortic recess, the lateral recess represents the pulmonary venous recess, and the retrocaval recess represents the postcaval recess. (Modified from McAlpine, W.: Heart and Coronary Arteries: An Anatomical Atlas for Clinical Diagnosis, Radiological Investigation, and Surgical Treatment. Heidelberg, Springer-Verlag, 1975, p. 132, with permission.)

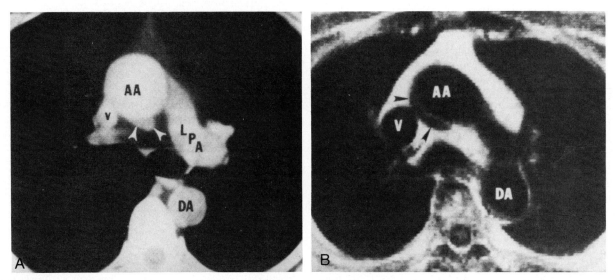

Figure 14–2. Pericardial sinuses and recesses. *A,* Computed tomography (CT) demonstrates the transverse sinus (superior aortic recess) as immediately posterior to the ascending aorta *(white arrowhead). B,* Because of fluid in motion in both the pericardial sinus and the aorta, signal void is present on the T_1-weighted magnetic resonance image (MRI) in both structures, simulating an aortic dissection *(black arrowhead).* LPA, Left pulmonary artery, AA, ascending aorta, V, superior vena cava, DA, descending aorta. (From Glazer, H.S., et al.: Pitfalls in CT recognition of mediastinal lymphadenopathy. AJR 144(2):267–274, 1985, with permission, © by American Roentgen Ray Society.)

that envelopes the major blood vessels is organized in the form of two tubes. The aorta and main pulmonary artery are enclosed within an anterosuperior pericardial tube, and the venae cavae and pulmonary veins are enclosed within an inferoposterior tube. The communicating passageway between the anterior and posterior tubes is the transverse sinus (Vesely and Cahill, 1986; Warwick and Williams, 1973).

The transverse sinus contains several recesses that extend as diverticula between the great vessels and the atria (Im et al., 1988; Vesely and Cahill, 1986). These recesses include the left pulmonic and right pulmonic recesses below the pulmonary arteries and the superior and inferior aortic recesses (Aronberg et al., 1984; Levy-Ravetch et al., 1985; Vesely and Cahill, 1986) (Fig. 14–2). The oblique sinus is posterior to the left atrium and medial to the inferior vena cava. It is separated from the transverse sinus by a double layer of serous pericardium, which connects the left and right superior pulmonary veins. Recesses of the pericardial cavity include the postcaval recess and the pulmonary venous recesses, which lie between the superior and inferior pulmonary veins (Vesely and Cahill, 1986).

DIAGNOSTIC IMAGING IN THE NORMAL PATIENT

Plain Film Radiography

On the frontal radiographic projection, the normal pericardium is rarely identifiable as a distinct structure, because it is in close proximity to the heart, and its attenuation values are similar to those of the heart. Occasionally, a normal pericardial line is visualized along the left ventricular border (Carsky et al., 1980; Kremens, 1955) (Fig. 14–3). The normal pericardium is more frequently identified on the lateral radiograph because of the contrast provided by the adjacent epicardial and anterior mediastinal fat planes. It appears as a curvilinear opacity that is 1 to 2 mm in thickness and is immediately posterior to the lower sternal segments; it may wrap around the cardiac apex and continue for several centimeters parallel to the inferior heart border (Carsky et al., 1980; Kremens, 1955; Lane and Carsky, 1968; Moncada et al., 1986) (Fig. 14–4).

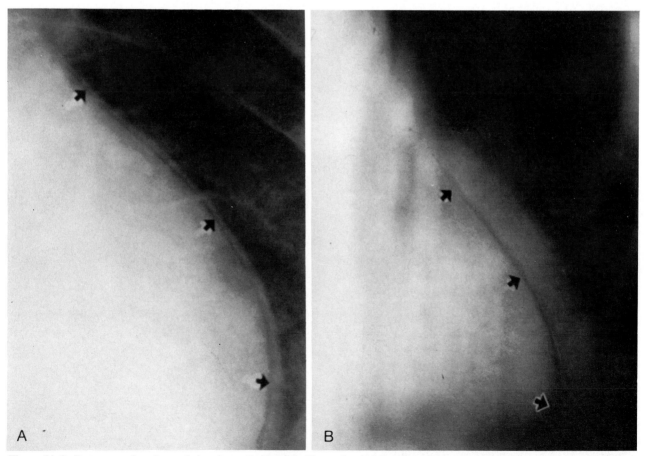

Figure 14–3. Posteroanterior views of the chest. *A,* Normal. The pericardial line is outlined by epicardial fat and lung *(arrows). B,* Pericardial effusion. The lucent fat stripe is separated from the left heart border as a result of pericardial effusion *(arrows).* (From Kremens, V.: Demonstration of the pericardial shadow on the routine chest roentgenogram. Radiology 64:72–80, 1955, with permission.)

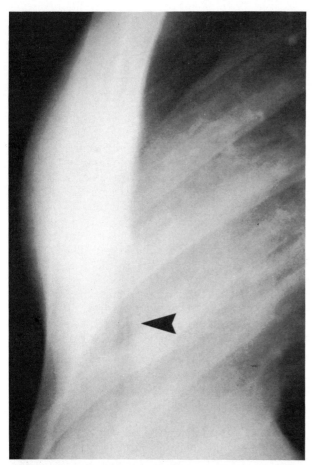

Figure 14–4. Lateral view of the chest shows a thin radiopaque line representing the normal pericardium in the retrosternal region *(arrowhead)*.

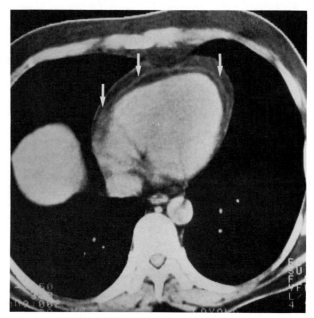

Figure 14–5. Computed tomography demonstrates the normal pericardium, which is anterior to the ventricles and lies along the left cardiac border *(arrows)*. (From Moncada, R., et al.: Multimodality approach to pericardial imaging. Cardiovasc. Clin. 17:409, 1986, with permission.)

Computed Tomography

The normal pericardium is commonly identified on CT images because of its superior contrast resolution and cross-sectional imaging format (Moncada et al., 1986; Silverman and Harell, 1983) (Fig. 14–5). As on chest radiographs, the anterior, preventicular pericardium is the most readily visualized region of the pericardium because of abundant retrosternal anterior mediastinal and epicardial fat (Paling and Williamson, 1987). The upper extent of the pericardium at the level of the great vessels is not usually visualized because of the relative lack of fat and the effect of pulsations of adjacent vessels. Inferior sternal and diaphragmatic pericardial insertions are occasionally identified and may be as thick as 3 to 4 mm (Silverman and Harell, 1983). The pericardial recesses may normally contain a small amount of fluid. The presence of this fluid permits visualization of the superior and inferior aortic recesses of the transverse sinus by cross-sectional imaging (Glazer et al., 1985) (see Fig. 14–2).

Small focal areas of pericardial thickening are normally visualized on CT scans in as many as 30% of cases. The most common site is anterior to the right

ventricle and is thought to be related to transmitted ventricular pulsations, technical artifact, or the angle of the pericardium in relation to the axial plane (Moncada et al., 1982, 1986) (Fig. 14–6).

Echocardiography

The diagnosis of pericardial disease, and particularly pericardial effusion is one of the most important

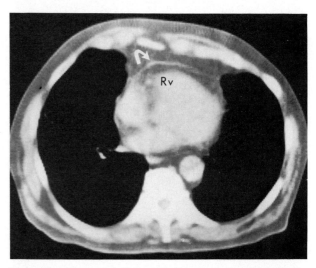

Figure 14–6. Computed tomography demonstrates mild thickening of the pericardium that is anterior to the right ventricle (RV) and is thought to be a normal finding *(curved arrow)*. (From Moncada, R., et al.: Multimodality approach to pericardial imaging. Cardiovasc. Clin. 17:409, 1986, with permission.)

contributions of echocardiography (ECHO) to clinical cardiology (Horowitz et al., 1974; Moncada et al., 1986). This noninvasive technique is exquisitely sensitive and can even detect normal amounts of pericardial fluid as a thin anechoic zone adjacent to the myocardium. Echocardiography is suitable for use in the intensive care unit because of its portability. The disadvantages of ECHO are its insensitivity to the presence of calcification, its difficulty in distinguishing myocardial from pericardial thickening (Silverman and Harell, 1983), and its technical limitations related to individual patient body habitus (Isner et al., 1983a; Rifkin et al., 1984; Yousem et al., 1987).

Magnetic Resonance Imaging

Magnetic resonance imaging clearly defines the pericardium as a structure of low signal intensity that surrounds the myocardium on T_1-weighted images and is separated from the higher-intensity epicardial and mediastinal fat (Im et al., 1988; Sechtem et al., 1986a; Tscholakoff et al., 1987; Westcott and Steiner, 1986) (Fig. 14–7). The pericardium is uniformly visible over the anterior border of the heart in front of the right ventricle and is visualized less often at the left ventricular apex, lateral left ventricular wall, and behind the heart, where it is contiguous with the low–signal-intensity lung parenchyma (Sechtem et al., 1986a). Magnetic resonance imaging may differentiate hemopericardium from other sources of abnormal pericardial fluid, may potentially distinguish inflammatory from noninflammatory effusions, and is valuable in differentiating restrictive cardiomyopathy from constrictive pericarditis (Kiat et al., 1989; Sech-

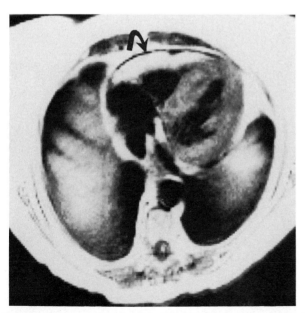

Figure 14–7. T_1-weighted MRI (TR600 TE30) of the normal pericardium which appears as a low–signal intensity line surrounded by high–signal-intensity epicardial and anterior mediastinal fat *(curved arrow)*.

tem et al., 1986b; Stark et al., 1984; Tscholakoff et al., 1987). Magnetic resonance imaging, however, is of less value than other imaging techniques in the critically ill patient, because of its limited availability, its lack of portability, and its incompatibility with pacemakers and other electronic equipment.

SPECIFIC PERICARDIAL DISORDERS

Pericardial Effusion

Pericardial fluid is regulated by the relative differences in hydrostatic and osmotic pressure between the pericardial capillaries and cavity fluid, by the permeability of the serous pericardium, and by lymphatic and venous clearance. Resorption of pericardial fluid is believed to be compromised by occlusion of epicardial lymphatic and venous drainage pathways, owing to inflammation or neoplasm (Miller et al., 1971).

Pericardial effusion is usually the result of acute or chronic pericarditis. The origin of acute pericarditis is often obscure but is presumably viral. Pericarditis may also result from bacterial or fungal infection as well as from a variety of noninfectious causes, including myocardial infarction, blunt thoracic trauma, surgical procedures, and aortic dissection. Chronic effusion may be caused by a variety of conditions, including infection, postpericardiotomy syndrome, collagen vascular disease, uremia, cardiogenic pulmonary edema, and malignancy.

When pericardial effusion is present, the radiographic appearance of the cardiac silhouette is that of a triangular, globular, or flask-shaped configuration in which the normal indentations of the cardiac borders are effaced (Ellis and King, 1973) (Fig. 14–8). Encroachment on the retrosternal space on the lateral projection and hilum overlay on the frontal projection are common features of pericardial effusion. These findings are to be differentiated from those of cardiomyopathy causing dilation, in which the hilar shadows are displaced laterally and the hilar vessels are not obscured (Baron, 1971). A widened pericardial stripe greater than 2 mm or a "positive epicardial fat pad sign" may be present when sufficient pericardial effusion or thickening causes visible separation of the epicardial and anterior mediastinal fat planes (Fig. 14–9). This sign is considered to be the most reliable plain film finding in pericardial effusion or thickening and has been reported in as many as 52% of cases (Carsky et al., 1980). Occasionally, a retrosternal extrapericardial hematoma or other fluid collection mimics a widened pericardial line and leads to a false diagnosis of pericardial effusion (Demos et al., 1983). The "differential density sign," an increase in lucency of the margin of the cardiac silhouette, is thought to be produced by the difference in tissue attenuation coefficients of the heart and of the pericardial fluid (Tehranzadeh and Kelley, 1979). Infrequently, asymmetric collections of fluid produce unusual cardiac

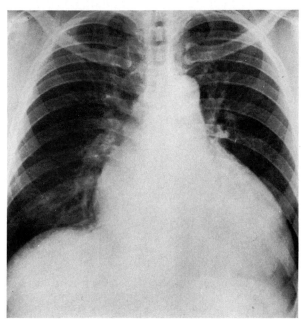

Figure 14–8. Posteroanterior chest radiograph demonstrates a globular configuration of the cardiac silhouette due to pericardial effusion.

Figure 14–9. Lateral chest radiograph shows separation of epicardial and anterior mediastinal fat planes *(arrows)* by a radiopaque band produced by pericardial effusion.

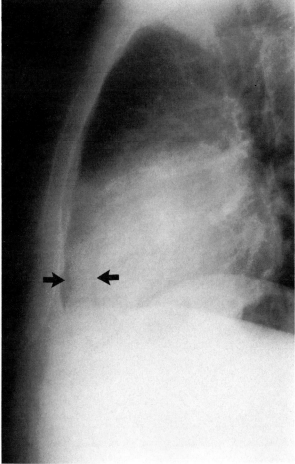

configurations, owing to loculation and uneven distensibility of the pericardial sac (Ellis and King, 1973).

Fluoroscopic evaluation of suspected pericardial effusion is of limited value and has been largely supplanted by other imaging techniques. Although chest fluoroscopy demonstrates a large, poorly contractile cardiac silhouette in patients with pericardial effusion, this finding is nonspecific and is more commonly due to restrictive myocardial disease. Fluoroscopy cannot characterize an effusion as bloody, chylous, or exudative, nor can it determine its size and extent. One valuable fluoroscopic clue to the diagnosis of effusion is vigorous "to and fro" motion of the epicardial fat or of calcified coronary arteries within a larger, immobile cardiac silhouette (Jorgens et al., 1962).

Echocardiography is the preferred initial examination for the diagnosis of pericardial effusion (Horowitz et al., 1974; Moncada et al., 1986; Plehn, 1989). A small effusion appears as an echo-free space between the left lung and posterior free wall of the left ventricle (Fig. 14–10A). Larger pericardial effusions are also found between the anterior wall of the right ventricle and the chest wall (see Fig. 14–10B). Occasionally, a false-positive diagnosis of pericardial effusion is due to large amounts of hypoechoic anterior mediastinal or epicardial fat, which may simulate a loculated anterior effusion (Demos et al., 1983; Rifkin et al., 1984). Pleural effusion (Moncada et al., 1986), atelectasis, and pneumonia (Erasmie and Lundell, 1987; Plehn et al., 1988) may also be mistaken for a posterior pericardial fluid collection (Yousem et al., 1987). On the other hand, a loculated or complex pericardial effusion may not be detected if it is located in an area inaccessible to the ultrasound beam. A complex effusion containing fibrotic strands, tumor, or thrombus may simulate an extrapericardial fluid collection.

Computed tomography is helpful in resolving many of the pitfalls of ECHO because of its superior contrast resolution. It can distinguish anterior mediastinal fat from pericardial collections when such distinction is not achieved by ECHO (Isner et al., 1983b; Rifkin et al., 1984; Yousem et al., 1987). Pleural effusions can be clearly differentiated from pericardial effusion (Wong et al., 1982), and pericardial calcifications are clearly identifiable. Perhaps CT is most valuable in locating small, loculated, or complex fluid collections containing septa, tumor, or thrombus (Moncada et al., 1986).

Computed tomography usually demonstrates small pericardial effusions in the dependent position, posteriorly to the left atrium and ventricle. Less often, pericardial fluid is identified in a high posterior location near the pulmonary veins. Larger anterior effusions may encircle the heart and protrude inferiorly toward the abdomen with increasing size (Gale et al., 1987; Isner et al., 1983b; Wong et al., 1982) (Fig. 14–11). Computed tomography may also suggest the nature of an effusion, because transudates and chylous effusions often have lower attenuation values than do exudates or bloody effusions (Moncada et al., 1982).

Pericardial effusion appears on T_1-weighted MRI as a low–signal-intensity zone around the cardiac chambers. Pericardial fluid appears as a bright signal-intensity zone on T_2-weighted spin-echo and gradient-refocused echo-pulse sequences. Complex or loculated pericardial effusions are well visualized because of the multiplanar capability of MRI. Inflamed pericardium can be distinguished by an abnormally high signal due to the high water content of the edematous tissue (Stark et al., 1984). At present, MRI is used

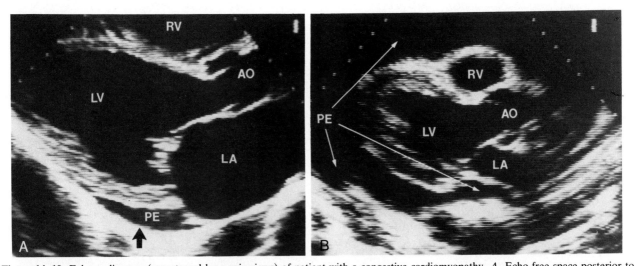

Figure 14–10. Echocardiogram (parasternal long-axis views) of patient with a congestive cardiomyopathy. *A,* Echo-free space posterior to left ventricular wall is produced by small pericardial effusion *(arrow). B,* Echo-free fluid of a large pericardial effusion surrounds the heart *(arrows).* LV, Left ventricle, RV, right ventricle, AO, aorta, LA, left atrium, PE, pericardial effusion. (From Moncada, R., et al.: Multimodality approach to pericardial imaging. Cardiovasc. Clin. 17:409, 1986, with permission.)

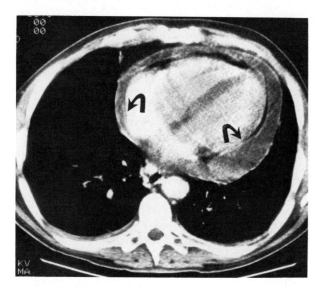

Figure 14–11. Contrast–enhanced CT demonstrates a large low-density effusion surrounding the heart *(curved arrows)*.

only occasionally in the diagnosis of pericardial effusion in the critically ill patient because of its lack of portability (Fig. 14–12).

Cardiac Tamponade

Cardiac tamponade is a serious disorder in the critically ill patient and may be rapidly fatal. It is defined as hemodynamically significant cardiac compression causing equalization of intrapericardial and ventricular diastolic pressures, which results in impaired diastolic ventricular filling and increased atrial pressure (Callaham, 1987; McKiernan, 1988; Spodick, 1983). Stroke volume, cardiac output, and systemic blood pressure are reduced, and pulmonary venous pressure increases. Pulsus paradoxus, defined as exaggeration of the normal inspiratory decrease in

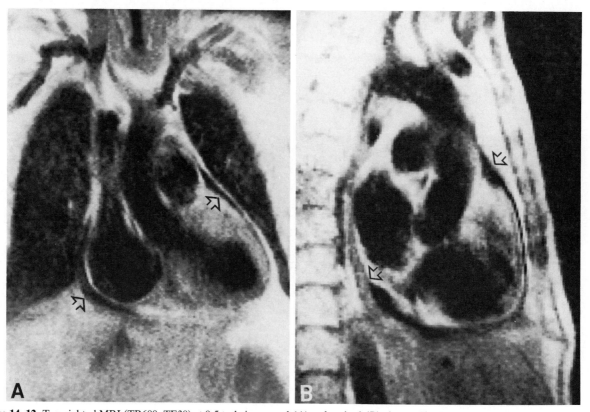

Figure 14–12. T$_1$-weighted MRI (TR600, TE30) at 0.5 tesla in coronal *(A)* and sagittal *(B)* planes. The low–signal-intensity region represents pericardial effusion *(open arrows)*.

systemic blood pressure, occurs with a large reduction in ventricular volume. The rapidity of fluid accumulation in the pericardial space is of major importance in determining whether cardiac tamponade will develop. When fluid accumulation is gradual, the pericardium expands to accommodate the increased volume with either no development or delayed development of tamponade (Baron, 1971).

Although cardiac tamponade is a clinical diagnosis, helpful ECHO features include right ventricular diastolic indentation and compression and fixed enlargement of the inferior vena cava (Gordon and Butler, 1989; Moncada et al., 1986). Right atrial compression may be a more sensitive indicator of cardiac tamponade than is ventricular compression, probably because the right atrium is more compliant and therefore more reflective of changes in pericardial pressure (Gordon and Butler, 1989). Similar features are demonstrated by CT and MRI.

Constrictive Pericarditis

Any disorder that produces pericardial inflammation can result in constriction. Constriction is usually initiated by an episode of acute pericarditis associated with effusion. Resorption of the fluid is followed by fusion of the visceral and parietal layers. The underlying cause of pericardial constriction may not be evident histologically, particularly after fibrous tissue and calcification replace the original inflammatory process. Although the inflammation is usually diffuse, focal pericardial fibrosis may occasionally obstruct the atrioventricular valve, the venae cavae, or the right ventricular outflow tract. The liver is usually enlarged, and ascites is common.

In the past, tuberculosis was thought to be the most common cause of constriction. Today, viral pericarditis, chronic renal disease, neoplasm, and irradiation are more frequently implicated. Less commonly, bacterial and fungal infection, connective tissue disorders, blunt or penetrating trauma, and drug effect may also cause constriction. Pericardial constriction affects cardiac function by limiting ventricular expansion during diastole, which results in equalization of diastolic pressures in all cardiac chambers, a typical feature of this condition.

Radiographically, the cardiac silhouette is usually normal, or slightly enlarged when a coexistent pericardial effusion is present. Pericardial calcification may be thin or thick, and patchy or continuous, and may be several millimeters or centimeters in length. The calcific deposits are most often found in the coronary sulcus between the left atrium and ventricle and along the diaphragmatic surface of the right ventricle (Agatston et al., 1984; Doppman et al., 1981; Rees et al., 1986) (Fig. 14–13). Pericardial calcification is present in 30% to 50% of patients with constriction and is best visualized on lateral (see Fig. 14–13B) and oblique radiographs. On the posteroanterior projection, calcification is often obscured because of underexposure of the mediastinum or imaging of the calcifications en face. Overpenetrated films may be helpful when calcification is suspected, but it is not clearly visualized on initial radiographs. CT may demonstrate calcium not seen on plain films (see Fig. 14–13C). When associated with the clinical features of constriction, the presence of calcification is diagnostic (Fig. 14–14). Absence of calcification does not exclude the diagnosis of constriction, however, and its presence alone does not establish it.

If restriction of diastolic filling is predominantly right-sided, dilatation of the azygous vein and vena cava may be observed. The right atrial border may be flattened if encased, or remain convex if atrial compliance remains normal. When constriction predominantly affects the left heart, left atrial enlargement and pulmonary venous hypertension may be present, resembling mitral stenosis.

Echocardiography is of limited value in the diagnosis of pericardial constriction, because pericardial thickening may be difficult to distinguish from adjacent myocardium (Agatston et al., 1984; Moncada et al., 1986). It is valuable, however, in detecting associated pericardial effusion and in assessing ventricular size and function. Echocardiography also differentiates mitral stenosis from constriction when the plain film findings are consistent with either diagnosis. Typical echocardiographic features of pericardial constriction include paradoxical septal motion, reduced diastolic posterior ventricular wall motion, and pericardial thickening. A lack of respiratory variation in the diameter of a dilated inferior vena cava when ventricular function is normal also suggests the diagnosis of pericardial constriction.

Computed tomography provides superior definition of the extent and location of pericardial thickening (Fig. 14–15) and calcification (see Fig. 14–14). It can distinguish diffuse from focal disease observed in a number of diverse conditions, including sarcoidosis, rheumatic heart disease, radiation fibrosis, and neoplasm. The most consistent CT finding of pericardial constriction is pericardial thickening. External deformity of the right heart border with reflux of contrast media into the coronary sinus (Doppman et al., 1981) (Fig. 14–16), systemic venous distention, ascites (see Fig. 14–13D), and pleural effusions are additional CT findings (Moncada et al., 1982). A normal pericardium demonstrated by CT in a patient exhibiting the signs and symptoms of constrictive pericarditis almost always indicates the diagnosis of restrictive cardiomyopathy (Isner et al., 1983b). When the myocardium and pericardium are both involved, as in radiation effect or following methysergide therapy, percutaneous endomyocardial biopsy is often indicated (Harbin et al., 1984; Moncada et al., 1986).

THE MEDICALLY ILL PATIENT

Acute nonspecific pericarditis is a common clinical entity and is often assumed to be viral in origin. In

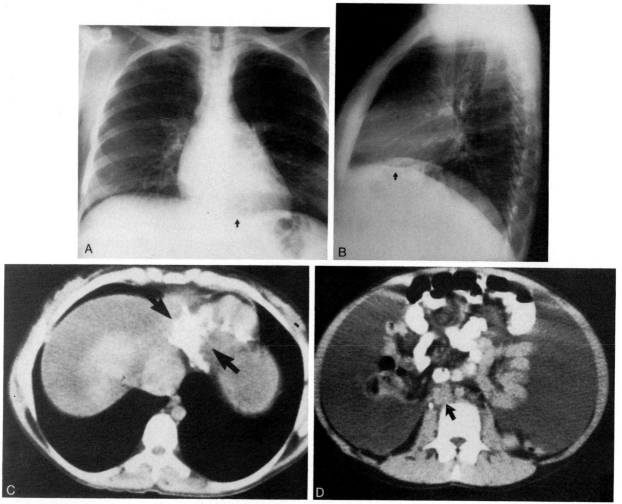

Figure 14–13. Calcific pericarditis with constriction. *A,* Posteroanterior radiograph shows a thin calcified line *(arrow)* at the diaphragmatic surface of the heart. *B,* Lateral radiograph. The pericardium is more clearly visualized *(arrow).* *C,* Computed tomography demonstrates the extent of the calcification *(arrows)* at the inferior cardiac margin. *D,* Abdominal CT. Ascites causes medial displacement of bowel segments, and a dilated inferior vena cava *(arrow)* due to pericardial constriction is present.

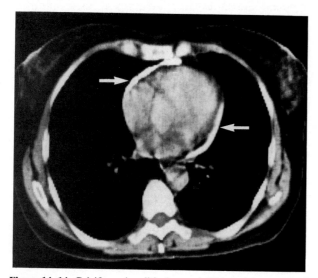

Figure 14–14. Calcific pericarditis *(arrows).* This patient presented with signs and symptoms of constriction. (From Moncada, R., et al.: Multimodality approach to pericardial imaging. Cardiovasc. Clin. 17:409, 1986, with permission.)

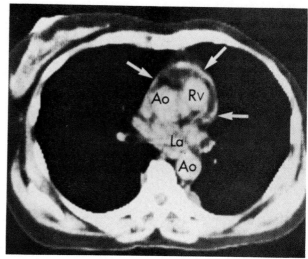

Figure 14–15. Computed tomography demonstrates focal areas of pericardial thickening *(arrows)* in a patient with clinical features of constriction. AO, Aorta, RV, right ventricle, LA, left atrium.

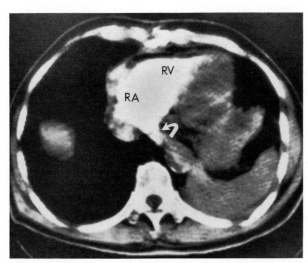

Figure 14–16. Pericardial constriction. Contrast-enhanced CT shows opacification of the right heart with retrograde flow into the coronary sinus due to elevated right atrial pressure *(curved arrow)*. RA, Right atrium, RV, right ventricle. (From Moncada, R., et al.: Multimodailty approach to pericardial imaging. Cardiovasc. Clin. 17:409, 1986, with permission.)

some cases, viral particles (usually of Coxsackie B virus) are actually isolated from pericardial fluid, or antibody titers suggest the causative agent. In most cases, however, a viral origin is not established with certainty. In this form of pericarditis, the patient often presents with the simultaneous onset of fever and precordial chest pain. This situation contrasts with that of myocardial infarction, in which fever usually follows the onset of pain. The pathognomonic physical finding is a pericardial friction rub, a high-pitched, scratchy, "to and fro" sound heard during precordial auscultation (Kusiak, 1985). Acute viral pericarditis usually has a short course of up to 2 weeks' duration, and coexistent pleural effusions and pneumonia are common. Purulent pericarditis is caused by extension of contiguous tuberculous or bacterial pneumonia, empyema, or myocarditis.

Acute noninfectious pericarditis with effusion may follow myocardial infarction. Postmyocardial infarction syndrome, or Dressler's syndrome, is manifested by high fever, precordial chest pain, arthralgia, and pericardial friction rub. It is thought to represent a hypersensitive reaction to an antigen originating from the necrotic myocardium. The pain usually begins within 2 to 4 weeks following myocardial infarction and lasts 1 to 2 weeks. Recurrences are common and may occur 2 or more years following the infarction (Levin and Bryk, 1966).

Pericardial effusion may also occur in association with cardiogenic pulmonary edema in the absence of pericardial inflammation. The mechanism of fluid accumulation is thought to be diminished myocardial venous and lymphatic drainage due to elevated central venous pressure (Spodick, 1983).

Chronic pericardial effusion commonly occurs in the terminal stages of renal failure and may be fibrinous, serous, or bloody (Hirshman, 1978). It is

associated with symptoms of pain, fever, and friction rub and may be complicated by pericardial constriction and cardiac tamponade. It develops in untreated patients as well as in 10% to 15% of patients on chronic dialysis.

Effusive pericarditis is a frequent occurrence in systemic lupus erythematosus. It may be associated with severe precordial chest pain or it may be incidentally detected because of an enlarged cardiac silhouette on a chest radiograph. Drug-induced lupus secondary to a wide variety of agents can produce identical manifestations. Among the commonly implicated pharmacologic agents are procainamide, hydralazine, diphenylhydantoin, and isoniazid (Lippman, 1977).

Radiation-induced pericarditis most commonly occurs in patients who have received a minimum of 40 Gy to the heart for treatment of mediastinal lymphoma (Hirshman, 1978). Pericardial constriction may develop several months or years following therapy and may be accompanied by chronic pericardial effusion (Schneider and Edward, 1979).

Primary pericardial neoplasms are rare and include teratomas, fibromas, and mesotheliomas. Pericardial metastases are common, however, and are usually derived from primary tumors of the lung or breast, melanoma, lymphoma, or leukemia. Diffuse pericardial thickening is typically accompanied by multiple nodules and a complex effusion. Effusions are usually slow in development and may attain a large size before producing symptoms (Moncada et al., 1982).

THE SURGICAL PATIENT

Pericardial Surgical Procedures

The tremendous increase in thoracic surgery in recent years has made transection of the pericardium commonplace. Today, the most frequently performed pericardial procedures occur in conjunction with coronary artery bypass graft or cardiac valve surgery. In both procedures, fenestration or partial resection of the pericardium is performed. Pericardial fenestrations are typically small retrosternal incisions that usually seal quickly after surgery following placement of sternal sutures. If sternal dehiscence is present, however, the pericardial communication may remain open or may reopen.

Primary pericardial surgical procedures include pericardiocentesis and pericardiotomy for the drainage of abscesses and relief of cardiac tamponade or pericardial constriction. Pericardial pneumonectomy is an infrequently performed procedure that widely exposes the vascular pedicle during the pneumonectomy (Iakasugi and Goodwin, 1989).

Complications of Pericardial Surgery

Hemorrhage is the most common complication of pericardial surgery. Hemopericardium usually occurs during the first 48 hours after surgery and should be suspected when the cardiac silhouette diffusely enlarges, or when a focal bulge is found on a postoperative plain film radiograph (Ellis and King, 1963; Ellis et al., 1971; Fyke et al., 1985). The definitive diagnosis may be made by ECHO (Fig. 14–17*A*), CT (Fyke et al., 1985) (see Fig. 14–17*B*), or in selected cases, by MRI (Ellis and King; 1963; Ellis et al., 1971; Fyke et al., 1985). Re-exploration and drainage may be indicated to prevent tamponade.

Pericardial effusion is common following cardiac surgery. In a series of 122 patients who underwent coronary bypass surgery, 85% developed pericardial effusion, although only one patient developed cardiac tamponade. The effusion attained maximum size by the tenth day in all patients in this series, but the

majority of patients developed some effusion within the first 2 to 5 days (Weitzman et al., 1984).

Postpericardiotomy syndrome is usually related to wide excision of the pericardium, but it may also follow cardiac trauma, pericardiocentesis, or minor pericardial surgery (Ellis and King, 1963; Kaminsky et al., 1982). It occurs in 10% to 40% of patients who undergo coronary bypass graft or valvular surgery. The onset of symptoms occurs 1 week to 6 months following the procedure, usually between 2 and 4 weeks. Fever, chest pain, friction rub, pleural and pericardial effusions, and small areas of parenchymal consolidation may be found. The syndrome is thought to be due to an immune reaction involving the necrotic visceral pericardium. It may alternatively be secondary to viral invasion of the visceral pericar-

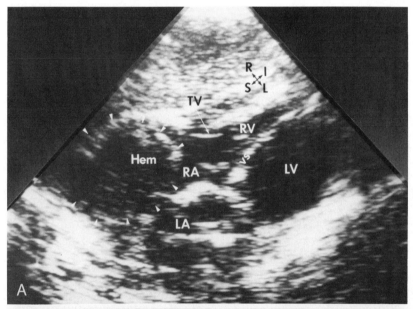

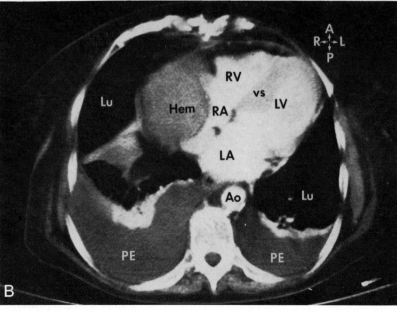

Figure 14–17. Intrapericardial hematoma after open heart surgery. *A,* Echocardiogram. Subcostal long-axis four-chamber view shows large hematoma compressing the right atrium. R, Right, I, inferior, S, superior, L, left. *B,* Contrast–enhanced CT. Hematoma is clearly shown to compress the right atrium *(arrowheads).* Hem, Hematoma, TV, tricuspid valve, RA, right atrium, VS, ventricular septum, LV, left ventricle, LA, left atrium, RV, right ventricle, PE, pleural effusion, LU, lung, A, anterior, R, right, P, posterior, C, left. (Reprinted with permission from the American College of Cardiology [Journal of the American College of Cardiology, 1985, 5:1496].)

dium. Symptoms usually last for 7 to 10 days and are relieved by anti-inflammatory agents, including corticosteroids and aspirin. Postpericardiotomy syndrome may be confused with sepsis, endocarditis, pneumonia, myocardial infarction, and aortic dissection. Pericardial constriction may eventually occur following postpericardiotomy syndrome (Ellis and King, 1963).

Cardiac tamponade occurs in 6% of patients who have undergone coronary bypass graft surgery (Steedman, 1986; Stevenson et al., 1984). The diagnosis is suspected when excessive blood loss through the drainage tubes is accompanied by an increase in central venous pressure, absence of pulmonary interstitial edema, decrease in systemic arterial pressure, tachycardia, and decreased urinary output. The differential diagnosis includes low output syndrome due to myocardial failure. Delayed tamponade may result from long-term anticoagulant therapy or, rarely, from perforation of the myocardium by a transvenous catheter. The development of postoperative chylopericardium following coronary bypass graft surgery has also been described in isolated case reports (Ellis and King, 1963; Periera et al., 1988).

Infectious pericarditis occurs in 1% of patients following cardiac surgery, often in association with sternal wound infections (Johnson et al., 1986). Radiographically, the mediastinum may be abnormally widened, and air may be present. Loculated collections may be found, and tracks to adjacent organs such as the pleura and peritoneum may develop.

Acute cardiac herniation may follow cardiac surgery, particularly when a defect has been created as part of a pericardial pneumonectomy (Arndt et al., 1978; Brady and Brogdon, 1986; Castillo and Oldham, 1985; Gates et al., 1970; Gurney et al., 1986; Hidvegi et al., 1981; Tschersich et al., 1976) (Fig. 14–18). Another predisposing cause of cardiac herniation is increased negative pleural pressure following thoracentesis. When herniation occurs following development of a right-sided pericardial defect, the cardiac apex usually also rotates to the right. The cardiac apex remains left-sided with a left-sided hernia (Takasugi and Goodwin, 1989), and the defect is often difficult to appreciate. A hernia may be suspected, however, by a mediastinal shift to the left with a prominent left heart border (Fig. 14–19) and main pulmonary artery. Air may enter the fixed portion of the pericardial sac if pneumothorax is present on the surgical side and if it freely communicates with the pericardial defect. Separation of the cardiac apex from the diaphragm by air in the pleural space is another clue to the diagnosis of cardiac herniation in the presence of pneumothorax.

The patient with cardiac herniation may be asymptomatic or may demonstrate catastrophic signs and symptoms when strangulation and myocardial ischemia occur in association with torsion of the great vessels. Cardiac strangulation is a rare occurrence and is found more often with smaller pericardial defects than with larger ones. Clinical findings of strangulation include chest pain accompanied by decreased blood pressure, venous distension, and cyanosis, which may be followed by shock and cardiac arrest. Impending herniation through a small pericardial defect may result in a "snow cone" appearance, characterized by a mound of soft tissue extending away from the cardiac border (Gurney et al., 1986).

PERICARDIAL TRAUMA

Blunt thoracoabdominal trauma is a well-recognized cause of pericardial disease. Intrapericardial

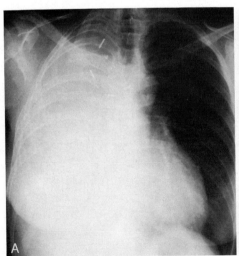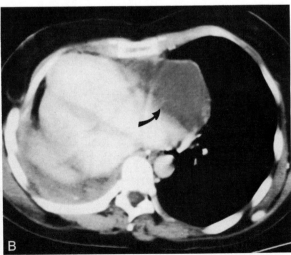

Figure 14–18. Right-sided pericardial defect following extrapleural pneumonectomy for treatment of mesothelioma. *A,* At 7 months after surgery, the right hemithorax is opacified and the cardiac apex appears to be in the normal position. *B,* Computed tomography shows the heart to be rotated into the right hemithorax through the defect. Pericardial fluid *(curved arrow)* creates the false impression of a left heart border on the plain film. (From Takasugi, J.E., and Godwin, J.D.: Surgical defects of the pericardium: Radiographic findings. AJR 152(5):951–954, 1989, with permission, © by American Roentgen Ray Society.)

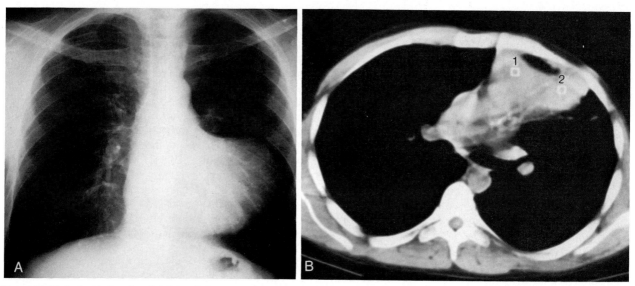

Figure 14–19. Left-sided pericardial defect following creation of a pericardial window for treatment of uremic pericarditis. *A,* Posteroanterior chest radiograph shows prominence of left heart border due to herniation of heart through pericardial defect. *B,* Computed tomography at level of the left coronary artery shows the abnormally high position of the right and left ventricles (1, right ventricle; 2, left ventricle). (From Takasugi, J.E., and Godwin, J.D.: Surgical defects of the pericardium: Radiographic findings. AJR 152(5):951–954, 1989, with permission, © by American Roentgen Ray Society.)

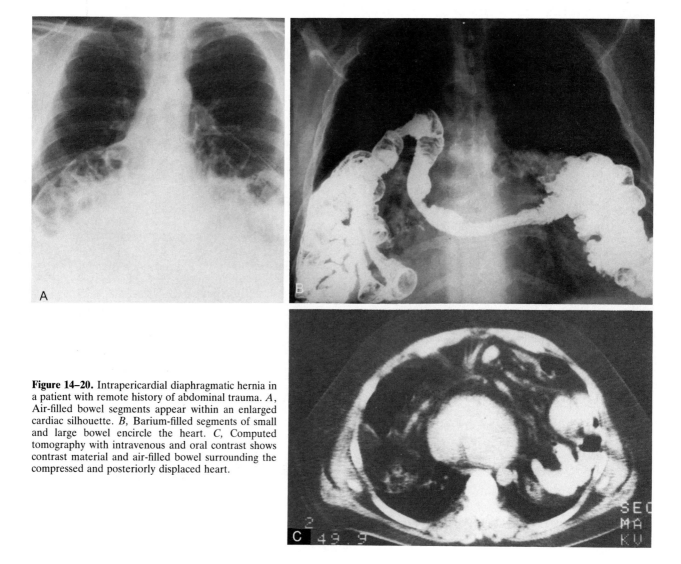

Figure 14–20. Intrapericardial diaphragmatic hernia in a patient with remote history of abdominal trauma. *A,* Air-filled bowel segments appear within an enlarged cardiac silhouette. *B,* Barium-filled segments of small and large bowel encircle the heart. *C,* Computed tomography with intravenous and oral contrast shows contrast material and air-filled bowel surrounding the compressed and posteriorly displaced heart.

diaphragmatic hernia (Van Loenhout et al., 1986) may occur when a defect is present in the transverse septum of the diaphragm, providing a passageway between the pericardium and the peritoneum. Patients with acute traumatic herniation of bowel into the pericardial space may present with hypovolemic shock, cardiac tamponade, and various respiratory and abdominal signs and symptoms. When the hernia develops slowly, the patient is relatively asymptomatic. The pattern of intrapericardial air may suggest bowel segments on plain film radiographs or CT (Fig. 14–20). Although a barium enema examination clearly demonstrates segments of bowel within the pericardial space, this study is contraindicated if strangulation is suspected. Acute hernias are surgically repaired by an abdominal approach, but chronic hernias generally require a thoracic incision to lyse adhesions prior to reduction of the hernia (Van Loenhout et al., 1986).

Pneumopericardium is occasionally a complication of blunt or penetrating chest trauma (Van Loenhout et al., 1986), surgical procedures (Takasugi and Goodwin, 1989; Westcott and Cole, 1983), or infection (Fig. 14–21). It may also be seen in the intensive care unit setting in patients who require high ventilatory pressures, and develop signs of thoracic barotrauma. Pneumopericardium may occasionally lead to cardiac tamponade. The air is thought to reach the pericardium by dissection along pulmonary interstitial planes into the mediastinum and then subsequently into the pericardial space. A check valve phenomenon must occur to produce significant pneumopericardium. Simultaneous tracheal or esophageal disruption and pericardial laceration may also produce pneumopericardium. Pneumopericardium may be extremely difficult to distinguish from pneumomediastinum; however, air that outlines the aortic knob or more than 1 to 2 cm of the superior vena cava lies outside the confines of the pericardium. Pericardial air may also demonstrate movement to the nondependent position with decubitus positioning, unlike pneumomediastinum which remains relatively fixed in position. A "small-heart" sign due to tension pneumopericardium has been described (Miruis et al., 1986). The treatment for pneumopericardium may necessitate drainage through the production of a subxiphoid window.

Hemopericardium may follow acute chest trauma and lead to cardiac tamponade which requires drainage for relief of symptoms and survival. Traumatic causes of hemopericardium include penetrating injury, aortic rupture due to blunt trauma, and occasionally aortic dissection (Ihde et al., 1987). The diagnosis is suggested by the appearance on plain film radiography of sudden enlargement of the cardiac silhouette. Computed tomography (Goldstein et al., 1989), MRI, and ECHO (Whye et al., 1988) help confirm the location and extent of hemorrhage and suggest the presence or absence of cardiac compromise.

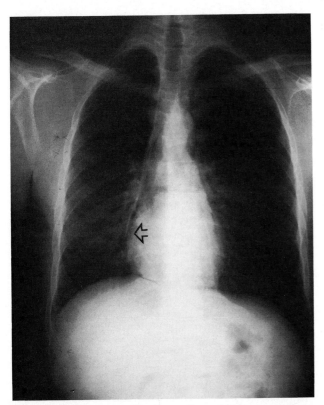

Figure 14–21. Posteroanterior chest radiograph shows pneumopericardium and pneumomediastinum *(arrow)*. Air within the pericardial space extends to the proximal half of the ascending aorta.

References

Agatston, A.S., Rao, A., Price, R.J., et al.: Diagnosis of constrictive pericarditis by pulsed Doppler echocardiography. Am. J. Cardiol. 54:929, 1984.

Arndt, R.D., Frank, C.G., Schmitz, A.L., et al.: Cardiac herniation with volvulus after pneumonectomy. AJR, 130:155, 1978.

Aronberg, D.J., Peterson, R.R., Glazer, H.S., et al.: The superior sinus of the pericardium: CT appearance. Radiology 153:489, 1984.

Baron, M.G.: Pericardial effusion. Circulation 44:294, 1971.

Brady, M.B. and Brogdon, B.G.: Cardiac herniation and volvulus: Radiographic findings. Radiology 161:657, 1986.

Callaham, M.L.: Current Therapy in Emergency Medicine. Toronto, B.C. Decker, 1987, p. 409.

Carsky, E.W., Mauceri, R.A., and Azimi, F.: The epicardial fat pad sign. Radiology 137:303, 1980.

Castillo, M., and Oldham, S.: Cardiac volvulus: Plain film recognition of an often fatal condition. AJR 145:271, 1985.

Chiles, C., Baker, M.E., and Silverman, P.M.: Superior pericardial recess simulating aortic dissection on computed tomography. J. Comput. Assist. Tomogr. 10:421, 1986.

Choe, Y.H., Im, J.G., Park, J.H., et al.: The anatomy of the pericardial space: A study of cadavers and patients. AJR 149:693, 1967.

Demos, T.C., Cardella, R.G., Moncada, R., et al.: Epicardial fat sign due to extrapericardial disease. AJR 141:289, 1983.

Doppman, J.L., Rienmuller, R., Lissner, J., et al.: Computed tomography in constrictive pericardial disease. J. Comput. Assist. Tomogr. 5:1, 1981.

Ellis, K., and King, D.L.: The pericardium. *In* Haskin, M. and Teplick, G. (eds.): Surgical Radiology. Philadelphia, W.B. Saunders, 1981, p. 1963.

Ellis, K., and King, D.L: Pericarditis and pericardial effusion. Rad. Clin. North Am. 11:393, 1973.

Ellis, K., Malm, J.R., Bowman, F.O. Jr., et al.: Roentgenographic findings after pericardial surgery. Radiol. Clin. North Am. 9:327, 1971.

Erasmie, U., and Lundell, B.: Pulmonary lesions mimicking pericardial effusion on ultrasonography. Pediatr. Radiol. 17:447, 1987.

Fyke III, F.E., Tancredi, R.G., Shub, C., et al.: Detection of intrapericardial hematoma after open heart surgery: The roles of echocardiography and computed tomography. J. Am. Coll. Cardiol. 5:1496, 1985.

Gale, M.E., Kiwak, M.G., and Gale, D.R.: Pericardial fluid distribution: CT analysis. Radiology 162:171, 1987.

Gates, G.F., Sette, R.S., and Cope, J.A.: Acute cardiac herniation with incarceration following pneumonectomy. Radiology 94:561, 1970.

Glazer, H.S., Aronberg, D.J., and Sagel, S.S.: Pitfalls in CT recognition of mediastinal lymphadenopathy. AJR 144:267, 1985.

Goldstein, L., Mirvis, S.E., Kostrubiak, I.S., et al.: CT diagnosis of acute pericardial tamponade after blunt chest trauma. AJR 152:739, 1989.

Gordon, S., and Butler, M.: Echocardiography in cardiac tamponade. Journal of Clinical Ultrasound 17:428, 1989.

Gurney, J.W., Arnold, S., and Goodman, L.R.: Impending cardiac herniation: The snow cone sign. Radiology 161:653, 1986.

Harbin, A.D., Gerson, M.C., and O'Connell, J.B.: Simulation of acute myopericarditis by constrictive pericardial disease with endomyocardial fibrosis. J. Am. Coll. Cardiol. 4:196, 1984.

Hidvegi, R.S., Abdulnour, E.M. and Wilson, J.A.S.: Herniation of the heart following left pneumonectomy. J. Can. Assoc. Radiol. 32:185, 1981.

Hirshman, J.V.: Pericardial constriction. Am. Heart J. 96:110, 1978.

Holt, J.P.: The normal pericardium. Am. J. Cardiol. 26:455, 1970.

Horowitz, M.S., Schultz, C.S., Stinson, E.B., et al.: Sensitivity and specificity of echocardiographic diagnosis of pericardial effusion. Circulation 50:239, 1974.

Ihde, J.K., Jacobsen, W.K., and Briggs, B.A.: Principles of Critical Care. Philadelphia, W.B. Saunders, 1987.

Im, J.G., Rosen, A., Webb, W.R. and Gamsu, G.: MR imaging of the transverse sinus of the pericardium. AJR 150:79, 1988.

Isner, J.M., Carter, B.L., Roberts, W.C., et al.: Subepicardial adipose tissue producing echocardiographic appearance of pericardial effusion. Am. J. Cardiol. 51:565, 1983a.

Isner, J.M., Carter, B.L., Bankoff, M.S., et al.: Differentiation of constrictive pericarditis from restrictive cardiomyopathy be computed tomographic imaging. Am. Heart J. 105:1019, 1983b.

Johnson, M.A., Hirji, M.K., Hennig, R.C., et al.: Pericardial abscess: Diagnosis using two-dimensional echocardiography and CT. Radiology 159:419, 1986.

Jorgens, J., Kundel, R. and Lieber, A.: The cine fluoroscopic approach to the diagnosis of pericardial effusion. AJR 87:911, 1962.

Kaminsky, M.E., Rodan, R.A., Osborne, D.R., et al.: Postpericardiotomy syndrome. AJR 138:503, 1982.

Kiat, H., Berman, D.S., and Maddahi, J.: Subepicardial fat mimicking pericardial effusion on radionuclide ventriculography: Diagnosis by magnetic resonance imaging. American Journal of Cardiac Imaging 3:57, 1989.

Kremens, V.: Demonstration of the pericardial shadow on the routine chest roentgenogram: Radiology 64:72, 1955.

Kusiak, V.: Pericarditis, myocarditis, and endocarditis. In Chung, E. (ed.): Cardiovascular Emergency Care, ed. 3. Philadelphia, Lea & Febiger, 1985, p. 268.

Lane, E.J., and Carsky, E.W.: Epicardial fat: Lateral plain film analysis in normals and in pericardial effusion. Radiology 91:1, 1968.

Levin, E.J., and Bryk, D.: Dressler syndrome (post–myocardial infarction syndrome). Radiology 87:731, 1966.

Levy-Ravetch, M., Auh, Y.H., Rubenstein, W.A., et al.: CT of the pericardial recesses. AJR 144:707, 1985.

Lippman, M.: Pulmonary reactions to drugs. Med. Clin. North Am. 61:1353, 1977.

Mangano, D.T., Van Dyke, D.C., Hickey, R.F., et al.: Significance of the pericardium in human subjects: Effects on left ventricular volume, pressure and ejection. J. Am. Coll. Cardiol. 6:290, 1985.

McKiernan, T.L.: The pericardium. In Civetta, J.M., et al. (eds.): Critical Care. Philadelphia, J.B. Lippincott, 1988.

Miller, A.J., Piek, R., and Johnson, P.J.: The production of acute pericardial effusion. Am. J. Cardiol. 28:463, 1971.

Mirvis, S.E., Indeck, M., Schorr, R.M., et al.: Post-traumatic tension pneumoperitoneum: The "small heart" sign. Radiology 158:663, 1986.

Moncada, R., Kotler, M.N., Churchill, R.J., et al.: Multimodality approach to pericardial imaging. Cardiovasc. Clin. 17:409, 1986.

Moncada, R., Baker, M., Salinas, M., et al.: Diagnostic role of computed tomography in pericardial heart disease: Congenital defects, thickening, neoplasms, and effusions. Am. Heart J. 1032:263, 1982.

Paling, M.R., and Williamson, B.R.J.: Epipericardial fat pad: CT findings. Radiology 165:335, 1987.

Pereira, W.M., Kalil, R.A., Prates, P.R., and Nesralla, I.A.: Cardiac tamponade due to chylopericardium after cardiac surgery. Ann. Thorac. Surg. 46:572, 1988.

Plehn, J.F.: Acute pericarditis and cardiac tamponade. In Heffernan, J.J., et al. (eds.): Clinical Problems in Acute Care Medicine. Philadelphia, W.B. Saunders, 1989, p. 83.

Plehn, J.F., Sager, J., Foster, E., et al.: Pericardial pseudotumor. Chest 94:837, 1988.

Rees, M., MacMillan, R., Flicker, S., et al.: Demonstration of chronic calcified pericardial constriction. CT 10:183, 1986.

Rifkin, R.D., Isner, J.M., Carter, B.L., et al.: Combined postero-anterior subepicardial fat simulating the echocardiographic diagnosis of pericardial effusion. J. Am. Coll. Cardiol. 3:1333, 1984.

Schneider, J.S., and Edward, J.E.: Irradiation-induced pericarditis. Chest 75:560, 1979.

Sechtem, U., Tscholakoff, D., and Higgins, C.B.: MRI of the normal pericardium AJR 147:239, 1986a.

Sechtem, U., Tscholakoff, D., and Higgins, C.B.: MRI of abnormal pericardium. AJR 147:245, 1986b.

Shabetai, R., Mangiardi, L., Bhargava, V., et al.: The pericardium and cardiac function. Prog. Cardiovasc. Dis. 22:107, 1979.

Shin, M.S., Jolles, P.R., and Ho, K.J.: CT evaluation of distended pericardial recess presenting as a mediastinal mass. J. Comput. Assist. Tomogr. 10:860, 1986.

Silverman, P.M., and Harell, G.S.: Computed tomography of the normal pericardium. Invest. Radiol. 18:141, 1983.

Spodick, D.: The normal and diseased pericardium: Current concepts of pericardial physiology, diagnosis and treatment. J. Am. Coll. Cardiol. 1:249, 1983.

Stark, D.D., Higgins, C.B., Lanzer, P., et al.: Magnetic resonance imaging of the pericardium: Normal and pathologic findings. Radiology 150:469, 1984.

Steedman, R.A.: Postoperative complications in the adult cardiac surgical patient. In Zschoche, D.A. (ed.): Comprehensive Review of Critical Care, ed. 3. St. Louis, C.V. Mosby, 1986, p. 369.

Stevenson, L.W., Child, J.S., Laks, H., et al.: Incidence and significance of early pericardial effusions after cardiac surgery. Am. J. Cardiol. 54:848, 1984.

Takasugi, J.E., and Goodwin, J.D.: Surgical defects of the pericardium: Radiographic findings. AJR 152:951, 1989.

Tehranzadeh, J., and Kelley, M.J.: Differential density sign of pericardial effusion. Radiology 133:23, 1979.

Tschersich, H.U., Slorapa, V., and Fleming, W.H.: Acute cardiac herniation following pneumonectomy. Radiology 120:546, 1976.

Tscholakoff, D., Sechtem, U., de Geer, G., et al.: Evaluation of pleural and pericardial effusions by magnetic resonance imaging. Eur. J. Radiol. 7:169, 1987.

Van Loenhout, R.M.M., Schiphorst, T.J., Wittens, C.H.A., et al.: Traumatic intrapericardial diaphragmatic hernia. J. Trauma 26:271, 1986.

Vesely, T.M., and Cahill, D.R.: Cross-sectional anatomy of the pericardial sinuses, recesses and adjacent structures. Surg. Radiol. Anat. 8:221, 1986.

Warwick, R., and Williams, P. (ed.): Gray's Anatomy, ed. 35. Philadelphia, W.B. Saunders, 1973, p. 598.

Weitzman, L.B., Tinker, W.P., Kronzon, I., et al.: The incidence and natural history of pericardial effusion after cardiac surgery—an echocardiographic study. Circulation 69:506, 1984.

Westcott, J.L., and Cole, S.: Barotrauma. *In* Herman, P.G. (ed.): Iatrogenic Thoracic Complications. New York, Springer-Verlag, 1983, p. 96.

Westcott, J.L., and Steiner, R.M.: Clinical applications of MRI of the heart. Cardiovasc. Clin. 17:323, 1986.

Whye, D., Barish R., Almquist, J., et al: Echocardiographic diagnosis of acute pericardial effusions in penetrating chest trauma. Am. J. Emerg. Med. 6:21, 1988.

Wong, B.Y.S., Lee, K.R., and MacArthur, R.I.: Diagnosis of pericardial effusion by computed tomography. Chest 81:177, 1982.

Yousem, D., Traill, T.T., Wheeler, P.S., et al.: Illustrative cases in pericardial effusion misdirection: Correlation of echocardiography and CT. Cardiovasc. Intervent. Radiol. 10:162, 1987.

15

Imaging After Cardiac Surgery

■

Lawrence R. Goodman

NORMAL POSTOPERATIVE APPEARANCE

Coronary artery bypass grafting (CABG) is the most frequently performed thoracic surgical procedure in the United States. Approximately 5.5 to 7.5 million people in this country suffer from symptomatic coronary artery disease. This disease leads to approximately 250,000 bypass grafts and approximately 250,000 coronary endotorectomies annually (Roberts, 1990).

Over the last decade, a major trend has arisen toward internal mammary artery (IMA) revascularization and away from venous bypass grafting (Rankin and Smith, 1990). Follow-up studies indicate an early patency of greater than 95% and a 10-year patency of about 90% for IMA grafts, compared with 90% and 25% to 50% for similar periods using venous bypass grafts. In major centers, the mortality rate for elective CABG is approximately 1%, and for urgent surgical procedures, it is approximately 3%. Preliminary data suggest an increased survival with the IMA procedure, although it is technically more difficult, and postoperative mediastinal infections and bleeding may be more frequent.

The second most common cardiac surgical procedure is valve replacement. With improved surgical techniques, improved prosthetic valves, and improved postoperative care, the hospital mortality rates for aortic and mitral valve surgery are approximately 3% and 9% respectively (Jacobs and Austin, 1990; Jones, et al., 1990, Spencer, 1990). The immediate postoperative clinical and radiographic problems are similar to those of CABG patients—atelectasis, edema, hemorrhage, pericardial effusion, and so forth. The incidence of postoperative complications increases when valve surgery is combined with CABG. Anticoagulation therapy for valve replacement patients is usually begun 2 to 3 days after surgery, resulting in more problems with bleeding in the ensuing days. Thromboembolic problems from air, calcium deposits, and thrombus are more frequent after valve surgery than after CABG.

Long-term complications may occur several months or years after discharge and may necessitate a return to the intensive care unit (ICU). Thromboembolic events lead to death at a rate of 1% per year and a slightly lower incidence after aortic surgery. Hemorrhagic events from anticoagulation occur at the rate of 1% to 4% per year and endocarditis occurs at a rate of approximately 1% to 3% per year. The latter complication has a 50% mortality rate. Valve malfunctions are another major long-term concern (Jones et al., 1990). Tissue valves have a 5%, 20%, and 50% failure rate at 5, 10, and 15 years, respectively. Metallic valves have a much lower failure rate but require permanent anticoagulation, and therefore hemorrhage is more frequent. The radiographic and echocardiographic evaluation of prosthetic valves is beyond the scope of this text. Recent reviews by Steiner and colleagues (1988) and by Soulen (1984) address this topic thoroughly.

Regardless of the procedure performed, the major postoperative radiographic changes result from the patient's underlying cardiovascular disease, the use of cardiopulmonary bypass, and the median sternotomy incision. The chest radiograph reflects a combination of the foregoing conditions, plus the expected sequelae of general anesthesia, which are discussed in Chapter 5. This chapter discusses primarily the radiographic changes of patients who have had coronary artery bypass operations, but the findings can be extrapolated to other conditions (Goodman, 1980; Henry et al., 1989a; Thorsen and Goodman, 1988). Proper radiographic evaluation in the immediate postoperative period requires a thorough understanding of the various support and monitoring apparatus inserted during the surgical procedure, the expected postoperative cardiopulmonary changes, and the complications frequently encountered postoperatively.

IMMEDIATE POSTOPERATIVE PERIOD

The first postoperative radiograph is usually obtained in the recovery room or ICU, shortly after the surgical procedure. At this point, the two major concerns are the appropriate positioning of various tubes and catheters and the state of the patient's cardiopulmonary system. Before the latter is assessed, all visible tubes and *expected* tubes should be sought, and their position verified (Landay et al., 1990).

The initial postoperative radiograph demonstrates numerous tubes, catheters, and sutures in the chest (Landay et al., 1990). Although the postoperative hardware varies from case to case and institution to institution, the following are the most frequently noted appliances:

1. An anterior mediastinal drainage tube parallel to the sternum. A second tube may be placed posteriorly to the heart (see Figs. 15–1, 15–2, and 15–4).

2. A right-angle drainage tube that is between the inferior heart border and the diaphragm, that points posterolaterally, and that drains the pericardium and posterior fluid collections (see Figs. 15–1 and 15–2).

3. An additional chest tube in the pleural space, or continuation of the mediastinal tube into the pleural space, if the pleural space is entered at the time of the operation (see Figs. 15–2 and 15–4).

4. A central venous pressure (CVP) catheter in the superior vena cava (see Fig. 15–1).

5. A thin epicardial pacing wire anchored in the myocardium on the right side of the heart and exiting through the anterior chest wall. Several centimeters of slack are often left in the pericardium (see Fig. 15–1).

6. A Swan-Ganz catheter, a thin left atrial catheter exiting through the chest wall, or both.

7. An endotracheal tube in the trachea.

8. An intra-aortic counterpulsation device when circulatory assistance is required (see Fig. 15–3).

9. Numerous mediastinal clips. A ring or opaque suture marks the proximal anastomosis with the aorta when a saphenous vein bypass graft is performed (see Figs. 15–8 and 15–9). When an IMA graft is performed, multiple clips are visualized along the mobilized internal mammary artery and along the stumps of the intercostal arteries behind the sternum (see Fig. 15–2).

10. Two interrupted steel wires closing the manubrium and three or four wires looping around the sternal body for closure of the sternum (see Figs. 15–1 and 15–3). More complex wires are usually used when the sternum is osteoporotic or otherwise diseased or following re-operations (see Fig. 15–2). Parham's bands, broad steel bands placed around the sternum, are used for problematic closures by some and routinely by others.

Under normal circumstances, the endotracheal tube is removed within 6 to 24 hours of the operation, and the mediastinal and pleural drains and various intravenous catheters are removed 1 to 2 days following the surgical procedure.

One seldom sees a "normal" radiograph after CABG. Atelectasis, pulmonary edema, pleural effusions, mediastinal widening, and extrapulmonary air collections are frequent, and if mild, they should almost be considered the expected surgical consequence rather than a complication. Other frequently encountered problems include increased cardiac size, pericardial disease, and thoracic cage lesions. As the patient progresses beyond the first postoperative week, other problems, such as postpericardiotomy syndrome and the major but infrequent complications of mediastinitis, osteomyelitis, dehiscence, constrictive pericarditis and aortic pseudoaneurysms, are encountered.

Atelectasis

Postoperative atelectasis is almost universal (see Chapter 5). The atelectasis ranges from mild elevation of the diaphragm or slightly increased lung density at the bases to consolidation and partial collapse of an entire lobe. Atelectasis is usually most severe and most frequent on the left side (Fig. 15–1). Carter and

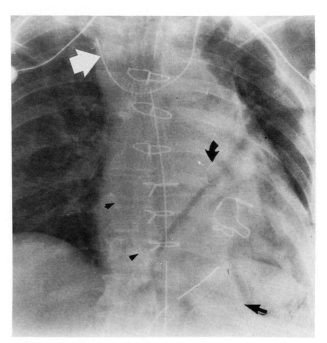

Figure 15–1. Post–mitral valve surgery. The endotracheal tube and the retrosternal and pericardial drainage tubes are in normal position. A left atrial catheter is barely visible over the spine (*arrowheads*). The central venous pressure (CVP) catheter, inserted via the left jugular vein, is heading cephalad, presumably in the right jugular vein (*white arrow*). The cardiac pacer wires are barely visible over the left hemidiaphragm (*straight black arrow*). The mitral valve prosthesis appears in normal position. Incidentally noted above the mitral prosthesis is a curvilinear radiodensity (*curved arrow*). This surgical needle, inadvertently left in the left atrium, eventually embolized to the abdominal aorta. Also, the superior mediastinum is moderately widened. The medial half of the left hemidiaphragm and the descending aorta are not visualized, owing to adjacent atelectasis.

colleagues (1983) found atelectasis in 84 of 99 patients: 40 of the cases were left-sided, 43 were bilateral, and only one was right-sided.

Several factors combine to make the left lower lobe more vulnerable to postoperative atelectasis. In topical, cardiac hypothermia (induced to decrease the metabolic needs of the heart during the surgical procedure), an ice slurry is used to cool the myocardium. The phrenic nerve is cooled in the process, which leads to paralysis or paresis of the diaphragm that may last for several days or weeks. Recent attempts at protecting the phrenic nerve from freezing appear to have decreased the frequency and severity of postoperative left lower lobe atelectasis (Wheeler et al., 1985; Wilcox et al., 1988). In addition, the enlarged heart often compresses the left lower lobe and distorts the bronchus, interfering with inflation and the clearing of secretions. Blind suctioning of the left lower lobe is also more difficult than that of the right lower lobe. Atelectasis often increases after weaning, when the lung volumes are no longer artificially supported by mechanical ventilation.

Edema

Pulmonary edema is present in the majority of patients in the immediate postoperative period. It is usually due to a combination of increased capillary permeability (from various factors related to cardiopulmonary bypass), and hemodilution and hypervolemia from excess fluid replacement. Intrinsic left ventricular problems may further aggravate the edema (Henry et al., 1989a). In the majority of patients, the edema is detectable only by decreased lung compliance or by widening of the oxygen gradient. In a significant minority of patients, the postoperative radiograph shows mild to moderate edema during the first 48 hours after the operation (Fig. 15–2).

The radiographic estimate of the severity of the edema is influenced by the level of positive end-expiratory pressure (PEEP) applied in the immediate postoperative period. By the second postoperative day, the cardiovascular system re-establishes autoregulation, the capillary integrity is restored, and edema is resorbed. Countering this improvement is the reabsorption of third space fluid that accumulated from preoperative cardiac failure or postoperative increased capillary permeability. This reabsorption often leads to hypervolemia, hemodilution, and persistent or recurrent edema.

Considerably less common but more serious is the situation in which the cardiac output is inadequate immediately after cardiopulmonary bypass or in the days that follow. This inadequacy is usually due to an intraoperative or postoperative myocardial infarction or arrythmia. These patients are frequently in severe pulmonary edema and require aortic counterpulsation balloon assistance to maintain adequate circulation (Fig. 15–3; see Chapter 4). Full-blown

adult respiratory distress syndrome (ARDS) from increased capillary permeability following cardiac bypass is uncommon. Iannuzzi and Pethy (1986) found the incidence to be less than 2% in patients without concomitant infection.

Pleural Disease

During the first 48 hours after the surgical procedure, the radiograph frequently suggests pleural effusion. As noted by C. E. Putman, M.D. (personal communication), however, decubitus films often fail to show an effusion. The overdiagnosis of effusion is probably due to a poor inspiration, basilar atelectasis, and perhaps lordotic angulation. Most true effusions regress within several days, often leaving minimal permanent blunting of the costophrenic angle (Kaminsky et al., 1982). Most effusions are probably due to the irritation caused by the surgical procedure, minor hemorrhage, or congestive heart failure. In addition, a close correlation has been noted between the severity of atelectasis and the size of effusions. With increasing atelectasis, the decreased transpleural pressure promotes effusion, and the atelectatic lung inhibits fluid resorption.

Large pleural effusions in the immediate postoperative period are usually due to intrapleural hemorrhage, a misplaced catheter that is pouring fluid into the pleural space, or an uncommon injury to the thoracic duct, causing a chylous effusion.

Mediastinal Bleeding

Mild, self-limited bleeding into the mediastinum is frequent after mediasternotomy and is usually of no consequence. Hemorrhage leading to re-exploration occurs in 2% to 5% of patients (Ikäheimo et al., 1988). Predisposing factors include coagulopathy, anticoagulation, repeat sternotomy, and perhaps IMA grafting (Fig. 15–4; see Figs. 15–1 and 15–3).

In the majority of cases requiring re-exploration, hemodynamic deterioration (e.g., low output due to cardiac tamponade or shock due to blood loss) or prolonged brisk bleeding through the chest tube determines the need for re-operation. The patient is usually re-explored if bleeding exceeds 1500 ml, if a sudden or delayed increase occurs in tube drainage, or if acute tamponade or hypotension from blood loss is clinically evident.

Rapid, acute widening of the mediastinum on the portable radiograph is a secondary indication for exploration. Judgment must be exercised because the width of the mediastinum does not correlate well with the need for surgery. Carter and co-workers (1983), studying 100 postoperative patients, found that seven required re-operation for hemorrhage. Four patients showed no significant radiographic widening of the mediastinum, two patients had apical caps and one patient demonstrated a wide mediastinum. Katzburg

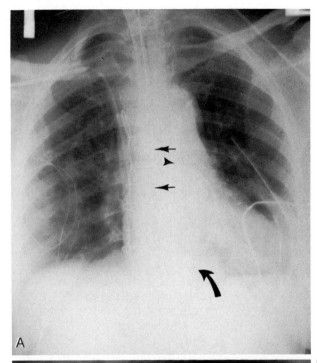

Figure 15–2. Immediate postoperative radiograph after coronary artery bypass grafting (CABG). *A,* Postoperative hardware includes an armored endotracheal tube at the tip of the midtrachea, a Swan-Ganz catheter with its tip in the right pulmonary artery (*arrowhead*), an anterior mediastinal tube (*small arrows*), and a right angle tube between the heart and the diaphragm (*curved arrow*). Also, a chest tube appears on the left.

The interstitial markings are slightly prominent, which represents a marked change from the preoperative radiograph and indicates interstitial edema. *B and C,* Because of pre-existing sternal disease, primary sternal closure was reinforced with a continuous wire woven between the right ribs. A similar wire is woven between the second and third ribs on the left. The interrupted sternal sutures are placed around these wires. The large vascular clip at the level of T10 on the left (*arrow*) represents the site of removal of the internal mammary artery. The smaller vascular clips directly above are on side branches along the chest wall. The clips in a more lateral location are on the internal mammary artery itself.

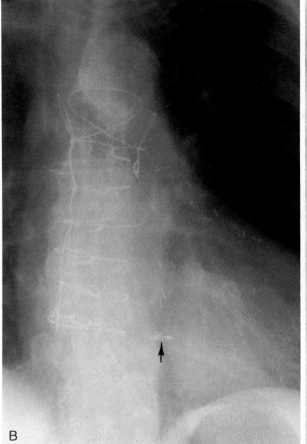

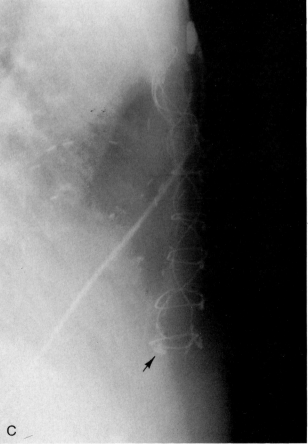

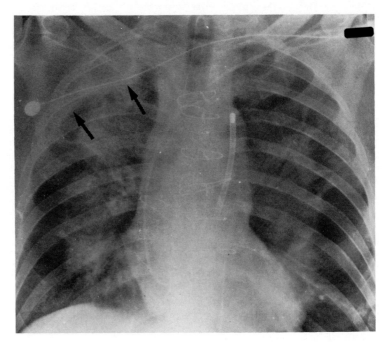

Figure 15–3. Postoperative heart failure. A butterfly pattern of pulmonary edema appears bilaterally. Because of the patient's intractable heart failure, an aortic counterpulsation catheter was inserted. The tip is at the aortic knob. Incidentally noted is a right apical cap indicative of extrapleural bleeding (*arrows*). In addition, some mild mediastinal widening has occurred. These changes regressed over several days.

and associates (1978) similarly documented that many seriously bleeding patients had relatively normal mediastinums, and that many patients with 60% widening postoperatively did not require re-operation. Occasionally, however, when the chest tube malfunctions or is obstructed by clot or once the chest tubes have been removed, radiographic evidence of progressive, widening does indicate the need for re-operation. Supine, expiratory radiographs may result in a 50% increase in mediastinal width from magnification alone. This apparent deterioration should not be mistaken for severe hemorrhage (see Chapter 2).

Cardiac Enlargement

An increase in the cardiac silhouette in the immediate postoperative period may be due to several conditions. Intraoperative or perioperative myocardial infarction or heart failure may cause the heart to enlarge. Hypervolemia from excess fluid administration or resorption of extravascular fluid may also dilate the heart. More frequently, the enlargement is due to fluid in the pericardium or mediastinal space (Fig. 15–5). Again, supine radiographs may cause marked magnification, which should not be mistaken for deterioration.

Extrapulmonary Air Collections

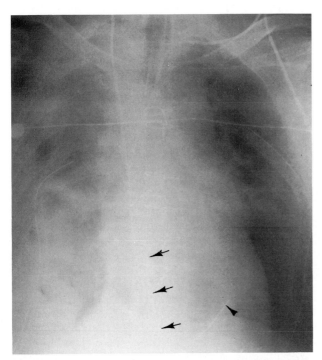

Figure 15–4. Postoperative hemorrhage. One day after CABG, there is marked widening of the mediastinum. There are also a right hemothorax and atelectasis. Neither the anterior drainage tube (*arrows*) nor the right thoracostomy tube drained excessive blood. A continuing fall in hematocrit, plus the radiographic changes, led to re-operation. In the mediastinum, the drainage tube was found to be at a site far removed from the mediastinal hemorrhage. Blood was found in the right hemithorax. (Note pericardial tube below the heart [*arrowhead*].)

Pneumothorax, pneumomediastinum, pneumopericardium, and subcutaneous emphysema are frequently present immediately following median sternotomy. These collections are usually due to the sternotomy itself and resolve over several days. Free air under the diaphragm is usually a benign postoperative condition caused by inadvertent entry into the peritoneal cavity during opening of the lower sternum

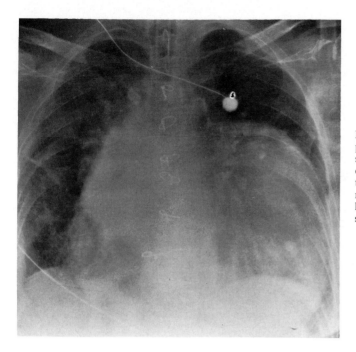

Figure 15–5. Hemopericardium following mitral surgery. The patient returned with severe fatigue following discharge. Clinical signs of cardiac tamponade were evident. The chest radiograph demonstrates a massive cardiac silhouette, which is approximately twice the size of the predischarge heart. Laboratory examination revealed the patient to be markedly overanticoagulated. Several hundred milliliters of blood were drained from the pericardial space, resulting in relief of symptoms.

(Fig. 15–6). Unless the patient has clinical findings of gastrointestinal perforation, abdominal air does not require further evaluation and usually disappears over several days (Glanz et al., 1978). A small collection of air or an air–fluid level in the anterior mediastinum is sometimes found on the initial lateral radiograph that is taken after the mediastinal drains have been removed. The majority of these air collections are benign and not associated with underlying infection. The air usually disappears over several days.

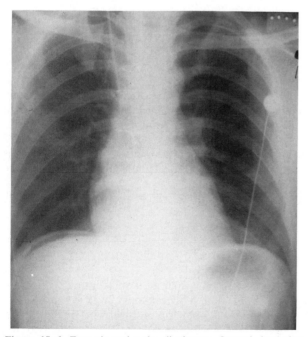

Figure 15–6. Free air under the diaphragm. Several days after CABG, free air was noted beneath the diaphragm on the first erect postoperative radiograph. The patient had no abdominal symptoms, and the air did not appear on a follow-up radiograph, 1 week later.

Pericardial Disease

Echocardiographic evidence of pericardial fluid is present in at least 50% of postoperative patients (Stevenson et al., 1984). The vast majority are asymptomatic, show a normal cardiac silhouette on the chest radiograph, and have an uneventful recovery. Cardiac tamponade, usually due to mediastinal hemorrhage, occurs in 2% to 3% of patients in the immediate postoperative period. The majority of cases of tamponade occur in the immediate postoperative period and result from bleeding at the graft suture lines or from arterial bleeders in the IMA bed or along the site of sternotomy. Coagulopathy may also contribute to this complication. Patients with early tamponade usually have evidence of excessive tube drainage or direct blood loss through the wound site. Tubes in the pericardium and pericardial windows do not guarantee protection from cardiac tamponade.

The patient usually presents with a combination of a low cardiac output syndrome and an equalization of right atrial, pulmonary artery diastolic, and pulmonary capillary wedge pressures. In approximately one half of the cases, the portable radiograph shows evidence of the enlargement of the cardiac silhouette (see Fig. 15–5). In the acute situation, a small amount of fluid may cause tamponade without apparent increase in cardiac size. Similarly, loculated pericardial or mediastinal fluid may cause single-chamber compression with or without evidence of radiographic abnormality. Free pericardial effusion is best diagnosed by echocardiography, whereas focal hematomas, seromas, and infections are best studied by computed tomography (CT) (Fyke et al., 1985). Computed tomography allows detection of focal intrapericardial hematomas as well as differentiation of mediastinal from pericardial fluid (Fig. 15–7). Scin-

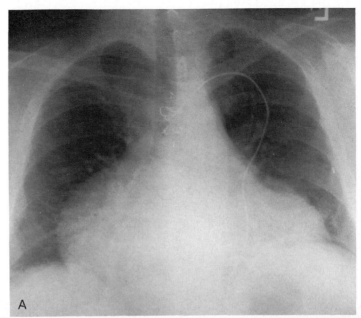

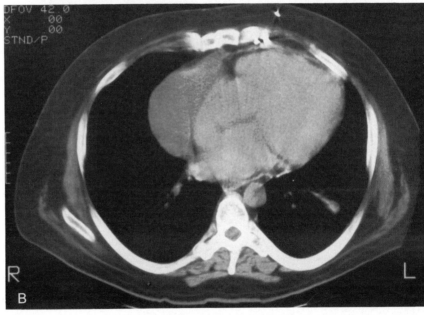

Figure 15–7. Approximately 1 year after cardiac transplantation, the patient experienced rapidly deteriorating exercise tolerance and weakness. *A,* The PA radiograph shows a huge cardiac silhouette, predominantly on the right. There is no evidence of heart failure. *B,* Computed tomography shows a large, loculated pericardial effusion compressing the lateral wall of the right atrium. The pericardium is normal elsewhere. The percutaneous aspiration of several hundred milliliters of straw-colored fluid caused dramatic relief. Symptoms recurred within a few weeks, however. The effusion was related to either the patient's cyclosporine therapy or a viral infection.

tigraphy may be helpful in evaluating right-sided compression (Bateman et al., 1982).

Postoperative pericardial defects may cause radiographic changes, acutely or chronically (Takasugi and Godwin, 1989). Acutely, air or fluid may pass between the pleural and pericardial cavities, producing several unusual radiographic appearances. For example, pneumothorax and a surgical defect on one side may result in visible air in the contralateral pericardium. Large pericardial defects after pericardial stripping or pneumonectomy may allow acute herniation of the heart through the defect (see Chapter 12). More often, a large pericardial defect allows partial protrusion of the heart with time. This protrusion may give a peculiar shape to the heart border but usually involves no symptoms. After CABG or

valve replacement, however, a visible defect or deformity is rare, because the pericardium is not resected but incised, healing is rather rapid, and the defect occurs in the retrosternal area.

Thoracic Cage Lesions

Most reviews indicate that fractures of the first or second rib are visible on 2% to 4% of postoperative radiographs. Greenwald and associates (1983) performed bone scans on 24 consecutive patients following median sternotomy. Thirty left and 14 right fractures were demonstrated. Even in retrospect, only four were visible on radiographs. Although routine postoperative bone scanning is not suggested, it may

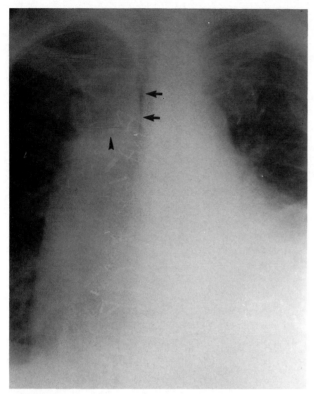

Figure 15–8. Sternal lucency after sternotomy. A thin linear lucency through the manubrium appears on this postoperative radiograph *(arrows)*. It was not present on subsequent films, and no postoperative sternal problems occurred. (Note round marker outlining the proximal anastomosis of the venous bypass graft [*arrowhead*]).

be helpful in patients with unexplained chest pain, chest wall pain, or brachial plexus symptoms.

In the early postoperative period, a lucent stripe that is 3 mm wide or thinner is often visible on at least one radiograph (Berkow and Demos, 1976; Ziter, 1977). This stripe represents a narrow gap in the sternum and is usually not a precursor to dehiscence (Fig. 15–8). A wider or progressively widening cleft strongly suggests dehiscence. Sternal instability and dehiscence are usually diagnosed clinically rather than radiographically. The only other reliable, albeit late, radiographic sign of dehiscence is the migration or re-orientation of sternal wires. As the sternum separates, the wires, rather than breaking, usually cut through the bone (Fig. 15–9). Thus, some wires migrate in one direction while others migrate in the opposite direction. Not infrequently, a routine radiograph demonstrates one or more broken sternal wires. The majority are not associated with sternal dehiscence.

DELAYED COMPLICATIONS

Postpericardiotomy Syndrome

The postpericardiography syndrome, which occurs several days to several months after cardiac surgery, is a febrile illness consisting of various combinations of pericarditis, pleuritis, and pneumonitis (Ebert and Nijafi, 1990; Kaminsky et al., 1982). It may elevate the sedimentation rate and white blood count and cause electrocardiographic (ECG) changes suggestive of pericarditis.

The radiograph may demonstrate an enlarging cardiac silhouette or a left pleural effusion, with or without patchy basilar infiltrates. In a group of 38 patients, Kaminsky and colleagues (1982) found pleural effusions alone in 11 patients, pericardial

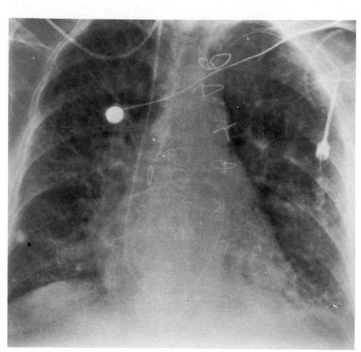

Figure 15–9. Postoperative sternal dehiscence. Sternal infection was noted on clinical examination approximately 10 days after surgery. A radiograph obtained several days later reveals that the first suture has unraveled. The upper two sutures are in the midline, and the lower three sutures have migrated to the left. (They had all been in line previously.) These changes are definitive evidence of sternal dehiscence. In addition, the patient appears to be in a state of mild congestive heart failure. Three rings over the spine mark the site of the proximal saphenous vein anastomosis.

effusions and pleural effusions in 11 patients, pericardial effusions alone in four patients, and pneumonitis with pleural or pericardial disease in four patients. (Echocardiography was not used routinely.) In no case was pulmonary consolidation the sole presenting sign. Eight patients had normal radiographs. The majority of radiographic changes surfaced within 1 or 2 days of the clinical symptoms. The syndrome is usually benign and self-limited but may lead to cardiac tamponade in 1% to 2% of patients, and to constrictive pericarditis in a smaller group of patients (Killian et al., 1989). Treatment usually consists of therapy with anti-inflammatory drugs.

The pathogenesis of this syndrome remains obscure. It most likely involves an autoimmune reaction to damaged pericardium or myocardium. Patients with postoperative pericardial and mediastinal hemorrhage are more prone to development of this syndrome (Ikäheimo et al., 1988). Other theories involve a recent or reactivated viral illness, which then triggers the autoimmune response.

Constrictive Pericarditis

Constrictive pericarditis complicates approximately 0.2% of median sternotomies and may surface several months or years after surgery (Killian et al., 1989; Kutcher et al., 1982). In approximately one half of the patients, a history of major mediastinal or pericardial bleeding or of postpericardiotomy syndrome is noted. The most frequent symptoms include dyspnea, chest pain, and leg swelling, and the most frequent signs include pedal edema, ascites, hepatomegaly, and jugular venous distention. On the chest radiographs, the heart is enlarged in only one half of the patients, and the superior vena cava and azygous vein may be dilated as well. Calcification of the pericardium is extremely unusual.

In the appropriate setting, pericardial thickening of 5 to 20 mm as demonstrated by CT strongly suggests constrictive pericarditis. Confirming CT signs include dilatation of the inferior vena cava, ascites, and pleural effusion. Following intravenous contrast injection, the intraventricular septum is usually visible and may be angulated, and pericardial thickening can be distinguished from pericardial effusions. The absence of pericardial thickening may not rule out constrictive pericarditis, as previously believed. In a series of 29 patients, 23 had positive CT scans but 6 had false-negative scans (Killian et al., 1989). The majority of false-negative scans occurred in the first year after surgery and the majority of true-positive scans occurred in the second year or beyond. Perhaps as the pericardial changes mature, the thickened pericardium is more visible on CT. In the same series, echocardiograms were positive in seven of 11 patients. The most definitive test for constrictive pericarditis remains cardiac catheterization. (Pericardial disease is discussed in Chapter 14.)

Postoperative Infection

The incidence of serious wound infections after median sternotomy is approximately 0.5% to 1.5% (Bor et al., 1983; Breyer et al., 1984; Cheung et al., 1985; Rutledge et al., 1985). These infections, which are difficult to eradicate, have been associated with markedly prolonged hospitalization and a mortality rate of approximately 50%. Over the last decade, a more aggressive surgical approach involving early use of extensive debridement and the use of muscle or omental pedicled flaps has resulted in a 75% decrease in both hospital time and mortality (Breyer et al., 1984; Cheung et al., 1985; Pairolero and Arnold, 1984; Rutledge et al., 1985). Major risk factors include prolonged ventilatory support of greater than 24 hours, combined coronary artery and valve surgery, re-exploration for bleeding, low cardiac output, and infection elsewhere.

Grossi and associates (1985) stressed that early diagnosis leads to more rapid treatment, less extensive surgery, and improved results. They also stressed the difficulty involved in making an early diagnosis. The most frequent clinical signs include fever, elevated white count, and drainage from a sternal wound or chest tube. In a significant minority of patients, clinical signs are not clear-cut, and the diagnosis is difficult. Patients may simply be febrile without an apparent source of infection or may simply "not be doing well." In others, especially obese patients, difficulty may arise in determining whether a clinically apparent infection is confined to the superficial tissues or is being fed by deeper osteomyelitis or anterior mediastinitis. Table 15–1 illustrates the variability of signs and symptoms. For suspected postoperative infection, conventional radiography, CT, ultrasonography, and nuclear medicine imaging may aid in establishing the diagnosis. In other cases, CT-guided percutaneous needle aspiration helps distinguish infected from noninfected fluid.

Mediastinitis. The majority of patients with postoperative mediastinitis or focal mediastinal abscess

Table 15–1. MANIFESTATIONS OF STERNAL WOUND INFECTION

Manifestation	Percentage (%) of Patients (n = 77)
Local	
Increased pain	40
Erythema and drainage	41
Sternal instability	75
Systemic	
Fever	70
Leukocytosis	48
Positive blood culture	58

Based on data from Grossir, E. A., et al.: A survey of 77 major infectious complications of median sternotomy: A review of 7,949 consecutive operative procedures. Ann. Thorac. Surg. 40:214, 1985.

have abnormal radiographs, but Carrol and colleagues (1987) found that the changes were often nonspecific and difficult to interpret. Sixty-three percent of patients had superior mediastinal widening, 54% had pleural effusions, 22% had focal or diffuse mediastinal gas, and only 9% had a focal mediastinal mass. In more than three quarters of the cases, "it was not possible on the basis of chest radiography alone to precisely characterize the mediastinal infection or to distinguish mediastinal abscess from cellulitis." Postoperative mediastinal hemorrhage, pericardial fluid, or pseudoaneurysm may also cause delayed or persistent mediastinal widening.

Over the last several years, several groups have evaluated the use of CT for postoperative infection (Breatnach et al., 1986; Carrol et al., 1987; Goodman et al., 1983b; Hélénon et al., 1987). The cross-sectional images clearly show the subcutaneous tissues, the muscles, the sternum, the mediastinum, and the pericardium, which are major areas of postoperative interest. Many of the changes that one might expect to see in infected patients are present in normal, noninfected patients in the week or two immediately following surgery. The following CT changes are present in patients scanned 1 to 2 weeks after uncomplicated median sternotomy (Goodman et al., 1983a):

1. The presternal soft tissues appear normal within 1 to 2 weeks. Occasionally, some mild subcutaneous edema persists (Fig. 15–10).
2. For 1 to 2 weeks after the surgical procedure, mediastinal abnormalities are *universal.* The anterior and middle mediastinal fat is usually indistinct or obliterated, owing to edema, inflammation, or blood. Focal, high-density fluid collections (presumably blood) are noted in a significant minority of patients. Small air bubbles or streaks without air–fluid levels are also frequent. By the third or fourth week, the mediastinum usually returns to normal.
3. Pericardial fluid or thickening is frequent during the first week or two after surgery. The epicardial fat and anterior mediastinal fat may be somewhat indistinct at this time, as well. An occasional dot of air remains in the pericardium (Fig. 15–11; see Fig. 15–10).
4. Perfect closure of the sternum is uncommon, even when no clinical problems exist. The sternum frequently contains gaps (1 to 3 mm), and the sternal tables are often at different levels (see Fig. 15–10). In the vast majority of patients, these step-offs "close" without incident, whereas in others, the segments appear open (i.e., no visible callus) for months or years, as demonstrated by CT.

Beyond the second or third postoperative week, findings of obliteration of fat planes or of diffuse or focal fluid collections in the mediastinum more strongly suggest infection. For example, a focal fluid collection at 1 week probably represents a benign serosanguinous collection, whereas this same CT appearance at 4 weeks would strongly suggest an ab-

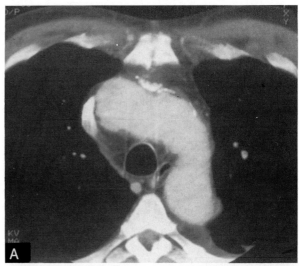

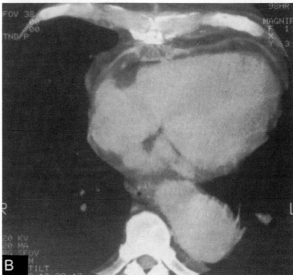

Figure 15–10. A normal postoperative CT scan, 8 days after surgery. *A,* Scan through the aortic arch showed minimal edema of the anterior mediastinal fat. A mild gap appears in the sternum. The posterior cortex of the manubrium is irregular, which represents a normal finding that should not be confused with osteomyelitis. *B,* At the level of the ventricles is a small loculated fluid collection in the pericardium. No adjacent inflammation is evident.

These changes are frequent in the first week or two after surgery and difficult to differentiate from a focal infection. Similar findings 1 month after surgery would suggest a loculated pericardial infection.

scess, especially in a febrile patient or in one with an elevated white count (Fig. 15–12). Hélénon and associates (1987), in a study of 69 CT examinations, emphasized that hypodense fluid collections are nonspecific and stressed the need for guided needle aspiration to establish the presence or absence of infection. In general, a normal or nearly normal CT scan essentially rules out a mediastinal infection requiring surgical intervention. Hélénon and co-workers (1987), however, found two cases of false-negative CT scans in which mediastinal drains were already in place. In other cases, in which ill-defined densities

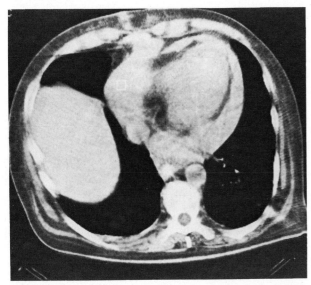

Figure 15–11. Computed tomography after CABG. This CT scan shows fluid in the pericardium and anterior mediastinal compartment several days after surgery. Neither tamponade nor infection was clinically evident. If infection had been suspected clinically, needle aspiration would have distinguished between a serosanguinous collection and an infected collection.

rather than focal collections are seen, and the clinical picture is equivocal, follow-up CT scans are often helpful in determining progression or regression of the abnormalities. Hélénon and co-workers (1987) felt that CT scanning was more helpful in detecting relapse following surgically treated mediastinitis than in the initial evaluation.

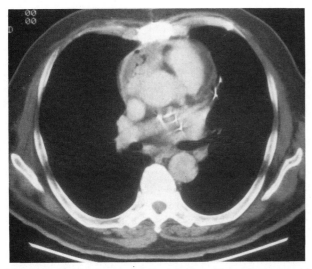

Figure 15–12. Focal postoperative infection. The patient returned to the hospital with a fever, several weeks after CABG. The chest radiograph was unchanged from the discharge radiograph. A CT scan shows a small loculated pericardial fluid collection anterior to the ascending aorta. Several small dots of air are present within. The pericardium is thickened and is enhanced with contrast. No abnormalities were seen elsewhere. With CT as a guide, the pericardial abscess was drained through a local incision, as an alternative to a repeat sternotomy.

Sternal Osteomyelitis. Sternal osteomyelitis may be a local infection or one associated with a deeper mediastinal infection. Conventional radiographs and tomograms are relatively insensitive indicators of osteomyelitis and of the condition of the anterior mediastinum. Computed tomography provides a potentially valuable depiction of both the sternum and the adjacent soft tissues. In the uncomplicated, postoperative patient, minor defects in sternal closure are frequent and are usually without clinical significance. In sternal osteomyelitis, the CT scan shows evidence of demineralization, destruction, and adjacent soft-tissue inflammation. The posterior cortex of the manubrium is often pitted and indistinct in normal patients. This sign should not be mistaken for one of osteomyelitis (see Fig. 15–10A). A CT scan is more sensitive than a tomogram, but it may be negative for several days after the onset of clinical symptoms. In early cases, demineralization may not be evident on the initial CT, whereas a follow-up examination several days later may show definite evidence of bone destruction. Conversely, CT may reveal evidence of clinically silent osteomyelitis when other lesions are being sought (Hélénon et al., 1987).

Gallium-67 (^{67}Ga) scanning of the postoperative sternum may aid in the early diagnosis of osteomyelitis. The normal postoperative sternum concentrates gallium in a thin line corresponding to the sternotomy. Salit and colleagues (1983) found that five of six patients with postoperative osteomyelitis showed an additional focal area of gallium uptake over the area of infection. Only one of 27 uninfected patients demonstrated similar focal uptake.

Pseudoaneurysm and Aortic Dissection

Although mediastinal infection is the major cause of delayed mediastinal widening, other lesions such as mediastinal hemorrhage, pseudoaneurysm, or pericardial fluid may also widen the mediastinum. Ascending aortic complications following cardiopulmonary bypass occur in less than 1% of patients. These problems usually occur at incision sites in the ascending aorta, namely, the site of cannulation for cardiopulmonary bypass, the site of aortotomy for aortic valve replacement, or the site of aortic anastomosis for a coronary artery bypass graft (Saffitz et al., 1983; Smith et al., 1983). Acute or chronic local infection, which weakens the suture lines, is present in approximately one half of the patients. In a review of 31 patients, Sullivan and colleagues (1988) found that the mean duration from operation to pseudoaneurysm presentation was 22 months (range 1 to 84 months), and that approximately one third of these patients died.

A pseudoaneurysm or aortic dissection should be considered in the differential diagnosis of any postoperative mediastinal widening or mass (Fig. 15–13).

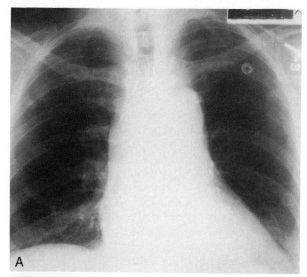

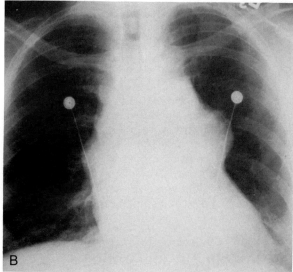

Figure 15–13. ■ Postoperative pseudoaneurysm. Patient had had coronary artery surgery 4 months earlier. The surgery was complicated by two bouts of sternal osteomyelitis requiring local excision. The patient returned to the hospital with evidence of colitis, a low-grade fever, and "tightness in the chest." *A,* Radiograph shows some mild mediastinal widening, an increase of approximately 1.5 cm over an earlier radiograph. While his colitis was evaluated, the patient was administered antibiotics in an attempt to control what was believed to be a mediastinal infection. *B,* Nine days later, the radiograph shows marked bilateral widening of the mediastinum. The patient was returned to the operating room with a diagnosis of recurrent mediastinal infection. During opening of the sternum, massive hemorrhage occurred, and the autopsy revealed a pseudoaneurysm with interruption of the left anterior descending graft. No organisms were cultured.

Dynamic contrast-enhanced CT or magnetic resonance imaging (MRI) helps separate pseudoaneurysms or dissection from other causes of mediastinal widening and helps determine the position of the ascending aorta or pseudoaneurysm in relation to the posterior table of the sternum (Moore et al., 1984; Nath and Soto, 1985; Thorsen et al., 1986) (Fig. 15–14). This information helps prevent an inadvertent

entry into the ascending aorta or pseudoaneurysm during re-exploration. When such a problem is anticipated, cardiopulmonary bypass via the femoral artery, hypothermia, and drainage of blood into the pump can be performed before the thorax is opened.

In summary, CT is a potentially valuable tool in evaluating the patient for poststernotomy problems. A flow chart summarizes our approach to these difficult problems (Goodman and Haasler, 1988) (Fig. 15–15).

CARDIAC TRANSPLANTATION

Cardiac transplantation is most frequently performed for end-stage cardiac failure resulting from cardiomyopathy or coronary artery disease. With improved surgical techniques, patient selection, and cyclosporine immunosuppression, the 1-year survival rate has risen to almost 90% and the 4-year survival to approximately 75% (Andreone et al., 1987; Goldstein and Wechsler, 1985; Reitz, 1987). Although cyclosporine immunosuppression has decreased the incidence of cardiac rejection and pulmonary infection in recent years, these complications remain the leading causes of morbidity and mortality.

In orthotopic cardiac transplantation, performed through a median sternotomy, the patient's heart is removed, leaving a cuff of both atria (containing the sinoatrial nodes, venae cavae, and pulmonary veins) and the severed ends of the ascending aorta and main pulmonary artery. The donor heart is then joined at both atria, the aorta, and the pulmonary artery. The donor superior vena cava stump is tied just above the right atrium, and the donor inferior vena cava is incorporated into the right atrial anastomosis.

Immediately following surgery, the complications are similar to those discussed previously. The cardiac silhouette frequently remains enlarged because of the discrepancy between the transplanted heart and the native pericardium (Guthaner et al., 1987). Because of the more extensive resection, postoperative mediastinal bleeding is more common, and mediastinal widening is universal (Florence et al., 1988). Left lower lobe atelectasis and effusions (greater on the right side than on the left) are frequent. The cardiac silhouette decreases in size over several months. One may see a double contour along the upper right border of the heart where the donor and recipient atria overlap (Shirazi, 1983).

Henry and associates (1989b) have outlined the following normal postoperative CT appearance of the heart and great vessels after transplantation (Fig. 15–16):

1. The main pulmonary artery is often high and adjacent to the aorta. It may be redundant and at right angles to the aorta. The pulmonary artery anastomosis may at times be recognized by a radiopaque band of synthetic material wrapping the anastomosis.

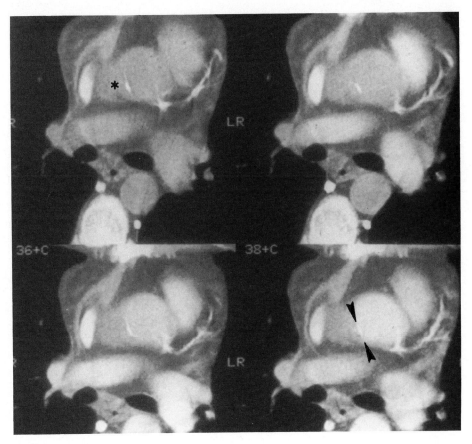

Figure 15–14. Postoperative pseudoaneurysm. Nine years after surgery, the patient returned to the hospital with fever, chills, malaise, and evidence of mediastinal widening appearing on the chest radiograph. A dynamic contrast-enhanced CT scan shows the aortic aneurysm (*asterisk*) projecting to the right. The fourth panel shows delayed opacification of the pseudoaneurysm. The neck of the aneurysm is visible (*arrowheads*). An angiogram demonstrated a large saccular aneurysm just proximal to the takeoff of the right innominate artery. (From Thorsen, M.K., et al.: Ascending aorta complications of cardiac surgery: CT evaluation. J. Comput. Assist. Tomogr. 10:219, 1986, with permission.)

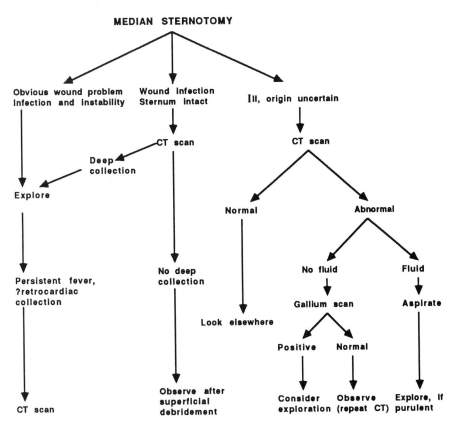

Figure 15–15. Imaging strategy for sternotomy complications. (From Goodman, L.R., and Haasler, G.B.: Mediastinal and sternal infection: Imaging strategies. Cardiac Surgery: State of the Art Reviews 2:445, 1988, with permission.)

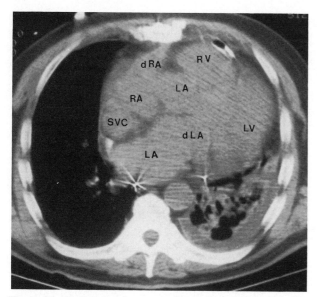

Figure 15–16. Computed tomography after cardiac transplantation—normal appearance of transplanted heart on axial scan through the atria. Note that both the recipient atria (LA, RA) and donor atria (dLA, dRA) are visible as discrete structures. The other structures are similar to a nontransplanted heart. LV, Left ventricle; RV, right ventricle; SVC, superior vena cava. (From Thorsen, M.K., and Goodman, L.R.: Extracardiac complications of cardiac surgery. Seminars in Roentgenology 23:32, 1988, with permission.)

2. A large space may exist between the recipient superior vena cava and the donor ascending aorta, and between the donor ascending aorta and the main pulmonary artery.

3. The ascending aorta may change caliber from recipient to donor, and a radiopaque synthetic patch may encircle this anastomosis as well.

4. The remnant of the donor superior vena cava may appear posterior to the donor ascending aorta and medial to the recipient superior vena cava. The left and right atrial anastomosis may cause a waste in the respective atria.

5. The host inferior vena cava may be large.

In addition to the usual postoperative problems, rejection and infection are potential complications during the weeks and months following the surgical procedure. Hyperacute rejection occurs within several hours or days postoperatively, acute rejection usually occurs between 2 weeks and 3 months postoperatively, and chronic rejection occurs 6 months to several years postoperatively (Andreone et al., 1987). Clinically, the patients experience dyspnea, lethargy, weakness, or hypotension and may appear to be in a state of heart failure. The radiograph may demonstrate cardiomegaly, but this sign is neither a sensitive nor a specific sign of rejection. Endomyocardial biopsy is required for diagnosis.

Approximately one third of patients have significant pulmonary infections, most occurring within the first several months. Infection accounts for about 40% of postoperative mortality (Andreone et al., 1987;

Austin et al., 1989). Approximately one half of the infections are bacterial and often gram-negative, and the remainder are divided between viral, fungal, and protozoan infections. Radiographic findings are often nonspecific and require invasive diagnostic methods (see Chapter 10).

As with heart–lung and lung transplants, additional delayed complications include a higher incidence of cancer and Epstein-Barr–induced lymphomas. Any increase in mediastinal width should be evaluated with CT to distinguish the more frequent steroid-induced lipomatosis from a lymphoma (Guthaner et al., 1987). Accelerated coronary atherosclerosis, perhaps a manifestation of chronic rejection, is a frequent problem beyond the second year (Andreone et al., 1987; Goldstein and Wechsler, 1985).

References

Andreone, P.A., Olivari, M.T., and Ring, W.S.: Clinical considerations of cardiac transplantation in organ transplantation: Preoperative and postoperative evaluation. Radiol. Clin. North Am. 25:357, 1987.

Austin, J.H., Schulman, L.L., and Matrobattista, J.D.: Pulmonary infection after cardiac transplantation: Clinical and radiologic correlations. Radiology 172:259, 1989.

Bateman, T., Gray, R., Chaux, A., et al.: Right atrial tamponade complicating cardiac operation: Clinical, hemodynamic, and scintigraphic correlates. J. Thorac. Cardiovasc. Surg. 84:413, 1982.

Berkow, A.E., and Demos, T.C.: The midsternal stripe and its relationship to postoperative sternal dehiscence. Radiology 121:525, 1976.

Bor, D.H., Rose, R.M., Modlin, J.F., et al.: Mediastinitis after cardiovascular surgery. Rev. Infect. Dis. 5:885, 1983.

Breatnach, E., Nath, P.H., and Delany, D.J.: The role of computed tomography in acute and subacute mediastinitis. Clin. Radiol. 37:139, 1986.

Breyer, R.H., Mills, S.A., Hudspeth, A.S. et al.: A prospective study of sternal wound complications. Ann. Thorac. Surg. 37:412, 1984.

Carrol, C.L., Jeffrey, R.B., Jr., Federle, M.P., and Vernacchia, F.S.: CT evaluation of mediastinal infections. J. Comput. Assist. Tomogr. 11:449, 1987.

Carter, A.R., Sostman, H.D., Curtis, A.M., and Swett, H.A.: Thoracic alterations after cardiac surgery. AJR 140:475, 1983.

Cheung, E.H., Carver, J.M., Jones, E.L., et al.: Mediastinitis after cardiac valve operations. J. Thorac. Cardiovasc. Surg. 90:517, 1985.

Ebert, P.A., and Nijafi, H.: The pericardium. In Sabiston, D.C., and Spencer, F.C. (eds.): Surgery of the Chest, ed. 5. Philadelphia, W.B. Saunders, 1990.

Florence, S.H., Hutton, L.C., McKenzie, F.N., and Kostuk W.J.: Cardiac transplantation: Postoperative chest radiographs. Can. Assoc. Radiol. J. 39:115, 1988.

Fyke III, F.E., Tancredi, R.G., Shub, C., et al.: Detection of intrapericardial hematoma after open heart surgery: The roles of echocardiography and computed tomography. J. Am. Coll. Cardiol. 5:1496, 1985.

Glanz, S., Ravin, C.E., and Deren, M.M.: Benign pneumoperitoneum following median sternotomy incision. AJR 131:267, 1978.

Goldstein, J.P., and Wechsler, A.S.: Heart transplantation. Invest. Radiol. 20:446, 1985.

Goodman, L.R.: Postoperative chest radiograph: II. Alterations after major intrathoracic surgery. AJR 134:803, 1980.

Goodman, L.R., and Haasler, G.B.: Mediastinal and sternal infection: Imaging strategies. Cardiac Surgery: State of the Art Reviews 2:445, 1988.

Goodman, L.R., Teplick, S.K., and Kay, H.R.: Computed tomography of the normal sternum. AJR 141:219, 1983a.

Goodman, L.R., Kay, H.R., Teplick, S.K., and Mundth, E.D.: Complications of median sternotomy: Computed tomographic evaluation. AJR 141:225, 1983b.

Greenwald, L.V., Baisden, C.E., and Symbas, P.N.: Rib fractures in coronary bypass patients: Radionuclide detection. Radiology 148:553, 1983.

Grossi, E.A., Culliford, A.T., Krieger, K.H., et al.: A survey of 77 major infectious complications of median sternotomy: A review of 7,949 consecutive operative procedures. Ann. Thorac. Surg. 40:214, 1985.

Guthaner, D.F., Schnittger, I., Wright, A., and Wexler, L.: Diagnostic challenges following cardiac transplantation. Radiol. Clin. North Am. 25:367, 1987.

Hélénon, O., Folinais, D., Cornud, F., et al.: Apport de la tomodensitométrie dans l'évolution des médiastinites après sternotomie pour chirurgie cardiaque. J. Radiol. 68:237, 1987.

Henry, D.A., Jolles, H., Berberich, J.J., and Schmelzer, V.: The post-cardiac surgery chest radiograph: A clinically integrated approach. J. Thorac. Imaging 4:20, 1989a.

Henry, D.A., Corcoran, H.L., Lewis, T.D., et al.: Orthotopic cardiac transplantation: Evaluation with CT. Radiology 170:343, 1989b.

Iannuzzi, M., and Pethy, T.L.: The diagnosis, pathogenesis, and treatment of adult respiratory distress syndrome. J. Thorac. Imaging 1:1, 1986.

Ikäheimo, M.J., Heikki, V.H., Airaksinen, K.E., et al.: Pericardial effusion after cardiac surgery: Incidence, relation to the type of surgery, antithrombotic therapy, and early coronary bypass graft patency. Am. Heart J. 116:97, 1988.

Jacobs, M.L., and Austin, W.G.: Acquired aortic valve disease. In Sabiston, D.C., and Spencer, F.C. (eds.): Surgery of the Chest, ed. 5. Philadelphia, W.B. Saunders, 1990.

Jones, E.L., Shwarzmann, S.W., Check, W.A., and Hatcher, C.R., Jr.: Infection, thrombosis, and emboli associated with intracardiac prosthesis. In Sabiston, D.C., and Spencer, F. C. (eds.): Surgery of the Chest, ed. 5. Philadelphia, W.B. Saunders, 1990.

Kaminsky, M.E., Rodan, B.A., Osborne, D.R., et al.: Postpericardiotomy syndrome. AJR 138:503, 1982.

Katzberg, R.W., Whitehouse, G.H., and deWeese, J.A.: The early radiologic findings in the adult chest after cardiopulmonary bypass surgery. Cardiovasc. Radiol. 1:205, 1978.

Killian, D.M., Furiasse, J.G., Scanlon, P.J., et al.: Constrictive pericarditis after cardiac surgery. Am. Heart J. 18:563, 1989.

Kutcher, M.A., King III, S.B., Alimurung, B.N., et al.: Constrictive pericarditis as a complication of cardiac surgery: Recognition of an entity. Am. J. Cardiol. 50:742, 1982.

Landay, M.J., Mootz, A.R., and Estrera, A.S.: Apparatus seen on chest radiographs after cardiac surgery in adults. Radiology 174:477, 1990.

Moore, E.H., Farmer, D.W., Geller, S.C., et al.: Computed tomography in the diagnosis of iatrogenic false aneurysms of the ascending aorta. AJR 142:1117, 1984.

Nath, P.H., and Soto, B.: Computed tomography in assessing a high risk patient for "redo" sternotomy. (Abstract.) Circulation 72:182, 1985.

Pairolero, P.C., and Arnold, P.G.: Management of recalcitrant median sternotomy wounds. J. Thorac. Cardiovasc. Surg. 88:357, 1984.

Rankin, J.S., and Smith, L.R.: Utilization of the internal mammary arteries for coronary artery bypass. In Sabiston, D.C., and Spencer, F.C. (eds.): Surgery of the Chest, ed. 5. Philadelphia, W.B. Saunders, 1990.

Reitz, B.A.: Cardiac and cardiopulmonary transplantation. Cardiovasc. Clin. 17:347, 1987.

Roberts, W.C.: Pathology of coronary athersclerosis. In Sabiston, D.C., and Spencer, F.C. (eds.): Surgery of the Chest, ed. 5. Philadelphia, W.B. Saunders, 1990.

Rutledge, R., Applebaum, R.E., and Kim, B.J.: Mediastinal infection after open heart surgery. Surgery 97:88, 1985.

Saffitz, J.E., Ganote, C.E., Peterson, C.E., and Roberts, W.C.: False aneurysm of ascending aorta after aortocoronary bypass grafting. Am. J. Cardiol. 52:907, 1983.

Salit, I.E., Detsky, A.S., Simor, A.E., et al.: Gallium-67 scanning in the diagnosis of postoperative sternal osteomyelitis: Concise communication. J. Nucl. Med. 24:1001, 1983.

Shirazi, K.K., Amendola, M.A., Tisnado, J., et al.: Radiographic findings in the chest of patients following cardiac transplantation. Cardiovasc. Intervent. Radiol. 6:1, 1983.

Smith, P., Qureshi, S., and Yacoub, M.: Dehiscence of infected aortocoronary vein graft suture lines: Cause of late pseudoaneurysm of ascending aorta. Br. Heart J. 50:193, 1983.

Soulen, R.L.: Cardiovascular system. In Schwartz, E.E. (ed.): The radiology of complications in medical practice. Baltimore University Park Press, 1984.

Spencer, F.C.: Acquired disease of the mitral valve. In Sabiston, D.C., and Spencer, F.C. (eds.): Surgery of the Chest, ed. 5. Philadelphia, W.B. Saunders, 1990.

Steiner, R.M., Mintz, G., Morse, D., et al.: The radiology of cardiac valve prostheses. Radiographics 8:277, 1988.

Stevenson, L.W., Child, J.S., Laks, H., and Kern, L.: Incidence and significance of early pericardial effusions after cardiac surgery. Am. J. Cardiol. 54:848, 1984.

Sullivan, K.L., Steiner, R.M., Smullens, S.N., et al.: Pseudoaneurysm of the ascending aorta following cardiac surgery. Chest 33:138, 1988.

Takasugi, E., and Godwin, J.D.: Surgical defects of the pericardium: Radiographic findings. AJR 152:951, 1989.

Thorsen, M.K., and Goodman, L.R.: Extracardiac complications of cardiac surgery. Semin. Roentgenol. 23:32, 1988.

Thorsen, M.K., Goodman, L.R., Sagel, S.S., et al.: Ascending aorta complications of cardiac surgery: CT evaluation. J. Comput. Assist. Tomogr. 10:219, 1986.

Wheeler, W.E., Rubis, L.J., Jones, C.W., and Harrah, J.D.: Etiology and prevention of topical cardiac hypothermia-induced phrenic nerve injury and left lower lobe atelectasis during cardiac surgery. Chest 88:680, 1985.

Wilcox, P., Baile, E.M., Hards, J., et al.: Phrenic nerve function and its relationship to atelectasis after coronary artery bypass surgery. Chest 93:693, 1988.

Ziter, F.M., Jr.: Major thoracic dehiscence: Radiographic considerations. Radiology 122:587, 1977.

16

Acute Aortic Disease and Peripheral Venous Disease

■

Elliot O. Lipchik
M. Kristin Thorsen

Radiology is no longer restricted to diagnostics. The interventional radiologist, with his or her special skills and knowledge of high-technology equipment, has become a vital team member in the assessment, care, and treatment of sick patients. The more critical the patient's illness, the greater the need for the most rapid and least interventional therapeutic procedure. The exact diagnosis and localization of a potentially life-threatening process—for example, propagation of a large thrombus from the calf veins to the large femoral vein—are requisites to the proper therapeutic procedure.

This chapter discusses the diagnosis and management of the diseases of the aorta, deep venous thrombosis, superior vena cava syndrome, inferior vena cava filter placement, and lung disease causing massive bleeding. The essential and interdependent nature of the roles of accurate, rapid diagnoses and interventional therapy is made obvious.

Rapid changes in both fields are occurring. For example, magnetic resonance imaging (MRI) has, to date, limited application in a critically ill patient and therefore limited mention in this chapter, but it has the potential to eventually replace angiography in several regions of the body. Therefore, the clinician should become more aware of the radiologist's skills and tools in the realms of both diagnostics and therapeutics. Conversely, radiologists have to be increasingly concerned with the clinical needs and must become more expert in the handling and usage of drugs and in understanding physiologic parameters.

AORTIC DISSECTION

Aortic dissection is a true medical emergency in which prompt diagnosis and treatment directly influ-

ence patient survival (Sorensen and Olsen, 1964). Approximately 2000 cases of acute aortic dissection are estimated to occur in the United States each year (Anagnostopoulos et al., 1972). In a series of 505 untreated cases of aortic dissection, 21% of patients died within 24 hours, 37% died within 48 hours, 49% died within 4 days, 74% died within 2 weeks, and more than 90% died within 3 months of diagnosis (Hirst et al., 1958). With the use of current methods of diagnosis and treatment, the mortality rate at 3 months has decreased significantly (DeBakey et al., 1955; Wheat, 1980; Wheat et al., 1965).

Aortic dissection usually begins as a tear in the intima. The tear allows blood to enter the aortic wall, separating the layers of the media. The tear most commonly starts either in the proximal ascending aorta near the aortic root, or in the descending aorta, distally in relation to the origin of the left subclavian artery. These two areas are thought to bear the maximum force of each systolic pulse. The increased mechanical stresses at these points and an underlying abnormality of the media are thought to be the dominant factors in the pathogenesis of aortic dissection (Dalen et al., 1980; Roberts, 1981). A small number of aortic dissections occur in the absence of an intimal tear. In 1920, Krukenberg postulated that rupture of the vasa vasorum within the aortic wall could cause an aortic dissection or dissecting hematoma.

Debakey and colleagues (1965) classified aortic dissections into three types, based on the site of the intimal tear and the extent of the false channel. Debakey Type I dissections involve the ascending aorta, extend around the aortic arch, and involve the descending aorta. Type II dissections involve only the ascending aorta, and Type III dissections begin at a site distal to the origin of the left subclavian artery and involve only the descending aorta. Daily and associates (1970) proposed a simpler classification, whereby Type A dissections involve only the ascending aorta and Type B dissections are limited to the descending aorta. Debakey Type I and II dissections or Type A dissections are considered surgical emergencies because they may dissect proximally to cause pericardial effusion and tamponade, acute aortic insufficiency, or acute myocardial infarction (Dalen et al., 1980; DeBakey et al., 1955, 1965). Type III or Type B aortic dissections are treated medically unless persistent pain, ischemia to major organs, or impending rupture occurs (Wheat, 1980).

Clinically, males are affected more commonly than females. Peak incidence occurs in the sixth or seventh decades, with hypertension as the most common predisposing condition. Other factors include cystic medial necrosis, coarctation, congenital aortic stenosis, bicuspid aortic valve, and pregnancy (Gore, 1953; Slater and DeSanctis, 1976). Iatrogenic injury secondary to thoracic surgery or cannulation for aortic bypass can also lead to aortic dissection (Saffitz et al., 1983; Thorsen et al., 1986a). The most common presenting symptom is chest pain, which occurs in greater than 90% of patients. Other, less common symptoms are syncope, transient stroke, congestive heart failure, symptoms of peripheral or intestinal ischemia, and hematuria (Slater, 1983; Weisman and Adams, 1944; Wolfe, 1980). On physical examination, the patient may appear to be in shock but may have markedly elevated blood pressure. Other patients are hypotensive. Pulses may be decreased or absent. Murmurs of aortic insufficiency, pericardial friction rub, or bruits may be noted (Lindsay and Hirst, 1967; Pate et al., 1976).

Plain chest radiographs are often nonspecific in the diagnosis of aortic dissection. Mediastinal widening is the most common abnormality encountered. Displacement of intimal calcification of more than 6 mm may be helpful in suggesting the diagnosis (Eyler and Clark, 1965) (Fig. 16–1). Other findings include disparity in size between the ascending and descending aorta, indistinct aortic contour, double aortic knob, or localized aneurysm formation. Displacement of mediastinal structures or pleural effusions may also occur (Dee et al., 1983; Kaufman and White, 1980; Smith and Jang, 1983; Wyman, 1957). Slater and DeSanctis (1976) noted normal chest radiographs in five of 116 patients with proven aortic dissections.

Numerous reports have described the value of two-dimensional echocardiography in the evaluation of patients with suspected aortic dissections (McLeod et al., 1983; Victor et al., 1981). Dee and co-workers (1985) evaluated 56 patients and identified all of 13 proximal dissections. Five Type B dissections were missed, and 38 cases were truly negative. The echocardiographic criteria of aortic dissection are (1) aortic dilatation in excess of 42 mm and (2) detection of an intimal flap, combined with high-frequency oscillation of this structure. Two-dimensional echocardiography combined with Doppler may detect differ-

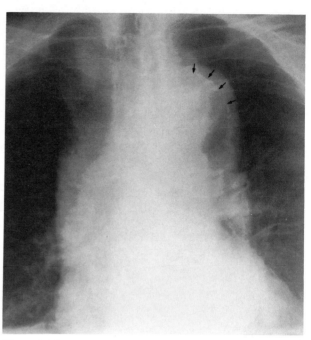

Figure 16–1. Type A aortic dissection. Chest radiograph shows enlarged aorta. Displacement of peripheral intimal calcification appears medially (*arrows*), suggesting the diagnosis.

ential flow in the true and false channels and may detect aortic regurgitation. The major limitation of two-dimensional echocardiography is that the study is operator-dependent. Also, problems in interpretation can result from reverberation artifacts and the lack of a suitable imaging window. In particular, the diagnosis of Type B dissections is extremely difficult (Jewitt, 1983).

Magnetic resonance imaging has been shown to be an effective imaging method of evaluating patients with aortic dissection. It is noninvasive and does not require contrast media. The sensitivity and specificity of MRI in evaluating patients with aortic dissection are 96% and 90%, respectively, for experienced observers (Kersting-Sommerhoff et al., 1988). The intimal flap appears as a linear structure of medium-signal intensity between the signal void of flowing blood in the true and false channels (Fig. 16–2). Thrombosed false channels and slow flow are the main problems in differentiating a dissection from a thrombosed aneurysm. Although MRI seems to be a reliable screening procedure, a major limitation is its inability to study the hemodynamically unstable patient requiring life-support equipment (Geisinger et al., 1985; White and Higgins, 1989).

Angiography and cineangiography are accurate techniques for evaluating patients with aortic dissections (Gutierrez et al., 1980; Stein and Steinberg, 1968). Angiographic findings can be divided into direct and indirect signs of aortic dissection. Direct signs include identification of two channels separated by an intimal flap (Fig. 16–3). Indirect signs include a thickening of the aortic wall greater than 5 to 6 mm, ulcer-like projections, spiraling of the true chan-

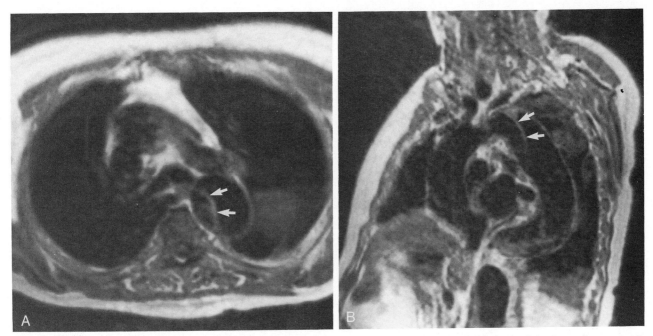

Figure 16–2. Type B aortic dissection. *A,* Axial magnetic resonance image (MRI) shows intimal flap (*arrows*) in descending aorta. *B,* Sagittal MRI also demonstrates intimal flap (*arrows*) in the descending aorta.

nel around the false channel, aortic regurgitation, abnormal catheter position, and aortic branch occlusions (Hayashi et al., 1974). Possible false-negative examinations can be obtained because of equal opacification of the true and false channels, nonopacification of the false channel due to delayed flow or thrombus, and incorrect positioning in visualizing the intimal flap in profile. False-positive results may be

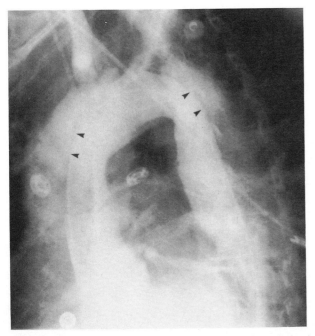

Figure 16–3. Type A aortic dissection. Aortogram shows intimal flap (*arrowheads*) in the ascending aorta and descending aorta.

caused by layering of contrast material within the aorta, thickening of the aortic wall, or branch occlusions from other pre-existing conditions (Hayashi et al., 1974). Angiography is invasive and not without complications. At present, angiography should be reserved for patients who have indeterminate computed tomographic examinations.

Currently, computed tomography (CT) is the diagnostic method of choice in the evaluation of patients with suspected aortic dissection. Several studies have documented the value of high-resolution CT used with dynamic scanning techniques (Godwin et al., 1980; Larde et al., 1980; Thorsen et al., 1983). Moncada and associates (1981) studied 16 patients with aortic dissection who underwent both CT and angiography, and they concluded that CT was as accurate as angiography in the diagnosis and classification of aortic dissection. Oudkerk and colleagues (1983) investigated 26 patients with suspected acute aortic dissection and found 21 dissections, with no false-positive or false-negative results. In two cases in the same series, CT indicated Type A dissections, while aortograms incorrectly indicated Type B dissections. In another series of 113 patients with suspected acute aortic dissection, one false-positive result and two false-negative results were obtained, with an overall accuracy of greater than 95% (Thorsen et al., 1986b). The false-negative CT results involved small focal dissections that were apparent on angiography as small ulcer-like projections from the aortic wall.

In evaluating patients with suspected aortic dissections, the CT technique is extremely important. First, an anteroposterior (AP) image of the chest is obtained to localize pre-contrast axial sections at the

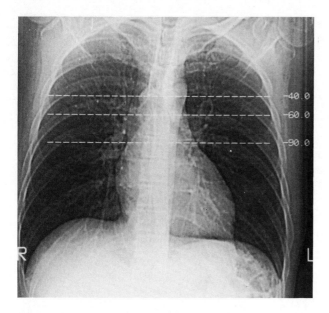

Figure 16–4. Digital radiograph is obtained in the CT evaluation of aortic dissection. Pre-contrast and post-contrast single-level dynamic scans are obtained at the level of the aortic arch, the midascending aorta, and the aortic root.

level of the aortic arch, mid–ascending aorta, and aortic root (Fig. 16–4). At each of these three preselected levels, a 50-ml bolus of 60% iodinated contrast material is injected with a power injector at a rate of 5 ml/sec. A series of eight fast (2-second) scans with a minimal interscan delay is obtained. Each single-level dynamic series is obtained on inspiration during a single breath. The diagnosis of aortic dissection is made if two contrast-filled channels separated by an intimal flap are identified within the aorta (Fig. 16–5). The differential flow of contrast in the true and false channels can also be identified using the single-level dynamic technique (Fig. 16–6).

Other less specific findings in aortic dissection include aortic widening, medial displacement of peripheral intimal calcification (Fig. 16–7), spiraling of the false lumen around the true lumen as it proceeds distally down the aorta (like the twisted ribbon sign in angiography), and extra-aortic fluid collections in the mediastinum, pericardium, retroperitoneum, or pleural spaces. Following the single-level dynamic sequences, survey scans are performed through the entire chest to detect pericardial effusions, or mediastinal or pulmonary parenchymal lesions. Pericardial effusions are found in approximately 50% of patients with Type A aortic dissections (Thorsen et al., 1983).

Proper clinical management of acute aortic dissection depends on prompt recognition and correct classification. At our institution, surgical management, medical management, or both are undertaken on the basis of the CT findings. Angiography is usually not performed except in cases of a strong clinical suspicion of aortic dissection and an equivocal CT exami-

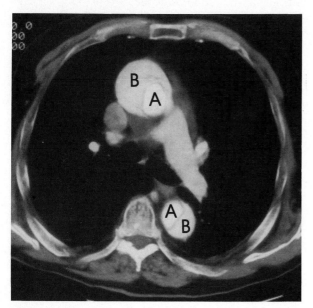

Figure 16–5. Type A aortic dissection. Contrast-enhanced scan at the level of the midascending aorta shows true (A) and false (B) lumens separated by an intimal flap.

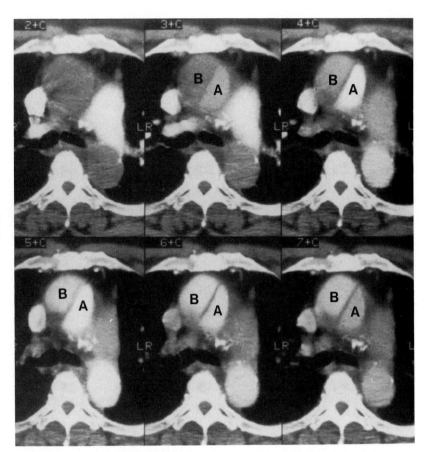

Figure 16–6. Type A aortic dissection. Single-level dynamic sequence shows the differential flow of contrast in the true (A) and false (B) channels. The true channel opacifies first.

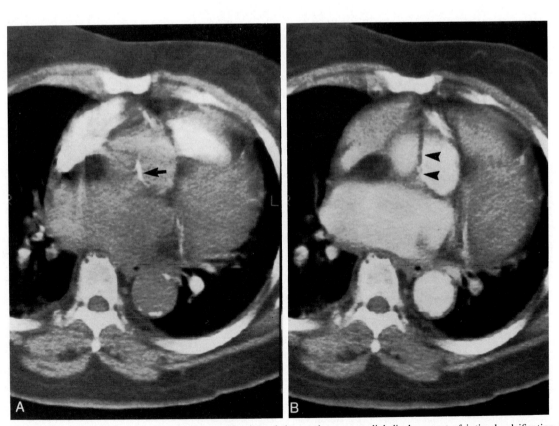

Figure 16–7. Type A aortic dissection. *A,* Prior to opacification of the aortic root, medial displacement of intimal calcification is noted (*arrow*). *B,* Following contrast enhancement, the intimal flap is well visualized (*arrowheads*). (Reprinted with permission from Thorsen, M.K., et al.: CT of aortic dissections. CRC Critical Reviews in Diagnostic Imaging. 26:291, 1986. Copyright CRC Press, Inc., Boca Raton, FL.)

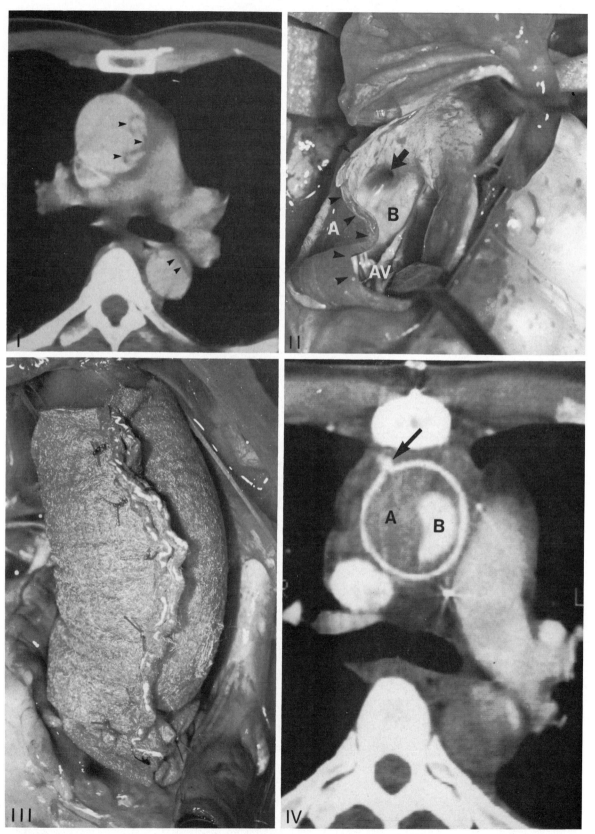

Figure 16–8. Type A dissection. *I,* Intimal flap is identified in the ascending and descending aorta (*arrowheads*). *II,* Intraoperative photograph shows false channel (A), true lumen (B), and intimal tear (*arrowheads*). Aortic valve (AV) and ostia of the coronary artery (*arrow*) are also shown. *III,* The intimal tear was repaired, and the aorta was wrapped with Teflon felt. *IV,* Postoperative scan shows Teflon felt and suture line (*arrow*) and persistence of two lumens A and B. (Reprinted with permission from Thorsen, M.K., et al.: CT of aortic dissections. CRC Critical Reviews in Diagnostic Imaging. 26:291, 1986. Copyright CRC Press, Inc., Boca Raton, FL.)

nation. Although CT does not depict the site of the intimal tear or the status of the aortic valve, these findings can be evaluated intraoperatively. Aortography detects the site of intimal tear in approximately only 60% of patients (Earnest et al., 1979).

Surgical repair of Type A dissections is aimed at preventing proximal extension, which may cause acute aortic insufficiency, pericardial tamponade, or acute myocardial infarction. The surgical approach to these patients consists of either (1) primary repair of the intimal tear, with oversewing of the true and false channels plus wrapping of the aorta with Teflon felt, or (2) resection of a segment of ascending aorta with interposition of a Dacron graft between the aortic valve and dissection. The aortic valve is resuspended or replaced if the valve is irreversibly damaged or bicuspid. Coronary artery bypass grafting may also be necessary to reconstitute coronary flow (Miller, 1983). Despite surgical repair, approximately 80% of patients have persistent patency of the false channel as demonstrated by postoperative CT and angiography (Godwin et al., 1981; Guthaner et al., 1979) (Fig. 16–8).

ACUTE AORTIC TRAUMA AND GREAT VESSEL INJURIES

The increasing incidence of traumatic aortic rupture has paralleled the increasing number of high-speed vehicular deceleration injuries. These injuries are being encountered more often in the hospital setting since the advent of regional trauma centers and rapid helicopter transportation systems. Prompt diagnosis and surgical treatment of these injuries are essential. Eighty-six percent of patients with traumatic aortic rupture are dead upon arrival at the hospital. Of the remaining 14% who arrive at the hospital alive, approximately one third die within 24 hours, and three fourths die within 15 days, if untreated (Parmley et al., 1958).

Traumatic aortic rupture or great vessel injury can result from vertical or horizontal deceleration injuries, or crush or blunt injuries. Shearing, bending, and torsion stresses are the major mechanical factors involved. The greatest strain placed on the aortic isthmus occurs where shearing stress results from the difference in deceleration between the fixed aortic arch and the mobile descending aorta. The indirect force of increased intravascular pressure may also play a role in aortic injuries.

An intriguing explanation of traumatic aortic rupture is pinching of the aorta between the spine and the anterior bony thorax during chest compression. Compression forces the manubrium, first rib, or the medial end of the clavicle to rotate, posteriorly and inferiorly, causing impact on the vertebral column. Thus, interposed vascular structures are compressed and cut. This mechanism would explain aortic tears proximal or distal to the aortic isthmus as well as give an explanation for the injuries to the origins of the great vessels (Crass et al., 1990).

Eighty percent to 90% of aortic ruptures occur at the aortic isthmus, just distally in relation to the origin of the subclavian artery. Other, less common locations are the ascending aorta, at a location proximal to the origin of the innominate artery; the aortic arch; and the distal descending aorta, at the aortic hiatus of the diaphragm.

Pathologically, the aortic tear is usually transverse or longitudinal, with the former being more common. Tears involve all layers of the aorta to varying degrees. Superimposed aortic dissection is rare but can result from intimal and medial laceration, with subsequent rupture through the adventitia. When the tear involves all layers of the aortic wall and surrounding structures, exsanguination occurs. When ruptures are contained by partially disrupted adventitia, parietal pleura, or mediastinal structures, a false aneurysm forms (Kirsh and Sloan, 1977).

Avulsion of the innominate artery from the aortic arch is the second most common arterial injury in the chest. Subclavian ruptures can also result from deceleration injuries. Rarely, subclavian rupture secondary to a fractured first rib or clavicle has been reported. The carotid arteries are rarely injured within the chest (Crawford and Crawford, 1984).

Clinically, one third to one half of patients with aortic rupture have no external evidence of thoracic injury at the time of presentation. The most common complaint is retrosternal or interscapular pain. Less frequently encountered symptoms include dysphagia from esophageal compression, stridor, dyspnea, hoarseness, and symptoms of ischemia. Other findings are the acute onset of upper-extremity hypertension, difference in pulse amplitude between the upper and lower extremities, and the presence of a harsh systolic murmur over the precordium or intrascapular area. In innominate artery avulsion, the brachial or radial pulse and blood pressure may be diminished. In transection of the subclavian artery, the radial pulse may be absent, or a pulsatile mass with a bruit in the root of the neck may be present. The most important clinical consideration in the evaluation of thoracic arterial injuries is the history of a deceleration injury (Kirsh and Sloan, 1977; Parmley et al., 1958).

In the setting of acute chest trauma, chest radiography can have an important triage role in determining which patients need further evaluation. Over the past 2 decades, numerous signs of aortic rupture have been reported. These include a widened mediastinum, depression of the left main bronchus, deviation of the trachea to the right, left pleural effusion, first rib fracture, deviation of a nasogastric tube, widened paravertebral stripe, and fractured spine, sternum, or clavicle (Mirvis et al., 1987a) (Fig. 16–9). Unfortunately, none of the signs has significant sensitivity or specificity to preclude the frequent use of angiography. In the presence of an abnormal mediastinum on chest radiographs, the positive yield of angiography for aortic rupture is usually between 10% and 20%

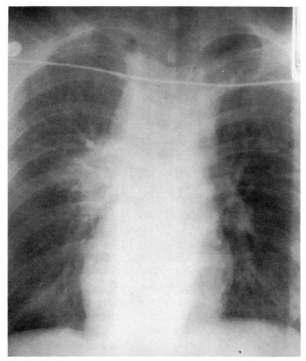

Figure 16–9. Aortic rupture. Chest radiograph demonstrates marked widening of the mediastinum in the setting of deceleration injury. A pulmonary contusion is also seen in the right midlung field.

(Gundry et al., 1982). Mirvis and colleagues (1987b) have shown that a normal supine chest radiograph in a patient with chest trauma has a negative predictive value for aortic rupture of 96%.

The role of CT in the diagnosis of traumatic thoracic arterial injuries is controversial. Heiberg and Wolverson (1985) evaluated 20 patients with suspected aortic rupture with CT and correctly identified six out of seven patients with aortic disruptions. Findings included, singly or in combination, a linear lucency, which represented the aortic tear; increased caliber of the aorta in comparison with the more proximal normal aorta; and deformity of the aortic luminal contour (Fig. 16–10). In Heiberg and Wolverson's series, the extent of mediastinal hemorrhage and pleural fluid collections seemed unrelated to the presence or absence of aortic injury.

Ishikawa and associates (1989) performed CT in 78 patients with abnormal mediastinal contours on chest radiographs. In 30 cases (38%), no evidence of mediastinal hematoma was demonstrated, and all of these patients had a benign clinical course. Forty-eight patients (62%) had mediastinal hematoma demonstrated on the CT scan. Of the remaining 48 patients, eight had aortic rupture, four had proximal great vessel injury, and 36 had negative angiograms. Contiguous peri-aortic or peri-arterial hematoma strongly suggested aortic rupture or proximal branch injury (Fig. 16–11). These investigators concluded that the patients can be followed without angiography when the CT results are negative for direct signs of great vessel injury or mediastinal hematoma, and that angiography should be performed when the CT scan demonstrates direct evidence of aortic rupture or peri-aortic, focal, or diffuse mediastinal hematoma.

Miller and co-workers (1989) used CT and angiography to evaluate 104 consecutive patients who had two features: mechanism of injury consistent with a major vessel injury and radiographic suspicion of an

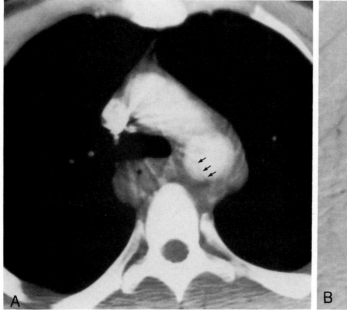
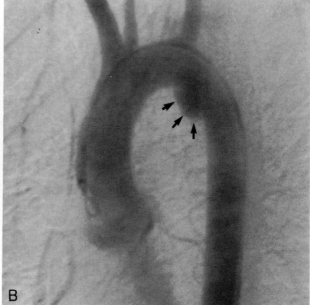

Figure 16–10. Aortic rupture. *A,* Computed tomography shows linear lucency through posterior wall of descending aorta, which represents an aortic tear (*arrows*). Hematoma adjacent to descending aorta also appears. *B,* Aortogram confirms aortic rupture (*arrows*), which is distal to origin of subclavian artery.

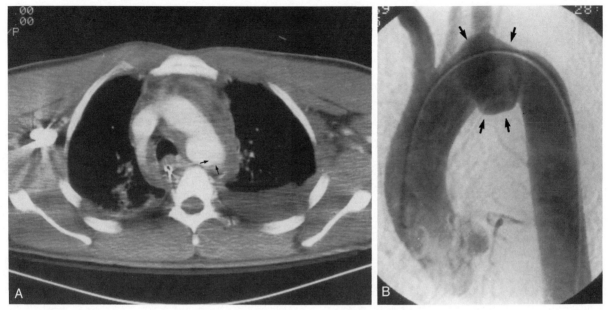

Figure 16–11. Aortic rupture. *A,* Extensive mediastinal hematoma and a left pleural effusion are present. Irregularity of the descending aorta with a linear lucency is present, indicating rupture (*arrows*). *B,* Aortogram confirms aortic rupture (*arrows*).

arterial injury on the plain chest roentgenogram. Eleven patients (10.6%) had positive angiograms for major vessel injury. Twenty-six patients had mediastinal hematomas detected by CT. Angiograms of six of these 26 patients were positive for aortic rupture. Sixty-seven CT scans were negative for mediastinal hematoma or vascular injury. The group with negative CT results included two patients with aortic transections, two with vertebral artery disruptions, and one with subclavian arterial injury. The sensitivity of chest CT for major thoracic vessel injury was 55%, with 65% specificity. Of the 11 injuries detected with angiography, five (45%) were missed by CT. This

study concluded that aggressive angiography should be used in patients with suspected aortic injuries.

At most centers, angiography continues to be the highest standard for the evaluation of patients with suspected aortic rupture and great vessel injuries (Fig. 16–12).

THORACIC AORTIC ANEURYSMS

Atherosclerotic aneurysms are the most common type of aneurysms involving the thoracic aorta. Other causes of aneurysm include cystic medial degenera-

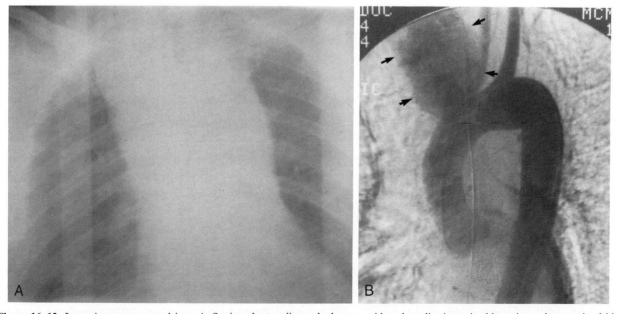

Figure 16–12. Innominate artery avulsion. *A,* Supine chest radiograph shows a widened mediastinum in this patient who sustained blunt trauma. *B,* Aortogram shows disruption of the innominate artery with a large false aneurysm (*arrows*).

tion, myxomatous degeneration, infection, trauma, poststenotic dilatation, and aortitis.

The majority of aneurysms involving the ascending aorta result from either cystic medial or myxomatous degeneration. These aneurysms are fusiform in nature and frequently involve the aortic root and proximal aortic arch. These types of aneurysms are often complicated by intimal tears and dissection. Although rare, luetic aneurysms also involve the proximal aorta. Atherosclerosis is an unusual cause of aneurysm formation in this location but is the primary cause of distal aortic arch aneurysms. These aneurysms are saccular and most often involve the inferior surface of the arch. The descending aorta is the most common site of aneurysm formation in the chest. All types of aneurysms can involve this segment, but atherosclerotic aneurysms are by far the most common. These aneurysms may be contiguous into the abdomen, although a second atherosclerotic aneurysm of the infrarenal aorta is seen in approximately 25% of patients (Crawford and Crawford, 1984; Pressler and McNamara, 1980).

The prognosis for untreated thoracic aneurysms is poor and is related to size at the time of diagnosis. Rupture occurs in 2% of aneurysms smaller than 5 cm in diameter, in 12% of aneurysms between 5 and 10 cm, and in 44% of aneurysms greater than 10 cm (Fomon et al., 1967).

Thoracic aneurysms are typically asymptomatic and are discovered on routine chest radiographs. When they are symptomatic, the most common presenting complaint is chest pain. Aneurysmal enlargement can also cause compression or obstruction of adjacent structures, resulting in postobstructive pneumonia, stridor, wheezing, dyspnea, dysphagia, hoarseness, or superior vena cava syndrome (Webb and Kelly, 1986).

Plain chest radiographic findings in symptomatic patients include fusiform or saccular dilatation of the aorta (Fig. 16–13). In some cases, linear calcification may clearly outline the walls, and plain films may be sufficient for diagnosis. Progressive enlargement of the aorta, a widened mediastinum, pleural effusion, or pericardial effusion, singly or in combination, may indicate rupture. Cardiomegaly and congestive heart failure may be secondary to aortic insufficiency. Other findings include atelectasis, airway narrowing, and elevation of the diaphragm from phrenic nerve compression.

Computed tomography may be helpful when chest radiographs cannot differentiate between a mediastinal mass and an aneurysm. Optimum scan technique should consist of contiguous 10-mm axial sections through the mediastinum with the use of rapid dynamic scanning and a bolus injection of approximately 150 ml of intravenous contrast, preferably with a power injector. The findings of thoracic aortic aneurysms on CT scans include fusiform dilatation of the aorta with an AP diameter greater than 4 cm, intraluminal thrombus, and peripheral intimal calcification (Fig. 16–14). Saccular aneurysms can be differen-

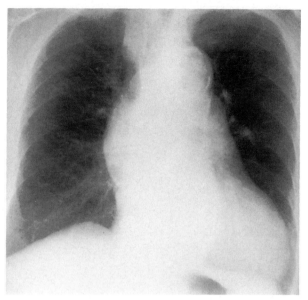

Figure 16–13. Chest radiograph shows a large aneurysm of the ascending and descending aorta with thin linear calcification.

tiated from mediastinal masses with the use of intravenous contrast. Even in the case of extensive thrombosis within the aneurysm, contrast-enhanced thin-section CT (slice thickness of 5 mm or 3 mm) can usually allow identification of the neck of the aneurysm (Fig. 16–15). Displacement of adjacent structures and bone erosion are also well demonstrated. Peri-aortic or mediastinal hematoma, or pleural and pericardial effusions, may indicate leakage (Godwin and Korobkin, 1983; Posniak et al., 1989).

Magnetic resonance imaging is an excellent method for evaluating stable patients with thoracic aneurysm. Its major advantage is that intravenous contrast is

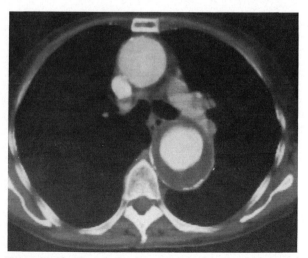

Figure 16–14. Thoracic aortic aneurysm. Computed tomography demonstrates descending aortic aneurysm, which contains intraluminal thrombus, a contrast-enhanced patent lumen, and peripheral intimal calcification.

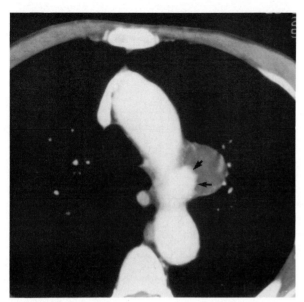

Figure 16–15. Saccular thoracic aneurysms. Computed tomography shows saccular aneurysm projecting off the inferior surface of the arch. The neck of the aneurysm fills with contrast material (*arrows*).

not necessary. Magnetic resonance imaging can assess size, shape, branch involvement, tracheobronchial compression, and peri-aortic hematoma; however, it cannot detect wall calcification (Fig. 16–16). It is an inappropriate technique for critically ill or unstable patients (White and Higgins, 1989).

Aortography can be helpful in preoperative planning. It can show the morphologic features and extent of a thoracic aneurysm, including its relationship to the coronary or brachiocephalic arteries, the presence of aortic valvular insufficiency, and aneurysm formation elsewhere in the aorta (Randall and Jarmolowski, 1983). Aortography may be limited in its ability to show adjacent structures, peri-aortic hematoma, and the extent of intraluminal thrombus.

ABDOMINAL AORTIC ANEURYSMS

Abdominal aortic aneurysm is a potentially lethal disease that is becoming more frequent as the general population ages. Atherosclerosis is the most common cause of aneurysm formation. Other causes include syphilis, cystic medial degeneration, trauma, and infection.

Most abdominal aortic aneurysms originate below the level of the renal arteries and extend into the common iliac arteries. Actual involvement of the renal or external iliac arteries is unusual. In a series of 170 abdominal aortic aneurysms, only three involved the renal arteries (Imparato and Riles, 1989).

Untreated abdominal aortic aneurysms are associated with a poor prognosis. In a series of 138 patients with untreated abdominal aortic aneurysms, 31% of patients with aneurysms less than 6 cm in diameter

and 43% of patients with aneurysms larger than 6 cm died from rupture within 2 years of diagnosis (Szilagyi et al., 1972). In an autopsy series of 473 patients with abdominal aortic aneurysm, 25% of patients died because of rupture. The frequency of rupture appeared to be related to size of the aneurysm; rupture occurs in 9.5% of patients with aneurysms less than 4 cm in diameter and 60.5% of patients with aneurysms greater than 10 cm in diameter (Darling et al., 1977). Because elective surgical mortality is relatively low (2% to 4%), as compared with a mortality greater than 50% in emergency operations, surgical intervention is recommended in suitable patients who have aneurysms larger than 4 cm in diameter (Crawford and Hess, 1989; Thompson et al., 1975).

Most patients with abdominal aortic aneurysms are asymptomatic, although abnormal abdominal pulsations or pain in the abdomen, back, flank, shoulder, or groin may be presenting symptoms. Symptoms from abdominal aortic aneurysms may mimic gastrointestinal or urologic abnormalities. The diagnosis can be made by physical examination in 75% of patients with palpation of a pulsatile midline abdominal mass. Gastrointestinal bleeding in a patient with an abdominal aortic aneurysm or a prior repair of an aneurysm may indicate an aortoduodenal fistula. Sudden vascular collapse and shock may indicate acute rupture (Crawford and Crawford, 1984).

Routine radiographs of the abdomen or lumbar spine in the AP, lateral, or oblique projections can often demonstrate a retroperitoneal mass. Linear calcifications outline the aneurysm on plain films in 55% to 83% of cases (Crane, 1955; Estes, 1950) (Fig. 16–17). For the diagnosis of asymptomatic aortic aneurysm, ultrasonography is the standard method,

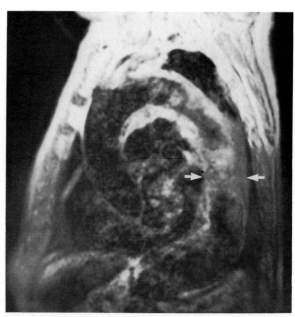

Figure 16–16. Thoracic aneurysm. Sagittal T_1-weighted MRI with cardiac gating shows atherosclerotic aneurysm of the aorta (*arrows*).

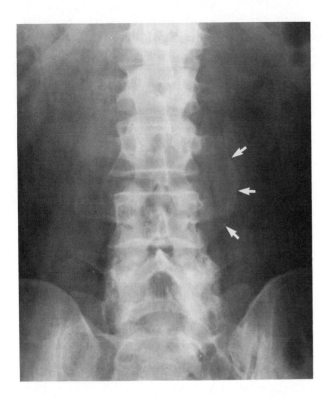

Figure 16–17. Plain-film abdominal radiograph shows a calcified abdominal aortic aneurysm (AAA) (*arrows*).

with an accuracy of nearly 100% (Shuman et al., 1988). The size, extent, and presence of intraluminal thrombus can all be evaluated by ultrasonography (Fig. 16–18). The patent lumen is anechoic and is usually surrounded by echogenic thrombus. Calcifications are visualized as high-amplitude echoes with acoustic shadowing. The value of ultrasonography is limited in obese patients and in patients with extensive bowel gas or ileus. In addition, the origin of the renal arteries and presence of extraluminal blood are difficult to identify by ultrasonography (Shuman et al., 1988).

For evaluation of the aorta, CT is a precise imaging technique that is not operator-dependent. Measurements of the aorta obtained by CT correlate well with those found surgically. Lateral and AP diameters, length, and relationship to the renal and iliac arteries are accurately demonstrated. Contrast-enhanced scans can differentiate the patent aortic lumen from adjacent intraluminal thrombus (Fig. 16–19). Irregu-

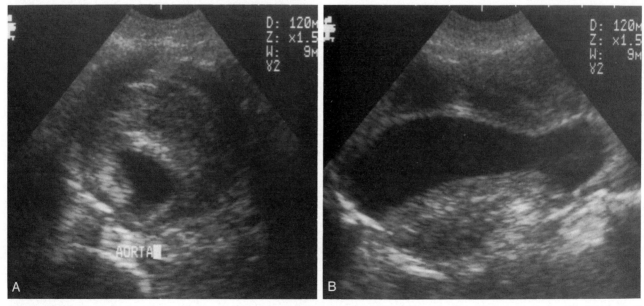

Figure 16–18. Abdominal aortic aneurysm. *A,* Transverse sonogram of the abdominal aorta shows large aneurysm with intraluminal thrombus. The anechoic patent lumen is crescent-shaped. *B,* The longitudinal view shows thrombus with patent lumen.

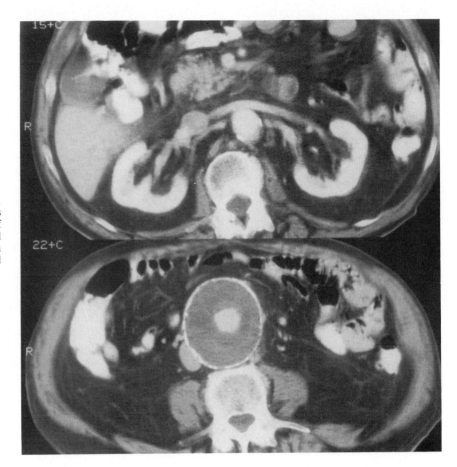

Figure 16–19. Abdominal aortic aneurysm. *Top,* Computed tomography demonstrates normal appearance of aorta at the level of the renal arteries. *Bottom,* Below the renal arteries is the abdominal aortic aneurysm which contains intraluminal thrombus and peripheral intimal calcification.

lar high-density collections adjacent to the aorta or extending into the retroperitoneal space, usually on the left, may indicate leaking or ruptured aneurysms (Fig. 16–20). Rupture may also occur anteriorly, directly into the peritoneal cavity or, rarely, into the duodenum, inferior vena cava, or iliac or renal veins (Crawford and Crawford, 1984; Lee, 1989).

Magnetic resonance imaging is also accurate in assessing abdominal aortic aneurysms. It can delineate the size and extent of the aneurysm plus its relationship to the renal arteries with the use of multiplanar imaging (Fig. 16–21). It cannot demonstrate small calcifications that may help differentiate displaced intimal calcification associated with aortic

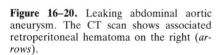

Figure 16–20. Leaking abdominal aortic aneurysm. The CT scan shows associated retroperitoneal hematoma on the right (*arrows*).

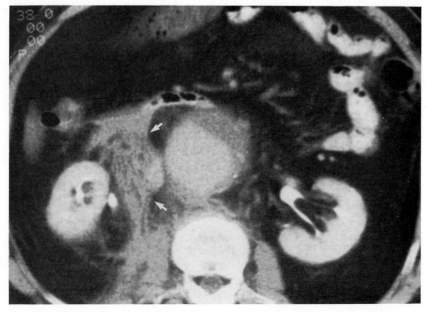

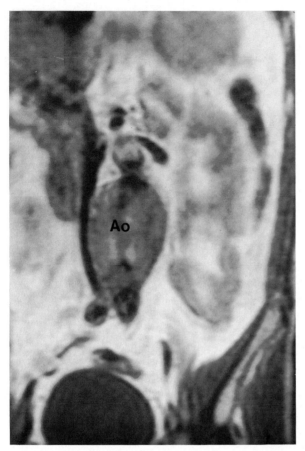

Figure 16–21. Abdominal aortic aneurysm. Coronal T_1-weighted image shows aneurysm (Ao) with slow flow.

dissection from thrombus within an aneurysm. Magnetic resonance imaging is not applicable to patients on life-support systems (LaRoy et al., 1989).

The routine use of angiography for preoperative evaluation of aneurysms, although safe, is controversial. Blood flow in the aorta may be extremely slow, resulting in poor opacification of the aneurysm and distal vessels. Increased contrast volumes and prolonged film sequences may be necessary (Lipchik and Rogoff, 1983). Angiography is usually performed if visceral branch compromise or occlusion is suspected, or if the aneurysm is thought to extend to or above the renal arteries (Fig. 16–22). Some surgeons require angiography for vessel mapping prior to surgery; however, angiography may underestimate the size and extent of the aneurysm if the aortic wall is not calcified and if only the patent lumen is opacified (Crawford and Crawford, 1984).

SUPERIOR VENA CAVA SYNDROME

Obstruction of the superior vena cava (SVC) can be caused by both benign and malignant disease. The most frequent cause of SVC syndrome is bronchogenic carcinoma, either secondary to direct invasion of the mediastinum by tumor or secondary to meta-

static lymphadenopathy. Lymphoma and metastatic disease from non-lung primary tumors, especially breast carcinoma, can also lead to obstruction of the SVC. Lochridge and associates (1979) reported that 82% of patients with SVC obstruction from malignant causes had bronchogenic carcinoma, 12% had lymphoma, and 6% had metastatic disease. Shimm and colleagues (1981) reported that 5% to 15% of lung cancers, 5% of lymphomas, and 1% of pulmonary metastases result in SVC obstruction. Twenty percent of cases result from benign causes such as fibrosing and granulomatous mediastinitis, usually from histoplasmosis. Methysergide maleate and radiation can also induce mediastinal fibrosis. Rarely, retrosternal goiters and aortic aneurysms can cause SVC obstruction. An ever-increasing cause is thrombosis of the SVC with obstruction secondary to indwelling catheters and pacemaker wires (Parish et al., 1981).

Clinically, SVC syndrome is manifested by dilatation of veins of the head, neck, arms, and upper trunk; swelling and plethora of the upper body; conjunctival edema; cerebral edema; dysphagia; and respiratory distress. The severity of the syndrome depends on the acuteness of the obstruction and on the development of collateral vessels. Some patients with complete SVC obstruction may have no symptoms if adequate collateral vessels develop over time (Ingram, 1987). These collateral pathways include the azygos, hemiazygos, internal mammary, vertebral,

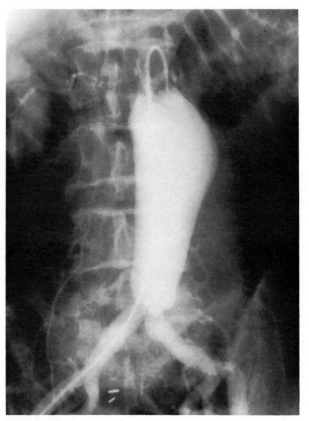

Figure 16–22. Abdominal aortic aneurysm. Aortogram shows infrarenal aneurysm that does not involve the renal arteries.

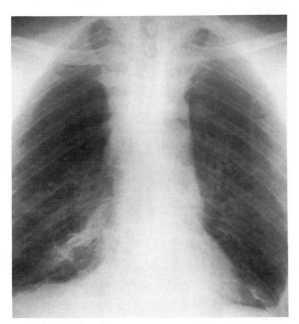

Figure 16–23. Superior vena cava obstruction. Chest radiograph shows widening of mediastinum secondary to tumor.

thoracoepigastric, lateral thoracic, superior intercostal, and paraesophageal veins (Okay and Bryk, 1969).

A normal chest radiograph can result in patients with the clinical diagnosis of SVC syndrome; however, the most common finding is mediastinal widening. Occasionally, an enlarged azygos or superior intercostal vein (the aortic nipple) may be noted on chest radiographs (Fig. 16–23). Esophagography may show downhill varices, which represent enlarged collateral paraesophageal veins.

In the past, venography and radionuclide imaging were employed to document SVC obstruction and to visualize the collateral vessels, but both of these techniques failed to provide information about the cause of the obstruction.

Contrast-enhanced CT is a rapid, noninvasive technique that can demonstrate clinically suspected abnormalities involving the SVC. Computed tomography can show collateral vessels, extrinsic compression of the SVC, or intraluminal thrombus (Fig. 16–24). Computed tomography can also depict the extent and the probable cause of the obstruction. In most cases, mediastinal tumor from a primary lung tumor, mediastinal adenopathy, calcific granulomatous mediastinitis, aneurysms, or retrosternal goiter can be differentiated by CT (Fig. 16–25). In addition, the information obtained from CT can be helpful in determining the safest route for obtaining histologic diagnosis. In cases involving the bronchi, bronchoscopy may be the method of choice, or CT-guided percutaneous needle-aspiration biopsy may be appropriate in some patients (Yedlicka et al., 1987) (Fig. 16–26).

Surgical venous bypass grafting or balloon angioplasty may be contemplated in cases of benign disease. In these cases, CT digital phlebography performed after the axial images are obtained provides the same information as standard venography. The technique involves simultaneous injection of both basilic veins with 25 ml of iodinated contrast agent during the CT digital radiography (Moncada et al., 1984) (Fig. 16–27).

Magnetic resonance imaging can demonstrate the same findings as CT and has the advantage of sagittal and coronal projections. It can also identify thrombus and slowly flowing blood. Fibrous mediastinitis may appear as a low-density mass on both partial-saturation and T_2-weighted images (Swensen et al., 1989). The disadvantage of MRI is its inability to demonstrate calcification, which may occur in granulomatous mediastinal fibrosis (Weinreb et al., 1986).

ACUTE VENOUS DISEASE

Acute venous thrombosis leading to pulmonary embolus is probably the most common preventable cause of death in hospitalized patients. The risk factors of stasis and trauma occur quite frequently in this group, particularly in the postoperative patient. Adenocarcinomas are well known to predispose patients to deep venous thrombosis (DVT).

Because the clinical manifestations of DVT are nonspecific and unreliable, finding tests that are reproducible and easy to perform has been the clinician's goal for many years (Hyers, 1989). Contrast venography, the accepted standard test, nicely defines the deep veins of the calf and thigh, and the iliac veins and lower inferior vena cava (IVC) (DeWeese and Rogoff, 1959). If properly performed, the study should be painless and without significant sequelae.

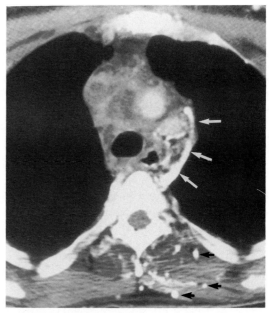

Figure 16–24. Superior vena cava obstruction—small-cell carcinoma. The CT scan shows soft-tissue tumor obliterating the superior vena cava (SVC). Collateral vessels appear in the back and in the mediastinum (*arrows*).

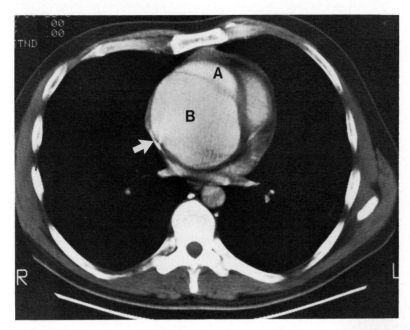

Figure 16–25. Superior vena cava obstruction. An ascending aortic dissection (A, true lumen; B, false lumen) in a patient with Marfan's syndrome causes marked compression of the SVC (*arrow*). (Reprinted with permission from Thorsen, M.K., et al.: CT of aortic dissections. CRC Critical Reviews in Diagnostic Imaging. 26:291, 1986. Copyright CRC Press, Inc., Boca Raton, FL.)

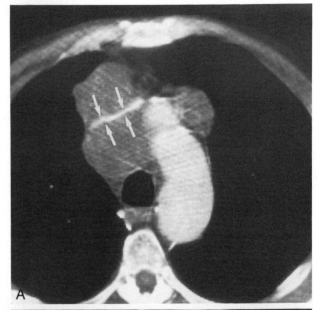

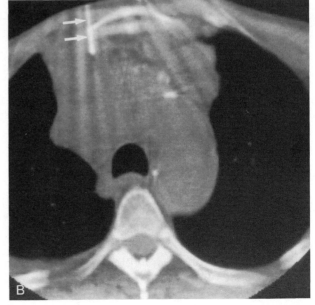

Figure 16–26. Superior vena cava syndrome—bronchogenic carcinoma. *A*, The SVC (*arrows*) is compressed between anterior and middle mediastinal tumor masses. *B*, Needle aspiration biopsy (*arrows*) was performed with CT guidance. Cytologic results were positive for large-cell undifferentiated bronchogenic carcinoma.

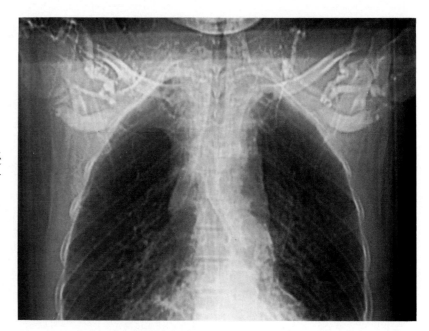

Figure 16–27. Superior vena cava obstruction. Numerous collateral vessels secondary to SVC obstruction are visualized by CT digital phlebography.

Complete lower limb phlebography should visualize all of the aforementioned veins. For a proper examination, the patient should be upright or semi-upright and non–weight-bearing on the affected extremity. To avoid causing the patient pain, iothalamate meglumine nova nonionic contrast medium should be injected, followed by saline washout solution. We recommend application of a tourniquet above the ankle to drive the contrast agent into the deep veins.

Contrast venography *is* an interventional test, is not feasible for repetition, and is often impossible to perform in sick or bedridden patients. Post-venography phlebitis (mostly superficial) has been documented in a small percentage of patients (Bettmann et al., 1987). Noninvasive tests are obviously needed, not only for diagnosis and screening, but also for repetitive follow-up for high-risk patients. The two noninterventional studies most commonly used and recommended are impedance plethysmography and Doppler ultrasonography.

Impedance Plethysmography. Impedance plethysmography measures changes in electrical impedance during inflation of and after release of a pneumatic cuff around the thigh (Gazzaniga et al., 1973). The change in impedance provides a record of the venous outflow and is therefore an *indirect* noninterventional test. With DVT, venous filling in the leg is decreased; thus, emptying of blood is decreased. Therefore, the test is insensitive to nonoccluding proximal thrombi as well as to calf vein thrombosis. It is a good screening procedure for relatively healthy outpatients but may have a high false-positive rate among sicker hospital inpatients. Muscle tension, congestive heart failure, and arterial insufficiency may all lead to false-positive results. Furthermore, in several series of prospective evaluations, patient selection was shown to be critical. For example, patients examined because of a clinical suspicion of DVT demonstrated

sensitivity of approximately 90%, whereas for the patients examined without overt clinical suspicion, the sensitivity for diagnosis of proximal vein thrombosis dropped to nearly 30% (Comerota et al., 1988). These studies, however, can be performed repetitively and can be useful for following ill, hospitalized patients (Hull et al., 1985).

Ultrasound Duplex Imaging. Duplex ultrasonography with color imaging is rapidly becoming the method of choice for the noninterventional diagnosis of DVT. The echogenic images and flow disturbances as well as the incompressibility of veins containing a thrombus are highly specific signs (Foley et al., 1989; Rose et al., 1990) (Fig. 16–28). Because plethysmography has a false-positive rate of 10% to 15% (Comerota et al., 1990), and because ultrasound equipment is portable, all patients, including those in the intensive care unit, should be studied with ultrasonography. Other causes of leg swelling that are possibly not detected by other studies, such as cysts or hematomas, can be detected by ultrasonography. A drawback of ultrasonography is that it does not demonstrate the iliac veins or the calf veins consistently (Rose et al., 1990). These studies are easy to perform repetitively and certainly more useful for ill, hospitalized patients (Hull et al., 1985). Some investigators even claim that in experienced hands, venous duplex imaging may be more sensitive than ascending phlebography (Comerota et al., 1990).

With recurrent DVT, ultrasonography is less reliable, but color Doppler ultrasonography may show the multiple channels of a recanalized vessel (Foley et al., 1989; Lipchik et al., 1976). Table 16–1 lists the indications for color Doppler imaging.

Treatment of Acute Deep Venous Thrombosis. The risk of pulmonary embolism is significant in patients with propagation of DVT from the calf (Philbrick and Becker, 1988). If patients with DVT

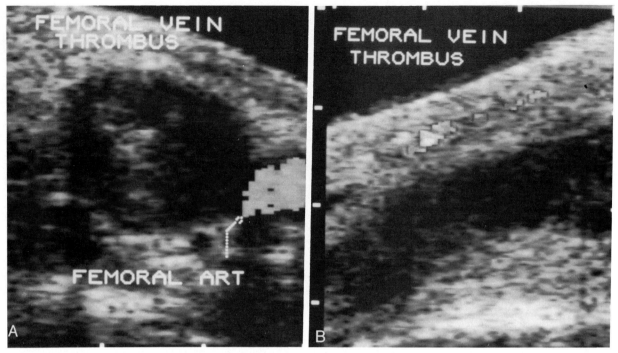

Figure 16–28. Ultrasound image of an occluding thrombus within the superficial femoral vein. This vessel was incompressible. *A* is transverse, and *B* is longitudinal to the axis of the vein. These black and white prints are from color Doppler images.

are treated with only 5 to 7 days of intravenous heparin, and if they are not placed on extended anticoagulation therapy, incidence of propagation is 10%, and the recurrence rate is almost 30% (Philbrick and Becker, 1988).

Much more frequent, but not yet as well understood or recognized, is the postphlebitic syndrome, which develops in the majority of patients who have recurrent DVT (Elliot et al., 1979; Immelman and Jeffery, 1984). If, however, patients are treated with thrombolytic therapy (first suggested by Dotter in 1972), the majority of patients followed during the same period remain asymptomatic. Three to four times as many patients treated with lytic therapy have their clots lysed as compared with those treated with heparin (Goldhaber et al., 1984). The signs and symptoms of DVT decline more rapidly following lytic therapy. Because lysis of acute thrombosis is

Table 16–1. INDICATIONS FOR COLOR DOPPLER ULTRASONOGRAPHY OF THE LOWER EXTREMITIES

Clinical suspicion of acute deep vein thrombosis.
Further evaluation of inadequate results of venography or other noninterventional study.
Suspected pulmonary embolus: screening to rule out need for pulmonary angiography if thrombosis is found.
Screening in high-risk patients (e.g., following orthopedic, neurosurgical, or prostatic surgery).
Follow-up of documented calf vein thrombus for detection of propagation if anticoagulation is not used.
Patency check of the femoral or jugular veins prior to interventional procedures performed through these veins.

essential in preventing postphlebitic syndrome, thrombolytic therapy is more forcibly recommended as the treatment of choice (Elliot et al., 1979; Immelman and Jeffery, 1984; Marder and Sherry, 1988).

In phlegmasia cerulea dolens (venous occlusion with secondary arterial compression and ischemia of tissues) (Lipchik and Altman, 1979) (Fig. 16–29), more rapid reperfusion may promote faster recovery (Elliot et al., 1979). In fact, in acute thrombosis of any system, whether it occurs in the extremity or in other organs, thrombolytic therapy, rather than heparin alone, may be indicated (Marder and Sherry, 1988).

FILTER PLACEMENTS FOR THE INFERIOR VENA CAVA

The prevention of pulmonary emboli following venous thrombosis has been a goal of clinicians for decades. Interruption of the inferior vena cava by either ligation or plication was a major surgical operation with high mortality and morbidity (Mobin-Uddin et al., 1967). The first IVC filter (umbrella) was described in 1967 (Mobin-Uddin et al., 1967). Other models of filters followed, and the Greenfield filter, still the most useful and popular filter, was first reported in 1973 (Greenfield et al., 1973). Today, percutaneous placement under fluoroscopic control is the standard procedure (Dorfman, 1990).

Until recently, the classic indications for filter placement have been the following:

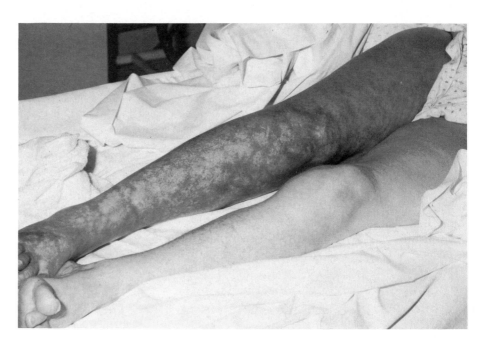

Figure 16–29. Phlegmasia cerulea dolens in a 55-year-old woman. This patient had metastatic bone involvement from carcinoma of the cervix. A venogram showed extensive thrombi filling the popliteal veins and extending upward into the superficial femoral vein. The venous occlusion involved the right common femoral vein, the right iliac system, and the proximal inferior vena cava. The patient rapidly improved following heparin therapy, and she was discharged to a nursing home. (From Lipchik, E.O., and Altman, D.P.: Phlegmasia cerulea dolens. Radiology, 133:81–82, 1979, with permission.)

1. Contraindication to anticoagulation in patients with proven pulmonary embolism.

2. Postpulmonary embolus with a complication of anticoagulation therapy.

3. Recurrent embolization during adequate anticoagulation.

4. Prophylactic insertion in patients with lower extremity thrombosis who may not receive anticoagulation.

5. Postsurgical pulmonary thromboendarterectomy for severe pulmonary hypertension.

6. Post-aspiration thrombectomy for massive pulmonary emboli.

Since the introduction of percutaneous, nonsurgical placement of filters (Rizk and Amplatz, 1973; Tadavarthy et al., 1984), the indications have widely expanded. An increasing number of high-risk patients are having filters placed as prophylaxis against pulmonary embolism in the *absence* of clinical evidence of acute thromboembolism (Rohrer et al., 1989). This group of patients may include those with multisystem trauma, malignancy or metastatic disease, pulmonary hypertension, recent surgery, especially lower extremity or hip orthopedic surgery, paraplegia from spinal cord injury, a prior history of DVT, or advanced age; many patients with extended immobility may have all of the foregoing conditions (Golueke et al., 1988; Tobin et al., 1989).

The ideal filter for the vena cava has not yet been developed. An effective filter should block significant emboli while maintaining patency of the inferior vena cava. The device should be easily and safely deliverable through a percutaneous technique. Most currently used filters are stable in a magnetic field (Teitelbaum et al., 1988). The simplest filter to insert percutaneously is the Vena Tech (Vena Tech Corporation, Evanston, Illinois) or the LGM filter (LG

Medical, Chasseneuil, France) (Ricco et al., 1988), which can be introduced through a 12 French (O.D.) sheath (Fig. 16–30), whereas the Greenfield filter (Medi Tech, Watertown, Massachusetts) (Greenfield and Michna, 1988) requires a 29 French (O.D.) sheath (Fig. 16–31). The Vena Tech filter may be inserted quite easily through either femoral vein or through the right jugular approach, whereas the Greenfield filter should not be introduced through the left femoral vein unless such a route is absolutely necessary, because the rigid holder cannot be easily manipulated through curved vessels. Recently, a new version of the Greenfield filter for percutaneous placement has been introduced; it requires a 14 French (O.D.) sheath.

Although these filters have been used for many years, no reports have been published of adequate in vivo, prospective studies or long-term follow-up examinations to state categorically which filter is better, or to rate how truly effective they are in preventing recurrent emboli. Morbidity and mortality rates for percutaneous filter placement are lower than those for surgical placement, although many series are not truly comparable (Dorfman, 1990). Most studies show approximately a 3% to 5% recurrence rate of pulmonary emboli and a 5% occlusion rate of the IVC with the Greenfield filter (Cimochowski et al., 1980). In addition, chronic venous stasis is more frequent, although it is perhaps a minor problem (Rohrer, 1989). One of the few studies that did prospectively evaluate the occurrence of thrombosis at the venous insertion site showed that this complication is much more frequent than has been clinically appreciated (Mewissen et al., 1989). Balloon distention for track dilation lessens the incidence of thrombosis as compared with multiple mechanical dilators. Deep venous thrombosis at the puncture site cannot be reliably diagnosed by clinical examination alone, and a sug-

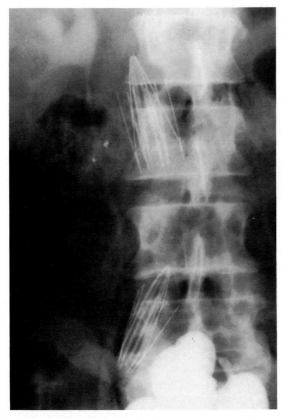

Figure 16–30. Two Vena Tech filters, one inadvertently placed into the right common iliac vein, and a second placed into the inferior vena cava below the renal veins. No sequelae to the filter in the iliac vein occurred. This patient had prior extensive right superficial femoral and common femoral vein thrombosis. Both filters were introduced via a right internal jugular percutaneous approach. The tilt of the superior filter is secondary to the anatomy of the inferior vena cava and not related to malposition, as judged by the preliminary inferior vena cavogram.

gestion has been made that a smaller sheath for filter delivery may be safer (Mewissen et al., 1989).

We believe that with meticulous and proper technique, whether surgical or percutaneous, most complications of improper placement, acute migration, or abnormal tilting can be avoided. We have observed that some filters may be more prone to tilting than others, and their positions and alignment have been reported to change with time (Berland et al., 1980). A tilted device loses its filtering capability. Preliminary vena cavagrams are essential for evaluating the width of the cava and the level of the renal veins, and for detecting the presence of clots (Fig. 16–32). For example, a Greenfield, Vena Tech, or Simon Nitinol (Simon et al., 1989) filter should not be placed in a vena cava wider than 28 mm, but rather the Bird's Nest filter (Cook, Inc., Bloomington, Indiana) (Roehm et al., 1988) may be used in venae cavae up to 40 mm in diameter. Preferably, all should be placed with their tips just below the renal veins (Fig. 16–33). A radiograph for documenting the position and alignment of the filter may prove important for future follow-up. If acute serious migration into the retro-

peritoneum or acute misplacement into the heart has occurred, operative intervention may be necessary. Most misplaced filters cannot be percutaneously retrieved, but anecdotal descriptions of success have been published (Guthaner et al., 1990).

We believe a more aggressive approach to filter placement is justified in an attempt to reduce the still unacceptably large number of preventable deaths resulting from pulmonary emboli. At present, numerous experiments are being performed, and filters are undergoing further development, so that in the future, these devices may be even simpler to use and may even be percutaneously removable.

MANAGEMENT OF MASSIVE HEMOPTYSIS

Massive hemoptysis is a terrifying emergency that often requires prompt lifesaving action. Conservative management may be associated with high mortality. Patients *can* undergo exsanguination, but most deaths and serious morbidity occur from asphyxiation with drowning, as aspirated blood fills the airways (Winter and Ingbar, 1988). The volume of the tracheal bronchial tree is approximately only 150 ml; thus, the more massive the hemorrhage, the higher the mortality, which may reach 70% in a 24-hour period if the expectorated blood is more than 600 ml (Conlan et al., 1983; Winter and Ingbar, 1988).

Tuberculosis, bronchiectasis, lung abscess, and lung cancer are the most common causes of massive bleeding. Patients with squamous-cell cancer, especially in the presence of cavitation, are much more likely to have massive hemoptysis than those with either adenocarcinoma or small-cell carcinoma (Tadavarthy et al., 1982). Intracavitary aspergilloma caused by colonization of pre-existent cavities from prior tuberculosis, sarcoid, lung abscess, or bronchiectasis is becoming more frequent as a cause of massive bleeding, particularly in immunosuppressed patients. Less se-

PUNCTURE SITE HOLE		INTRODUCER	
		O.D.	I.D.
GF	●	29	24
BNF	●	14	12
VTF	●	12	10
SNF	●	9	7

Figure 16–31. A comparison of puncture site holes and filter introducers. O.D., Outer diameter; I.D., inner diameter; GF, Greenfield filter; BNF, Bird's Nest filter; VTF, Vena Tech filter; SNF, Simon Nitinol filter (Nitinol Medical Technologies Inc., Woburn, Massachusetts).

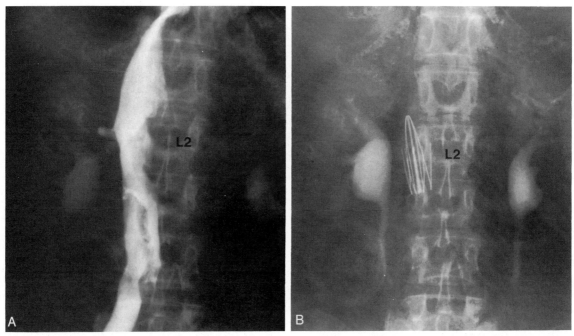

Figure 16–32. *A*, Inferior vena cavogram demonstrating a free-floating thrombus extending from the left iliac vein into the inferior vena cava up to the middle of the third lumbar vertebral body. *B*, Uncomplicated placement of a Vena Tech filter just above the floating thrombus but partially straddling the renal veins. The filter was inserted by a percutaneous right femoral vein approach. A jugular approach would have been safer and was attempted, but it was precluded because of technical problems.

Figure 16–33. The radiographic appearance of a Greenfield filter placed with its tip just below the renal veins. The clamp is an external marker placed during fluoroscopy to denote the position of the inferior border of the left renal vein. The entrance of the renal veins is determined by a preceding vena cavogram. Vena cavograms are always obtained prior to the insertion of any filter to evaluate the patient for intraluminal thrombi and the position of the entrances of the renal veins, to check for anomalous position of any draining renal vein, usually on the left, and to measure the width of the vena cava at the level at which the filter is to be placed.

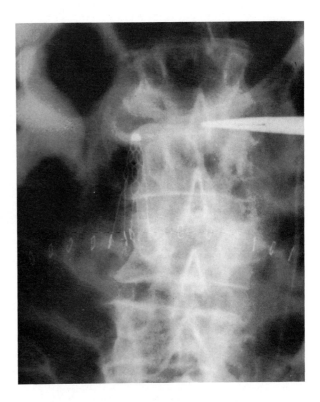

vere bleeding in patients with cystic fibrosis may have more disastrous implications for pulmonary function because of the already compromised pulmonary status of these patients (Cohen et al., 1990).

During massive hemoptysis, when the patient's life is at stake, interventional bronchoscopy with saline lavage, balloon occlusion techniques of the bronchus, or both may be lifesaving prior to the institution of definitive treatment. Surgical procedures performed during peak hemorrhage may be associated with mortality as high as 35% (Magilligan et al., 1981). Bronchial artery catheterization and embolization constitute safe, rapid, and effective treatment.

Of prime diagnostic importance is the localization of the site of bleeding. Bronchoscopy may be helpful for localizing the side and site of the bleeding and may facilitate the angiographic search for the proper artery if bilateral disease is present. A recent chest radiograph would be important in unilateral disease but most often does not help in localizing the bleeding when diffuse, severe, bilateral abnormalities are present. Also, in our experience, most patients know which lung is involved.

Bronchial artery embolization has met with increasing success since it was first introduced in 1974 (Remy et al., 1974). The long-term efficacy of bronchial embolization is uncertain, but the short-term success is striking: it approaches 90%. The recurrence rate within 8 months, however, has been reported as varying from 5% to 30% (Katoh et al., 1990; Rabkin et al., 1987; Remy et al., 1977; Uflacker et al., 1985; White, 1984). Recurrence of bleeding may occur because of incomplete embolization, collateralization and hypertrophy of other vessels, recanalization, or

pulmonary artery involvement. The most frequent cause of recurrence is the presence of cavitary disease associated with aspergilloma (Katoh et al., 1990). In the largest series of patients managed by transcatheter embolization, 12% of the cases of bleeding recurred, and of this group, one quarter of the patients eventually underwent operation (Rabkin et al., 1987). Almost one half of patients with recurrent bleeding had successful surgical procedures in another series (Katoh et al., 1990). Surgical treatment, therefore, does remain an elective option in a suitable candidate if bleeding recurs. In our experience, however, most patients are inoperable, owing to extensive diffuse lung disease, active tuberculosis, or invasive carcinoma. Thus, long-term follow-ups are difficult to achieve in these extremely sick patients.

Patients with bleeding secondary to tuberculosis (Rasmussen's aneurysm), arteriovenous malformations, or invasive carcinoma should undergo pulmonary arteriography in addition to bronchial angiography because erosions or pseudoaneurysms of the pulmonary arteries are more common in these conditions (Plessinger and Jolly, 1949; Thompson, 1954). Those patients with a history of chronic inflammatory disease, such as bronchiectasis or cystic fibrosis, can be solely evaluated by bronchial artery studies, because pulmonary abnormalities are rare in such cases. In one series, 8% of the patients bled from the pulmonary artery (Rabkin et al., 1987).

Unfortunately, in contradistinction to gastrointestinal bleeding, the actual extravasation of contrast is usually not visualized in massive hemoptysis. One must rely on the angiographic abnormalities of hypervascularity, increased tortuosity, shunts between

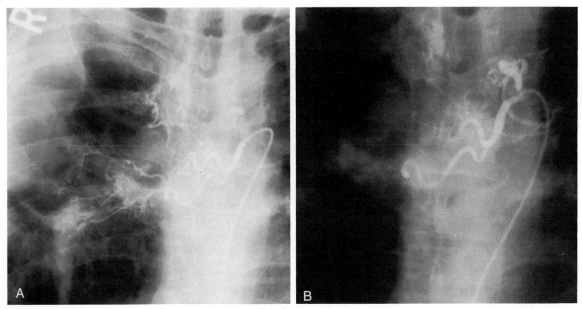

Figure 16–34. *A,* A 50-year-old male with cystic sarcoid and aspergillosis superinfection presented clinically with massive bleeding on the right side. Bronchial arteriography demonstrates coiled, tortuous hypervascularity, originating from all the branches of the right bronchial artery. *B,* After successful embolization with absorbable gelatin sponge, the patient gradually stopped bleeding over a 2-day period. Note opacification of the left bronchial artery from a common trunk with the right artery, which represents one of the more frequent anatomic patterns. The position of the catheter tip was too proximal, precluding placement of a coil.

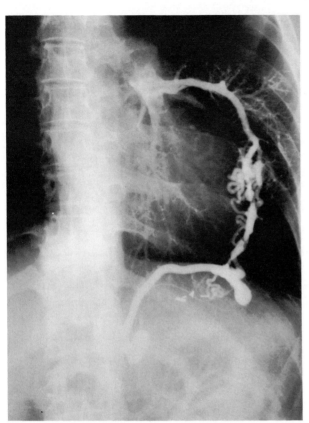

Figure 16–35. Anteroposterior and lateral angiograms illustrate development of huge transpleural and parenchymal collateral vessels. Enormous dilatation of the phrenic artery and its collateralization to the left pulmonary artery are shown. This patient had a history of Hodgkin's disease, splenectomy, and pleural adhesions. (Courtesy of Dr. H. Bradley, Milwaukee, Wisconsin.)

the bronchial artery and the pulmonary artery, aneurysms, abnormally dilated vessels, and so forth for a presumptive diagnosis and localization (Fig. 16–34).

Seventy percent of the bronchial arteries arise from the descending thoracic aorta between T5 and T6, and 20% arise from above or below those levels (Cauldwell et al., 1948). Ten percent of the bronchial arteries arise from aberrant origins such as the subclavian, internal thoracic, and other arteries from the brachiocephalic system, and even from the phrenic arteries. All of the bronchial arteries arise from the anterior surface of the aorta, except for a right common intercostobronchial trunk, which arises from the medial surface of the aorta (Cauldwell et al., 1948).

In our experience, the best catheter shape is a 5F cobra or a shepherd's crook. Small amounts of nonionic contrast agents should be used; about 2 to 5 ml is usually sufficient. *All* vessels that may contribute to the bleeding should be embolized. If significant chronic pleural parenchymal disease is present, subclavian and other nonbronchial systemic angiograms may be indicated to localize aberrant vessels and transpleural collaterals (Keller et al., 1987; Vujic et al., 1982) (Fig. 16–35). Successful bronchial artery

embolization can be performed with small bits of absorbable gelatin sponge, with the embolization performed as peripherally as possible. We almost always follow with a minicoil to achieve a more permanent occlusion (Fig. 16–36). Polyvinyl alcohol sponge (Ivalon) may also be used; in fact, any nonresorbable particulate embolic material can be used. Despite isolated successful reports in the literature, absorbable gelatin sponge powder, sclerosing agents, and alcohol are *not* recommended because of the risk of tissue necrosis and bronchial infarction (Hickey et al., 1988; Ivanick et al., 1983).

Serious complications are uncommon when good technique is used. The proximal bronchi have poor collateral circulation, and bronchial infarction and necrosis have been reported (Remy et al., 1977). Some branches of bronchial arteries supply a portion of the esophagus, and dysphagia may result (Uflacker

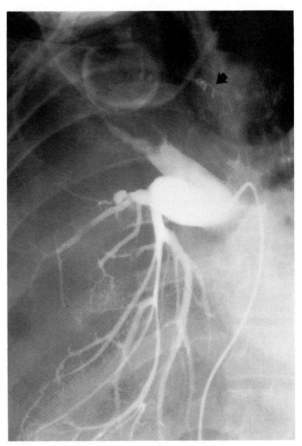

Figure 16–36. A 63-year-old woman, several years following laryngectomy, who now has bronchogenic carcinoma. She presented acutely with near drowning by blood welling up into the tracheostomy tube. Particles of absorbable gelatin sponge and a coil (*arrow*) were placed into the involved right upper lobe bronchial artery. The hemorrhage rapidly abated, and the patient died peacefully and suddenly 1 week later. The pulmonary angiogram obtained at the time of bronchial embolization shows malignant cutoff of the upper lobe pulmonary artery and a small aneurysm (possibly a pseudoaneurysm) in one of the arteries to the middle lobe. The "circle" overlying the upper chest on the right is an extrinsic device.

et al., 1985). Transverse myelitis or spinal cord infarction should not occur if proper care is taken to avoid the spinal artery.

References

Anagnostopoulos, C.E., Prabhakar, M.J., and Kittle, C.F.: Aortic dissections and dissecting aneurysms. Am. J. Cardiol. 30:263, 1972.

Berland, L.L., Maddison, F.E., and Bernhard, V.M.: Radiologic follow-up of vena cava filter devices. AJR 134:1047, 1980.

Bettmann, M.A., Robbins, A., Braun, S.D., et al.: Contrast venography of the leg: Diagnostic efficacy, tolerance, and complication rates with ionic and nonionic contrast media. Radiology 165:113, 1987.

Cauldwell, E. W., Siekert, R.G., Lininger, R.E., and Anson, B.J.: The bronchial arteries: An anatomic study of 150 human cadavers. Surg. Gynecol. Obstet. 86:395, 1948.

Cimochowski, G.E., Evans, R.H., Zarins, C.K., et al.: Greenfield filter versus Mobin-Uddin umbrella: The continuing quest for the ideal method of vena caval catheterization. J. Thorac. Cardiovasc. Surg. 79:358, 1980.

Cohen, A.M., Doershuk, C.F., and Stern, R.C.: Bronchial artery embolization to control hemoptysis in cystic fibrosis. Radiology 175:401, 1990.

Comerota, A.J., Katz, M.L., Greenwald, L.L., et al.: Venous duplex imaging: Should it replace hemodynamic tests for deep venous thrombosis? J. Vasc. Surg. 11:53, 1990.

Comerota, A.J., Katz, M.L., Grossi, R.J., et al.: The comparative value of noninvasive testing for diagnosis and surveillance of deep vein thrombosis. J. Vasc. Surg. 7:40, 1988.

Conlan, A.A., Hurwitz, S.S., Krige, L., et al.: Massive hemoptysis: Review of 123 cases. J. Thorac. Cardiovasc. Surg. 85:120, 1983.

Crane, C.: Arteriosclerotic aneurysm of the abdominal aorta: Some pathological and clinical correlations. N. Engl. J. Med. 253:954, 1955.

Crass, J.R., Cohen, A.M., Motta, A.O., et al.: A proposed new mechanism of traumatic aortic rupture: The osseous pinch. Radiology 176:645, 1990.

Crawford, E.S., and Crawford, J.L.: Diseases of the Aorta Including an Atlas of Angiographic Pathology and Surgical Technique. Baltimore, Williams & Wilkins, 1984.

Crawford, E.S., and Hess, K.R.: Abdominal aortic aneurysm. (Editorial comment.) N. Engl. J. Med. 321:1040, 1989.

Daily, P.O., Trueblood, H.W., Stinson, E.B., et al.: Management of acute aortic dissections. Ann. Thorac. Surg. 10:237, 1970.

Dalen, J.E., Pape, L.A., Cohn, L.H., et al.: Dissection of the aorta: Pathogenesis, diagnosis and treatment. Prog. Cardiovasc. Dis. 23:237, 1980.

Darling, R.C., Messina, C.R., Brewster, D.C., and Ottinger, L.W.: Autopsy study of unoperated abdominal aortic aneurysms: The case for early resection. Circulation 56:161, 1977.

DeBakey, M.E., Cooley, D.A., and Creech, O., Jr.: Surgical considerations of dissecting aneurysm of the aorta. Ann. Surg. 142:586, 1955.

DeBakey, M.E., Henly, W.S., Cooley, D.A., et al.: Surgical management of dissecting aneurysms of the aorta. J. Thorac. Cardiovasc. Surg. 49:130, 1965.

Dee, P., Granato, J.E., and Gibson, R.S.: The CT and ultrasound diagnosis of aortic dissection. Seminars in Ultrasound, CT and MR 6:146, 1985.

Dee, P., Martin, R., Oudkerk, M., and Overbosch, E.: The diagnosis of aortic dissection. Curr. Probl. Diagn. Radiol. 12:3, 1983.

DeWeese, J.A., and Rogoff, S.M.: Functional ascending phlebography of the lower extremity by serial long film techniques. AJR 81:841, 1959.

Dorfman, G.S.: Percutaneous inferior vena caval filters. Radiology 174:987, 1990.

Dotter, C.T., Rösch, J., Seaman, A.J., et al.: Streptokinase treatment of thromboembolic disease. Radiology 102:283, 1972.

Earnest, F., Muhm, J.R., and Sheedy, P.F.: Roentgenographic findings in thoracic aortic dissection. Mayo Clin. Proc. 54:43, 1979.

Elliot, M.S., Immelman, E.J., Jeffery, P., et al.: The role of thrombolytic therapy in the management of phlegmasia cerulea dolens. Br. J. Surg. 66:422, 1979.

Estes, J.E., Jr.: Abdominal aortic aneurysm: A study of 102 cases. Circulation 2:258, 1950.

Eyler, W.R., and Clark, M.D.: Dissecting aneurysms of the aorta: Roentgen manifestations including a comparison with other types of aneurysms. Radiology 85:1047, 1965.

Foley, W.D., Middleton, W.D., Lawson, T.L., et al.: Color Doppler ultrasound imaging of lower-extremity venous disease. AJR 152:371, 1989.

Fomon, J.J., Kurzweg, F.T., and Broadaway, F.K.: Aneurysms of the aorta: A review. Ann. Surg. 165:557, 1967.

Gazzaniga, A.B., Bartlett, R.H., and Shobe, J.B.: Bilateral impedance rheography in deep venous thrombosis: Role of respiratory maneuvers and saphenous occlusion. Arch. Surg. 106:835, 1973.

Geisinger, M.A., Risius, B., O'Donnell, J.A., et al.: Thoracic aortic dissections: Magnetic resonance imaging. Radiology 155:407, 1985.

Godwin, J.D., Herfkens, R.I. Skiöldebrand, C.G., et al.: Evaluation of dissections and aneurysms of the thoracic aorta by conventional and dynamic CT scanning. Radiology 136:125, 1980.

Godwin, J.D., and Korobkin, M.: Acute disease of the aorta: Diagnosis by computed tomography and ultrasonography. Radiol. Clin. North Am. 21:551, 1983.

Godwin, J.D., Turley, K., Herfkens, R.J., and Lipton, M.J.: Computed tomography for follow-up of chronic aortic dissections. Radiology 139:655, 1981.

Goldhaber, S.Z., Buring, J.E., Lipnick, R.J., and Hennekens, C.H.: Pooled analyses of randomized trials of streptokinase and heparin in phlebographically documented acute deep venous thrombosis. Am. J. Med. 76:393, 1984.

Golueke, P.J., Garrett, W.V., Thompson, J.E., et al.: Interruption of the vena cava by means of the Greenfield filter: Expanding the indications. Surgery 103:111, 1988.

Gore, I.: Dissecting aneurysms of the aorta in persons under forty years of age. AMA Arch. Path. 55:1, 1953.

Greenfield, L.J., and Michna, B.A.: Twelve-year clinical experience with the Greenfield vena caval filter. Surgery 104:706, 1988.

Greenfield, L.J., McCurdy, J.R., Brown, P.P., and Elkins, R.C.: A new intracaval filter permitting continued flow and resolution of emboli. Surgery 73:599, 1973.

Gundry, S., Williams, S., Burney, R., et al.: Indications for aortography in blunt thoracic trauma: A reassessment. J. Trauma 22:664, 1982.

Guthaner, D.F., Wyatt, J.O., and Mehigan, J.T.: Monorail system for percutaneous repositioning of the Greenfield vena cava filter. Radiology 176:872, 1990.

Guthaner, D.F., Miller, D.C., Silverman, J.F., et al.: Fate of the false lumen following surgical repair of aortic dissections: An angiographic study. Radiology 133:1, 1979.

Gutierrez, F.R., Gowda, S., Ludbrook, P.A., and McKnight, R.C.: Cineangiography in the diagnosis and evaluation of aortic dissection. Radiology 135:759, 1980.

Hayashi, K., Meaney, T.F., Zelch, J.V., and Tarar, R.: Aortographic analysis of aortic dissection. AJR 122:769, 1974.

Heiberg, E., and Wolverson, M.K.: CT of traumatic injuries of the aorta. Seminars in Ultrasound, CT and MR 6:172, 1985.

Hickey, N.M., Peterson, R.A., Leech, J.A., et al.: Percutaneous embolotherapy in life-threatening hemoptysis. Cardiovasc. Intervent. Radiol. 11:270, 1988.

Hirst, A.E., Jr., Johns, V.J., Jr., and Klime, S.W., Jr.: Dissecting aneurysm of the aorta: A review of 505 cases. Medicine 37:217, 1958.

Hull, R.D., Carter, C.J., Jay, R.M., et al.: Diagnostic efficacy of impedance plethysmography for clinically suspected DVT: A randomized evaluation. Ann. Intern. Med. 102:21, 1985.

Hyers, T.M.: Deep vein thrombosis: Selecting the best diagnostic method for in-hospital screening. Journal of Critical Illness 4:37, 1989.

Immelman, E.J., and Jeffery, P.C.: The postphlebitic syndrome: Pathophysiology, prevention and management. Clin. Chest Med. 5:537, 1984.

Imparato, A.M., and Riles, T.S.: Peripheral arterial disease. In Schwartz, S.I., et al. (eds.): Principles of Surgery. New York, McGraw-Hill, 1989, p. 981.

Ingram, R.H., Jr.: Diseases of pleura, mediastinum and diaphragm. In Braunwald, E., et al. (eds.): Harrison's Principles of Internal Medicine, ed. 11. New York, McGraw-Hill, 1987, p. 1123.

Ishikawa, T., Nakajima, Y., and Kaji, T.: The role of CT in traumatic rupture of the thoracic aorta and its proximal branches. Semin. Roentgenol. 24:38, 1989.

Ivanick, M.J., Thorwarth, W., Donohue, J., et al.: Infarction of the left mainstem bronchus: A complication of bronchial artery embolization. AJR 141:535, 1983.

Jewitt, D.E.: Diagnosis of acute aortic dissection by M-mode and cross-sectional echocardiography: A five-year experience. Eur. Heart. J. 4:196, 1983.

Katoh, O., Kishikawa, T., Yauada, H., et al.: Recurrent bleeding after arterial embolization in patients with hemoptysis. Chest 97:541, 1990.

Kaufman, S.L., and White, R.I., Jr.: Aortic dissection with "normal" chest roentgenogram. Cardiovasc. Intervent. Radiol. 3:103, 1980.

Keller, F.S., Rosch, J., Loflin, T.G., et al.: Nonbronchial systemic collateral arteries: Significance in percutaneous embolotherapy for hemoptysis. Radiology 164:687, 1987.

Kersting-Sommerhoff, B.A., Higgins, C.B., White, R.D., et al.: Aortic dissection: Sensitivity and specificity of MR imaging. Radiology 166:651, 1988.

Kirsh, M.M., and Sloan, H.: Blunt chest trauma: General principles of management. Boston, Little, Brown, 1977.

Krukenberg, E.: Beitrage zur frage des aneurysma dissecans. Beitrage zur Pathologische Anatomie 67:329, 1920.

Larde, D., Belloir, C., Vasile, N., et al.: Computed tomography of aortic dissection. Radiology 136:147, 1980.

LaRoy, L.L., Cormier, P.J., Matalon, T.A., et al.: Imaging of abdominal aortic aneurysms. AJR 152:785, 1989.

Lee, J.K.T.: Retroperitoneum. In Lee, J.K.T., et al.: (eds.): Computed Body Tomography with MRI Correlation. New York, Raven Press, 1989, p. 711.

Lindsay, J., Jr., and Hurst, J.W.: Clinical features and prognosis in dissecting aneurysms of the aorta: A re-appraisal. Circulation 35:880, 1967.

Lipchik E.O., Altman D.P. Phlegmasia cerulea dolens. Radiology 133:81, 1979.

Lipchik, E.O., and Rogoff, S.M.: Aneurysms of the abdominal aorta. In Abrams, H.L. (ed.): Abrams' Angiography: Vascular and Interventional Radiology, ed. 3. Boston, Little, Brown, 1983, p. 1029.

Lipchik, E.O., Deweese, J.A., and Rogoff, S.M.: Serial long-term phlebography after documented lower leg thrombosis. Radiology 120:563, 1976.

Lochridge, S.K., Knibbe, W.P., and Doty, D.B.: Obstruction of the superior vena cava. Surgery 85:14, 1979.

Magilligan, D.J., Jr., Ravitati, S., Zayat, P., et al.: Massive hemoptysis: Control by transcatheter bronchial artery embolization. Ann. Thorac. Surg. 32:392, 1981.

Marder, V.J., and Sherry, S.: Thrombolytic therapy: Current status. N. Engl. J. Med. 318:1585, 1988.

McLeod, A.A., Monaghan, M.J., Richardson, P.J., et al.: Diagnosis of acute aortic dissection by M-mode and cross-sectional echocardiography. A five year experience. Eur. Heart J. 4:196, 1983.

Mewissen, M.W., Erickson, S.J., Foley, W.D., et al.: Thrombosis at venous insertion sites after inferior vena caval filter placement. Radiology 173:155, 1989.

Miller, D.C.: Surgical management of aortic dissections: Indications, perioperative management and long-term results. In Doroghazi, R.M., and Slater, E.E. (eds.): Aortic Dissection. New York, McGraw-Hill, 1983, p. 193.

Miller, F.B., Richardson, J.D., Thomas, H.A., et al.: Role of CT in diagnosis of major arterial injury after blunt thoracic trauma surgery. Surgery 106:596, 1989.

Mirvis, S.E., Bidwell, J.K., Buddemeyer, E.U., et al.: Imaging diagnosis of traumatic aortic rupture: A review and experience at a major trauma center. Invest. Radiol. 22:187, 1987a.

Mirvis, S.E., Bidwell, J.K., Buddemeyer, E.U., et al.: Value of chest radiography in excluding traumatic aortic rupture. Radiology 163:487, 1987b.

Mobin-Uddin, K., Smith, P.E., Martinez, L.O., et al.: A vena caval filter for the prevention of pulmonary embolus. Surg. Forum 18:209, 1967.

Moncada, R., Cardella, R., Demos, T.C., et al.: Evaluation of superior vena cava syndrome by axial CT and CT phlebography. AJR 143:731, 1984.

Moncada, R., Salinas, M., Churchill, R., et al.: Diagnosis of dissecting aortic aneurysm by computed tomography. Lancet 1:238, 1981.

Okay, N.H., Bryk, D.: Collateral pathways in occlusion of the superior vena cava and its tributaries. Radiology 92:1493, 1969.

Oudkerk, M., Overbosch, E., and Dee P.: CT recognition of aortic dissection. AJR 141:671, 1983.

Parish, J.M., Marschke, R.F., Jr., Dines, D.E., et al.: Etiologic considerations in superior vena cava syndrome. Mayo Clin. Proc. 56:407, 1981.

Parmley, L.F., Mattingly, T.W., Manron, W.C., and Jahnke, E.J., Jr.: Nonpenetrating traumatic injury of the aorta. Circulation 17:1086, 1958.

Pate, J.W., Richardson, R.L., and Eastridge, C.E.: Acute aortic dissections. Am. Surg. 42:395, 1976.

Philbrick, J.T., and Becker, D.M.: Calf deep vein thrombosis: A wolf in sheep's clothing? Arch. Intern. Med. 148:2131, 1988.

Plessinger, V.A., and Jolly, P.N.: Rasmussen's aneurysms and fatal hemorrhage in pulmonary tuberculosis. Am. Rev. TB 60:589, 1949.

Posniak, H.V., Demos, T.C., and Marsan, R.E.: Computed tomography of the normal aorta and thoracic aneurysms. Semin. Roentgenol. 24:7, 1989.

Pressler, V., and McNamara, J.J.: Thoracic aortic aneurysm: Natural history and treatment. J. Thorac. Cardiovasc. Surg. 79:489, 1980.

Rabkin, J.E., Astafjev, V.I., Gothman, L.H., and Grigorjev, Y.G.: Transcatheter embolization in the management of pulmonary hemorrhage. Radiology 163:361, 1987.

Randall, P.A., and Jarmolowski, C.R.: Aneurysms of the thoracic aorta. In Abrams, H.L. (ed.): Abrams' Angiography: Vascular and Interventional Radiology, ed. 3. Boston, Little, Brown, 1983, p. 417.

Remy, J., Arnaud, A., Fardou, H., et al.: Treatment of hemoptysis by embolization of bronchial arteries. Radiology 122:33, 1977.

Remy, J., Viosin, C., Dupois, C., et al.: Treatement des hemoptysies par embolization de la circulation systemique. Ann. Radiol. 17:5, 1974.

Ricco, J.B., Crochet, D., Sebilotte, P., et al.: Percutaneous transvenous caval interruption with the "LGM" filter: Early results of a multicenter trial. Ann. Vasc. Surg. 2:242, 1988.

Rizk, G.K., and Amplatz, K.: A percutaneous method of introducing the caval umbrella. AJR 117:903, 1973.

Roberts, W.C.: Aortic dissection: Anatomy, consequences, and causes. Am. Heart J. 101:195, 1981.

Roehm, J.O., Jr., Johnsrude, I.S., Barth, M.H., and Gianturco, C.: The bird's nest inferior vena cava filter: Progress report. Radiology 168:745, 1988.

Rohrer, M.J., Scheidler, M.G., Wheeler, H.B., and Cutler, B.S.: Extended indications for placement of an inferior vena cava filter. J. Vasc. Surg. 10:44, 1989.

Rose, S.C., Zwiebel, W.J., Nelson, B.D., et al.: Symptomatic lower extremity deep venous thrombosis: Accuracy, limitations, and role of color duplex flow imaging in diagnosis. Radiology 175:639, 1990.

Saffitz, J.E., Ganote, C.E., Peterson, C.E., and Roberts, W.C.: False aneurysm of ascending aorta after aortocoronary bypass grafting. Am. J. Cardiol. 52:907, 1983.

Shimm, D.S., Logue, G.L., and Rigsby, L.C.: Evaluating the superior vena cava syndrome. JAMA 245:951, 1981.

Shuman, W.P., Hastrup, W., Jr., Kohler, T.R., et al.: Suspected leaking abdominal aortic aneurysm: Use of sonography in the emergency room. Radiology 168:117, 1988.

Simon, M., Athanasoulis, C.A., Ducksoo, K., et al.: Simon Nitinol inferior vena cava filter: Initial clinical experience. Radiology 172:99, 1989.

Slater, E.E.: Aortic dissection: Presentation and diagnosis. *In* Doroghazi, R.M., and Slater, E.E. (eds.): Aortic Dissection. New York, McGraw-Hill, 1983.

Slater, E.E., and DeSanctis, R.W.: The clinical recognition of dissecting aortic aneurysm. Am. J. Med. 60:625, 1976.

Smith, D.C., and Jang, G.C.: Radiological diagnosis of aortic dissection. *In* Doroghazi, R.M., and Slater, E.E. (eds.): Aortic Dissection. New York, McGraw-Hill, 1983.

Sorensen, H.R., and Olsen, H.: Ruptured and dissecting aneurysms of the aorta: Incidence and prospects of surgery. Acta Chir. Scand. 128:644, 1964.

Stein, H.L., and Steinberg, I.: Selective aortography, definitive technique for the diagnosis of dissecting aneurysm of the aorta. AJR 102:333, 1968.

Swensen, S.J., Ehman, R.L., and Brown, L.R.: Magnetic resonance imaging of the thorax. J. Thorac. Imaging 4:19, 1989.

Szilagyi, D.E., Elliott, J.P., and Smith, R.F.: Clinical fate of the patient with asymptomatic abdominal aortic aneurysm and unfit for surgical treatment. Arch. Surg. 104:600, 1972.

Tadavarthy, S.M., Castaneda-Zuniga, W., Salomonowitz, E., et al.: Kimray-Greenfield vena cava filter: Percutaneous introduction. Radiology 151:525, 1984.

Tadavarthy, S.M., Klugman, J., Castaneda-Zuniga, W.R., et al.: Systemic-to-pulmonary collaterals in pathological states: A review. Radiology 144:55, 1982.

Teitelbaum, G.P., Bradley, W.G., Jr., and Klein, B.D.: MR imaging artifacts, ferromagnetism and magnetic torque of intravascular filters, stents, and coils. Radiology 166;65, 1988.

Thompson, J.R.: Mechanisms of fatal pulmonary hemorrhage in tuberculosis. Diseases of the Chest 25:193, 1954.

Thompson, J.E., Hollier, L.H., Patman, R.D., and Persson, A.V.: Surgical management of abdominal aortic aneurysms: Factors influencing mortality and morbidity—a 20-year experience. Ann. Surg. 181:654, 1975.

Thorsen, M.K., Lawson, T.L., and Foley, W.D.: CT of aortic dissections. CRC Crit. Rev. Diagn. Imaging 26:291, 1986b.

Thorsen, M.K., Goodman, L.R., Sagel, S.S., and Olinger, G.N.: Ascending aorta complications of cardiac surgery: CT evaluation. J. Comput. Assist. Ionogr. 10:219, 1986a.

Thorsen, M.K., San Dretto, M.A., Lawson, T.L., and Foley, W.D.: Dissecting aortic aneurysms: Accuracy of computed tomographic diagnosis. Radiology 148:773, 1983.

Tobin, K.D., Pais, S.O., and Austin, C.B.: Reevaluation of indications for percutaneous placement of the Greenfield filter. Invest. Radiol. 24:115, 1989.

Uflacker, R., Kaemmerer, A., Picon, P.D., et al.: Bronchial artery embolization in the management of hemoptysis: Technical aspects and long-term results. Radiology 157:637, 1985.

Victor, M.F., Mintz, G.S., Kotler, M.N., et al.: Two-dimensional echocardiographic diagnosis of aortic dissection. Am. J. Cardiol. 48:1155, 1981.

Vujic, I., Pyle, R., Hungerford, G.D., and Griffin, C.N.: Angiography and therapeutic blockade in the control of hemoptysis: The importance of nonbronchial systemic arteries. Radiology 143:19, 1982.

Webb, W.R., and Kelly, J.P.: Aneurysms of the thoracic aorta. *In* Sabiston, D.C., Jr. (ed.): Textbook of Surgery: The Biological Basis of Modern Surgical Practice, ed. 13. Philadelphia, W.B. Saunders, 1986, p. 1816.

Weinreb, J.C., Mootz, A., and Cohen, J.M.: MRI evaluation of mediastinal and thoracic inlet venous obstruction. AJR 146:679, 1986.

Weisman, A.D., and Adams, R.D.: Neurological complications of dissecting aortic aneurysm. Brain 67:69, 1944.

Wheat, M.W., Jr.: Acute dissecting aneurysms of the aorta: Diagnosis and treatment—1979. Am. Heart J. 99:373, 1980.

Wheat, M.W., Jr., Palmer, R.F., Bartley, T.D., et al.: Treatment of dissecting aneurysms of the aorta without surgery. J. Thorac. Cardiovasc. Surg. 50:364, 1965.

White, R.I.: Embolotherapy in vascular disease. AJR 142:27, 1984.

White, R.D., and Higgins, G.B.: Magnetic resonance imaging of thoracic vascular disease. J. Thorac. Imaging 4:34, 1989.

Winter, S.M., and Ingbar, D.H.: Massive hemoptysis: Pathogenesis and management. Journal of Intensive Care Medicine 3:171, 1988.

Wolfe, W.G.: Acute ascending aortic dissection. Ann. Surg. 192:658, 1980.

Wyman, S.M.: Dissecting aneurysm of the thoracic aorta: Its roentgen recognition. AJR 78:247, 1957.

Yedlicka, J.W., Jr., Cormier, M.G., Gray, R., and Moncada, R.: Computed tomography of superior vena cava obstruction. J. Thorac. Imaging 2:72, 1987.

ACUTE ABDOMINAL DISEASE

PART V

17

Acute Gastrointestinal Disorders

∎

Steven K. Teplick
Jeffrey C. Brandon
Hemendra R. Shah
Richard McKenzie
Roberta L. Itzkoff
David L. Harshfield

Although plain radiographs of the chest and abdomen are still the forefront of the imaging studies used in acutely ill patients, advances in computed tomography (CT) and real-time ultrasonography have significantly increased our ability to detect disease.

The following discussion reviews many of the disease entities related to gastrointestinal (GI) tract, abdomen, and spleen that may be encountered in the acutely ill patient.

ESOPHAGUS

Radiographic Localization of Support Apparatus

A variety of tubes are placed in the upper alimentary tract of patients in intensive care units (ICUs). These include nasogastric (NG) tubes for gastric decompression, long tubes (e.g., Cantor tubes) for small bowel decompression, and feeding tubes (e.g., Dobhoff tubes) (Fig. 17–1). Malpositions of these tubes are readily detected on the plain radiograph since most are radiopaque (Fig. 17–2). The NG tube generally passes into the stomach without impediment. However, because of local anatomic variations, cervical abnormality, or a number of other causes, NG tubes can inadvertently pass into the tracheobronchial tree, most commonly into the right mainstem bronchus. It is obligatory to confirm the position of these tubes radiographically before undertaking any further tube manipulation, since physical findings supporting successful gastric placement of the distal tube tip can be deceptive. Feedings through a tube inadvertently placed in a bronchus or through its wall can cause severe pneumonitis, hydrothorax, empyema, mediastinitis, and possibly death (McWey et al., 1988). A less common cause of NG tube malposition is curling within the esophagus itself or within esophageal diverticula, especially if they are large. Some patients with diverticula may have histories of esophageal complaints that alert the clinician to potential difficulties in passing an NG tube (Eterline and Thompson, 1984). Pre-existing esophageal inflammatory disease with stricture and esophageal neoplasm can also make the passage of NG tubes difficult or impossible. Rarely, a tube knots itself and tightens if attempts are made to withdraw it. Under these circumstances an experienced endoscopist or interventional radiologist can often successfully unravel the tube or recover the knot through a perorally placed sheath.

Because the distal 10 cm of most NG tubes are fenestrated, at least this length of tubing should be seen past the area of the gastroesophageal (GE) junction on a plain radiograph of the upper abdomen. In patients without hiatus hernia, this generally is located at or just below the level of the left cardiophrenic sulcus. Tubes placed more proximally may predispose the patient to aspiration of any contents placed through the tube since sideholes will be present in the distal esophagus. In the ICU a small amount

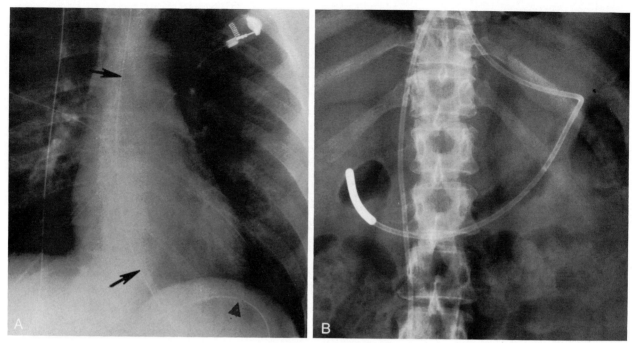

Figure 17–1. Nasogastric and Dubhoff tubes. *A,* A nasogastric tube is seen coiled in the fundus of the stomach *(arrows).* A sidehole is seen on the stomach *(arrowhead).* No sideholes are seen above the gastroesophageal junction. *B,* A Dubhoff feeding tube is in good position in the duodenal bulb. Gastroesophageal reflux is less likely when positioned beyond the pylorus.

of barium can be placed through the tube to confirm its proper position. If contrast is injected, a dilute barium mixture should be used. Water-soluble contrast, if aspirated, is toxic to lung tissue. The typical soft single-lumen feeding tube with its tungsten-filled tip also has sideholes about 7 cm from its end, so at least this length should be seen distal to the GE junction. These types of tubes are often equipped with a stiffening wire that is removed after successful tube placement. Reinsertion of this wire for tube repositioning can cause esophageal perforation if the stiffener inadvertently exits a sidehole. The radiographic position of an NG tube can be helpful in determining the integrity of normal mediastinal vascular structures in acutely injured patients. Deviation of the NG tube to the right, beyond the level of the pedicle of the thoracic vertebrae, is highly suggestive of mediastinal hemorrhage from an aortic tear and is an indication for angiography (Fig. 17–3).

Esophageal Stricture and Perforation

Complications of NG intubation include esophagitis, stricture formation, and perforation. Although uncommon, strictures develop most often in patients who have been intubated for 3 to 15 days, but strictures can develop in less than 48 hours (Graham et al., 1959) (Fig. 17–4). Some investigators believe that disruption of the integrity of the lower esophageal sphincter caused by the tube and subsequent GE reflux is related to the pathogenesis of the esophageal

injury (Graham et al., 1959). Others believe that the trauma of intubation or the irritant effect of the tube itself may cause a direct contact-type of esophagitis leading to stricture formation (Waldman and Berlin, 1965).

Whereas endoscopy accounts for most iatrogenic perforations, the esophagus can also be perforated by any of the various NG tubes (Levine, 1989) (Fig. 17–5). A leaking esophageal anastomosis may present as a pneumomediastinum. The increasing use of endoscopic sclerotherapy for bleeding esophageal varices has substantially reduced the use of balloon tamponade with the Sengstaken-Blakemore tube, which in itself causes a high incidence of complications (Fig. 17–6). Nevertheless, esophageal perforation does occur in 1% to 6% of patients after endoscopic sclerotherapy (Korula et al., 1989; Perino et al., 1987). Other complications following esophageal sclerotherapy are ulceration, stricture, and hematoma (Low and Patterson, 1988) (Fig. 17–7). Perforation of the esophagus may also be caused by severe vomiting against a resistance in the upper esophagus and glottis (Boerhaave's syndrome) (Fig. 17–8). Boerhaave's syndrome involves all layers of the esophageal wall and most commonly occurs on the left posterolateral aspect of the lower esophagus just above the diaphragm. Less commonly, the midesophagus is torn, usually on the right side close to the level of the azygos arch. Mallory-Weiss tears are also caused by vomiting but do not result in a complete disruption of the wall. Unlike patients with Boerhaave's syndrome, in whom hemorrhage can escape

Text continued on page 320

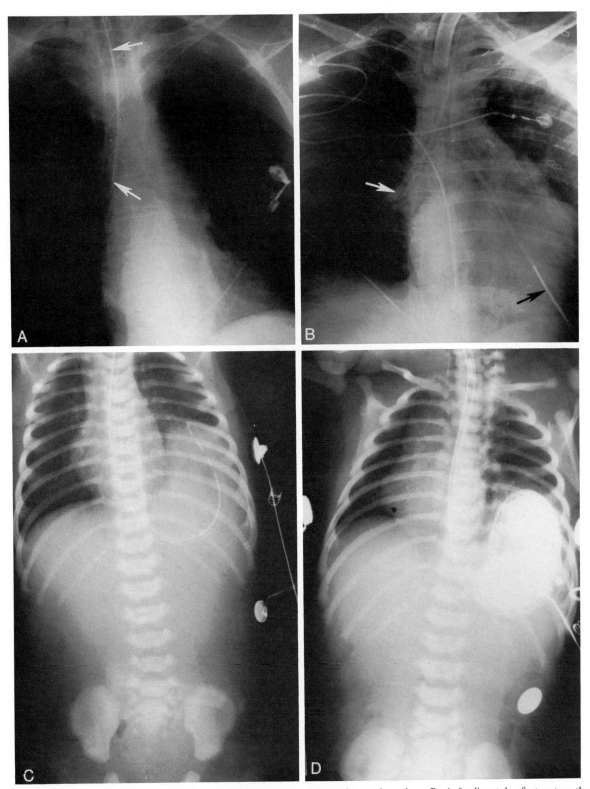

Figure 17–2. Malpositioned tubes. *A,* Nasogastric tube *(arrows)* in right mainstem bronchus. *B,* A feeding tube first enters the right bronchus *(white arrow),* then crosses over to enter the left bronchus. The tip *(black arrow)* is in the lung periphery. Tube feedings would cause pneumonia, which could be fatal. *C* and *D,* A newborn with respiratory distress and an abnormal density in the left chest. A nasogastric tube passed easily into the density *(C).* Barium through the nasogastric tube *(D)* demonstrates malposition of the stomach caused by a diaphragmatic eventration.

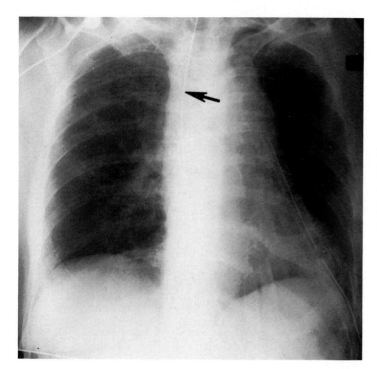

Figure 17–3. Mediastinal hemorrhage. A portable chest radiograph in a 60-year-old man who had a recent motor vehicle accident demonstrates widening of the mediastinum and a poorly defined aortic knob. The nasogastric tube *(arrow)* is deviated to the right. At surgery a laceration of the aorta contained by the adventitia was found. A left chest tube is in place.

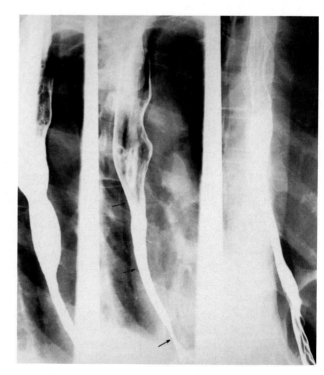

Figure 17–4. Esophageal stricture. After 10 days of nasogastric tube therapy, this patient complained of dysphagia. The barium swallow shows a long distal esophageal stricture *(arrows)* present in all three views and presumably caused by the nasogastric tube.

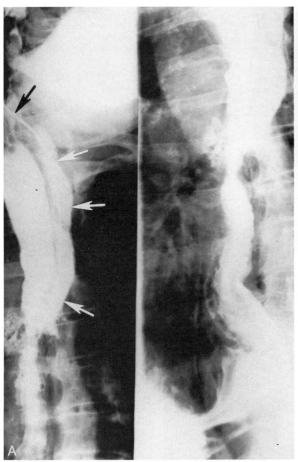

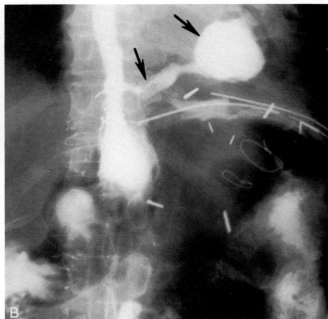

Figure 17–5. Esophageal injuries. *A,* Oblique and lateral views of a Gastrografin swallow in a patient with chest pain after nasogastric tube insertion shows a dissection of the upper esophagus. The nasogastric tube *(black arrow)* is in the false lumen *(white arrows). B,* A Gastrografin swallow in a different patient shows a free perforation *(arrows)* of the esophagus into the left pleural space after attempted nasogastric tube insertion. Two chest tubes are also in place.

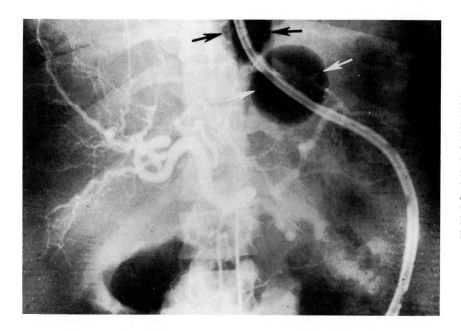

Figure 17–6. Sengstaken-Blakemore tube. Hepatic angiogram in a patient with bleeding esophageal varices. The Sengstaken-Blakemore tube is a double-balloon system with an additional lumen for gastric suction. The proximal balloon *(black arrows)* is inflated in the esophagus to tamponade the varices and the distal balloon *(white arrows)* is in the stomach. The complication rate from balloon tamponade is as high as 15% (esophageal perforation and pulmonary aspiration).

Figure 17–7. Esophageal submucosal hematoma. A 47-year-old man complained of chest pain 4 hours after sclerotherapy for varices. A barium swallow showed a large submucosal mass *(arrows)* consistent with a hematoma.

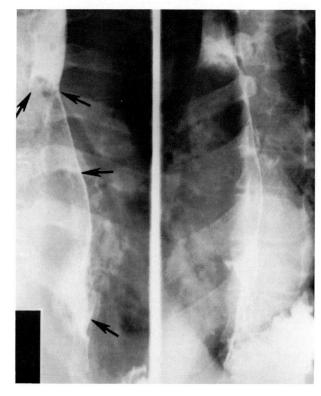

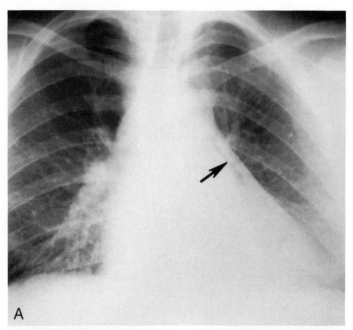

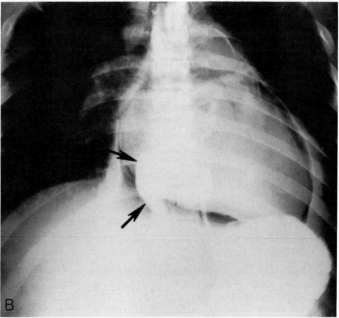

Figure 17–8. Boerhaave's syndrome. *A,* A 23-year-old man with a 1-day history of severe vomiting. Chest radiograph shows enlarged cardiac silhouette and air along the left upper cardiac border *(arrow)*. *B,* A barium swallow 24 hours later shows barium in the pericardiaum and mediastinum *(arrows)*. There is now more air in the pericardium. At surgery there was an esophagopericardial fistula. In most cases of Boerhaave's syndrome, the esophagus ruptures into the mediastinum or pleural space.

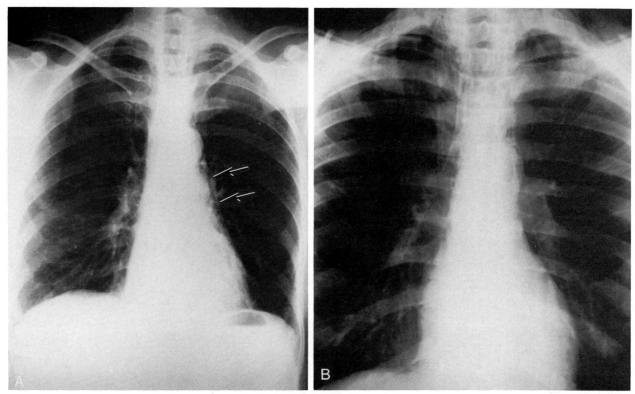

Figure 17–9. Perforation of esophagus. *A,* A chest radiograph after endoscopy shows a pneumomediastinum *(arrows)* from a distal esophageal perforation. *B,* A follow-up chest radiograph shows the air has dissected into the neck.

into adjacent mediastinal structures, patients with Mallory-Weiss tears present with hematemesis.

Findings of esophageal perforation on plain radiographs depend on the site and extent of injury. Perforation of the cervical esophagus results in cervical subcutaneous emphysema with subsequent dissection of the air along fascial planes into the mediastinum. Thoracic esophageal perforation can cause mediastinal widening or a pneumomediastinum, which may later extend superiorly and cause subcutaneous emphysema in the neck (Levine, 1989) (Fig. 17–9). Most thoracic esophageal perforations are associated with either a hydropneumothorax or pleural effusion. In ICU patients, however, these findings on plain radiographs are also commonly encountered in other conditions, such as subclavian line placement. Because of this, contrast studies may be necessary to determine the cause. The initial contrast evaluation is performed with a water-soluble agent, because it absorbed and nontoxic in the pleural space and mediastinum. If the initial study is negative and there remains a strong clinical suspicion of perforation, or if the patient is prone to aspiration, a dilute barium suspension with an approximately 30% to 50% weight-to-volume suspension can be used. If there is still concern that the injury is not well defined, a CT examination of the chest may be helpful.

STOMACH

Gastric Intubation

The resurgence of long-term nutritional support provided by gastrostomy (G) tubes has reduced the reliance on NG tubes for enteral feedings (Fig. 17–10). Whether introduced surgically, endoscopically, or percutaneously, some degree of free intraperitoneal air is usually present immediately after G-tube placement and does not imply gastric leakage. This is particularly true for percutaneously placed G tubes, which require a distended stomach for insertion. After percutaneous placement, abdominal wall or gastric hematomas are common and usually resolve without difficulty, unless accompanied by subcutaneous emphysema or evidence of free or loculated peritoneal fluid, which suggests fascitis or leakage (Wojtowycz et al., 1988). Other complications of G tubes include tube dislodgment and tract breakdown with peritonitis, GI hemorrhage, and cologastric fistula (Wolf et al., 1986; Stefan et al., 1989). Balloon-tipped tubes also can migrate to the gastric outlet or beyond and cause obstruction (Fig. 17–11). Foley catheters used as G tubes placed percutaneously have been associated with more complications than other nonballoon types of self-retaining tubes (Hicks et al.,

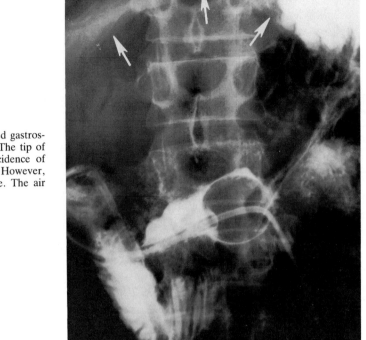

Figure 17–10. Gastrostomy tube. A percutaneously inserted gastrostomy tube is anchored to the gastric wall with a balloon. The tip of the catheter is in the duodenum, which reduces the incidence of aspiration. Injected contrast shows that there is no leak. However, free peritoneal air *(arrows)* is present from the procedure. The air was reabsorbed in several days.

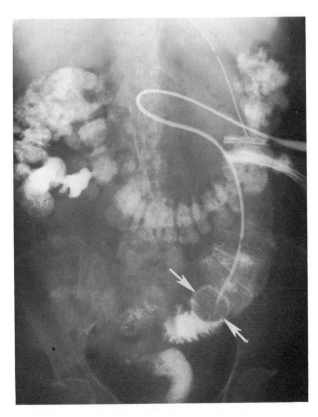

Figure 17–11. Gastrostomy tube causing obstruction. The gastrostomy tube has migrated into the small bowel. The inflated balloon *(arrows)* is causing partial small bowel obstruction. A nasogastric tube is also present. Contrast in the colon is from a previous CT.

1990), but their larger caliber provides easier instillation of feedings and medications. Catheters with anchoring devices consisting of mushroom tips or closed pigtail loops are smaller in caliber but rarely obstruct should they migrate to the pylorus or duodenum. Because of increasing use of these more sophisticated anchoring devices within the stomach, in concert with similar devices designed to firmly position the external portion of the catheter to the skin, complications arising from tube migration should diminish. If the position of a G tube is uncertain or leakage is suspected, a small quantity of water-soluble contrast can be injected through the tube. Leakage into the peritoneal cavity demonstrates contrast around the walls of the stomach and bowel in the paracolic gutters. A gastrocolic fistula is present if contrast simultaneously fills the colon and stomach. Patients receiving G-tube feedings are at higher risk for GE reflux and aspiration pneumonia, particularly those with recent histories of previous pneumonia (Cogen and Weinry, 1989; Grunow et al., 1989). In these patients a longer tube should be used and advanced into the small bowel.

Gastritis and Gastric Ulcers

The reported incidence of stress-related mucosal damage to the upper GI tract shortly after admission to the ICU is from 60% to 100%; if complicated by perforation and massive hemorrhage requiring surgical intervention, mortality can approach 80% (Peora, 1987). These statistics have prompted several investigations into the efficacy of the prophylactic use of histamine receptor antagonists or antacids (Noseworthy et al., 1987; Poleski and Spanier, 1986). The more severe the underlying illness, the greater the likelihood of developing mucosal damage with certain subgroups at higher risk—patients with extensive burns (Curling's ulcer) or sepsis; those with renal, respiratory, or hepatic failure; and those sustaining central nervous system injury (Cushing's ulcer) or multiple trauma (Peora, 1987). The initial lesions tend to be multiple and begin in the gastric fundus and body, but they can ultimately involve the distal esophagus, antrum, and proximal duodenum.

Bleeding may be heralded by the onset of bloody return through the NG tube. Endoscopy is usually successful in pinpointing the site and nature of the hemorrhage, but angiography sometimes is necessary for localization and possibly treatment. Although contrast studies are capable of demonstrating even superficial mucosal lesions, such examinations are not practical in ICU patients and serve little purpose in pinpointing hemorrhage. Nevertheless, water-soluble contrast studies can be used in patients with suspected perforation. CT is particularly helpful to look for abscess formation in patients with suspected perforation. Free abdominal air is readily detected subdiaphragmatically on upright abdominal radiographs.

Because many critically ill patients cannot be positioned upright, a left lateral decubitus or cross-table lateral view shows even small amounts of free air. Moderately large amounts of free air are necessary before it can be visualized on supine abdominal radiographs (Fig. 17–12). Air in the lesser sac may be best seen on the supine abdominal radiograph. The diagnosis of abscess can be suspected when a mottled gas pattern is seen on the plain radiographs. The diagnosis can be confirmed by CT. Visualization of a bubbly gas collection within the stomach wall is nearly diagnostic for bacterial emphysematous gastritis in acutely ill patients and is associated with a 60% to 80% mortality (Kussin et al., 1987) (Fig. 17–13). This entity must be distinguished from the more benign condition, gastric interstitial emphysema (Fig. 17–14). Predisposing factors for emphysematous gastritis include recent abdominal surgery, GI infarction, alcohol abuse, and corrosive material ingestion (Monteferrante and Shimkin, 1989). Patients with emphysematous gastritis present with acute abdomens, whereas gastric interstitial emphysema is usually asymptomatic and generally follows known gastric outlet obstruction or gastric instrumentation.

Acute Gastric Dilatation

Acute gastric dilatation was originally believed to be caused by obstruction of the duodenum (von Rokitansky, 1842). Current opinion points to a multifactorial etiology including aerophagia, lower esophageal sphincter dysfunction, neural reflex gastric inhibition, and atony secondary to excessive potassium and chloride losses in the traumatized, immobilized, or postoperative patient (Byrne and Cahill, 1961; Clearfield and Stahlgren, 1985; Dragstedt et al., 1931; Morris et al., 1947). Unfortunately, resuscitation techniques used in the field for trauma victims can aggravate gastric distention (Moyers, 1957). If not decompressed, the acutely distended stomach can cause profound hypotension and respiratory distress by restricting inferior vena caval flow and diaphragmatic motion, interfering with physical examination and diagnostic peritoneal lavage (Passi et al., 1969). Other complications of acute gastric dilatation are aspiration, post-decompressive gastric hemorrhage, prolonged ileus, and, rarely, perforation. Diagnosis of acute gastric dilatation is easily made from the abdominal plain film and is treated by NG intubation (Fig. 17–15). Early NG tube insertion for gastric decompression is recommended for patients recovering from major abdominal surgery and for acutely traumatized patients. This is particularly true for those with spinal injuries or who require endotracheal intubation, since the incidence of gastric distention is greater in these subgroups (Duncan and Milnes, 1969). A confirmatory radiograph showing proper placement of the NG tube is mandatory.

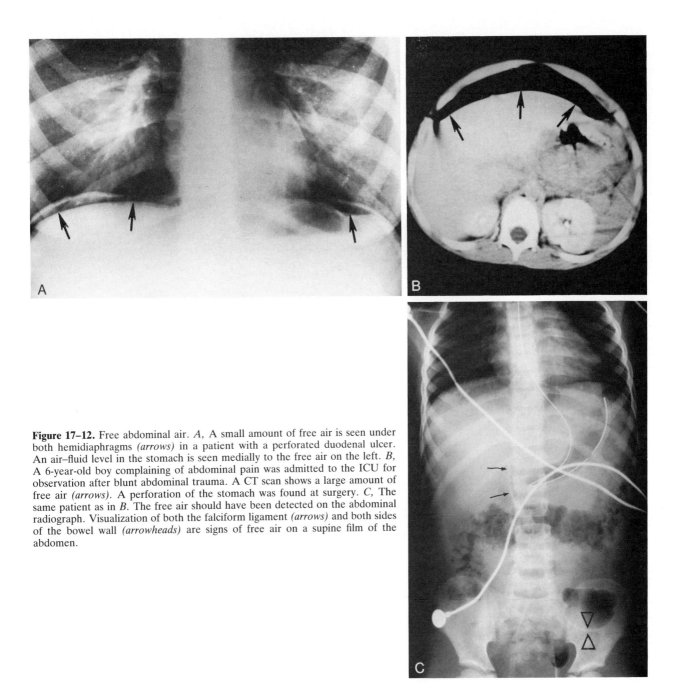

Figure 17–12. Free abdominal air. *A,* A small amount of free air is seen under both hemidiaphragms *(arrows)* in a patient with a perforated duodenal ulcer. An air–fluid level in the stomach is seen medially to the free air on the left. *B,* A 6-year-old boy complaining of abdominal pain was admitted to the ICU for observation after blunt abdominal trauma. A CT scan shows a large amount of free air *(arrows).* A perforation of the stomach was found at surgery. *C,* The same patient as in *B.* The free air should have been detected on the abdominal radiograph. Visualization of both the falciform ligament *(arrows)* and both sides of the bowel wall *(arrowheads)* are signs of free air on a supine film of the abdomen.

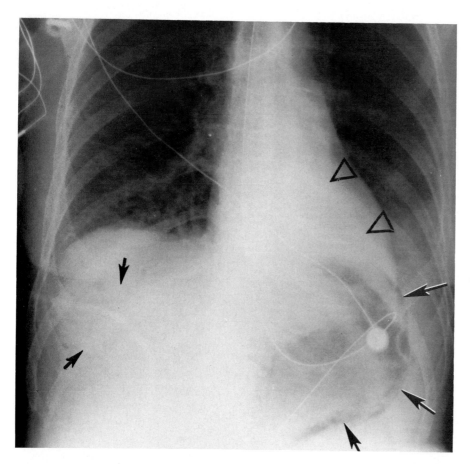

Figure 17–13. Emphysematous gastritis. A bubbly gas pattern is seen in the gastric wall *(large arrows)* of a patient who ingested a caustic agent. Air is also visible in the portal venous system *(small arrows)* and left lower lobe atelectasis *(arrowheads)*. At autopsy the stomach was necrotic.

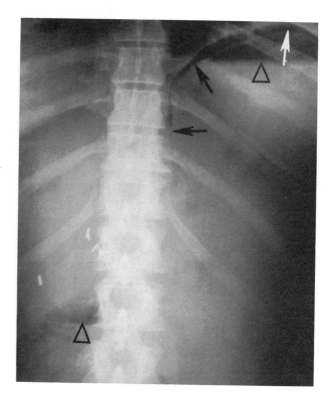

Figure 17–14. Gastric interstitial emphysema. A linear collection of air can be seen in the wall of the stomach *(arrows)* of a patient with gastric outlet obstruction from ulcer disease. The intramural air does not change in location as the patient is placed in different positions. The stomach is distended with fluid and a small amount of air *(arrowheads)*.

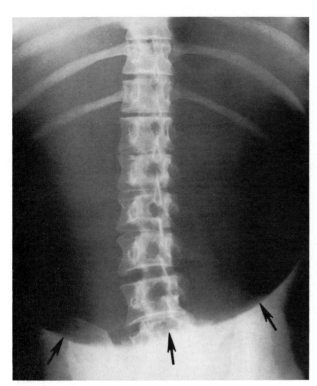

Figure 17–15. Acute gastric dilatation. A patient admitted with severe body burns experienced massive gastric distention *(arrows)*. A nasogastric tube was subsequently inserted, and the stomach was uneventfully decompressed.

SMALL INTESTINE

The most common small intestinal abnormalities that occur in critically ill patients include obstruction, adynamic ileus, and ischemia. These conditions occur as either the primary problem that necessitates ICU care or secondary to surgery or other disease processes while the patient is already in the ICU. In the latter circumstance, these small bowel abnormalities may be difficult to diagnose because their occurrence may be masked by the patient's underlying condition. Radiographic studies such as plain abdominal radiographs, contrast studies, CT, and angiography can help establish the diagnosis.

Obstruction and Adynamic Ileus

Small bowel obstruction is defined as either complete or partial blockage of the intestinal lumen.

In the United States, 75% of small bowel obstructions are caused by adhesions. Adhesions are usually a result of previous abdominal surgery. About 5% to 20% of patients undergoing abdominal surgery experience small bowel obstruction from adhesions, and the obstruction can occur shortly after surgery or many years later (Jones and Munro, 1985). Most adhesions are found in the lower abdomen and cause distal small bowel obstruction. Other causes of small

bowel obstruction include hernias, volvulus, intussusception, and trauma.

The diagnosis of small bowel obstruction can usually be made on plain radiographs. It is important to try to distinguish partial small bowel obstruction from complete and closed-loop obstructions, since the latter two conditions usually require imminent surgery. Closed-loop obstructions result in a high incidence of ischemia with subsequent perforation and peritonitis. In incomplete obstruction abdominal radiographs show air in the colon, but the small bowel is disproportionately distended. In complete obstruction there is no colonic air after 24 to 48 hours. Closed-loop obstruction may be difficult to diagnose on plain radiographs but should be suspected if a fixed and dilated loop of small intestine is seen on several radiographs (Fig. 17–16). CT may be useful to diagnose closed-loop obstructions (Cho et al., 1989) and also may be useful to detect the causes of small bowel obstruction other than adhesions such as hernias or intussusceptions (Ghahremani and Gove, 1989) (Fig. 17–17).

The value of oral barium studies to diagnose small bowel obstruction is controversial, but contrast studies can be useful when plain radiographs are equivocal or unable to distinguish complete from partial obstruction (Cheadle et al., 1988; Ericksen et al., 1990; Riveron et al., 1989) (Fig. 17–18). Enteroclysis can be used instead of the routine small intestinal follow-through (Dehn and Nolan, 1989). Water-soluble contrast medium is generally not used in small bowel obstruction because of the poor-quality images obtained and because its hypertonicity can aggravate pre-existing fluid and electrolyte imbalance. Nonionic contrast agents, however, result in better radiographic visualization of the small intestine. Both ionic and nonionic contrast media have been reported to relieve partial small bowel obstruction caused by adhesions (Stordaht et al., 1988).

Small bowel obstruction in the early postoperative period (Frykberg and Phillips, 1989; Pickleman and Lee, 1989; Stewart et al., 1987) may be difficult to recognize because of the normal decrease in bowel function after abdominal surgery. The average onset is 4 to 10 days after surgery, and it is particularly common after colorectal surgery. Most cases are due to adhesions. It is important to consider small bowel obstruction in the differential diagnosis of patients whose bowel function is not recovering properly after abdominal surgery because the mortality rate is high (7% to 18%). The diagnosis can usually be made by plain abdominal radiographs. Barium small bowel studies may be helpful when the plain films are not diagnostic. Most patients can be successfully treated by suction and supportive methods. Occasionally, surgical intervention is required.

In general, untreated small bowel obstruction has a mortality rate of about 60%; with treatment the rate drops to less than 5%. Specific treatment of small bowel obstruction consists of tube decompression or surgery (Helmkamp and Kimmel, 1985; Richards and

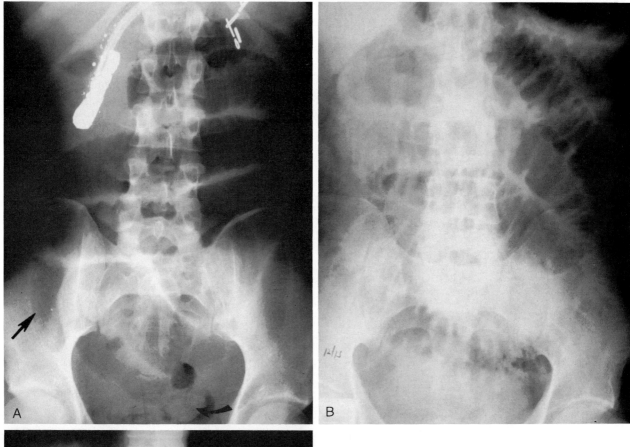

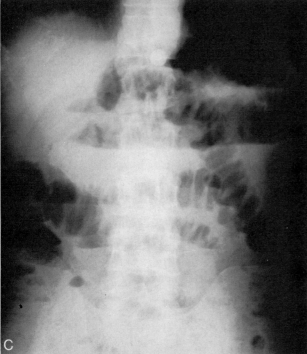

Figure 17–16. Several different small bowel obstructions from adhesions. *A,* Partial small bowel obstruction. The patient had previous surgery *(clips in left upper quadrant).* A small bowel tube for decompression is in the descending duodenum, and multiple dilated, centrally located small bowel loops are also present. This is a partial obstruction because of the presence of air in the cecum *(arrow)* and air and stool in the rectum *(curved arrow)* several days after the onset of symptoms. *B* and *C,* Complete small bowel obstruction consisting of multiple dilated small bowel loops with air–fluid levels. There is no air in the colon. *D,* Closed-loop obstruction consisting of a single dilated small bowel loop with air–fluid levels. This finding was present on serial abdominal films. *E,* Partial small bowel obstruction—CT findings. A patient with a known ovarian tumor presents with abdominal distention. A CT scan shows a large amount of ascites *(white arrows),* dilated small bowel loops *(black arrows),* and a normal caliber colon *(arrowheads)* that contains air. The findings are consistent with an incomplete small bowel obstruction.

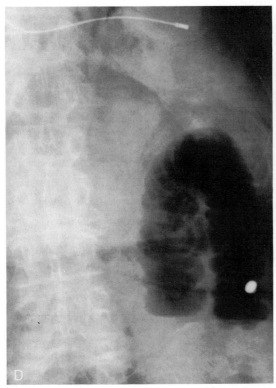

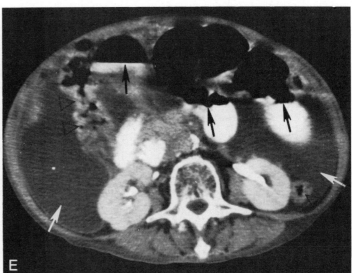

Figure 17–16. *Continued.* See legend on opposite page

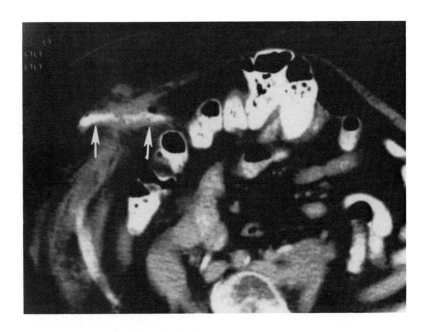

Figure 17–17. Spigelian hernia. A CT scan shows a loop of small bowel herniating through the lateral border of the right rectus muscle *(arrows)* in a patient who has symptoms consistent with intermittent small bowel obstruction. This diagnosis can be difficult to make on conventional barium studies.

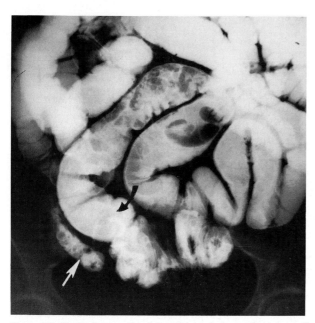

Figure 17–18. Barium studies in small bowel obstruction. A small bowel follow-through shows a transition between a dilated small bowel loop *(curved arrow)* and the more distally located normal caliber loop *(arrow)*. This finding indicates a partial small bowel obstruction, in this patient due to adhesions *(arrowheads)*.

Williams, 1988; Tanphiphat et al., 1987). Tube decompression can be accomplished by the use of long tubes (e.g., Cantor tubes), which are inserted perorally into the small intestine near the site of the obstruction (Fig. 17–19) or by NG tubes that are inserted into the stomach. Controversy exists as to which type of decompression is best. Patients who respond best to tube decompression therapy are usually those who experience early postoperative small bowel obstruction and those with partial small bowel obstruction. Complete and closed-loop obstructions usually require surgery.

Adynamic ileus is classically defined as generalized distention of the GI tract (stomach, small intestine, and colon) and absent peristalsis without underlying mechanical blockage. The most common cause is abdominal surgery, particularly surgery that involves extensive bowel manipulations. The exact etiology is unknown but is probably due to the interaction of neural, humoral, and metabolic factors. The causes of paralytic ileus are legion. Common causes besides surgery include electrolyte imbalance (especially low potassium), drugs such as narcotics and phenothiazines, pneumonia and systemic infections, and trauma.

The diagnosis of generalized adynamic ileus can usually be made on supine and upright abdominal radiographs (Fig. 17–20). Difficulties arise when bowel dilatation is not uniform or when there is a localized ileus (Fig. 17–21). Under these circumstances, the differential diagnosis between adynamic ileus and partial small bowel obstruction may not be possible on routine plain radiographs. Additional

plain radiographs, such as a prone abdomen or a left lateral view of the rectum and serial plain films, may help in the diagnosis. When plain radiograph diagnosis is equivocal, contrast studies are useful. A barium small bowel study looking for the absence of a "transition zone" (a change in caliber of the lumen from dilated to normal size) is probably the procedure of choice (Fig. 17–22). A barium enema with reflux into the small intestine is faster and may provide the necessary information.

Paralytic ileus after abdominal surgery is common and usually subsides after 2 or 3 days (Livingston and Passaro, 1990). A persistent ileus is abnormal, and although it may be a result of the surgery with no apparent cause, underlying causes such as infection or electrolyte imbalance should be sought. Additionally, it is important to distinguish persistent ileus from postoperative small bowel obstruction. As indicated, this differentiation can usually be made by plain abdominal radiographs or contrast studies.

The standard treatment of postoperative ileus is intubation usually with an NG tube and intravenous

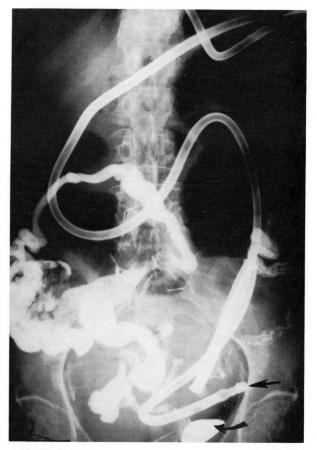

Figure 17–19. Cantor tube decompression. These dilated proximal small bowel loops are consistent with small bowel obstruction. Residual contrast in the colon is from a previous barium enema. A Cantor tube with the mercury-filled balloon at its distal end is located in the distal small bowel. The separation between the end of the tube *(arrow)* and the mercury-filled balloon *(curved arrow)* is commonly seen and is normal.

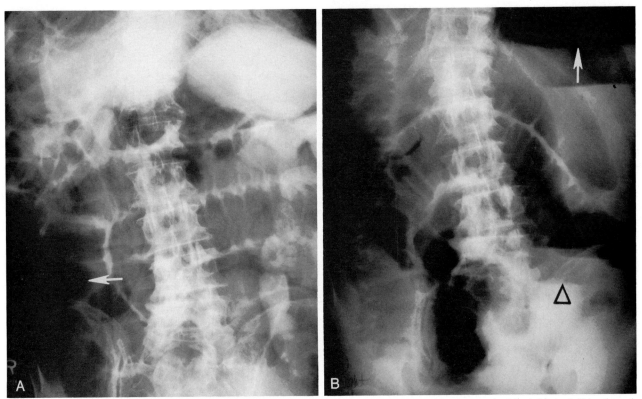

Figure 17–20. Generalized adynamic ileus. A 75-year-old man with left lower lobe pneumonia presented with abdominal distention. *A,* The supine abdomen shows distention of the stomach, small bowel (central loops), and colon *(arrow)*. There is residual contrast in the stomach and descending colon from a prior CT scan. *B,* An upright abdomen 1 day later shows air–fluid levels in the stomach *(arrow),* small bowel *(arrowhead),* and colon (not shown). Generalized bowel distention is consistent with an adynamic ileus. As the pneumonia subsided, the ileus resolved.

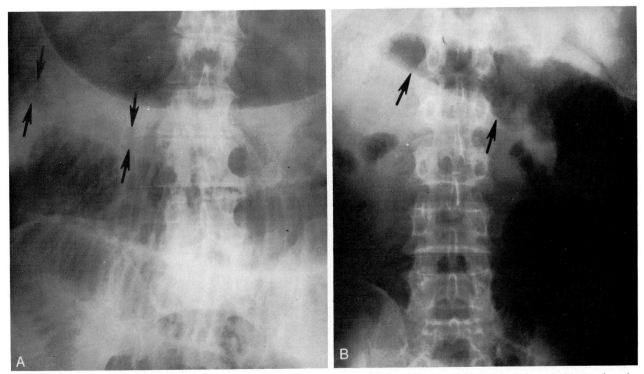

Figure 17–21. Nonuniform and localized ileus characterized by *A,* generalized distention of the small bowel and stomach, but not the colon *(arrows)*. This could be a small bowel obstruction, but gastric distention does not occur often in small bowel obstruction. *B,* There is sequential dilatation of the horizontal portion of the duodenum (sentinel loop sign; *arrows*) in a patient with pancreatitis.

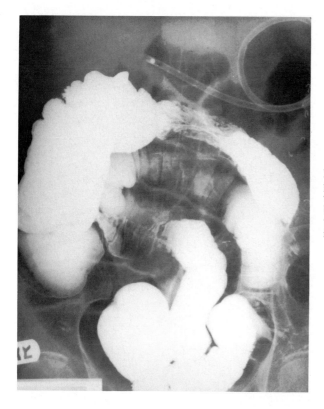

Figure 17–22. Adynamic ileus contrast study. A patient who had previous surgery experienced abdominal distention. On plain films it was difficult to distinguish ileus from partial small bowel obstruction. A barium small bowel study shows dilatation of the small bowel but no transition zone. The colon is opacified to the splenic flexure, and there is an area of spasm in the mid–transverse colon.

hydration until the ileus subsides. Occasionally, if the ileus is severe, long intestinal tubes or even surgical decompression may be necessary. Resolution of postoperative ileus after administration of water-soluble contrast agents by mouth has been reported (Watkins and Robertson, 1985).

Air in the peritoneal cavity is normally seen on abdominal films after abdominal surgery. The amount of free air is variable and in itself of no significance. Normally the amount of air decreases daily, and in most instances it is totally reabsorbed in 7 to 10 days. Increasing amounts of free air on serial radiographs

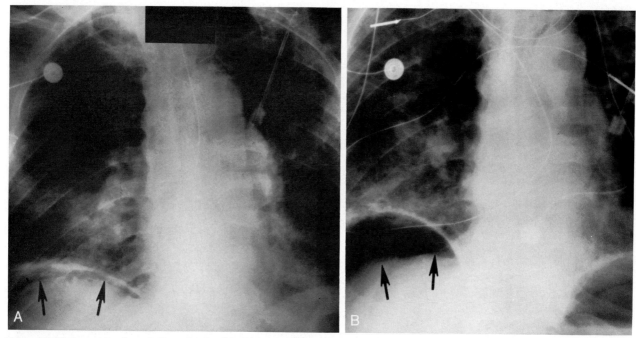

Figure 17–23. Increasing free air from duodenal leakage. *A,* A 60-year-old man had a recent partial gastrectomy and gastrojejunostomy for carcinoma of the stomach. An upright radiograph several days after surgery shows a small amount of free air under the right hemidiaphragm *(arrows).* There are also patchy areas of pneumonitis at the right lung base and left lung laterally. *B,* Two days later there is an increase in the amount of free air *(arrows).* At surgery there was a leak at the duodenal stump.

suggest bowel perforation or leakage from a surgical anastomosis (Fig. 17–23).

Ischemia

Ischemia of the small intestine may occur as a complication of small bowel obstruction or may be primary, due to vascular disease. In either case the diagnosis is often difficult and the clinical manifestations often protean. Early diagnosis is important, and mortality rates range from 30% to 70% (Merine et al., 1989; Nemcek, 1989; Stordahl, 1989). Many patients present with severe abdominal pain disproportionate to their physical findings. The causes of primary vascular ischemia are generally classified as due to arterial disease such as from emboli or atherosclerosis; nonocclusive disease presumably due to diseased arterial perfusion; and venous occlusive disease that may occur in malignancies or hypercoagulation states. The length of small intestine affected depends on the size and number of vessels involved, and the layers of the bowel wall involved depends on the completeness of the occlusion. The mucosa is involved first, since it is the most sensitive part of the wall to diminished blood flow.

The radiologic diagnosis should center on abdominal plain radiographs, CT, and angiography (Fig. 17–24). GI contrast studies should be avoided if possible, since contrast in the GI tract negates the usefulness of angiography or CT. On plain radiographs and even CT, findings are often nonspecific, resembling ileus or partial small bowel obstruction. More specific signs such as thumbprinting, air in the bowel wall, or air in the portal vein are uncommon but are better visualized on CT than on plain radiographs (Nemcek, 1989). CT scans may also show occluded veins or arterial thrombosis or emboli. Angiography has the advantages of better visualization of the vessels and can be used therapeutically, as with vasodilators or thrombolytic agents. Water-soluble contrast agents may leak through the damaged bowel wall (even without frank perforation) and be absorbed by the peritoneum and subsequently excreted by the kidneys into the bladder. Segmental ischemia usually resolves in 1 or 2 weeks but may cause a stricture with subsequent small bowel obstruction.

Treatment of small bowel ischemia usually requires surgical resection of the involved small intestine.

Trauma

Penetrating injuries to the abdomen generally require immediate surgery, and radiology has no major role. Five to 15% of the cases of severe blunt abdominal trauma result in intestinal injuries (colon, small intestine, and mesentery). In some series, especially with seat belt injuries, the proximal jejunum and the ileum are more commonly involved than is the duodenum (Christophi et al., 1985; Dauterive et al.,

1985). Small bowel injuries often present with vague signs and symptoms and are difficult to diagnose. Free intraperitoneal air may or may not be present, or it may develop several hours after the trauma. Injury to the mesentery may cause distal small bowel ischemia. If undetected these injuries have a high mortality from peritonitis.

Because most of the duodenum is fixed in the retroperitoneum, it is susceptible to injury from blunt trauma to the upper abdomen. This is particularly true for the third portion of the duodenum, where it crosses the spine. Less severe trauma may result in a duodenal hematoma from submucosal vascular tears. The hematoma may cause varying degrees of duodenal obstruction. The diagnosis can usually be made by upper GI series (Fig. 17–25). If possible, treatment should be conservative, using NG suction, since most cases resolve in 1 or 2 weeks. More severe trauma may cause duodenal rupture and concomitant pancreatic injuries. Rupture generally occurs in the third part of the duodenum, along the posterior wall and extends into the retroperitoneum. When the anterior wall ruptures, spillage is into the peritoneal cavity. Plain radiographs are diagnostic in fewer than half of the cases (Fig. 17–26). CT is more sensitive than plain radiography and has the added advantage of showing any additional injuries. Even with treatment, the mortality rate is as high as 50%.

COLON

Ileus and Obstruction

The terms *acute colonic ileus, pseudo-obstruction of the colon,* and *Ogilvie's syndrome* refer to the presence of clinical and radiographic evidence of colonic distention without obstruction. Colonic ileus usually occurs as part of a generalized ileus, but may occur without small bowel or gastric involvement. Although the pathogenesis remains unknown, the widely held view is that colonic ileus results from an imbalance between sympathetic and parasympathetic stimulation with resultant inhibition of bowel peristalsis.

Colonic ileus may be seen in postsurgical patients, after blunt abdominal trauma or myocardial infarction, with prolonged bed rest, and in association with sepsis, shock, pancreatitis, inflammatory bowel disease, malignancy, orthopedic injury or surgery, metabolic abnormalities, and retroperitoneal hematoma. It is also associated with respiratory failure, including lower lobe pneumonia, in which case it requires mechanical ventilatory support (Golden and Chandler, 1975). Steroid-induced colonic ileus has been reported as a complication of renal transplantation (Stratta et al., 1988).

Patients with ileus must be distinguished from those with true colonic obstruction due to malignancy, hernia, or volvulus. Clinically, ileus and obstruction present with abdominal distention and the inability

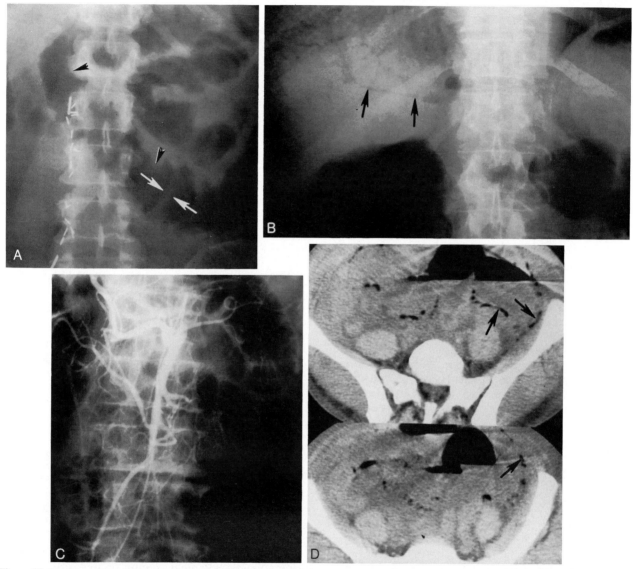

Figure 17–24. Several examples of small bowel ischemia. *A,* A plain radiograph of the abdomen shows mild dilatation of several small bowel loops with thickening of the valvulae conniventes *(white arrows).* There is scalloping of the bowel wall contour (thumbprints; *arrowheads).* These findings were present on serial radiographs and represent submucosal edema and hemorrhage. *B,* A different patient demonstrating air in the portal veins *(arrows).* This finding usually indicates bowel necrosis and carries a poor prognosis. The patient subsequently died. *C,* A CT scan in a patient with unexplained abdominal pain shows multiple predominantly fluid-filled small bowel loops with air in the bowel wall *(arrows).* The plain abdominal radiographs showed mildly dilated small bowel loops but no bowel wall air. At surgery there was extensive small bowel ischemia. *D,* A superior mesenteric angiogram shows a paucity of jejunal vessels in the left midabdomen in a patient surgically proved to have small bowel ischemia.

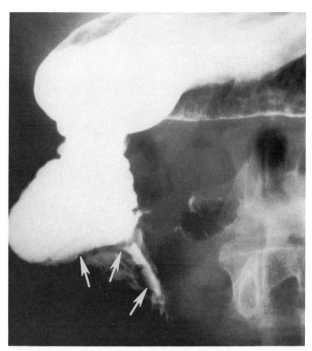

Figure 17–25. Duodenal hematoma. An upper GI series on an adult man after blunt upper abdominal trauma shows a submucosal mass *(arrows)* causing obstruction at the junction of the second and third parts of the duodenum. The findings are consistent with a hematoma. After several days of nasogastric suction, there was considerable resolution.

to pass flatus and stool. The distention in obstruction, especially when due to malignancy, can be insidious. The onset is more acute and is associated with pain when obstruction is caused by volvulus or intussusception.

On plain radiographs, the usual finding in colonic obstruction is dilatation of the colon proximal to the point of obstruction and a paucity of colonic gas distal to the obstruction. The distention with ileus may be segmental or may involve the entire colon. With low colonic obstruction, the left lateral decubitus view of the rectum is useful, and gaseous distention of the rectum indicates the absence of mechanical obstruction (Laufer, 1976). Although plain radiographs of the abdomen demonstrate what segments of the colon are dilated, they often cannot be used exclusively to distinguish ileus from mechanical obstruction. Barium enema and colonoscopy are often necessary to distinguish the two (Figs. 17–27 and 17–28).

Both colonic ileus and obstruction can lead to infarction and perforation. Because the cecum has the thinnest wall, it is most susceptible to perforation. When the cecal diameter approaches 14 cm, it is in danger of perforating and should be decompressed. Cecal perforation as a result of colonic obstruction has been reported in 1.5% to 14.8% of cases (Casola et al., 1986). The incidence of cecal perforation in colonic ileus is unknown. Perforation of cecum has a mortality rate of nearly 50% (Stroder et al., 1983). In general, the treatment of colonic obstruction,

regardless of the cause, is surgery. Various methods besides surgical decompression have been tried for colonic ileus. These include the insertion of rectal tubes and, recently, endoscopic decompression. In the past few years, CT-guided percutaneous cecostomy has been used to treat cecal distention due to ileus or obstruction (Haaga et al., 1987).

Ischemia

The blood supply to the colon is from branches of the superior mesenteric artery (SMA), which perfuses the right and transverse colon, and the inferior mesenteric artery (IMA), which perfuses to the left side of the colon.

Ischemia of the colon usually affects elderly patients. The classical clinical presentation is bloody diarrhea and acute abdominal pain. Ischemia most commonly involves the distal left colon and the cecum. Contrary to earlier descriptions, the "watershed zone," or the splenic flexure area, is not the most commonly involved segment (Jeffrey, 1989). The rectum is often spared because of its dual blood

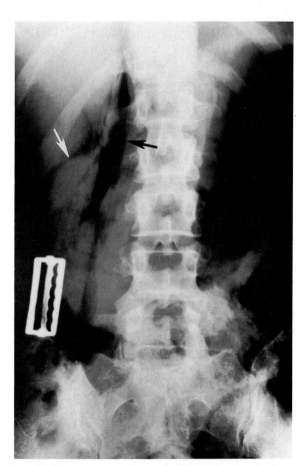

Figure 17–26. Duodenal rupture. A patient who sustained major trauma to the upper abdomen was found at surgery to have a ruptured horizontal portion of the duodenum. The abdominal film showed retroperitoneal air along the psoas muscle *(black arrow)* and around the right kidney *(white arrow)*.

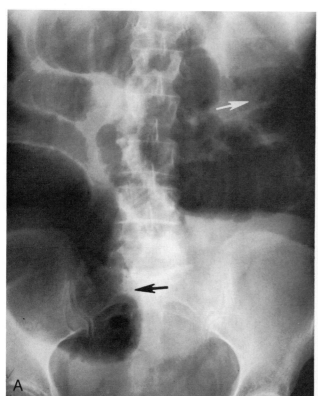

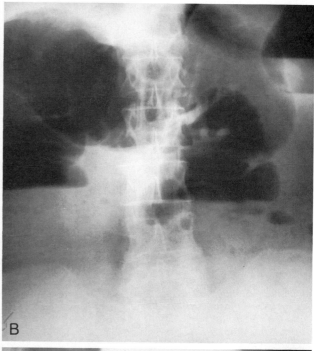

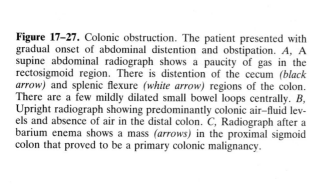

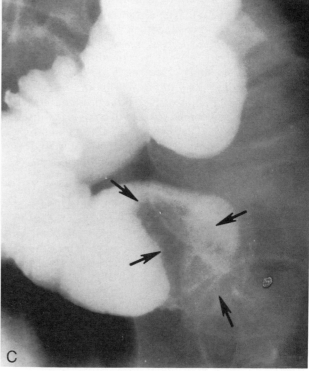

Figure 17–27. Colonic obstruction. The patient presented with gradual onset of abdominal distention and obstipation. *A,* A supine abdominal radiograph shows a paucity of gas in the rectosigmoid region. There is distention of the cecum *(black arrow)* and splenic flexure *(white arrow)* regions of the colon. There are a few mildly dilated small bowel loops centrally. *B,* Upright radiograph showing predominantly colonic air–fluid levels and absence of air in the distal colon. *C,* Radiograph after a barium enema shows a mass *(arrows)* in the proximal sigmoid colon that proved to be a primary colonic malignancy.

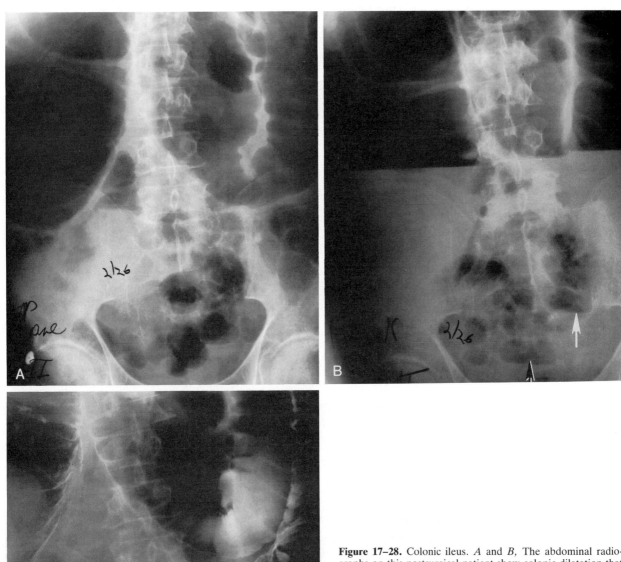

Figure 17–28. Colonic ileus. *A* and *B*, The abdominal radiographs on this postsurgical patient show colonic dilatation that is most prominent in the transverse and ascending colon. There are multiple air–fluid levels, even in the distal colon *(arrows in B)*, which is only minimally distended. *C*, A partial barium enema shows that there is no obstruction.

supply. Any section of the large intestine may be affected, however.

Causes of ischemia include embolism, thrombosis, and perfusion defects. Acute ischemia is due to reduction or abolition of blood flow, usually to a limited area supplied by a single branch of the SMA or IMA (Meyers, 1986). As opposed to ischemia of the small bowel, colonic ischemia is usually not the result of major vaso-occlusive disease but probably is due to low-flow states and rarely results in transmural infarction (Bailey et al., 1986). Although the exact mechanism of ischemic colitis remains unproved, evidence suggests that the colon may be unusually sensitive to vasoconstriction from low-flow states or hypotension, especially in the elderly (Bailey et al., 1986; Jeffrey, 1989). In addition to low-flow states, ischemia changes may also be due to local hemodynamic disturbances secondary to increased luminal pressure, as may be seen proximal to an obstruction.

On plain abdominal radiograph or contrast studies, the bowel wall is generally thickened with mural scalloping (thumbprints) due to submucosal edema and hemorrhage (Fig. 17–29). Occasional patients with colonic ischemia may progress to transmural infarction. With loss of mucosal integrity, intestinal gas may enter the bowel wall (Fig. 17–30). Pneumatosis intestinalis is not, however, pathognomonic for infarction; it may be seen with infectious or inflammatory colitis. Spasm may also be noted. CT scans show findings similar to the plain films or contrast enema but are better for demonstrating bowel wall thickening. Because ischemic colitis is often limited to the mucosa, radiographic studies may be normal or nonspecific. Consequently, colonoscopy can be helpful in making the diagnosis. In a series of 15 patients with ischemic colitis, all had abnormal colonoscopic results, whereas barium enema results were abnormal and suggestive of ischemic colitis in 6 of the 15 patients (Scowcraft et al., 1981). Angiography has proved to be of little value in the evaluation of patients with colonic ischemia. Selective arteriography of the IMA generally shows findings of an inflammatory process with hypervascularity of the bowel wall and intense opacification of draining veins. These findings are nonspecific. Intra-arterial infusion of vasodilatory drugs has no role in these patients (Athanasoulis et al., 1982).

The clinical symptoms of ischemic colitis usually subside within 7 to 10 days, and the radiographic changes are usually reversible. Treatment is supportive with bed rest and antibiotics. If symptoms of peritonitis (secondary to bowel infarction and gangrene) develop, surgical intervention is warranted.

Most patients with ischemic colitis recover fully. Fibrous stricture may develop, however, resulting in colonic obstruction (Fig. 17–31).

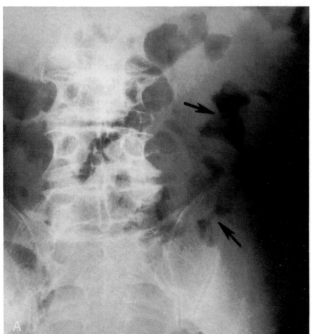

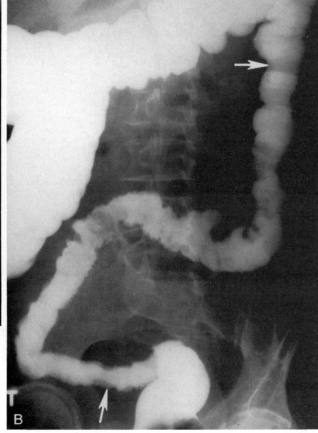

Figure 17–29. Ischemia. *A,* Mural scalloping (submucosa edema and hemorrhage) of the descending colon *(arrows)* is visible in a patient with bloody diarrhea. *B,* A barium enema 2 days later in the same patient shows findings consistent with ischemia of the sigmoid and descending colon. The haustral pattern is distorted and thickened *(arrows)*. Because of its dual blood supply, the rectum is spared.

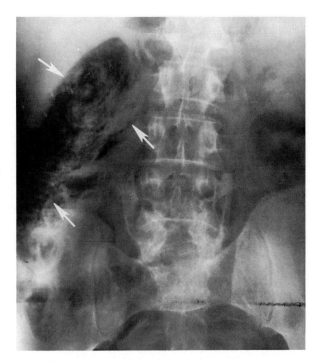

Figure 17–30. Ischemia. A patient with transmural infarction of the ascending colon. The abdominal radiograph shows air in the bowel wall *(arrows)* and absence of the normal haustral pattern.

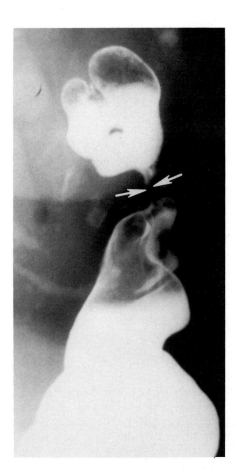

Figure 17–31. Ischemic stricture. A barium enema shows a tight stricture *(arrows)* of the sigmoid colon in a patient with previous ischemic colitis.

Colitis

The major causes of inflammatory changes in the colon are ulcerative colitis, Crohn's disease, ischemia, and infection. These processes are often difficult to distinguish radiographically because of overlapping findings. The clinical presentation is also similar and includes abdominal pain, diarrhea, bleeding, fever, and leukocytosis. Knowledge of the patient's age, underlying medical condition, and travel and exposure history may suggest a diagnosis, but frequently other diagnostic tests, including stool culture, serologic tests, endoscopy, and biopsy are needed for confirmation.

Pseudomembranous colitis is an acute colonic inflammation characterized by yellowish brown plaques that may occur in ICU patients taking antibiotics. The main cause is antibiotic treatment, usually from clindamycin, which destroys the bowel flora and allows overgrowth of *Clostridium difficile,* which produces an enterotoxin. The plain abdominal radiographs in pseudomembranous colitis are similar to those seen with other inflammatory bowel diseases. Contrast enemas should be performed carefully to avoid perforation, and water-soluble contrast agents should be used (Fig. 17–32). The findings on CT are nonspecific. Sigmoidoscopy usually shows characteristic mucosal pseudomembranes. A high serologic titer for *C. difficile* is diagnostic. Complete recovery is usually obtained with vancomycin therapy.

Toxic megacolon is an acute colitis accompanied by systemic toxicity and colonic dilatation. It is most frequently seen with ulcerative colitis but may occur

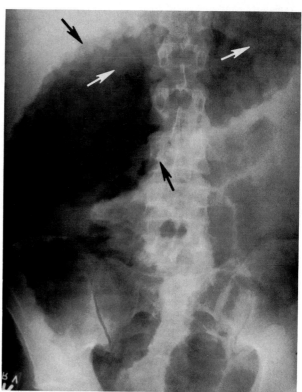

Figure 17–33. Toxic megacolon. A patient with acute ulcerative colitis presented initially with a toxic megacolon. On the supine radiograph, the findings are most evident in the transverse colon. The colon is dilated *(black arrows).* The haustra are absent, and there are multiple intraluminal polypoid excrescences *(white arrows).*

with any colitis. It occurs in 2% of people with ulcerative colitis and may be the initial presentation of the disease. Toxic megacolon indicates transmural extension of the inflammatory process with involvement of the neural elements. The supine film of the abdomen reveals a dilated colon, which is generally most pronounced in the transverse portion of the colon (Fig. 17–33). Contrast enema should not be performed in patients suspected of having toxic megacolon, since the risk of perforation is high. If the diagnosis is not certain, proctoscopy is usually diagnostic. Therapy involves fluid and electrolyte correction, antibiotics, long-tube intubation, steroids, and cessation of opiates and anticholinergics. Failure to respond in several days should prompt a colectomy.

Blunt Trauma

Injury to the colon after blunt abdominal trauma is rare and accounts for less than 5% of colonic injuries (Howell et al., 1976). Blunt trauma to the colon accounts for only 3% to 12% of all intra-abdominal injuries (Jeffrey, 1989). The cecum, transverse, and sigmoid colons are the most commonly involved sites (Fig. 17–34). Lap-type seat belts and steering wheel compression of the abdomen are two factors responsible for large bowel injury.

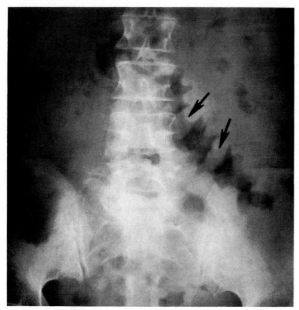

Figure 17–32. Pseudomembranous colitis. There is submucosal edema (thumbprints; *arrows*) of the sigmoid and descending colon. The appearance is nonspecific and can be seen with ischemia or any colitis. The specific diagnosis was made by endoscopic visualization of the pseudomembranes.

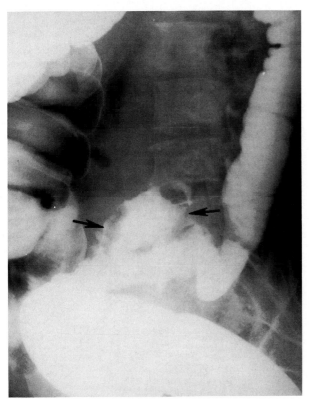

Figure 17–34. Trauma. A lap-type seat belt injury to the sigmoid colon. The barium enema shows a confined perforation *(arrows)* of the sigmoid colon.

Mesenteric laceration is the most frequent large bowel injury from blunt trauma. If major vessels are torn, bowel ischemia may occur. Barium enema may demonstrate changes compatible with ischemic colitis. Delayed stricture may result as the ischemic bowel heals.

Intramural hematoma is also associated with blunt abdominal trauma. It probably becomes symptomatic only if it causes bowel obstruction. Acute and chronic obstructing hematoma of the colon usually involves the sigmoid and descending colon.

Blunt trauma resulting in rectal injury usually is seen with severe fractures of the pelvic bones in which bony fragments perforate the extraperitoneal segments of the colon. This is associated with genitourinary injuries and massive blood loss (Howell et al., 1976).

Laceration of the large intestine, either complete or incomplete, also occurs after blunt trauma. Incomplete tears involve the serosa and muscularis. Perforation results when all layers are torn. Acute perforations and transections are more common in the transverse and sigmoid colons. Retroperitoneal or intraperitoneal air visible on radiographs of the abdomen may suggest colon perforation. With a colonic transection, however, there does not have to be free air, because the bowel ends may seal. Barium enema can confirm the resultant mechanical obstruction, the symptoms and diagnosis of which may be delayed. Surgical intervention is necessary in these cases.

HEMORRHAGE (INTRAPERITONEAL AND RETROPERITONEAL)

In critically ill patients, hemorrhage can occur in either the peritoneal cavity or the retroperitoneum. The clinical presentation usually is not typical but may consist of sudden abdominal pain, tenderness, a drop in hematocrit, and an abdominal mass. Often the patient has only vague abdominal pain (Alexander and Clark, 1982; Sagel et al., 1977).

Most intraperitoneal hemorrhages are secondary to trauma (Alexander and Clark, 1982). Other causes include bleeding from tumors, ectopic pregnancy, pancreatitis, rupture of aneurysms, and anticoagulant therapy (Alexander and Clark, 1982; Lewin and Patterson, 1980). Hemorrhage presents as free intraperitoneal fluid or as a subcapsular or intraparenchymal hematoma (e.g., spleen, liver, kidney) (Alexander and Clark, 1982; Swensen et al., 1984). Trauma is also the most common cause of retroperitoneal hemorrhage, including iatrogenic trauma such as after surgery, biopsy, or arteriography (Illescas et al., 1986). Other causes include anticoagulant therapy, bleeding diathesis, leaking or ruptured aortic aneurysm, neoplasms (e.g., renal, adrenal), arteriovenous malformations, and severe sepsis (Alexander and Clark, 1982; Lewin and Patterson, 1980; Sagel et al., 1977; Swensen et al., 1984).

Plain radiographs of the abdomen are nonspecific and may include evidence of ascites with fluid around the dome of the bladder ("rabbit ears"), a mass, or loss of retroperitoneal structures (Figs. 17–35 and 17–36). Ultrasound can be used to evaluate hematomas, but it does not provide a detailed evaluation of the intra-abdominal organs and retroperitoneal structures. CT is the method of choice because it not only detects, quantitates, and localizes the hematomas, but it may also provide the cause, thus directing appropriate clinical management (Sagel et al., 1977; Swensen et al., 1984). Radionuclide bleeding scans and angiography are used only to localize actual bleeding sites. Intraperitoneal hemorrhage appears similar to ascites on CT and collects in Morrison's pouch, around the liver and spleen, in the paracolic gutters, and in the pelvis (Alexander and Clark, 1982; Federle and Jeffrey, 1983) (Fig. 17–37). The density of the blood measures 20 to 80 Hounsfield units (HU). The higher-density fluid collections, which represent clotted blood, are usually near the source of the bleeding (Alexander and Clark, 1982; Federle and Jeffrey, 1983; Lewin and Patterson, 1980). Subcapsular hematomas appear as low-density collections contiguous to the organ and, because they may be isodense with the organ, may be missed if only noncontrast scans are obtained (Federle and Jeffrey, 1983; Swensen et al., 1984). Intraparenchymal hematomas are linear, irregular, low-density lesions within the organ on contrasted CT scans (Fig. 17–38).

Retroperitoneal hemorrhage presents as a mass on CT and may extend into more than one retroperito-

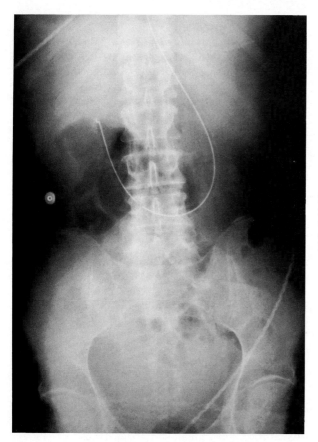

Figure 17–35. Intraperitoneal hemorrhage. A patient with hemorrhage from a ruptured spleen. The abdominal radiograph with a nasogastric tube in place shows a mass in the left upper quadrant displacing the stomach medially and increased soft tissue density in the pelvis caused by blood.

Figure 17–36. Retroperitoneal hemorrhage. Spontaneous hemorrhage from anticoagulation therapy. The abdominal radiograph shows a left flank mass displacing the colon medially *(arrows)* and loss of the left psoas margin.

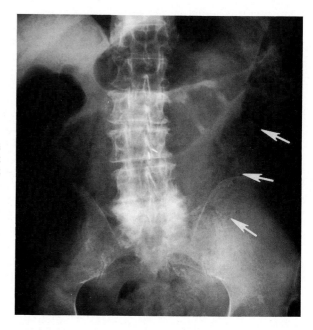

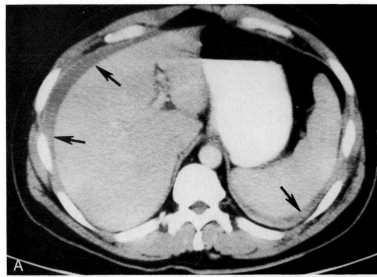

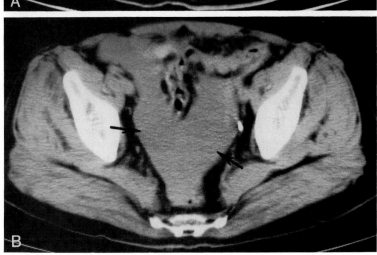

Figure 17–37. Intraperitoneal hemorrhage on CT. *A,* Intraperitoneal hemorrhage from a recent bleed shows fluid around the liver and spleen *(arrows).* On contrasted scans, the blood appears similar to ascites but has a higher HU number. *B,* Same patient as *A.* Fresh blood in the pelvis *(arrows)* is slightly less dense than adjacent muscle.

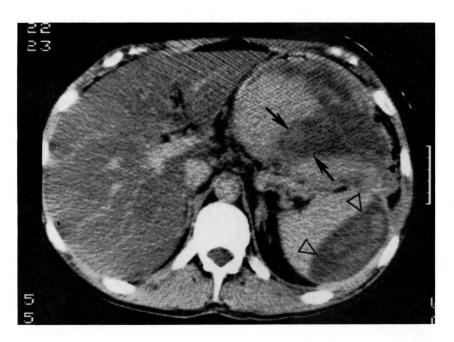

Figure 17–38. Subcapsular and intrasplenic hematomas. Trauma to the spleen caused a predominantly low-density subcapsular hematoma *(arrowheads).* An intrasplenic hematoma is also visible *(arrows).* The areas of higher density within the hematomas probably represent clotted blood.

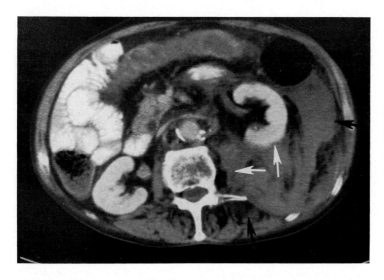

Figure 17-39. Retroperitoneal hemorrhage. The same patient as Figure 17-36. The CT scan shows blood in the anterior and posterior pararenal spaces *(black arrows).* Blood in the perirenal space is obliterating the left psoas muscle *(white arrow)* and displacing the kidney anteriorly *(white arrow).*

neal space (Fig. 17–39). Acute bleeding is usually isointense with adjacent muscles but becomes hyperdense (60 to 80 HU) in 48 to 72 hours (Sagel et al, 1977; Swensen et al., 1984). As the hematoma ages, it gets less dense but may be heterogeneous as a result of rebleeding or irregular resorption (Alexander and Clark, 1982; Swensen et al., 1984). Contrast medium extravasation is rarely seen (Swensen et al., 1984). A chronic hematoma may form a pseudocapsule, is of low density (30 HU), and cannot be differentiated from abscess or urinoma (Alexander and Clark, 1982; Swensen et al., 1984).

Treatment of abdominal hemorrhage depends on the stability of the patient. Supportive measures are used in stable patients. Unstable patients usually require surgical intervention. Angiographic embolization can occasionally be used.

ABSCESSES (INTRAPERITONEAL AND RETROPERITONEAL)

The diagnosis of intra-abdominal abscess can be a challenge, particularly in ICU patients who are usually critically ill or have had recent abdominal surgery or trauma (Callen, 1979; Mintz et al., 1983). Mortality of the untreated intra-abdominal abscess is 80% to 100%, and it is as high as 30% in treated patients (Altemier et al., 1973; Ariel and Kazarian, 1971). Many radiologic examinations to diagnose abscesses are available. Conventional radiographs and contrast studies in general are not very helpful (Callen, 1979; Ferrucci and vanSonnenberg, 1981; Mintz et al., 1983). Plain radiographic findings of an extraluminal gas collection, although pathognomic, are clearly seen prospectively in about half of the cases (Connell et al., 1980; Halber et al., 1979) (Fig. 17–40). CT, ultrasound, and nuclear medicine studies help to diagnose abscesses in more than 90% of the patients. Radionuclide studies, such as gallium-67– and indium-111–labeled leucocytes, are sensitive but not specific (Connell et al., 1980). They are used in patients who are not critically ill because of the 24- to 48-hour delay in obtaining diagnostic information (Ferrucci and vanSonnenberg, 1981; Sones, 1984).

Ultrasound and CT are the preferred modalities. Both are noninvasive, rapid, and highly accurate. Ultrasound has a few disadvantages, such as being operator-dependent. In addition, it is difficult to perform in postoperative patients and in patients who are obese, have open wounds, external catheters, and dressings. With real-time equipment, however, good studies can often be obtained. An advantage is that critically ill patients who cannot be moved can be studied at the bedside (Cooperberg et al., 1980; Crass and Karl, 1982). Some abscesses can also be drained at the bedside under ultrasound guidance. CT is probably more accurate than ultrasound in the detection of abscesses (Callen, 1979; Ferrucci and vanSonnenberg, 1981; Mintz et al., 1983; Sones, 1984; Wolverson et al., 1979). Abscesses can be missed, however, if the bowel is not adequately opacified with contrast. Most of the abscesses appear as low-density fluid collections with attenuation numbers around 20 to 30 HU and may have a well-defined wall (Fig. 17–41). Gas can be visualized in 30% to 50% of the cases (Callen, 1979; Ferrucci and vanSonnenberg, 1981).

Diagnostic Aspiration and Drainage

Unless air is present within the fluid collection, an abscess cannot be distinguished on imaging studies from other sterile fluid collections. Diagnostic aspiration of the fluid is needed to confirm the abscess. This is usually performed using 22- to 20-gauge needles. If infection is present, percutaneous drainage of the abscesses is considered a safe and widely accepted procedure (Callen, 1979; Crass and Karl, 1982; Ferrucci and vanSonnenberg, 1981; Gerzof et al., 1981; Haaga and Weinstein, 1980; Mintz et al., 1983; Sones, 1984; vanSonnenberg et al., 1982).

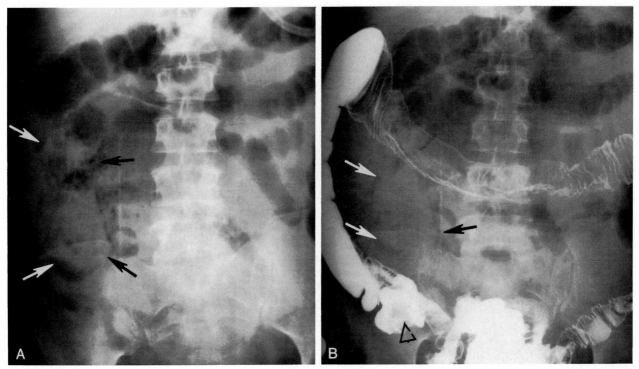

Figure 17–40. Right intra-abdominal abscess. *A,* Mottled radiolucencies are visible in the right midabdomen *(arrows)* in a patient with right lower quadrant pain and temperature elevations. This mottled appearance could be mistaken for stool in the ascending colon. *B,* A barium enema radiograph shows that the mottled gas pattern *(arrows)* is outside the colon. The ascending colon is displaced laterally, and a mass is visible at the base of the cecum *(arrowhead).* An appendiceal abscess was found at surgery.

Early on, indications for percutaneous drainage included a well-defined, unilocular collection with a safe, direct access route. Further, the tract should not traverse a sterile cavity (pleural or peritoneal), organ, or bowel loop (Gerzof et al., 1981; vanSonnenberg et al., 1982). With experience, the initial considerations were expanded to include multiple abscesses, multiloculated abscesses, complex abscesses, abscesses with enteric fistulae or whose drainage routes traversed normal organs (Casola et al., 1987; Gerzof et al., 1985; Mueller et al., 1984; Neff et al., 1987; vanSonnenberg et al., 1984, 1987; vanWaes et al., 1983). As the complexity of the abscess increases, however, the cure rate decreases and the complication rate increases (Casola et al., 1986).

The techniques for percutaneous drainage and subsequent catheter care have been well described (Gerzof et al., 1981; Haaga and Weinstein, 1980; Mueller et al., 1984; vanSonnenberg et al., 1982; vanWaes et al., 1983). In most instances, 12 or 14 French catheters are used. Catheters can be placed using ultrasound, CT, or fluoroscopic guidance. Large superficial collections can be drained under ultrasound guidance, but deeper abscesses are best drained using CT alone or CT combined with fluoroscopic guidance.

There are few complications from abscess drainage procedures (Gerzof et al., 1981, 1985; Haaga and Weinstein, 1980; vanSonnenberg et al., 1982, 1984). Major complications include hemorrhage and septi-

cemia. The average success rate is over 80%. In addition to obtaining a cure, abscess drainage can be used to stabilize a surgically poor-risk patient so he or she can tolerate surgery at a later date.

SPLEEN

Trauma

The spleen is the most commonly affected organ in cases of blunt abdominal trauma, and splenic injury is a leading cause of morbidity and mortality (Delany and Jason, 1981; Pearl, 1988; Stivelman et al., 1963; Trunkey, 1982). Twenty-five percent of the patients with splenic lacerations have associated lower rib fractures, 10% have left kidney injuries, and 2% have left hemidiaphragmatic injuries (Federle et al., 1987). Clinical signs include severe abdominal pain and intraperitoneal hemorrhage. There are several reports of delayed rupture of the spleen in which the initial CT evaluation was normal (Fabian et al., 1986; Fagelman et al., 1985; Pappas et al., 1987; Taylor and Rosenfeld, 1984) (Fig. 17–42). These patients may have small intrasplenic hematomas or lacerations that are not detected on the initial CT, and the hyperosmolar effect produces expansion of the hematoma with tearing of the splenic tissue (Pappas et al., 1987).

Plain film findings are usually absent or nonspecific (Johnson and Rice, 1985; Rolfer and Ross, 1990).

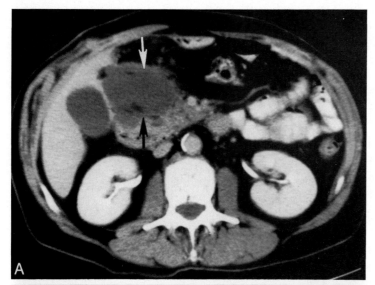

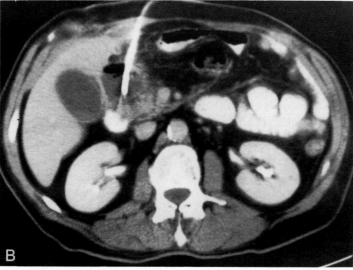

Figure 17–41. Subhepatic abscess with percutaneous drainage. *A,* CT scan shows a fluid collection in the right subhepatic region *(arrows)* in a patient who had recent gastric surgery. A few collections of air are seen within the fluid collection. *B,* The abscess was drained percutaneously. An immediate post-drainage CT scan shows the catheter in the abscess cavity, which is considerably smaller.

Suggestive findings include fractures of the left lower ribs, medial displacement of the gastric air bubble, inferior displacement of the splenic flexure of the colon, elevation of the left hemidiaphragm, and enlargement of the spleen (Johnson and Rice, 1985; Rolfer and Ross, 1990) (see Fig. 17–35). Hemoperitoneum can be suspected by separation of the flank stripe from the descending colon and presence of fluid in the pelvis, above the bladder (rabbit ear sign) (Johnson and Rice, 1985). Other imaging modalities, such as CT, ultrasound, or radionuclide scintigraphy, provide much better information (Berger and Kuhn, 1981; Federle et al., 1987; Freeman et al., 1985; Jeffrey et al., 1981; Kaufman et al., 1984; Leopold, 1985; Pearl, 1988; Rolfer and Ross, 1990; Wing et al., 1985).

CT is probably the method of choice for evaluation of splenic trauma. Its accuracy is as high as 96% to 98% (Jeffrey et al., 1981; Wing et al., 1985). Because many cases of splenic injury are treated nonsurgically, radiologists need not only to diagnose the splenic injury but also to determine the extent of the injury

(Brick et al., 1987; Douglas and Simpson, 1971; Ein et al., 1978; Mirvis et al., 1989). The decision to operate should not be based solely on the extent of injury seen on CT, however, but on the hemodynamic status of the patient (Brick et al., 1987; Mirvis et al., 1989). To avoid false-negative studies, intravenous contrast, preferably given dynamically, is a necessity (Federle et al., 1987). An improper contrast injection may make the hematoma isodense with the spleen (Federle et al., 1987). Because associated injuries are common, the whole abdomen, including the pelvis, should be examined. On CT, splenic injury appears as intrasplenic hematoma, subcapsular hematoma, minor splenic lacerations, fractured spleen, or vascular pedicle injury (Fig. 17–43; see Fig. 17–38). Most splenic lacerations are associated with a perisplenic hematoma, which may have a higher CT density than blood elsewhere in the peritoneum. This was recently described as the *sentinel clot sign* (Federle et al., 1987) (see Fig. 17–42). Intrasplenic hematomas are low-density lesions within the contrasted spleen; if the blood has clotted, they may become isodense (Federle et al., 1987; Rolfer and Ross, 1990). A subcapsular hematoma causes indentation or flattening of the splenic contour and is usually present on the lateral aspect (Federle et al., 1987). Chronic subcapsular hematomas present as low-density cystic masses. The splenic laceration is a linear low-density lesion that may be branching or stellate in appearance (Federle et al., 1987). A fractured spleen shows multiple areas of fragmentation intermixed with intrasplenic and perisplenic hematomas. Injury to the vascular pedicle may manifest as partial lack of enhancement of the lower three fourths of the spleen, since the upper part of the spleen may get its blood supply from the short gastric arteries. CT pitfalls include a normal cleft in the spleen that is usually situated near the upper medial pole, streak artifacts caused by ribs or the patient's arms if they cannot be elevated, and a prominent left lobe of the liver that may occasionally extend laterally adjacent to the spleen and may resemble a fracture (Federle et al., 1987; Rolfer and Ross, 1990) (Fig. 17–44). In patients in hypovolemic shock, the entire spleen may appear hypodense (Berland and Vandylce, 1985). Splenic arteriography has become less important in diagnosis because of the wide use of CT (Rolfer and Ross, 1990). It can be used therapeutically, however, to control bleeding (Buntain et al., 1986; Rolfer and Ross, 1990).

Abscess

Splenic abscesses are uncommon. They have been found to occur in 0.14% to 0.70% of several autopsy series (Chun et al., 1980; Freund, et al., 1982). If untreated, the mortality is 100% (Linos et al., 1983; Pickelman et al., 1970; Simpson, 1980). With modern imaging modalities, especially CT, it is possible to make an early diagnosis, and with appropriate intervention, the survival rate has been reported as high as 93% (Freund et al., 1982; Linos et al., 1983).

The more common causes of splenic abscess include trauma, sepsis, emboli, infarction, or local extension of infection (Beakman et al., 1983; Chulay and Lan-

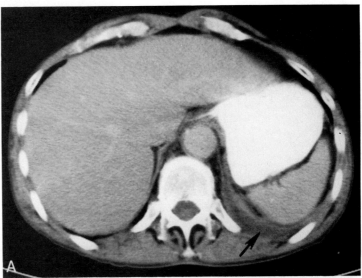

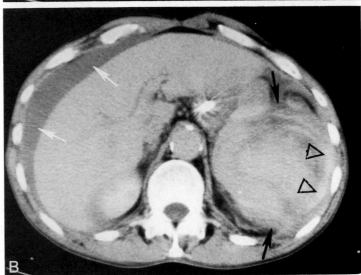

Figure 17–42. Delayed rupture of the spleen. *A*, A contrasted CT scan shortly after trauma shows a normal spleen and a left pleural effusion *(arrow)*. *B*, One week later, a large splenic hematoma *(black arrows)* with increased density (80 HU) is visible at the periphery of the mass *(arrowheads)*, and low-density blood is seen in the peritoneal cavity around the liver *(white arrows)*. High-density blood is often seen adjacent to the organ that is bleeding (sentinal clot sign).

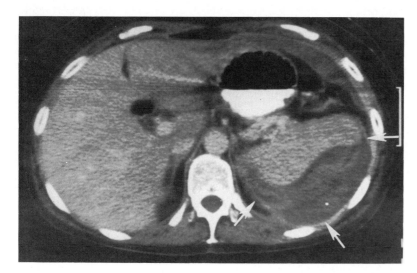

Figure 17–43. Subcapsular hematoma. CT scan in a young woman after an automobile accident shows high- and low-density blood in the splenic subcapsular space *(arrows)*. The hematoma is displacing the normal splenic tissue anteriorly and medially. The small white dot is a cursor.

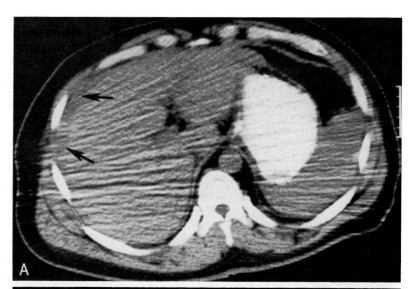

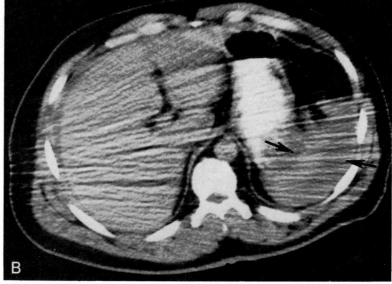

Figure 17–44. Artifacts and isodense hematoma. *A*, Precontrast CT scan after trauma shows multiple streak artifacts caused by the patient's right arm in the scanning field. There is fluid (blood) around the liver *(arrows)*, but the liver and spleen are not well seen. *B*, Post-contrast CT scan shows lower density subcapsular and intrasplenic hematomas *(arrows)*.

kenrani, 1976; Chun et al., 1980; Linos et al., 1983). The most common cause is hematogenous spread of infection (e.g., bacterial endocarditis). The clinical symptoms and signs are often nonspecific (Chun et al., 1980; Linos et al., 1983). The classic findings of fever, chills, left upper quadrant tenderness, and splenomegaly are present in only half of the patients (Chun et al., 1980; Linos et al., 1983).

The plain film findings are nonspecific and include elevation of the left hemidiaphragm, left pleural effusion, left lower lobe atelectasis or infiltration, and left upper quadrant mass (Freund et al., 1982; Pawar et al., 1982; Rolfer and Ross, 1990). Gallium-67 nuclear medicine scans are useful for detecting splenic abscesses, but CT and ultrasound are the two most widely used imaging modalities (Beakman et al., 1983; Jeffrey, 1989; Johnson et al., 1981; Lerner and Spataro, 1984; Pawar et al., 1982; Ralls et al., 1982; Rolfer and Ross, 1990). CT is probably the best modality. It evaluates not only the spleen but also the rest of the abdomen, which can be important in

critically ill patients who may have more than one abnormality. Ultrasound has an advantage over CT in that it can be performed at the bedside for both diagnosis and as a guide for percutaneous catheter insertion.

Splenic abscesses can be treated by splenectomy or percutaneous drainage (Beakman et al., 1983; Chulay and Lankenrani, 1976; Chun et al., 1980; Freund et al., 1982; Johnson et al., 1981; Lerner and Spataro, 1984; Linos et al., 1983). Recent radiologic literature states that percutaneous drainage of splenic abscesses is a safe procedure (Beakman et al., 1983; Lerner and Spataro, 1984; Rolfer and Ross, 1990). There is less emphasis to remove the spleen because of concern over potential immunologic abnormalities that may occur after splenectomy (Hekeler et al., 1982). Splenic abscesses can be drained using CT, ultrasound, or fluoroscopic guidance. After localization by CT or ultrasound, a diagnostic aspiration is done using a 20-gauge needle. Once the abscess is confirmed, a 10 or 12 French catheter is inserted using

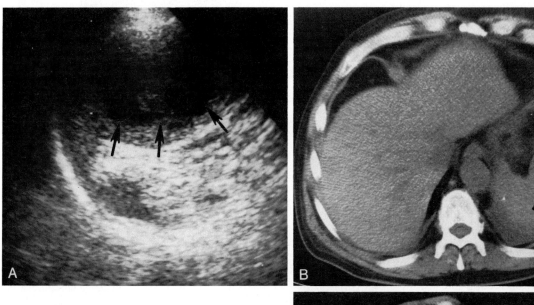

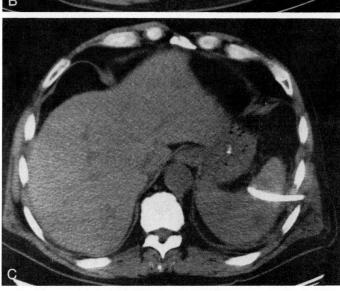

Figure 17–45. Splenic abscess. *A,* An ultrasound of the spleen in a patient with subacute bacterial endocarditis and fever shows a complex cystic mass *(arrows). B,* The CT scan shows a low-density mass (20 HU; *arrows*) in the spleen consistent with an abscess. *C,* The abscess was drained under CT guidance. The follow-up CT shows that the fluid is almost completely gone.

the Trochar or Seldinger technique (Chun et al., 1980; Johnson et al., 1981; Ralls et al., 1982; van-Sonnenberg et al., 1986) (Fig. 17–45). CT has the advantage of defining precisely the relationship of the splenic abscess to the colon, pleura, kidney, and pancreas (Jeffrey, 1989). Because the spleen is often situated high in the left upper abdomen, triangulation methods may be necessary to avoid entering the pleura. No major complications have been reported in the literature, and we have not encountered any major complications in the cases treated at our institution.

GASTROINTESTINAL BLEEDING

Esophagus

The most common causes of clinically significant esophageal bleeding are varices and Mallory-Weiss tears (Cutler and Mendeloff, 1981). Rarely tumors of the esophagus present with upper GI bleeding (Welch and Hedberg, 1973).

Because the venous drainage of the lower esophagus is into the portal vein, esophageal varices are caused by elevated portal vein pressure. High portal pressures are usually due to liver disease (most commonly cirrhosis) and less commonly portal vein thrombosis or other vascular anomalies (Conn, 1974). Less commonly, varices can occur in the upper third of the esophagus without involving the lower esophagus. These "downhill" varices occur when the superior vena cava is obstructed, since the venous drainage of the upper esophagus is by means of the azygos vein into the superior vena cava. Variceal bleeding may stop spontaneously, continue to bleed slowly, or bleed massively. There is a 50% mortality with the first bleed and even higher mortality in patients who experience rebleeding (Hanna et al., 1981).

Esophageal varices can be demonstrated by barium swallow (Fig. 17–46), but endoscopy is the more sensitive method for detection and can also be used for sclerotherapy treatment (Galambos, 1979). Angiography has been used to diagnose and treat varices but is not used as much currently (Athanasoulis et al., 1976).

The treatment of varices is usually either a surgical shunt procedure or endoscopic sclerotherapy (Conn, 1974). Intravascular vasoconstrictors, transhepatic portal vein embolizations, and the use of Sengstaken-Blakemore tubes have not proved to be definitive methods of treatment but may serve to stop bleeding or temporize until the patient is stabilized for surgery (Hermann and Traul, 1970).

The Mallory-Weiss syndrome is characterized by esophageal tears limited to the mucosal surface and not extending through the wall, as is seen in Boerhaave's syndrome. This condition is caused by strenuous vomiting and can present as massive upper GI bleeding. The mucosal disruption is usually not visu-

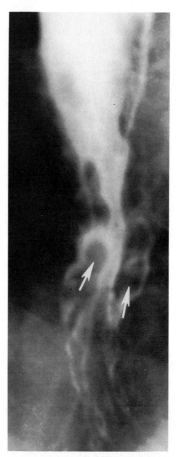

Figure 17–46. Lower esophageal varices. A barium swallow demonstrates large varices *(arrows)*. The larger the varices, the more likely they are to bleed.

alized on barium swallow. Endoscopy can detect these lesions with high sensitivity, and occasionally the bleeding site can be demonstrated with arteriography (Erickson and Glick, 1986). The bleeding from these mucosal tears may stop spontaneously. Intravenous vasopressin can be used in these patients, however, and intra-arterial vasopressin therapy occasionally is required (Baum, 1982). Surgical therapy is seldom necessary.

Stomach and Small Intestine

Bleeding from the stomach and small intestine is usually arterial or capillary in origin. The most common sites are in the stomach and duodenum and are usually due to peptic ulcers and gastritis (Goldman, 1983) (Fig. 17–47). Benign and malignant neoplasms may bleed but usually do so intermittently, causing chronic rather than acute blood loss. Bleeding from the small bowel can be caused by tumors, Meckel's diverticuli, and inflammatory diseases. In most patients who experience GI bleeding during anticoagulation therapy, the bleeding emanates from the upper GI tract and is usually secondary to peptic ulcer

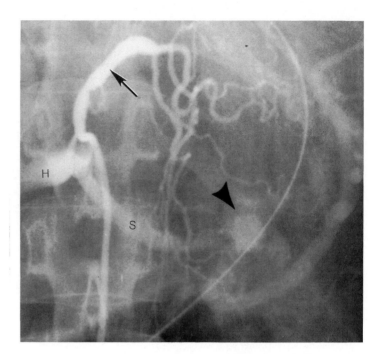

Figure 17–47. Gastric bleed. A selective left gastric artery *(arrow)* injection in a patient with an upper GI bleed shows a bleeding site in the stomach from an ulcer *(arrowhead)*. There is some backflow of contrast into the splenic *(S)* and hepatic *(H)* arteries. An earlier nonselective injection into the celiac artery did not demonstrate the bleeding site (not shown).

disease (Nusbaum and Baum, 1963). Upper GI endoscopy is the diagnostic procedure of choice for detecting bleeding from the stomach and duodenum, and barium studies should have no role in the acute upper GI bleed (Morris et al., 1975). Diagnosing a bleeding site in the small intestine distal to the ligament of Treitz is difficult. In general, endoscopy is of limited usefulness. Angiography or technetium-labeled red blood cells may show the site if the patient is actively bleeding (Alavi and McLean, 1980). In cases of chronic intermittent bleeding, the patient may require surgery.

Bleeding from gastric and duodenal ulcers can be treated by endoscopic methods, angiography, or surgery (Morris et al., 1975). In most cases, the bleeding can be stopped by endoscopic electrocoagulation (Silverstein et al., 1971). If endoscopy is not successful and the patient is stable, angiographic methods can be used. Many bleeding ulcers do not respond to intra-arterial vasoconstrictors but can often be successfully managed by embolization. Management of small bowel bleeding often requires surgery, but vasoconstrictors and arterial embolizations can be successfully employed (Baum, 1982).

Lower Gastrointestinal Bleeding

Although tumors, especially polyps, may bleed, they generally bleed intermittently and cause chronic anemia (Carmie and Goldstein, 1975). Significant acute colonic bleeding is usually secondary to diverticular disease and, less commonly, angiodysplasias (Smith, 1981). Barium studies and colonoscopy readily detect colonic neoplasms but often fail to detect the site of an acute bleed. Radionuclide scans are highly sensitive and can provide localization of the site of acute colonic bleeding (Markisz et al., 1982) (Fig. 17–48). Angiography also may be helpful in patients who are actively bleeding and can be used for therapy as well as diagnosis (Doreman et al., 1987).

Diagnosing the site of colonic bleeding is important because operative morbidity in patients undergoing emergency colectomy without determining the site is 38%, whereas in those patients in whom the bleeding site is located, the morbidity rate is less than 10% (Boley et al., 1979).

Although diverticula are more common in the left side of the colon, two thirds of bleeding diverticuli occur from the right-sided colonic diverticuli (Todd and Forde, 1979). Vasopressin has been shown to control diverticular hemorrhage successfully in 80% to 90% of patients (Athanasoulis et al., 1976).

Angiodysplasias (vascular ectasias) are generally located in the cecum or ascending colon and, unless large, may not be visualized by endoscopy or barium enema. On angiography they have a characteristic cluster of vessels seen during the arterial phase, may demonstrate intense staining during the capillary phase, and may have early draining veins (Wolff et al., 1977) (Fig. 17–49).

Angiodysplasias may present as chronic anemia with episodes of recurrent GI bleeding or, less commonly, as life-threatening hemorrhage. Of interest is the associated incidence of aortic stenosis in patients with unexplained GI bleeding (Boley et al., 1977). As many as one fourth of patients with colonic angiodysplasia have aortic stenosis (Boley et al., 1977). It has been hypothesized that these patients have concurrent development of these two diseases related to an underlying endothelial defect.

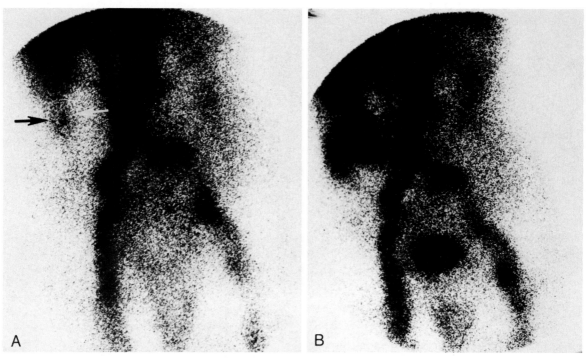

Figure 17–48. Lower GI bleed. A technetium-99m–labeled RBC nuclear medicine scan in an acute colonic bleed from an ascending colon diverticulum shows an area of increased radiotracer activity in the region of the right colon *(arrows)* on the initial scan *(A)*. A scan at 25 minutes *(B)* shows increasing intensity in the same area.

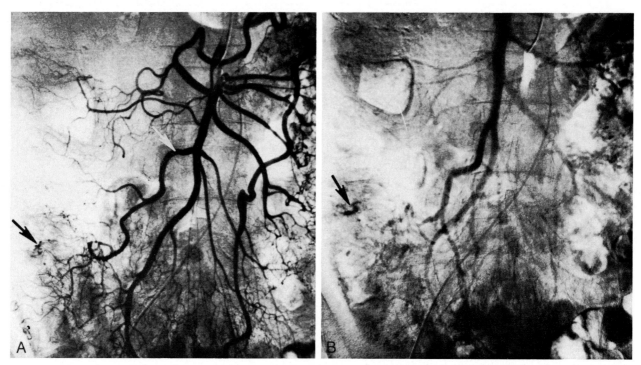

Figure 17–49. Colonic angiodysplasia. *A*, A superior mesenteric angiogram in a patient with acute GI bleeding shows a cluster of vessels in the cecal region *(black arrow)* supplied by the ileocecal artery *(white arrow)*. *B*, Subsequently there is intense staining *(arrow)*. At surgery this was a cecal angiodysplasia.

References

Alavi, A., and McLean, G.K.: Radioisotopic detection of gastrointestinal bleeding: An integrated approach with other diagnostic and therapeutic modalities. *In* Freeman, L.M., Weissman, H.S. (eds.): Nuclear Medicine Annual 1980. New York, Raven Press, 1980, p. 177.

Alexander, E.S., and Clark, R.A.: Computed tomography in the diagnosis of abdominal hemorrhage. JAMA 248(9):1104, 1982.

Altemier, W.A., Culbertson, W.R., Fuller, W.D., et al.: Intra-abdominal abscesses. Am. J. Surg. 125:70, 1973.

Ariel, I.M., and Kazarian, K.K.: Diagnosis and Treatment of Abdominal Abscesses. Baltimore, Williams & Wilkins, 1971.

Athanasoulis, C.A., Pfister, R.C., Greene, R.E., and Roberson, G.H.: Interventional Radiology. Philadelphia, W.B. Saunders, 1982.

Athanasoulis, C.A., Waltman, A.C., Novelline, R.A., et al.: Angiography: Its contribution to the emergency management of gastrointestinal hemorrhage. Radiol. Clin. North Am. 14:265, 1976.

Bailey, R.W., Buckley, G.B., Hamilton, S.R., et al.: Pathogenesis of nonocclusive ischemic colitis. Ann. Surg. 203:590, 1986.

Baum, C.: Angiography and the gastrointestinal bleeder. Radiology 143:569, 1982.

Beakman, W.A., Harris, S.A., and Bernardino, M.E.: Nonsurgical drainage of splenic abscess. AJR 141:395, 1983.

Berger, P.E., and Kuhn, J.P.: CT of blunt abdominal trauma in childhood. AJR 136:105, 1981.

Berland, L.L., and Vandylce, J.A. Decreased splenic enhancement on CT in traumatized hypotensive patients. Radiology 156:469, 1985.

Boley, S.J., DiBiase, A., Brandt, L.J., and Sammartand, R.J.: Lower intestinal bleeding in the elderly. Am. J. Surg. 137:57, 1979.

Boley, S.J., Sammartand, R., Adams, A., et al.: On the nature and etiology of vascular ectasis of the colon: Degenerative lesions of aging. Gastroenterology 72:650, 1977.

Brick, S.H., Taylor, G.A., Potter, B.M., et al.: Hepatic and splenic injury in children: Role of CT in the decision for laparotomy. Radiology 165:643, 1987.

Buntain, W.L., Gould, H.R., and Maule, K.I.: Predictability of splenic salvage by computed tomography. J. Trauma 28:24, 1986.

Byrne, J.J., and Cahill, J.M.: Acute gastric dilatation. Am. J. Surg. 101:301, 1961.

Callen, P.W.: Computed tomographic evaluation of abdominal and pelvic abscesses. Radiology 131:171, 1979.

Carmie, D.R., and Goldstein, H.M.: Angiographic management of bleeding following transcolonic polypectomy. Am. J. Dig. Dis. 20:1196, 1975.

Casola, G., vanSonnenberg, E., Neff, C.C., et al.: Abscesses in Crohn disease: Percutaneous drainage. Radiology 163:19, 1987.

Casola, G., Withers, C., vanSonnenberg, E., et al.: Percutaneous cecostomy for decompression of the massively distented cecum. Radiology 158:793, 1986.

Cheadle, W.G., Garr, E.E., and Richardson, J.D.: The importance of early diagnosis of small bowel obstruction. Am. Surg. 54:565, 1988.

Cho, K.C., Hoffman-Tretin, J.C., and Alterman, D.D.: Closed-loop obstruction of the small bowel: CT and sonographic appearance. J. Comput. Assist. Tomogr. 13(2):256, 1989.

Christophi, C., McDermott, F.T., McVey, I., et al.: Seat belt–induced trauma to the small bowel. World J. Surg. 9:794, 1985.

Chulay, J.D., and Lankenrani, M.R.: Splenic abscess: Report of 10 cases and review of the literature. Am. J. Med. 61:513, 1976.

Chun, C.H., Raff, M.J., Contreras, L., et al.: Splenic abscess. Medicine 59(1):50, 1980.

Clearfield, H.R., and Stahlgren, L.H.: Acute dilatation, volvulus, and torsion of the stomach. *In* Berk, J.E. (ed.): Bockus: Gastroenterology. Philadelphia, W.B. Saunders, 1985, p. 1373.

Cogen, R., and Weinry, B.J.: Aspiration pneumonia in nursing home patients fed via gastrostomy tubes. Am. J. Gastroenterol. 84(12):1509, 1989.

Conn, H.: The rational evaluation and management of portal hypertension. *In* Schaffner, F., Sherlock, S., Leevy, C.M. (eds.).: The Liver and Its Diseases. New York, Intercontinental Medical Books, 1974, p. 289.

Connell, T.R., Stephens, D.K., Carlson, H.C., et al.: Upper abdominal abscess: A continuing and deadly problem. AJR 134:759, 1980.

Cooperberg, P.L., Li, D.K.B., and Sauerbrei, E.E.: Abdominal and peripheral applications of realtime ultrasound. Radiol. Clin. North Am. 18:59, 1980.

Crass, J.R., and Karl, R.: Bedside drainage of abscesses with sonographic guidance in the desperately ill. AJR 139:183, 1982.

Cutler, J.A., and Mendeloff, A.I.: Upper gastrointestinal bleeding: Nature and magnitude of the problem in the U.S. Dig. Dis. Sci. 26(Suppl):90, 1981.

Dauterive, A.H., Flancbaum, L., and Cox, E.F.: Blunt intestinal trauma: A modern-day review. Ann. Surg. 201(2):198, 1985.

Delany, H.M., and Jason, R.S.: Abdominal Trauma: Surgical and Radiological Diagnosis. New York, Springer-Verlag, 1981.

Dehn, T.C.B., and Nolan, D.J.: Enterolysis in the diagnosis of intestinal obstruction in the early postoperative period. Gastrointest. Radiol. 14:15, 1989.

Doreman, G.S., Croven, J.J., and Staundinger, K.M.: Scintigraphic signs and pitfalls in lower gastrointestinal hemorrhage: The continued necessity of angiography. Radiographics 7:543, 1987.

Douglas, G.J., and Simpson, J.S.: The conservative management of splenic trauma. J. Pediatr. Surg. 6:565, 1971.

Dragstedt, L.R., Montgomery, M.L., Ellis, J.C., et al.: The pathogenesis of acute dilation of the stomach. Surg. Gynecol. Obstet. 52:1975, 1931.

Duncan, J.W., and Milnes, R.F.: Subacute gastric dilatation in air evacuated combat injuries. Milit. Med. 134:57, 1969.

Ein, S.H., Shandling, B., Simpson, J.S., and Stephens, C.A.: Nonoperative management of the traumatized spleen in children: How and why. J. Pediatr. Surg. 13:117, 1978.

Erickson, R., and Glick, M.: Why have controlled trials failed to demonstrate a benefit of esophagogastroduodenoscopy in acute upper gastrointestinal bleeding? Dig. Dis. Sci. 31(7):760, 1986.

Ericksen, A.S., Krasna, M.J., Mast, B.A., et al.: Use of gastrointestinal contrast studies in obstruction of the small and large bowel. Dis. Colon Rectum 33(1):56, 1990.

Eterline, H., and Thompson, J.: Diverticula and diverticulosis. *In* Pathology of the Esophagus. New York, Springer-Verlag, 1984, p 43.

Fabian, T.C., Mangiante, E.C., White, T.J., et al.: A prospective study of 91 patients undergoing both computed tomography and peritoneal lavage following blunt abdominal trauma. J. Trauma 26(7):602, 1986.

Fagelman, D., Hertz, M.A., and Ross, A.S.: Delayed development of splenic subcapsular hematoma. J. Comput. Assist. Tomogr. 9:815, 1985.

Federle, M.P., Griffiths, B., Minagi, H., et al.: Splenic trauma: Evaluation with CT. Radiology 162:69, 1987.

Federle, M.P., and Jeffrey, R.B.: Hemoperitoneum studied by computed tomography. Radiology 148:187, 1983.

Ferrucci, J.T., Jr., vanSonnenberg, E.: Intra-abdominal abscess: Radiological diagnosis and treatment. JAMA 246(23):2728, 1981.

Freeman, L.M., Lutzker, L.G., and Weissmann, H.S.: The acute abdomen: Radionuclide imaging. Radiographics 5(2):285, 1985.

Freund, R., Pichi, J., Heyder, N., et al.: Splenic abscess: Clinical symptoms and diagnostic possibilities. Am. J. Gastroenterol. 77(1):35, 1982.

Frykberg, E.R., and Phillips, J.W.: Obstruction of the small bowel in the early postoperative period. South Med. J. 82(2):169, 1989.

Galambos, J.T.: Evaluation and therapy of portal hypertension. *In* Cirrhosis (Major Problems in Internal Medicine). Philadelphia, W.B. Saunders, 1979, p. 253.

Gerzof, S.G., Johnson, W.C., Robbins, A.H., et al.: Expanded criteria for percutaneous abscess drainage. Arch. Surg. 120:227, 1985.

Gerzof, S.G., Robbins, A.H., Johnson, W.C., et al.: Percutaneous catheter drainage of abdominal abscesses. N. Engl. J. Med. 305:653, 1981.

Ghahremani, G.G., and Gore, R.M.: CT of postoperative abdominal complications. Radiol. Clin. North Am. 27(4):787, 1989.

Golden, G.T., and Chandler, J.B.: Colonic ileus and cecal perforation in patients requiring mechanical ventilatory support. Chest 68:661, 1975.

Goldman, L.: The enigma of endoscopy: Does it really improve the outcome? Mod. Med. May;11, 1983.

Graham, J., Barnes, M., and Rubenstein, A.S.: The nasogastric tube as a cause of esophagitis and stricture. Am. J. Surg. 98:116, 1959.

Grunow, J.E., al-Hafidh, A., and Tunell, W.P.: Gastroesophageal reflux following percutaneous endoscopic gastrostomy in children. J. Pediatr. Surg. 24(1):42, 1989.

Haaga, J.R., Bick, R.J., Zollinger, R.M. Jr.: CT-guided percutaneous catheter cecostomy. Gastrointest. Radiol. 12:166, 1987.

Haaga, J.R., and Weinstein, A.J.: CT-guided percutaneous aspiration and drainage of abscesses. AJR 135:1187, 1980.

Halber, M.D., Daffner, R.H., Morgan, C.L., et al.: Intra-abdominal abscess: Current concepts in radiologic evaluation. AJR 133:9, 1979.

Hanna, S., Warren, W.D., Galambos, J.T., et al.: Bleeding varices. I. Emergency management. Canadian Medical Association J. 124:29, 1981.

Hebeler, R.F., Ward, R.E., Miller, P.W., et al.: The management of splenic injury. J. Trauma 22(6):492, 1982.

Helmkamp, B.F., and Kimmel, J.: Conservative management of small bowel obstruction. Am. J. Obstet. Gynecol. 152(6):677, 1985.

Hermann, R.E., and Traul, D.: Experience with the Sengstaken-Blakemore tube for bleeding esophageal varices. Surg. Gynecol. Obstet. 130:879, 1970.

Hicks, M.E., Surratt, R.S., Picus, D., et al.: Fluoroscopically guided percutaneous gastrostomy and gastroenterostomy: Analysis of 158 consecutive cases. AJR 154(4):725, 1990.

Howell, H.S., Bartizal, J.F., and Freeark, R.J.: Blunt trauma involving the colon and rectum. J. Trauma 16:624, 1976.

Illescas, F.F., Baker, M.E., McCann, R., et al.: CT evaluation of retroperitoneal hemorrhage associated with femoral arteriography. AJR 146:1289, 1986.

Jeffrey, R.B., Jr.: CT and Sonography of the Acute Abdomen: Splenic Abscesses. New York, Raven Press, 1989, p. 93.

Jeffrey, R.B., Laing, F.C., Federle, M.P., and Goodman, P.C. Computed tomography of splenic trauma. Radiology 141:729, 1981.

Johnson, W.C., Gerzof, S.G., Robbins, A.H., et al.: Treatment of abdominal abscesses: Comparative evaluation of operative drainage versus percutaneous catheter drainage guided by computed tomography or ultrasound. Ann. Surg. 194(4):510, 1981.

Johnson, C.D., and Rice, R.P.: The acute abdomen: Plain radiologic evaluation. Radiographics 5(2):259, 1985.

Jones, P.F., Munro, A.: Recurrent adhesive small bowel obstruction. World J. Surg. 9:868, 1985.

Kaufman, R.A., Towbin, R., Babcock, D.S., et al.: Upper abdominal trauma in children: Imaging evaluation. AJR 142:449, 1984.

Korula, J., Pandya, K., and Yameda, S.: Perforation of esophagus after variceal sclerotherapy: Incidence and clues to pathogenesis. Dig. Dis. Sci. 34(3):324, 1989.

Kussin, S.Z., Henry, C., Navarro, C., et al.: Gas within the wall of the stomach: Report of a case and review of the literature. Dig. Dis. Sci. 27:949, 1982.

Laufer, I.: The left lateral view in the plain-film assessment of abdominal distention. Radiology 119:265, 1976.

Leopold, G.R.: The acute abdomen: Ultrasonography. Radiographics 5(2):273, 1985.

Lerner, R.M., and Spataro, R.F.: Splenic abscess: Percutaneous drainage. Radiology 153:643, 1984.

Levine, M.S.: Radiology of the Esophagus. Philadelphia, W.B. Saunders, 1989, p. 213.

Lewin, J.R., and Patterson, E.A.: CT recognition of spontaneous intraperitoneal hemorrhage complicating anticoagulant therapy. AJR 134:1271, 1980.

Linos, D.A., Nagorney, D.M., and McIlrath, D.C.: Splenic abscess: The importance of early diagnosis. Mayo Clin. Proc. 58:261, 1983.

Livingston, E.H., and Passaro, E.P., Jr.: Postoperative ileus. Dig. Dis. Sci. 35(1):121, 1990.

Low, D.E., and Patterson, D.J.: Complete esophageal obstruction secondary to dissecting intraluminal hematoma after endoscopic variceal sclerotherapy. Am. J. Gastroenterol. 83(1):135, 1988.

Markisz, J.A., Front, D., Romal, H.D., et al.: An evaluation of ^{99m}Tc labelled red blood cell scintigraphy for the detection and localization of gastrointestinal bleeding sites. Gastroenterology 83:394, 1982.

McWey, R.E., Curry, N.S., Schabel, S.L., et al.: Complications of nasoenteric feeding tubes. Am. J. Surg. 155(2):253, 1988.

Merine, D., Fishman, E.K., and Jones, B.: CT of the small bowel and mesentery. Radiol. Clin. North Am. 27(4):707, 1989.

Meyers, M.A. (ed.): Computed Tomography of the Gastrointestinal Tract. New York, Springer-Verlag, 1986.

Mintz, M.C., Arger, P.N., and Icressel, H.Y.: An algorithmic approach to the radiologic evaluation of a suspected abdominal abscess. Sem. Ultrasound 4(2):80, 1983.

Mirvis, S.E., Whitley, N.O., and Gens, D.R.: Blunt splenic trauma in adults: CT-based classification and correlation with prognosis and treatment. Radiology 171:33, 1989.

Monteferrante, M., and Shimkin, P.: CT diagnosis of emphysematous gastritis. AJR 153(1):191, 1989.

Morris, C.R., Ivy, A.C., and Maddock, W.G.: Mechanism of acute abdominal distension. Arch. Surg. 55:101, 1947.

Morris, D.W., Levine, G.M., Soloway, P.D., et al.: Prospective randomized study of diagnosis and outcome in acute upper-gastrointestinal bleeding: Endoscopy versus conventional radiography. Am. J. Dig. Dis. 20:1103, 1975.

Moyers, J.: Acute gastric dilatation. Postgrad. Med. 21:149, 1957.

Mueller, P.R., vanSonnenberg, E., and Ferrucci, J.T., Jr.: Percutaneous drainage of 250 abdominal abscesses and fluid collections. II. Current procedural concepts. Radiology 151:343, 1984.

Neff, C.C., vanSonnenberg, E., Casola, G., et al.: Diverticular abscesses: Percutaneous drainage. Radiology 163:15, 1987.

Nemcek, A.A., Jr.: CT of acute gastrointestinal disorders. Radiol. Clin. North Am. 27(4):773, 1989.

Noseworthy, T.W., Shustack, A., Johnston, R.G., et al.: A randomized clinical trial comparing ranitidine and antacids in critically ill patients. Crit. Care. Med. 15(9):817, 1987.

Nusbaum, M., and Baum, S.: Radiographic demonstration of unknown site of gastrointestinal bleeding. Surg. Forum 14:374, 1963.

Pappas, D., Mirvis, S.E., and Crepps, J.T.: Splenic trauma: False negative CT diagnosis in cases of delayed rupture. AJR 149:727, 1987.

Pawar, S., Kay, C.J., Gonzalez, R., et al.: Sonography of splenic abscess. AJR 138:259, 1982.

Passi, R.B., Kraft, A.R., and Vasko, J.S.: Pathophysiologic mechanisms of shock in acute gastric dilatation. Surgery 65:298, 1969.

Pearl, M.: Evaluating patients with multiple injuries. Hosp. Physician May:63, 1988.

Peora, D.A.: Stress-related mucosal damage: An overview. Am. J. Med. 83(Suppl 6A):3, 1987.

Perino, L.E., Gholson, C.F., and Goff, J.S.: Esophageal perforation after fiberoptic variceal sclerotherapy. J. Clin. Gastroenterol. 9(3):386, 1987.

Pickleman, J., Lee, R.M.: The management of patients with suspected early postoperative small bowel obstruction. Ann. Surg. 210(2):216, 1989.

Pickleman, J.R., Paloyan, E., and Block, G.E.: The surgical significance of splenic abscess. Surgery 68(2):287, 1970.

Poleski, M.H., and Spanier, A.H.: Cimetidine versus antacids in the prevention of stress erosions in critically ill patients. Am. J. Gastroenterol. 81(2):107, 1986.

Ralls, P.W., Quinn, M.F., Collitti, P., et al.: Sonography of pyogenic splenic abscess. AJR 138:523, 1982.

Richards, W.O., and Williams, L.F.: Obstruction of the large and small intestine. Surg. Clin. North Am. 68(2):355, 1988.

Riveron, F.A., Obeid, F.N., Horst, H.M., et al.: The role of contrast radiography in presumed bowel obstruction. Surgery 106(3):496, 1989.

Rolfer, R.J., and Ross, P.R.: The spleen: An integrated imaging approach. Crit. Rev. Diagn. Imag. 30(1):41, 1990.

Sagel, S.S., Siegel, M.J., Stanley, R.J., and Jost, G.: Detection of retroperitoneal hemorrhage by computed tomography. AJR 129:403, 1977.

Scowcroft, C.W., Sanowski, R.A., and Kozarek, R.A.: Colonoscopy in ischemic colitis. Gastrointest. Endosc. 27(3):156, 1981.

Silverstein, F.E., Gilbert, D.D., and Auth, D.C.: Endoscopic hemostasis using laser photocoagulation and electrocoagulation. Dig. Dis. Sci. 26(Suppl):31, 1981.

Simpson, J.N.L.: Solitary abscess of the spleen. Br. J. Surg. 67:106, 1980.

Smith, G.W.: Lower GI bleeding in the elderly: Diverticulosis and angiodysplasia as dominant causes. Postgrad. Med. 69(3):36, 1981.

Sones, P.J.: Percutaneous drainage of abdominal abscess. AJR 142:35, 1984.

Stefan, M.M., Holcomb, G.W. III, Ross, A.J. III: Cologastric fistula as a complication of percutaneous endoscopic gastrostomy. JPEN 13(5):554, 1989.

Stewart, R.M., Page, C.P., Brender, J., et al.: The incidence and risk of early postoperative small bowel obstruction: A cohort study. Am. J. Surg. 154:643, 1987.

Stivelman, R.L., Glaubitz, J.P., and Crampton, R.S.: Lacerations of the spleen due to nonpenetrating trauma: One hundred cases. Am. J. Surg. 106:888, 1963.

Stordahl, A.: Water-soluble contrast media in obstructed and in ischemic small intestine: A clinical and experimental study. J. Oslo City Hosp. 39:3, 1989.

Stordahl, A., Laerum, F., Gjolberg, T., et al.: Water-soluble contrast media in radiography of small bowel obstruction: Comparison of ionic and non-ionic contrast media. Acta Radiol. 29:53, 1988.

Stratta, R.J., Starling, J.R., D'Alessandro, A.M., et al.: Acute colonic ileus (pseudo-obstruction) in renal transplant recipients. Surgery 104(4):616, 1988.

Stroder, W.E., Nostrant, T.T., Eckhauser, F.E., and Dent, T.L.: Therapeutic and diagnostic colonoscopy in non-obstructive colonic dilatation. Ann. Surg. 197:416, 1983.

Swensen, S.J., McLeod, R.A., and Stephens, D.H.: CT of extracranial hemorrhage and hematomas. AJR 143:907, 1984.

Tanphiphat, C., Chittmittrapap, S., and Prasopsunti, K.: Adhesive small bowel obstruction: A review of 321 cases in a Thai hospital. Am. J. Surg. 154:283, 1987.

Taylor, C.R., and Rosenfield, A.T.: Limitations of computed tomography in the recognition of delayed splenic rupture. J. Comput. Assist. Tomogr. 9:1205, 1984.

Todd, G.J., and Forde, K.A.: Lower gastrointestinal bleeding with negative or inconclusive radiographic studies: The role of colonoscopy. Am. J. Surg. 138:627, 1979.

Trunkey, D.D.: The spleen. In Blaisdell, F.W., and Trunkey, D.D. (eds.): Abdominal Trauma. New York, Thieme-Stratton, 1982, p. 185.

vanSonnenberg, E., Casola, G., Wittich, G.R., et al.: Interventional radiology of spleen. Radiology 161:289, 1986.

vanSonnenberg, E., Ferrucci, J.T., Jr., Mueller, P.R., et al.: Percutaneous drainage of abscesses and fluid collections: Techniques, results, and applications. Radiology 142:1, 1982.

vanSonnenberg, E., Mueller, P.R., Ferrucci, J.T., Jr.: Percutaneous drainage of 250 abdominal abscesses and fluid collections. I. Results, failures, and complications. Radiology 151:337, 1984.

vanSonnenberg, E., Wittich, G.R., Casola, G., et al.: Periappendiceal abscesses: Percutaneous drainage. Radiology 163:23, 1987.

vanWaes, P.F.G.M., Feldberg, M.A.M., Mali, W.P.T.M., et al.: Management of loculated abscesses that are difficult to drain: A new approach. Radiology 147:57, 1983.

vonRokitansky, K.: Handbuch de Spezlellen Pathologischen Anatomie, vol. 3, ed. 3. Wein, Braunmuller v. Siedel, 1842, p. 178.

Waldman, I., and Berlin, L.: Stricture of the esophagus due to nasogastric intubation. AJR 94:321, 1965.

Watkins, D.T., and Robertson, C.L.: Water-soluble radiocontrast material in the treatment of postoperative ileus. Am. J. Obstet. Gynecol. 152(4):450, 1985.

Welch, C.E.A., and Hedberg, S.: Gastrointestinal hemorrhage. I. General considerations of diagnosis and therapy. Adv. Surg. 7:95, 1973.

Wing, V.M., Federle, M.P., Morris, J.A., Jr., et al.: The clinical impact of CT for blunt abdominal trauma. AJR 145:1191, 1985.

Wolf, E.L., Frager, D., and Benevenato, T.C.: Radiological demonstration of important gastrostomy tube complications. Gastrointest. Radiol. 11:20, 1986.

Wolff, W.I., Grossman, M.B., and Shinya, H.: Angioplasia of the colon: Diagnosis and treatment. Gastroenterology 72:329, 1977.

Wolverson, M.K., Jagannadharao, B., Sundaram, M., et al.: CT as a primary diagnostic method in evaluating intraabdominal abscess. AJR 133:1089, 1979.

Wojtowycz, M.M., Arata, J.A., Jr., Micklos, T.J., et al.: CT findings of uncomplicated percutaneous gastrostomy. AJR 151(2):307, 1988.

18

Acute Hepatobiliary and Pancreatic Disease

■

R. Brooke Jeffrey, Jr.

ACUTE PANCREATITIS

Clinical Overview

Acute pancreatitis has been defined by the International Cambridge Symposium as an acute inflammatory disorder resulting in abdominal pain and elevation of serum or urinary pancreatic enzymes (Sarner and Cotton, 1984). The specific criteria to establish the diagnosis include a tenfold elevation of plasma levels of pancreatic enzymes and direct evidence of acute pancreatitis derived from either imaging studies, laparotomy or autopsy (Sarner and Cotton, 1984). In addition to this clinical definition, the Marseilles Symposium of 1984 outlined two broad pathologic classifications of pancreatitis: (1) a mild form (edematous pancreatitis) characterized by peripancreatic fat necrosis and parenchymal interstitial edema; and (2) a severe form (necrotizing pancreatitis) associated with extensive peripancreatic and interpancreatic fat necrosis, parenchymal necrosis, and hemorrhage. Both forms of acute pancreatitis may be either focal or diffuse. After a clinical episode of acute pancreatitis and resolution of any associated complications such as a pseudocyst, the pancreas generally reverts to normal and only rarely progresses to chronic pancreatitis.

Although these definitions are helpful guidelines in many cases, acute pancreatitis is a complex and clinically challenging disorder, and there are no pathognomic physical signs or laboratory features that can serve in every instance to establish the diagnosis. In patients who are acutely ill and who represent diagnostic dilemmas, noninvasive imaging of the pancreas with sonography and computed tomography (CT) is essential not only to establish the diagnosis of pancreatitis in questionable cases but to suggest an alternate diagnosis if the pancreas appears normal. Although extensive research has attempted to predict the clinical outcome of patients presenting with acute pancreatitis, the prognosis is highly variable and ranges from a benign self-limited disorder to progressive multi-organ failure. In severe forms of acute pancreatitis, survival often depends greatly on early imaging diagnosis of complications such as infected necrosis and on prompt intervention with appropriated surgical or percutaneous therapy.

Imaging Strategy in Patients With Acute Pancreatitis

Plain abdominal radiographs and conventional contrast studies of the gastrointestinal (GI) tract are unable to image the pancreas directly and thus provide only limited information about the nature and extent of pancreatic inflammation. Abdominal CT and sonography are the primary imaging methods for evaluation of the pancreas and peripancreatic anatomic compartments in patients with suspected acute pancreatitis. In general, patients with mild clinical symptoms compatible with edematous pancreatitis need not undergo urgent imaging, because no immediate intervention is required and conservative, supportive therapy is the only treatment available. In these patients, sonography is often performed electively to evaluate the gallbladder for calculi in possible biliary pancreatitis and to detect residual peripancre-

355

atic phlegmons or fluid collections. Patients who either fail to respond to initial conservative therapy or who have severe clinical pancreatitis based on prognostic signs, howevever, should undergo urgent evaluation with abdominal CT. This is first to establish firmly the diagnosis of pancreatitis and to exclude other entities that may mimic the diagnosis such as mesenteric infarction or intra-abdominal abscess, and secondly to detect early complications of pancreatitis such as infected necrosis, pseudocysts, and hemorrhage.

When compared with sonography, CT has several specific diagnostic advantages in evaluation of the pancreas and peripancreatic compartments in patients with severe pancreatitis. CT is superior to sonography in defining complex retroperitoneal anatomic relationships. Unlike sonography, CT can directly visualize fascial planes and can readily demonstrate extrapancreatic spread of acute fluid collections, phlegmons, or abscesses. In addition, the ability to perform bolus-enhanced CT of the pancreas provides information about vascular perfusion, thus permitting accurate identification of focal or diffuse areas of avascular pancreatic necrosis. The extent of pancreatic necrosis may be of important prognostic value in assessing the potential for overall mortality and development of specific complications in severe pancreatitis (Balthazar et al., 1990).

CT and Sonographic Features

Edematous Pancreatitis

Alteration of the parenchymal echogenicity of the pancreas in acute pancreatitis is variable (Jeffrey, 1989b). In mild cases of acute edematous pancreatitis, the pancreas may appear relatively normal on sonography. In some patients, however, diffuse edema results in an enlarged, relatively hypoechoic gland (Fig. 18–1). Decreased echogenicity of the pancreas occurs in about one third of patients with acute pancreatitis (Jeffrey, 1989b). A number of factors may affect the parenchymal echogenicity in acute pancreatitis. This includes not only the timing of the sonographic study but also the extent of intrapancreatic hemorrhage, necrosis, or extrapancreatic fluid. In patients with diffuse interstitial edema from pancreatitis, the pancreas demonstrates the greatest decrease in echogenicity about 2 to 5 days after the onset of an attack of abdominal pain (Freise, 1987). The echogenicity of the pancreas is generally compared to the parenchymal echogenicity of the liver. In patients with increased echogenicity of the liver secondary to fatty infiltration from alcoholic liver disease, however, this internal comparison may not be valid. Without reference to previous scans, subtle enlargement of the pancreas may be difficult to detect with either sonography or CT. Furthermore, the size of the normal pancreas varies with age because of the normal aging phenomena of parenchymal atrophy and fatty infiltration. Thus, the determination of mild

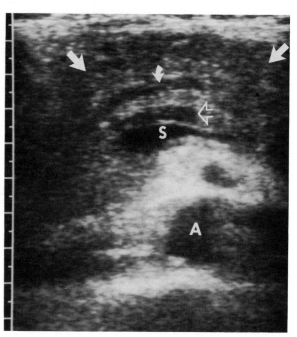

Figure 18–1. Sonographic demonstration of acute edematous pancreatitis. A transverse sonogram of the pancreas demonstrates a diffusely enlarged hypoechoic gland *(arrows)*. Note the slightly dilated main pancreatic duct *(curved arrow)* and retropancreatic fluid *(open arrow)* compressing the splenic vein *(S)*. *A*, Aorta. (From Jeffrey, R.B.: CT and Sonography of the Acute Abdomen. New York, Raven Press, 1989, p. 125, with permission.)

pancreatic enlargement acute pancreatitis is somewhat subjective when it is borderline. Often one of the most reliable and objective types of imaging evidence to establish the diagnosis of acute pancreatitis by sonography is the demonstration of acute peripancreatic fluid collections (Fig. 18–2).

In addition to diffuse parenchymal changes, focal intrapancreatic masses may be present as a result of areas of hemorrhage or phlegmon. At times it may be difficult to distinguish focal pancreatitis from carcinoma by imaging criteria alone. Either clinical follow-up or percutaneous biopsy may be required. Peripancreatic hemorrhage is uncommon in patients believed clinically to have edematous pancreatitis, but it may appear sonographically as a focal echogenic mass (Hashimoto et al., 1984). Noncontrast CT is of significant value in demonstrating high attenuation values of acute hematoma, which are generally greater than 30 Hounsfield units (HU).

CT is superior to sonography in defining the anatomic extent of acute extrapancreatic fluid collections (Jeffrey et al., 1986). With careful attention to real-time scanning technique, however, it is possible to define many extrapancreatic fluid collections by sonography. The three most common anatomic compartments involved with acute pancreatic fluid collections are the lesser sac, anterior pararenal space, and transverse mesocolon. Lesser sac fluid collections can readily be demonstrated sonographically using an anterior transgastric approach. Sagittal views are

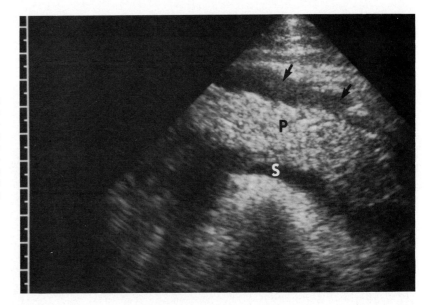

Figure 18–2. Extrapancreatic fluid as a main diagnostic criteria for acute pancreatitis. Transverse sonogram of the pancreas *(P)* demonstrates fluid anterior to the pancreas within the anterior pararenal space *(arrow)*. The echogenicity of the pancreas is normal. The peripancreatic fluid is the main abnormal finding. *S*, splenic vein. (From Jeffrey, R.B.: CT and Sonography of the Acute Abdomen. New York, Raven Press, 1989, p. 125, with permission.)

often useful in defining extension of fluid into the superior recess of the lesser sac (Fig. 18–3). Identification of fluid collections in the anterior pararenal spaces, however, requires coronal imaging from a lateral flank approach to identify fluid collections in proximity to the lateral aspect of the kidney (Jeffrey et al., 1986). Extrapancreatic involvement of the transverse mesentery is often difficult to visualize with sonography. Gaseous distention of the transverse colon from an associated ileus often precludes optimal imaging of the transverse mesocolon. Fluid collections in the transverse mesocolon can occasionally be identified with sonography because of their proximity to the mesenteric vasculature (Falkoff et al., 1986). In general, however, CT is superior to sonography in visualizing mesenteric involvement (Jeffrey et al., 1983).

Perivascular spread of acute pancreatitis may occur with inflammatory reaction encasing the portal, splenic, or superior mesenteric veins. This spread appears sonographically as a hypoechoic area dissecting along the course of the portal venous system (Jeffrey et al., 1986). Perivascular spread of acute fluid collections may amount for the well-known association of portal venous thrombosis in acute pancreatitis.

Any discrete cystic mass seen in the region of the pancreatic bed should be analyzed with deep Doppler sonography to exclude a pancreatic pseudoaneurysm (Falkoff et al., 1986). Arterial pulsations may not be readily apparent by real-time imaging alone, and thus Doppler is essential so that a pseudoaneurysm is not misinterpreted as a pseudocyst (Gooding, 1981).

On CT, patients with clinical and laboratory findings of mild edematous pancreatitis may demonstrate a relatively normal-appearing pancreas. As with sonography there may be diffuse enlargement of the gland or a focal inflammatory mass. There often is subtle peripancreatic edema or fluid involving the anterior pararenal space with thickening of Gerota's

fascia (Fig. 18–4). Because sonography is superior to CT in evaluating the gallbladder for calculi, sonography is still a useful adjunct to CT in possible cases of biliary pancreatitis.

Necrotizing Pancreatitis

CT is the imaging method of choice in patients with clinical features of severe pancreatitis (Jeffrey, 1983; Siegelman et al., 1980). Careful attention to CT technique is essential for optimal diagnosis. Initial

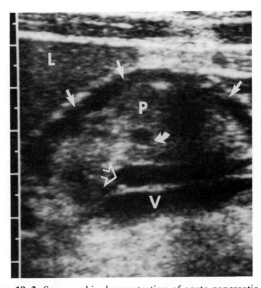

Figure 18–3. Sonographic demonstration of acute pancreatic fluid collection in the lesser sac. Sagittal scan of the pancreas *(P)* demonstrates hypoechoic fluid collection *(arrows)* extending above the pancreas into the superior recess of the lesser sac. Slight dilatation of the main pancreatic duct *(curved arrow)* and inferior pancreatic fluid collection *(open arrow)* is visible adjacent to the superior mesenteric vein *(V)*. *L*, liver. (From Jeffrey, R.B.: CT and Sonography of the Acute Abdomen. New York, Raven Press, 1989, p. 118, with permission.)

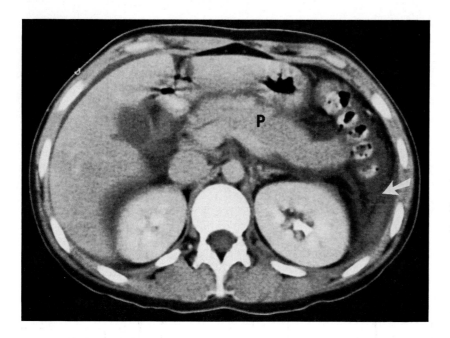

Figure 18–4. CT demonstration of mild edematous pancreatitis. Contrast-enhanced CT demonstrates a normal-appearing pancreas *(P)*. The only CT evidence of pancreatitis is the extrapancreatic fluid collection extending into the anterior pararenal space *(arrow)*. (From Jeffrey, R.B.: CT and Sonography of the Acute Abdomen. New York, Raven Press, 1989, p. 126, with permission.)

scans performed without intravenous contrast through the upper abdomen are helpful to identify focal areas of high-density (greater than 30 HU) hematoma in the pancreatic bed. Intravenous contrast enhancement administered as a sustained bolus, however, is essential for identification of avascular areas within the pancreas. These areas of relative nonperfusion correspond to areas of pancreatic necrosis (Balthazar, 1989; Balthazar et al., 1990). Because pancreatic fluid collections may extend from the mediastinum to the inguinal area, the entire abdomen should be scanned with dynamic incremental bolus technique.

Pancreatic or extrapancreatic fluid collections are exceedingly common in patients with necrotizing pancreatitis and occur in up to 54% of patients undergoing CT (Siegelman et al., 1980). Although many acute pancreatic fluid collections resolve spontaneously, about 3% of patients ultimately develop encapsulated pseudocysts (Balthazar, 1989). Acute fluid collections are characterized by CT as ill-defined, low attenuation areas (less than 20 HU) often confined to a specific anatomic compartment (e.g., lesser sac, anterior pararenal space) (Fig. 18–5). It is important to draw a clear distinction between acute pancreatic fluid collections and an actual pseudocyst. The time of development and imaging appearance of these two lesions are quite different. Pseudocysts generally develop several weeks after the acute onset of pancreatitis,

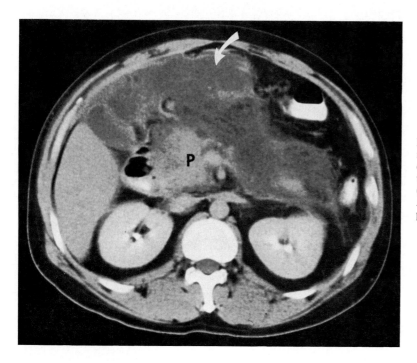

Figure 18–5. Acute pancreatic fluid collection in necrotizing pancreatitis. Contrast-enhanced CT demonstrates extensive fluid collection involving the transverse mesocolon *(arrow)*. *P*, pancreas. (From Jeffrey, R.B.: CT and Sonography of the Acute Abdomen. New York, Raven Press, 1989, p. 130, with permission.)

are of fluid density, and appear rounded or oval in configuration. Pseudocysts have a well-defined fibrous pseudocapsule that enhances after contrast CT (Fig. 18–6). Pseudocysts often demonstrate significant mass effect on adjacent organs and bowel loops. It is not possible by imaging criteria alone to determine whether a pancreatic fluid collection or pseudocyst is infected without diagnostic needle aspiration.

Pancreatic Abscess and Infected Pancreatic Necrosis

Sepsis after necrotizing pancreatitis is a feared complication and may be due to infected acute fluid collections, infection within a pancreatic pseudocyst, or infected necrosis. It is important to distinguish with imaging criteria these three entities because the treatment and prognosis are different. Infected pancreatic necrosis is often a diffuse process that is poorly defined, composed of both necrotic pancreatic parenchyma and retroperitoneal fat. The term *pancreatic abscess* as used in the surgical literature most often refers to infected necrosis. In the era before CT, infected pancreatic necrosis was notoriously difficult to diagnose and carried mortality often in excess of 70% (Jeffrey et al., 1987). Fortunately, only a small percentage of patients (1% to 9%) with acute pancreatitis ultimately have infected necrosis. Infected necrosis generally develops insidiously 2 to 4 weeks after the onset of an attack of acute pancreatitis. Because patients are febrile with severe pancreatitis alone without underlying infection, it may be difficult

to establish the diagnosis of infected necrosis on the basis of clinical findings alone. Delay in diagnosis has been one of the major factors in the high morbidity and mortality of this lesion.

The CT findings in patients with pancreatic abscess and infected necrosis are somewhat valuable. The presence of underlying infection often cannot be excluded by imaging criteria alone (Balthazar, 1989; Federle et al., 1981; Hiatt et al., 1987; Jeffrey et al., 1987). A high degree of clinical suspicion must be combined with an aggressive approach to CT-guided needle aspiration to permit early diagnosis of pancreatic infection. Gas-forming pancreatic abscesses are relatively uncommon and occurred in only 5 of 23 patients with proven pancreatic abscesses at San Francisco General Hospital (Jeffrey et al., 1987) (Fig. 18–7). Most patients demonstrate ill-defined areas of low or heterogenous attenuation suggesting a combination of phlegmon and/or fluid collection. In patients with persistent fever, CT is particularly valuable in defining a safe access route for diagnostic needle aspiration of any pancreatic fluid collections. A transhepatic, transgastric, or lateral flank approach that avoids traversing the colon and prevents contamination from colonic bacteria may be used (Fig. 18–8). In general, guided needle aspiration is a safe and effective method of determining the presence of infected pancreatic fluid collections (Federle et al., 1981; Hiatt et al., 1987). The needle aspiration can be performed with either a 20- or 22-gauge needle, since pancreatic abscesses most often contain thin turbid fluid rather than thick, viscous pus. In patients with diffuse involvement of the pancreatic bed, multiple sites of peripancreatic fluid often must be aspirated to ensure that there is no underlying infection.

Early diagnosis and prompt surgical débridement is essential for survival of patients with infected pancreatic necrosis. Percutaneous catheter drainage is generally not effective in treating these patients with necrosis, since the solid tissue within the pancreatic bed must be resected with early diagnosis. With CT-guided needle aspiration and emergency surgery, the overall mortality from infected necrosis has declined to an historical low of below 20% (Jeffrey et al., 1987). In patients with well-encapsulated pseudocysts, however, percutaneous drainage may provide a safe and effective alternative method of treatment. Preliminary data suggest that as experience grows, percutaneous drainage may become the treatment of choice for infected pseudocysts. Pseudocysts can either be punctured directly under CT or ultrasound guidance or approached by means of a transgastric or transhepatic route (Fig. 18–9). Advocates of the transgastric route of percutaneous pseudocyst drainage claim that it more closely approximates actual surgical cystogastrostomy (Jeffrey, 1989a). Residual fluid collections in the pancreas could potentially drain into the stomach through a fistulous connection created by an indwelling transgastric catheter after several weeks. Actual patency of this connection to the stomach has not been

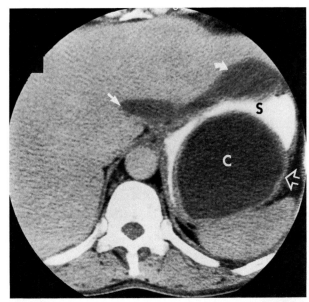

Figure 18–6. Typical pancreatic pseudocyst. Lesser sac pseudocyst *(C)* is noted posterior to contrast-filled stomach *(S)*. Note mass effect on the posterior wall of the stomach and well-defined enhancing fibrous pseudocapsule *(open arrow)*. White arrows correspond to other pancreatic fluid collections. (From Jeffrey, R.B.: CT and Sonography of the Acute Abdomen. New York, Raven Press, 1989, p. 128, with permission.)

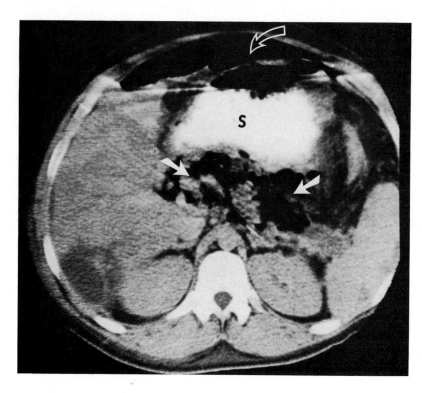

Figure 18–7. Gas-forming pancreatic abscess. Extensive gas-forming abscess is seen throughout the pancreatic bed *(white arrows)*. Extension of gas through the foramen of Winslow associated with pneumoperitoneum *(open arrow)*. *S*, stomach. (From Jeffrey, R.B.: CT and Sonography of the Acute Abdomen. New York, Raven Press, 1989, p. 137, with permission.)

documented clinically. Generally 10 to 14 French catheters are effective in adequately draining well-defined infected pseudocysts.

The role of CT-guided percutaneous drainage of infected acute pancreatic fluid collections in patients without infected necrosis remains more controversial. Although often technically feasible, percutaneous catheter drainage of acute fluid collections may involve a protracted course requiring multiple catheter exchanges, abscess sinograms, and repeated CT scans (Freeny et al., 1988; Steiner et al., 1988; vanSonnenberg et al., 1985). After percutaneous drainage, abscess sinography is essential to determine the presence of an occult fistula to either the pancreatic duct or GI tract. If there is an underlying fistula to the pancreatic duct, the percutaneous catheter cannot be removed until the fistula closes. When there is proximal ductal obstruction, this often neces-

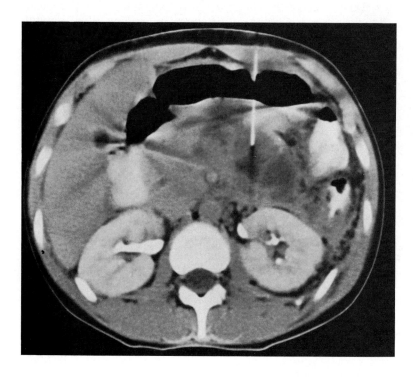

Figure 18–8. Transgastric needle aspiration of infected pancreatic fluid collection. Aspiration revealed coliform bacteria on Gram's stain and prompted emergency surgery. (From Jeffrey, R.B.: CT and Sonography of the Acute Abdomen. New York, Raven Press, 1989, p. 137, with permission.)

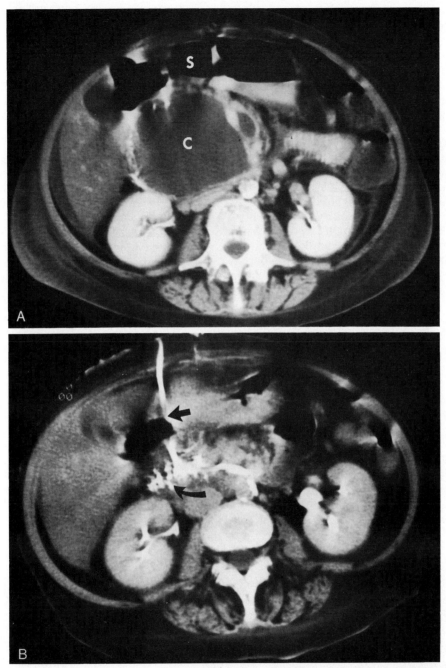

Figure 18–9. Transgastric drainage of infected pancreatic pseudocyst. *A,* Large pseudocyst in the head of the pancreas *(C). S,* stomach. *B,* After percutaneous catheter *(arrow)* placement under CT guidance, the pseudocyst was completely evacuated. Curved arrow indicates pancreatic calcifications from associated chronic pancreatitis. The pseudocyst resolved after 2 weeks of catheter drainage. (From Jeffrey, R.B. CT and Sonography of the Acute Abdomen. New York, Raven Press, 1989, p. 134, with permission.)

sitates prolonged (2 or 3 months) catheter drainage (Freeny et al., 1988). There has been no randomized prospective trial comparing surgical drainage with percutaneous drainage of acute pancreatic fluid collections. Therefore, the ultimate utility of percutaneous drainage versus surgery remains somewhat speculative. Nevertheless, in patients who are poor candidates for operation, CT-guided percutaneous catheter drainage often can be used as a temporizing measure before more definitive surgery (vanSonnenberg et al., 1984).

Vascular Complications of Necrotizing Pancreatitis

Erosion of peripancreatic vessels by activated proteolytic enzymes in pancreatitis may result in either pseudoaneurysm formation or pancreatic hemorrhage. Exsanguinating retroperitoneal hemorrhage may occur, or bleeding may be contained within the cavity of a pseudocyst. Rarely, GI bleeding results from direct extension of a pseudoaneurysm into the pancreatic duct or erosion directly into intestine.

Patients with obvious hemodynamic instability and GI or intra-abdominal hemorrhage generally undergo urgent visceral angiography to define the source of pancreatic hemorrhage. Not uncommonly, lesser degrees of pancreatic hemorrhage are clinically unsuspected. This is particularly true of hemorrhage contained within a pancreatic pseudocyst.

Diagnostic imaging with CT and sonography may detect clinically occult pancreatic hemorrhage on the basis of characteristic features (Fig. 18–10). On sonography, pancreatic hematomas appear as focal echogenic masses with enhanced sound transmission (Hashimoto et al., 1984; Jeffrey, 1989a). On CT, pancreatic hemorrhage is best recognized on noncontrast scans. Acute hematoma generally has an attenuation value generally greater than 30 HU, which is significantly higher than other biologic fluid collections. If only contrast-enhanced CT scans are performed, it may be difficult to distinguish a soft-tissue

inflammatory mass (phlegmon) from a focal area of pancreatic hemorrhage.

Both duplex sonography and contrast-enhanced CT may be of value in identifying larger pseudoaneurysms resulting from acute pancreatitis (Falkoff et al., 1986; Jeffrey, 1989a; Lim et al., 1989). (Fig. 18–11). Smaller pseudoaneurysms can be diagnosed only by selective visceral arteriography. Arterial pulsation confirmed by Doppler within a "cystic" mass is diagnostic of a pseudoaneurysm with duplex sonography (Falkoff et al., 1986). On bolus-enhanced CT, the inner lumen of the pseudoaneurysm demonstrates similar enhancement to adjacent arterial structures (Jeffrey, 1989a). Many visceral pseudoaneurysms are surgically difficult to approach, and therefore transcatheter embolization of peripancreatic pseudoaneurysms is generally the treatment of choice (Mandel et al., 1987).

Other vascular complications of acute pancreatitis

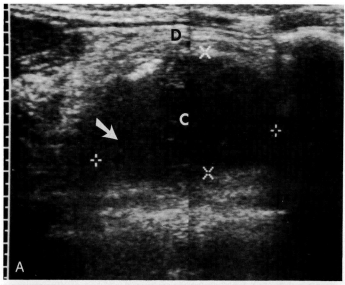

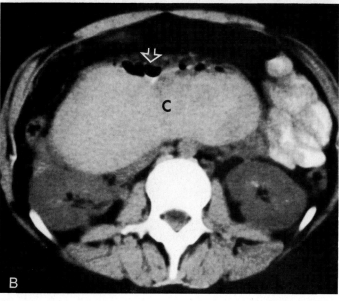

Figure 18–10. Hemorrhagic intramural pseudocyst of the duodenum. *A,* Transverse sonogram of the duodenum demonstrating a large cystic mass containing echogenic fluid *(white arrow).* Note anterior displacement of transverse duodenum *(D). B,* Noncontrast scan demonstrating high-density fluid (48 HU) consistent with blood. Hemorrhagic intramural pseudocyst was drained surgically. Open arrow indicates transverse duodenum. (From Jeffrey, R.B. CT and Sonography of the Acute Abdomen. New York, Raven Press, 1989, p. 130, with permission.)

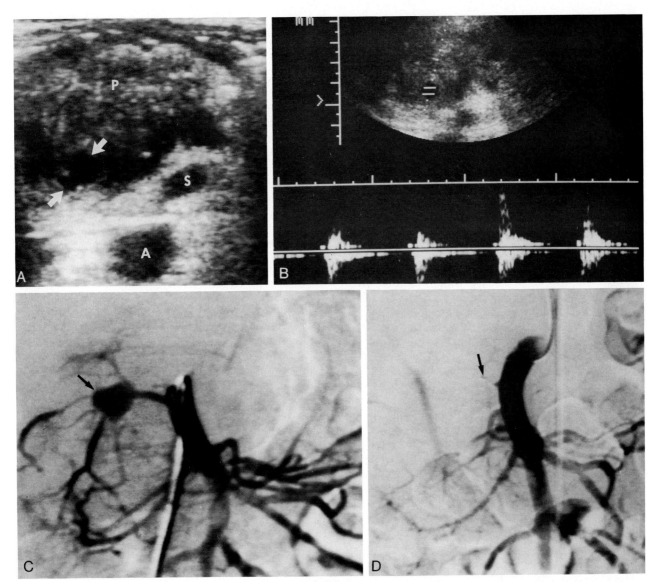

Figure 18–11. Duplex sonographic diagnosis of pancreatic pseudoaneurysm with transcatheter embolization. *A,* Transverse sonogram of the head of the pancreas demonstrating a lobulated cystic mass *(arrows). P,* Pancreas; *S,* superior mesenteric vein; *A,* aorta. *B,* Doppler analysis of cystic mass reveals arterial flow within cystic mass, diagnostic of a pseudoaneurysm. *C,* Superior mesenteric artery arteriogram confirming the presence of a pancreatic pseudoaneurysm arising from the inferior pancreatic duodenal arcade. *D,* Repeat superior mesenteric artery arteriogram after transcatheter embolization of the aneurysm with a stainless steel coil. Arrow indicates coil. (From Jeffrey, R.B.: CT and Sonography of the Acute Abdomen. New York, Raven Press, 1989, p. 122, with permission.)

include thrombosis of the splenic portal venous system with resultant splenomegaly and gastric varices. Acute superior mesenteric vein thrombosis may result in mesenteric bowel infarction. CT and duplex sonography may be of considerable value in the diagnosis of mesenteric venous thrombosis and its complications.

GI Complications of Acute Pancreatitis

Plain abdominal radiographs, conventional barium studies, and endoscopy are generally the most effective methods for demonstrating ileus, small bowel obstruction, or mucosal abnormalities of the GI tract accompanying acute pancreatitis. However, mesenteric mass or other extrinsic lesions caused by pancreatic phlegmons, pseudocysts, or abscesses often may be demonstrated only by CT or sonography. Localized inflammatory changes of the bowel wall characterized by bowel wall thickening, spasm, and edema occur commonly when extrinsic inflammation from acute pancreatitis encases adjacent loops of intestine. Because of the proximity of the pancreas to the small bowel mesentery and transverse mesocolon, dissection of pancreatic inflammation may occur along these mesenteric pathways. Acute fluid collections in the anterior pararenal space are often in proximity to the splenic or hepatic flexures. Pancreatic inflammatory masses may ultimately cause obstruction or GI fistualization. Spontaneous decompression of pancreatic pseudocysts may occur into the stomach or adjacent loops of intestine, and thus it is important to document the persistent nature of the pseudocyst before laparotomy for cyst drainage (Fig. 18–12).

BLUNT TRAUMA TO THE PANCREAS

Clinical Features

Blunt trauma to the pancreas is relatively uncommon, but may be associated with severe multi-organ injury necessitating urgent laparotomy. In stable patients with isolated pancreatic trauma, delay in diagnosis is a significant factor contributing to the high morbidity and mortality of this injury (Bach and Frey, 1971; Frey, 1982; Northrup and Simmons, 1972). The clinical diagnosis of pancreatic trauma may be challenging, because there are often no pathognomonic physical or laboratory findings that establish the diagnosis. Because of the lack of peritoneal irritation, a high clinical index of suspicion is essential for diagnosis of pancreatic injuries. Often there is a history of a direct blow to the midepigastrium, and the abdominal pain experienced by the patient is clinically out of proportion to the degree of abdominal tenderness detected by physical examination.

Pancreatic injuries may be classified according to their degree of parenchymal injury and extent of involvement of the main pancreatic duct (Jeffrey et al., 1983). Most severe injuries (grades III and IV) involve deep lacerations of the parenchyma with disruption of the duct of Wirsung (Jeffrey et al.,

1983). Serum amylase values may be elevated in patients with pancreatic injuries, but this is not invariably the case. There are well-documented episodes of pancreatic fracture occurring in patients with normal serum amylase for 24 hours (Frey, 1982). Second, the overall numeric value of the rise of the serum amylase does not correlate well with the degree of parenchymal disruption, and the highest levels of serum amylase may occur in patients with contusions rather than fractures (Frey, 1982).

CT Diagnosis of Pancreatic Trauma

Dynamic bolus CT is the imaging method of choice in evaluating stable patients with possible pancreatic trauma after blunt injury (Jeffrey et al., 1983). Sonography may be falsely negative in a significant number of patients (Jeffrey et al., 1986). The CT diagnosis is based not only on the direct visualization of an intrapancreatic laceration but also on the detection of indirect evidence such as post-traumatic pancreatitis. On contrast CT, lacerations of the pancreas result in areas of nonperfusion and appear as linear low-attenuation abnormalities (Fig. 18–13). The CT findings of post-traumatic pancreatitis include focal pancreatic enlargement and infiltration of the peripancreatic soft-tissue planes with thickening of Gerota's fascia (Jeffrey et al., 1983). Because the development of post-traumatic pancreatitis is somewhat time-dependent, subtle but significant pancreatic injuries may be missed on CT scan in patients who undergo scanning immediately after trauma. In some patients the only abnormality is slight thickening of

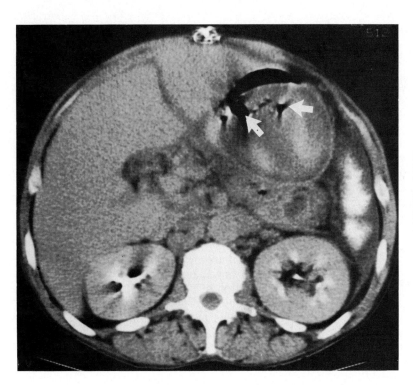

Figure 18–12. Spontaneous fistualization of lesser sac pseudocyst into the stomach. Gas is noted within a lesser sac pseudocyst *(arrows)* from surgically proven pseudocyst erosion into the posterior wall of the stomach. (From Jeffrey, R.B.: CT and Sonography of the Acute Abdomen. New York, Raven Press, 1989, p. 146, with permission.)

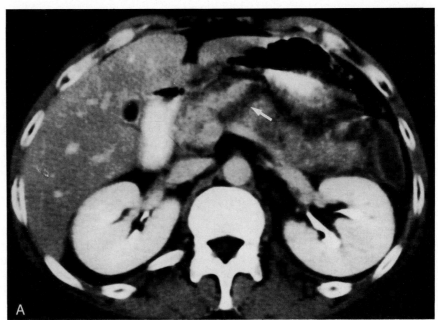

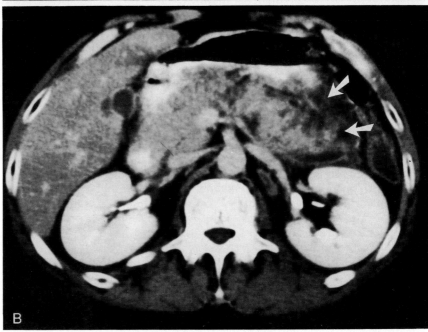

Figure 18–13. Blunt trauma to the pancreas after motor vehicle accident. *A,* Linear laceration at the juncture of the body and tail of the pancreas, representing a pancreatic fracture *(arrow). B,* Evidence of post-traumatic pancreatitis *(arrows)* with soft tissue infiltration in the adjacent anterior pararenal space in proximity to the tail of the pancreas. (From Jeffrey, R.B.: CT and Sonography of the Acute Abdomen. New York, Raven Press, 1989, p. 113, with permission.)

the anterior reflection of Gerota's fascia caused by dissection of blood or inflammation, and thus a high index of suspicion for pancreatic injury must be maintained if this abnormality is present. When CT is equivocal, endoscopic retrograde cholangeopancreatography (ERCP) may be of considerable value in determining the integrity of the main pancreatic duct. In patients without main ductal disruption, conservative therapy without surgery may be indicated. In patients treated nonoperatively, serial follow-up examinations with sonography or CT are useful for determining the presence of post-traumatic pancreatic pseudocysts and for guiding percutaneous drainage where appropriate.

GALLBLADDER AND BILE DUCTS

Acute Calculous Cholecystitis

High-resolution, real-time sonography and biliary scintigraphy are both sensitive techniques for the diagnosis of acute calculous cholecystitis with accuracy exceeding 90% (Cooperberg and Gibney, 1987; Jeffrey et al., 1983; Laing et al., 1981; Madrazo et al., 1982; Mauro et al., 1982; Ralls et al., 1985; Simeone et al., 1989; Weissmann et al., 1979). In general, sonography is often the initial imaging method of choice in patients with acute right upper quadrant pain and possible acute cholecystitis. Sonography can reliably diagnose or exclude acute cholecystitis, and it permits rapid real-time evaluation of the upper abdomen to detect other acute abdominal disorders that may simulate the clinical presentation of acute biliary tract disease. In addition, in selected patients sonography can distinguish between uncomplicated cholecystitis and gangrenous cholecystitis with perforation. In patients with uncomplicated acute calculous cholecystitis, CT has not been used as a primary imaging modality. Biliary scintigraphy is often used if sonography is equivocal in patients with complicated cholecystitis such as emphysematous cholecystitis or pericholecystic abscesses; CT may provide clinically useful information that is complementary to sonography.

Calculous obstruction of the cystic duct is the primary pathologic mechanism leading to acute cholecystitis in some 90% to 95% of patients. Cystic duct obstruction results in acute gallbladder distention and clinical symptoms of biliary colic. As the inflammatory process evolves, there is mucosal irritation by concentrated bile salts within the lumen and associated ischemic changes in the gallbladder wall secondary to prolonged gallbladder distention and vascular compromise. If secondary infection ensues, the inflammatory process may extend to the serosa of the gallbladder and involve adjacent omentum, pericholecystic fat, or other peritoneal surfaces.

The clinical signs and symptoms of acute cholecystitis are not always straightforward. In fact, only one third of patients clinically suspected of having acute cholecystitis are found to have surgically proved acute cholecystitis (Laing et al., 1981). In addition to the physical findings of abdominal guarding and localized right upper quadrant rebound tenderness, one third of patients with acute cholecystitis have positive Murphy signs. The Murphy sign relates to focal tenderness illicited on palpation of the gallbladder with inspira-

tory arrest. A wide variety of other acute abdominal disorders can clinically mimic acute cholecystitis such as pancreatitis, appendicitis, hepatitis, hepatic abscess, neoplasm, and retroperitoneal abnormalities like acute ureteral obstruction and pyelonephritis (Laing et al., 1981). Superdiaphragmatic processes such as pneumonia or myocardial infarction can also on occasion mimic the clinical presentation of acute cholecystitis. Diabetic and elderly patients with gangrenous cholecystitis may often have deceptively benign clinical presentations despite extensive transmural inflammation of the gallbladder.

Sonographic technique is important to optimize the diagnosis of acute cholecystitis. In general, high-resolution real-time images are performed with a 3.5-mHz sector scanner; in thin patients, however, a 5-mHz transducer often provides higher resolution. The examination is performed in both the supine and left posterior oblique positions. Careful attention should be directed toward imaging of the gallbladder neck for an impacted stone (Fig. 18–14).

The two primary sonographic criteria for diagnosis of acute cholecystitis are the presence of calculi and focal tenderness over the gallbladder illicited by direct pressure from the transducer (i.e., the sonographic Murphy sign) (Laing et al., 1981; Ralls et al., 1985). Ralls and associates (1985) noted that 99% of patients with acute cholecystitis demonstrated both gallbladder calculi and a positive sonographic Murphy sign. The spectrum of other sonographic features that may be visualized in patients with acute cholecystitis includes gallbladder distention, sludge, subserosal edema, intraluminal membranes or debris, and pericholecystic fluid.

Gangrenous cholecystitis is associated with significantly increased morbidity and mortality from associated perforation and subsequent peritonitis. A number of sonographic features are highly suggestive of

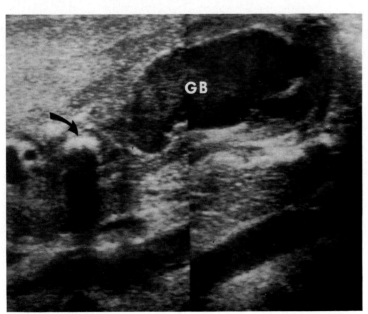

Figure 18–14. Sonographic diagnosis of acute cholecystitis with gallstone impacted in the cystic duct. Sagittal sonogram demonstrates markedly distended gallbladder (GB) with thickened wall. A stone is impacted in the region of the cystic duct *(curved arrow)*. (From Jeffrey, R.B.: CT and Sonography of the Acute Abdomen. New York, Raven Press, 1989, p. 58, with permission.)

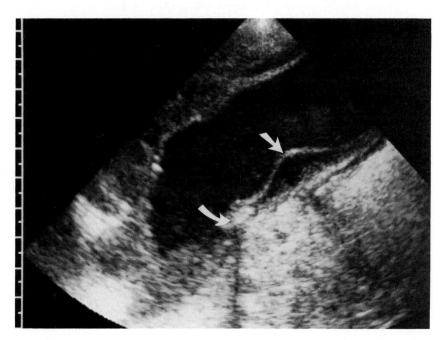

Figure 18–15. Sonographic diagnosis of gangrenous cholecystitis. Sagittal scan of the gallbladder demonstrates calculous within the gallbladder *(curved arrow)*. Intraluminal membrane *(arrow)* represents either mucosal debris, intraluminal clot, or fibrinous strand of exudate. Gangrenous cholecystitis was confirmed surgically. (From Jeffrey, R.B.: CT and Sonography of the Acute Abdomen. New York, Raven Press, 1989, p. 60, with permission.)

gangrenous cholecystitis in the appropriate clinical setting. These include asymmetric gallbladder wall thickening, intraluminal membranes, coarse debris, and pericholecystic fluid (Jeffrey et al., 1983) (Fig. 18–15). Intraluminal membranes may be due to sloughing of the gallbladder mucosa, fibrinous strands of exudate from empyema, or mucosal hemorrhage. The mural changes accompanying gangrenous cholecystitis may be due to intramural abscesses or hemorrhage. Simeone and colleagues (1989) noted that in two thirds of patients with gangrenous cholecystitis, the sonographic Murphy sign may be absent because of denervation of sensory fibers in the gallbladder wall from ischemia (Jeffrey et al., 1983; Madrazo et al., 1982). In the absence of a positive sonographic

Murphy sign, imaging features of gangrenous cholecystitis take on even greater importance. Early surgery should be performed in patients with sonographic evidence of gangrenous cholecystitis to minimize the risk of peritonitis from perforation. Sonographically guided percutaneous cholecystostomy may be an effective alternative to surgical cholecystectomy in high-risk patients (Fig. 18–16). The combination of both sonography and fluoroscopic control is frequently used to perform percutaneous cholecystostomy with a guide wire exchange technique.

On CT and sonography, pericholecystic abscesses are complex fluid collections containing septations, debris, or gas. Often there is significant mass effect

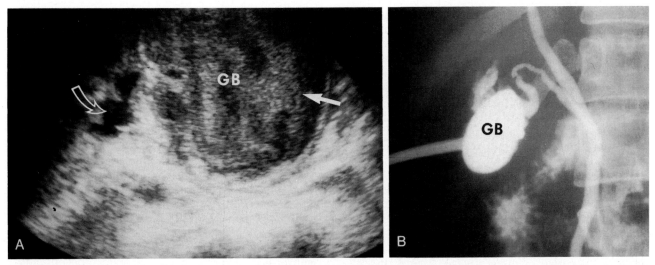

Figure 18–16. Sonographically guided percutaneous cholecystostomy. *A,* Markedly distended gallbaldder *(GB)* containing diffuse low level echoes representing pus *(white arrow)*. Open arrow indicates pericholecystic fluid from perforation. *B,* Cholangiogram through percutaneous catheter after resolution of empyema of gallbladder *(GB)*. Note patent cystic duct and slight perforation along the superior margin of the gallbladder. (From Jeffrey, R.B.: CT and Sonography of the Acute Abdomen. New York, Raven Press, 1989, p. 61, with permission.)

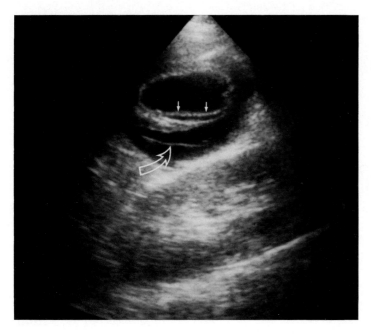

Figure 18–17. Sonographic diagnosis of pericholecystic abscess. Sagittal sonogram demonstrates intraluminal membranes within the gallbladder *(small arrows)* from gangrenous cholecystitis. Complex pericholecystic fluid is noted with intraluminal membranes seen within pericholecystic abscess *(open arrow)*. (From Jeffrey, R.B.: CT and Sonography of the Acute Abdomen. New York, Raven Press, 1989, p. 60, with permission.)

on adjacent organs (Fig. 18–17). Although often walled off or localized by inflamed omentum, pericholecystic abscesses may extend to the hepatorenal fossa, right subphrenic paces or occasionally cause generalized peritonitis. In patients too ill for surgery, percutaneous drainage of pericholecystic abscesses may be useful as a temporizing measure prior to elective cholecystectomy.

Acalculous Cholecystitis

About 5% of all patients with acute cholecystitis have acalculous cholecystitis (Glen and Becker, 1982). A variety of clinical conditions may predispose to the development of acalculous cholecystitis including burns, sepsis, major trauma, hyperalimentation, and diabetes. Although the exact pathophysiology of acalculous cholecystitis is incompletely understood, ischemia and mucosal injury from concentrated bile salts appear to be factors in the development of acalculous cholecystitis (Howard, 1981). Acalculous cholecystitis is often extremely difficult to prospectively diagnose clinically, particularly in obtunded or postoperative patients. Because of difficulties in early diagnosis, acalculous cholecystitis is associated with a higher incidence of both gangrenous cholecystitis and perforation.

There are few reliable imaging criteria to establish the diagnosis of acalculous cholecystitis early in its clinical course (Shuman et al., 1984). Serial sonograms demonstrating progressive changes in the gallbladder wall with development of subserosal edema are suggestive of the diagnosis (Fig. 18–18). Other features indicative of more advanced cases of acalculous cholecystitis include visualization of intraluminal membranes, asymmetric wall thickening, and pericholecystic fluid. Although biliary scintigraphy

has a high sensitivity (90% to 95%) for the diagnosis of calculous cholecystitis due to cystic duct obstruction, the sensitivity is substantially lower in patients with acalculous cholecystitis (Shuman et al., 1984). Positive studies with biliary scintigraphy must be interpreted cautiously because of the fact that prolonged illness, hepatocellular dysfunction, and recent postoperative state may predispose to nonfilling of the gallbladder with radionuclide agents (Fig et al., 1990; Radons et al., 1990).

CT may occasionally be of potential value in patients with possible acalculous cholecystitis and inconclusive sonograms. CT may demonstrate subtle mural changes, omental edema, or soft-tissue infiltration of the fat in the pericholecystic space. Although CT-guided percutaneous needle aspiration may be helpful in patients with an empyema of the gallbladder, there are substantial numbers of false-negative aspirates in patients with early acalculous cholecystitis (McGahan and Walter, 1985).

Ascending Cholangitis

The two common pathophysiologic features of ascending cholangitis are biliary obstruction and secondary bacterial infection. Ascending cholangitis is frequently associated with common duct stones or iatrogenic biliary strictures, and less commonly with neoplastic biliary obstruction. However, any form of biliary obstruction may result in bacterial cholangitis. The classic clinical triad consists of pain, jaundice, and fever and chills (Way and Sleisenger, 1983). Patients with suppurative cholangitis often present with profound sepsis, hypotension, mental obtundation, and cardiovascular collapse. Prompt drainage of the biliary tree is essential to minimize mortality from this disease.

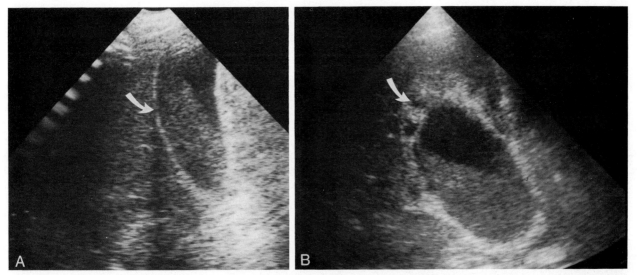

Figure 18–18. Sonographic diagnosis of acalculous cholecystitis by serial sonograms. *A,* Sagittal sonogram of the gallbladder demonstrating intraluminal sludge but a normal gallbladder wall *(arrow)*. *B,* Follow-up sonogram 3 days later demonstrates marked asymmetric thickening of the gallbladder wall with subserosa edema *(arrow)*. Acalculous cholecystitis was proved at surgery. (From Jeffrey, R.B.: CT and Sonography of the Acute Abdomen. New York, Raven Press, 1989, p. 63, with permission.)

CT and sonography can reliably demonstrate biliary ductal dilatation. The main advantage of sonography in this setting is that it can be performed at the bedside and without intravenous contrast enhancement. CT, however, has a number of potential advantages in assessing patients with suspected cholangitis. This is particularly true if there is an associated gas-forming abscess or if percutaneous abscess or biliary drainage is contemplated. In patients with intrahepatic calculi, the distribution of involvement may be better depicted by CT (Fig. 18–19). Gas

within the biliary tree often precludes adequate imaging for sonography but can be readily appreciated by CT.

In patients with mild forms of cholangitis, direct cholangiography either by ERCP or percutaneous transhepatic cholangiography may be required for accurate definition of ductal anatomy and diagnosis of small calculi or strictures. However, the need for these more invasive imaging procedures must be tempered by the slightly higher risk of inducing sepsis in patients with underlying bacterial cholangitis, since

Figure 18–19. CT diagnosis of intrahepatic calculi in a patient with ascending cholangitis. Contrast-enhanced CT demonstrates multiple dilated intrahepatic bile ducts. Note intrahepatic calculus in left ductal system *(arrow)*. (From Jeffrey, R.B.: CT and Sonography of the Acute Abdomen. New York, Raven Press, 1989, p. 69, with permission.)

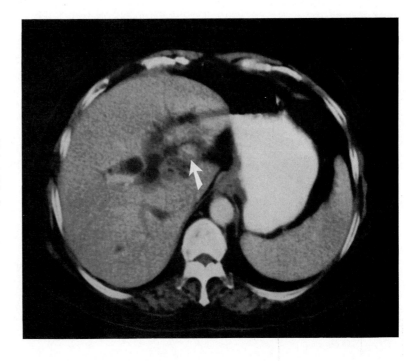

the injection of positive contrast agents into an obstructed biliary tree may be associated with transient bacteremia.

Biliary Trauma

Minor lacerations of the intrahepatic biliary tree after blunt hepatic parenchymal trauma are common. Generally these lesions are insignificant lesions and heal without direct intervention (Penn, 1962; Way and Sleisenger, 1983). Rarely biliary duct injury leads to development of post-traumatic bile collections (bil-

omas) either within the hepatic parenchyma or the peritoneal cavity. The clinical symptoms associated with bilomas vary depending on the size and location of the lesion. It is not uncommon, however, for large bilomas to occur in asymptomatic patients in the absence of infection.

Both CT and sonography may suggest the diagnosis of postoperative or post-traumatic biloma because of its characteristic water density. However, an abscess, pancreatic pseudocyst, or seroma may have similar appearance and tissue density. Guided intervention may be useful for drainage of bilomas (Posner and Moore, 1985) (Fig. 18–20). In the absence of distal

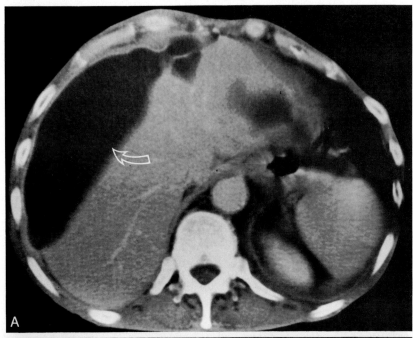

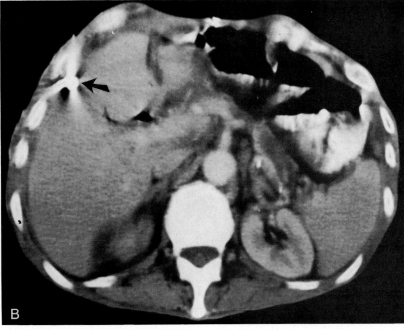

Figure 18–20. Percutaneous drainage of post-traumatic biloma. *A,* Large perihepatic water-density biloma *(arrow). B,* Repeat CT scan after insertion of a percutaneous catheter drain *(arrow).* The biloma was successfully drained by percutaneous techniques alone. (From Jeffrey, R.B.: CT and Sonography of the Acute Abdomen. New York, Raven Press, 1989, p. 56, with permission.)

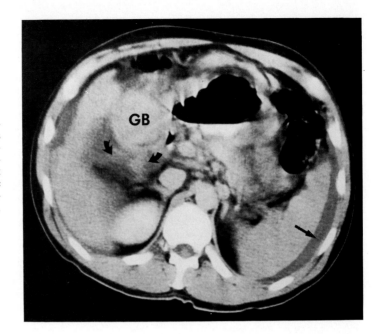

Figure 18–21. Laceration of gallbladder *(GB)* with intraluminal clot after blunt trauma. High-density hematoma is seen within a distended gallbladder. Note subhepatic hemoperitoneum *(curved arrow)* and lower attenuation hemoperitoneum adjacent to the spleen *(straight arrow)*. At laparotomy, laceration of the gallbladder wall and cystic artery was apparent. (From Jeffrey, R.B.: CT and Sonography of the Acute Abdomen. New York, Raven Press, 1989, p. 57, with permission.)

biliary obstruction, guided percutaneous drainage is often highly effective for intrahepatic or intraperitoneal bilomas (Posner and Moore, 1985).

Direct trauma to the gallbladder after blunt injury is rare and is seen in only 2% of all visceral injuries (Way and Sleisenger, 1983). A variety of injuries to the gallbladder may occur including laceration (Fig. 18–21), perforation, evulsion, or intramural contusion or hematoma (Way and Sleisenger, 1983). In unstable patients in whom further diagnostic information is required after blunt trauma, CT is the imaging method of choice. Pericholecystic hemorrhage may be noted in patients with laceration or avulsion of the gallbladder (Jeffrey et al., 1986). In patients with bile peritoneal leakage, however, the clinical course may be indolent, and bile peritonitis may not be clinically apparent for several days (Jeffrey et al., 1986).

References

Bach, R.D., and Frey, C.F.: Diagnosis and treatment of pancreatic trauma. Am. J. Surg. 121:20–29, 1971.

Balthazar, E.J.: CT diagnosis and staging of acute pancreatitis. Radiol. Clin. North Am. 27:19–37, 1989.

Balthazar, E.J., Robinson, D., Megibow, A.J., et al.: Acute pancreatitis: Value of CT in establishing prognosis. Radiology 174:331–336, 1990.

Cooperberg, P.L., and Gibney, R.G.: Imaging of the gallbladder, 1987. Radiology 163:605–613, 1987.

Falkoff, G.E., Taylor, K.J.W., and Morse, S.: Hepatic artery pseudoaneurysms: Diagnosis with real-time and pulsed Doppler US. Radiology 158:55–56, 1986.

Federle, M.P., Jeffrey, R.B., Crass, R.A., et al.: Computed tomography of pancreatic abscesses. AJR 136:879–882, 1981.

Fig, L.M., Wahl, R.L., Stewart, R.E., et al.: Morphine-augmented hepatobiliary scintigraphy in the severely ill: Caution is in order. Radiology 175:467–473, 1990.

Freeny, P.C., Lewis, G.P., Traverso, L.W., and Ryan, J.A.: Infected pancreatic fluid collections: Percutaneous catheter drainage. Radiology 167:435–441, 1988.

Freise, J.: Evaluation of sonography in the diagnosis of acute pancreatitis. *In* Beger, H.G., and Buchler, M. (eds.): Acute Pancreatitis. Berlin, Springer-Verlag, 1987, pp. 118–131.

Frey, C.: Trauma to the pancreas and duodenum. *In* Blaisdell, F.W., and Trunkey, D.D. (eds.): Abdominal Trauma. New York, Thieme-Stratton, 1982, pp. 87–122.

Glen, F., and Becker, C.: Acute acalculous cholecystitis. Ann. Surg. 195:131–136, 1982.

Gooding, G.: Ultrasound of a superior mesenteric aneurysm secondary to pancreatitis: A plea for real-time ultrasound of sonolucent masses in pancreatitis. J. Clin. Ultrasound 9:255–256, 1981.

Gyr, K.E., Singer, M.V., and Sarles, H.: Pancreatitis: Concepts and classification. Amsterdam, Excerpta Medica, 1984.

Hashimoto, B.E., Laing, F.C., Jeffrey, R.B., Jr, et al.: Hemorrhagic pancreatic fluid collections examined by ultrasound. Radiology 150:803–808, 1984.

Hiatt, J.R., Fink, A.S., King, W., III, et al.: Percutaneous aspiration of peripancreatic fluid collections: A safe method to detect infection. Surgery 101:523–530, 1987.

Howard, R.J.: Acute acalculous cholecystitis. Am. J. Surg. 141:194–198, 1981.

Jeffrey, R.B.: CT and Sonography of the Acute Abdomen. New York, Raven Press, 1989a, pp. 111–147.

Jeffrey, R.B., Jr.: Sonography in acute pancreatitis. Radiol. Clin. North Am. 27:5–17, 1989b.

Jeffrey, R.B., Jr., Federle, M.P., and Crass, R.A.: Computed tomography of pancreatic trauma. Radiology 147:491–494, 1983.

Jeffrey, R.B., Federle, M.P., and Laing, F.C.: Computed tomography of mesenteric involvement in fulminant pancreatitis. Radiology 147:185–188, 1983.

Jeffrey, R.B. Jr., Federle, M.P., Laing, F.C., and Wing, V.W.: Computed tomography of blunt trauma to the gallbladder. J. Comput. Assist. Tomogr. 10:756–758, 1986.

Jeffrey, R.B., Jr., Grendell, J.H., Federle, M.P., et al.: Improved survival with early CT diagnosis of pancreatic abscess. Gastrointest. Radiol. 12:26–30, 1987.

Jeffrey, R.B., Laing, F.C., and Wing, V.W.: Extrapancreatic spread of acute pancreatitis: New observations with real-time US. Radiology 159:707–711, 1986.

Jeffrey, R.B., Laing, F.C., and Wing, V.W.: Ultrasound in acute pancreatic trauma. Gastrointest. Radiol. 11:44–46, 1986.

Jeffrey, R.B., Jr., Laing, F.C., Wong, W., and Callen, P.W.: Gangrenous cholecystitis: Diagnosis by ultrasound. Radiology 148:219–221, 1983.

Laing, F.C., Federle, M.P., Jeffrey, R.B., Jr., and Brown, T.W.:

Ultrasonic evaluation of patients with acute right upper quadrant pain. Radiology 140:449–455, 1981.

Lim, G.M., Jeffrey, R.B., Jr., and Tolentino, C.S.: Pancreatic pseudoaneurysm: Monitoring the success of transcatheter embolization with duplex sonography. J. Ultrasound Med. 8:643–646, 1989.

Madrazo, B.L., Francis, I., Hricak, H., et al.: Sonographic findings in perforation of the gallbladder. Radiology 139:491–496, 1982.

Mandel, S.R., Jacques, P.J., Mauro, M.A., et al.: Nonoperative management of peripancreatic arterial aneurysms: A 10-year experience. Ann. Surg. 205:126, 1987.

Matzinger, F.R.K., Ho, C.S., Yee, A.C., and Gray, R.R.: Pancreatic pseudocysts drained through a percutaneous transgastric approach: Further experience. Radiology 167:431–434, 1988.

Mauro, M.A., McCartney, W.H., and Melmed, J.R.: Hepatobiliary scanning with 99mTc-PIPIDA in acute cholecystitis. Radiology 142:193–197, 1982.

McGahan, J.P., and Walter, J.P.: Diagnostic percutaneous aspiration of the gallbladder. Radiology 155:619–622, 1985.

Northrup, W.F., and Simmons, R.L.: Pancreatic trauma: A review. Surgery 1971:27–43, 1972.

Penn, I.: Injuries of the gallbladder. Br. J. Surg. 49:636–641, 1962.

Posner, M.C., and Moore, E.E.: Extrahepatic biliary tract injury: Operative management plan. J. Trauma 25:833–837, 1985.

Raduns, R., McGahan, J.P., and Beal, S.: Cholecystokinin sonography: Lack of utility in diagnosis of acute acalculous cholecystitis. Radiology 175:463–466, 1990.

Ralls, P.W., Colletti, P.M., Lapin, S.A., et al.: Real-time sonography in suspected acute cholecystitis. Radiology 155:767–771, 1985.

Sarner, M., and Cotton, P.B.: Classification of pancreatitis. Gut 25:756–759, 1984.

Shuman, W.P., Rogers, J.V., Rudd, T.G., et al.: Low sensitivity of sonography and cholescintigraphy in acalculous cholecystitis. AJR 142:531–534, 1984.

Siegelman, S.S., Copeland, B.E., Saba, G.P., et al.: CT of fluid collections associated with pancreatitis. AJR 134:1121–1132, 1980.

Simeone, J.F., Brink, J.A., Mueller, P.R., et al.: The sonographic diagnosis of acute gangrenous cholecystitis: Importance of the Murphy sign. AJR 152:289–290, 1989.

Steiner, E., Hahn, P.F., Saini, S., et al.: Complicated pancreatic abscesses: Problems and interventional management. Radiology 167:443–446, 1988.

vanSonnenberg, E., Wing, V.W., Casola, G., et al.: Temporizing percutaneous drainage of complicated abscesses in critically ill patients. AJR 142:821–826, 1984.

vanSonnenberg, E., Wittich, G.R., Casola, G., et al.: Complicated pancreatic inflammatory disease: Diagnostic and therapeutic role of interventional radiology. Radiology 155:335–340, 1985.

Vasquez, J.L., Thorsen, M.K., Dodds, W.J., et al.: Evaluation and treatment of intraabdominal bilomas. AJR 144:933–938, 1985.

Way, L.W., and Sleisenger, M.H.: Biliary obstruction, cholangitis, and choledocholithiasis. *In* Sleisinger, M.H., Fordtran, J.S. (eds.): Gastrointestinal Disease. Philadelphia, W.B. Saunders, 1983, pp. 1389–1403.

Weissmann, H.S., Frank, M.S., Bernstein, L.H., and Freeman, L.M.: Rapid and accurate diagnosis of acute cholecystitis with 99mTc-HIDA cholescintigraphy. AJR 132:523–528, 1979.

19

Acute Genitourinary Disease

■

N. Reed Dunnick

Imaging of the urinary tract must always be done with an appreciation for the clinical setting of the patient. Elective studies are designed to arrive at the most appropriate diagnosis in a timely, yet cost-effective, fashion. In patients with acute problems, however, it is often more appropriate to go immediately to the study most likely to be diagnostic, regardless of cost. In hospitalized patients it is likely that a rapid diagnosis will expedite therapy and be more cost-effective in the long run. The methods chosen must always reflect the available equipment and expertise in any given institution.

INFECTION

Acute Pyelonephritis

Acute bacterial pyelonephritis is usually acquired as an ascending infection from the bladder in patients with vesicoureteral reflux. Diabetes mellitus is an important predisposing factor, and women are affected more often than men.

The renal infection may be global, involving the entire kidney, or may be localized to one or more segments of the kidney. This localized form may appear as a renal mass without liquefaction and has been described as acute "lobar nephronia" (Rosenfield et al., 1979).

Most patients with acute pyelonephritis do not require imaging studies. The diagnosis is based on clinical and laboratory findings, and antibiotic treatment is usually effective. Radiographic imaging is usually reserved for patients who do not respond to medical therapy or who have more severe illnesses that suggest renal or perinephric abscesses.

An enlarged, poorly functioning kidney is seen with excretory urography (Fig. 19–1). The affected kidney is swollen by inflammation and edema. Decreased renal function is reflected in the poor opacification of the collecting system. The calyces remain delicately cupped, and there may be attenuation of the calyces and infundibulae by the enlarged kidney. The presence of gas suggests emphysematous pyelonephritis, which is seen most often in diabetic patients infected with *Escherichia coli*. In many patients, however, the urogram may be normal (Silver et al., 1976).

Poorly defined hypoechoic regions are demonstrated with sonography. The corticomedullary junction may be blurred. The primary value of sonography in this setting is to exclude obstruction (Edell and Bonavita, 1979). This is relatively easy to do, because the collecting system is not dilated but compressed by the swollen kidney.

Contrast-enhanced computed tomographic (CT) scans demonstrate a characteristic striated appearance (Fig. 19–2). This consists of linear or wedge-shaped lucent areas interspersed between normally enhancing portions of renal parenchyma (Gold et al., 1983). These low-density bands radiate from the renal hilum to the periphery of the kidney in a lobar distribution. This appearance is presumably due to interstitial edema but may also be seen in patients with acute tubular necrosis or vascular infarction.

Most patients respond to appropriate antibiotic therapy (Morgan and Nyberg, 1985). In some patients, however, the amount of renal damage is too great for the kidney to recover. In these patients tissue necrosis may lead to renal abscess.

Abscess

Most renal abscesses arise from a urinary tract infection. The most common organisms are *E. coli* and *Proteus* and *Pseudomonas* species. Severe or inadequately treated bacterial nephritis may cause sufficient tissue necrosis to undergo cavitation and develop into a renal abscess. Patients with renal abscesses are typically febrile, complain of flank pain, and have marked leukocytosis.

Imaging studies are needed to identify an abscess,

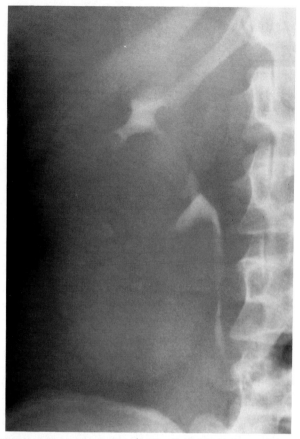

Figure 19–1. Acute pyelonephritis. Excretory urogram demonstrates a swollen kidney with diminished function and attenuation of the collecting system.

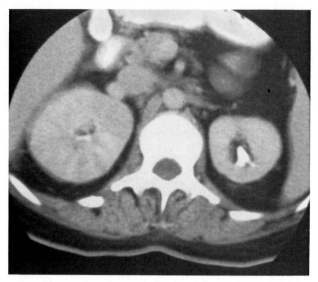

Figure 19–2. Acute pyelonephritis. The right kidney is enlarged and has a striated nephrogram.

since they will not respond to medical therapy alone. If the remainder of the kidney is relatively unaffected, there may be sufficient renal function to identify a focal mass. An abscess can be distinguished from a simple renal cyst by the presence of a thick wall.

Sonography demonstrates a cystic cavity with increased through transmission. Multiple echoes reflect pus and debris within the abscess cavity. Gas is present in only about 10% of renal abscesses.

A low-attenuation cystic mass is seen on CT (Fig. 19–3). A thick enhancing rim defines the abscess. There is often soft-tissue stranding and thickening of the adjacent perirenal fascia (Hoddick et al., 1983). CT also defines any retroperitoneal extension that may be present.

Percutaneous drainage combined with appropriate antibiotic coverage is often effective treatment. Either CT or ultrasound may be used to guide percutaneous aspiration and placement of the drainage catheter.

Pyonephrosis

Pyonephrosis refers to the accumulation of pus within an infected collecting system. There is usually an underlying ureteral obstruction, often due to stone disease. If the obstruction has been long-standing,

there is unlikely to be sufficient renal function to excrete contrast material.

Excretory urography is used to identify radiopaque calculi on the preliminary radiographs and to evaluate the contralateral kidney. Sonography is most useful for identifying dilatation of the collecting system, but it may also detect the obstructing calculus. Echoes from pus and debris are appreciated within the dilated renal pelvis. This may occasionally layer out to a fluid–debris level.

An unenhanced CT scan may be useful, because even "radiolucent" stones are readily detected by CT. Intravenous contrast injection demonstrates enhancement of the vascular renal parenchyma, but renal function is seldom sufficient for renal contrast excretion.

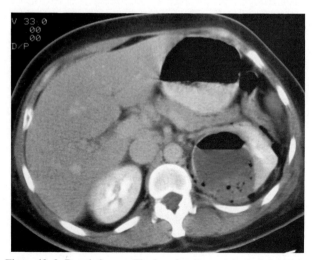

Figure 19–3. Renal abscess. The low-density mass in the left kidney has a thick wall and contains gas. Percutaneous aspiration revealed frankly purulent material.

Xanthogranulomatous pyelonephritis is an uncommon form of pyonephrosis. The diagnosis is based on the demonstration of lipid-laden macrophages, which compose the xanthomatous tissue. Although the diagnosis is pathologic, it can often be suggested by the typical radiographic appearance of an obstructing stone in a patient with pyonephrosis (Tolia et al., 1981) (Fig. 19–4).

Xanthogranulomatous pyelonephritis is typically seen in women with histories of multiple urinary tract infections. The most common organisms are *Proteus* and *E. coli.* Most patients have obstructing branched calculi with marked hydronephrosis.

Most patients have no renal function on the affected side. There is, however, a focal form of xanthogranulomatous pyelonephritis that involves only a portion of the kidney. Xanthogranulomatous pyelonephritis may also extend into the perinephric space (Goldman et al., 1984) and occasionally involves adjacent organs. The treatment is nephrectomy.

OBSTRUCTION

One of the most common acute genitourinary problems is ureteral obstruction. The most common cause is a ureteral calculus, but occasionally a tumor, blood clot, fungus ball, or even a sloughed papilla may result in ureteral obstruction. Typically, patients complain of flank pain that radiates to the groin. It is usually sufficiently intense that patients seek medical attention. Thus, the degree of dilatation of the collecting system is mild.

Hematuria is commonly seen in patients in whom obstruction is due to stone disease. The absence of hematuria, however, does not exclude a ureteral calculus, especially when there is complete ureteral obstruction.

Excretory urography remains the modality of choice to screen patients for suspected ureteral ob-

struction. The plain abdominal radiograph must be carefully scrutinized to identify calculi. Many times it is not clear whether a calcification represents a ureteral stone or any number of other possible causes, especially vascular calcifications. If good-quality preliminary radiographs are not obtained, it may be impossible to determine whether a density seen after contrast injection represents excreted contrast material or a urinary tract calculus.

With contrast injection there is delayed excretion from the ipsilateral kidney into a mildly dilated collecting system (Fig. 19–5). The nephrogram is delayed and increased in density. In the acute setting, renal function is sufficient to excrete contrast material, even in patients with high-grade ureteral obstruction. However, delayed films (to 24 or even 36 hours) may be required to demonstrate the site of obstruction.

Sonography is often valuable in patients with urolithiasis. Mild ureteropelvocaliectasis can often be detected, but sonography is less sensitive than excretory urography for this purpose. A calculus is seen as an echogenic structure with shadowing (Fig. 19–6). In patients with histories of adverse contrast reactions, ultrasound may be a good alternative to urography. When nonionic contrast materials are used for excretory urography, ultrasound may also be a cost-effective choice.

Because the degree of dilatation of the collecting system is usually mild, it is more difficult for ultrasound than excretory urography to distinguish these patients from normal. In a series of 41 patients with acute ureteral obstruction (Hill et al., 1985), excretory urography identified 85%, and sonography correctly diagnosed only 66% of patients.

CT may be a useful adjunct, particularly for identifying nonradiopaque renal calculi. As many as 10% of stones are not dense enough to be detected by abdominal radiography. These are primarily uric acid stones or, rarely, xanthine stones. Cystine stones are usually sufficiently opaque to be detected by plain radiography. Even these "lucent" uric acid stones are readily detected on CT, where their density is well above 100 Hounsfield units (Federle et al., 1981). If the stone is small, however, multiple contiguous sections are required for identification.

CT is particularly useful in patients in whom filling defects are identified on excretory urography (Fig. 19–7). Calculi are readily identified by their high density. Blood clots usually undergo lysis from the urokinase produced normally by the kidney, such that their appearance changes from day to day.

RENAL FAILURE

Acute renal failure may be due to a wide variety of causes, including prerenal and postrenal causes, as well as renal parenchymal disease. Prerenal causes include hypotension due to either low cardiac output or hypovolemia. Postrenal causes are usually due to

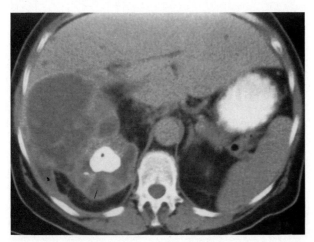

Figure 19–4. Xanthogranulomatous pyelonephritis. An obstructing central calculus is seen on CT. There is hydronephrosis with only a thin rim of parenchyma.

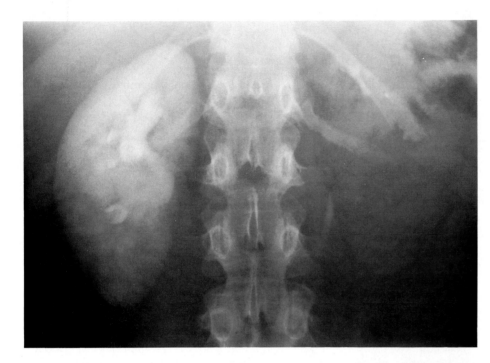

Figure 19–5. Right ureteral obstruction. There is delayed contrast excretion into a dilated intrarenal collecting system. The nephrogram is delayed but intense.

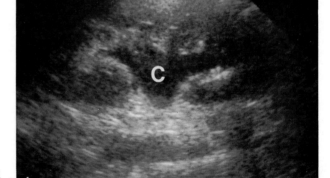

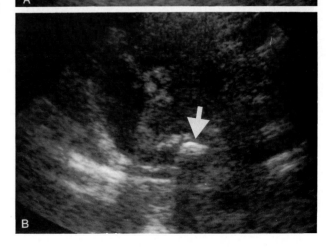

Figure 19–6. Ureteral obstruction. *A,* A mildly dilated intrarenal collecting system *(C)* is detected by sonography. *B,* An obstructing ureteral stone *(arrow)* is seen as an echogenic mass with shadowing.

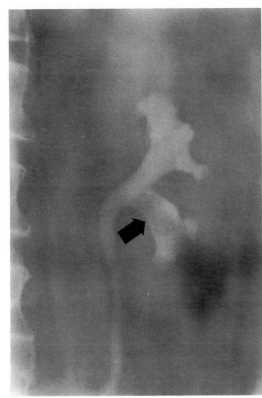

A

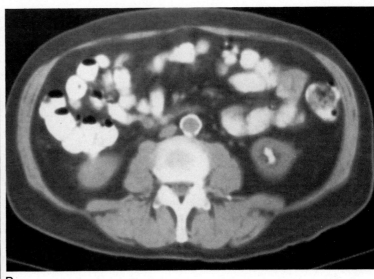

B

Figure 19–7. Lucent stone. *A*, A filling defect *(arrow)* is seen in the lower pole infundibulum of the left kidney on urography. *B*, The high density of this filling defect on unenhanced CT clearly identifies it as a renal calculus.

acute ureteral obstruction. Intrarenal causes of acute renal failure include medical renal diseases, bilateral cortical necrosis, and interstitial or vascular diseases. Acute tubular necrosis may be due to hemolysis, myolysis, antibiotics (e.g., aminoglycosides or amphotericin), or contrast-induced renal failure.

The primary role of radiology in this setting is to identify patients whose renal failure is due to acute ureteral obstruction (Dunnick et al., 1991). Unless there is only a single functioning renal unit or a prior transureteroureterostomy, ureteral obstruction must be bilateral to cause acute renal failure.

Excretory urography is not helpful in this setting, since it depends on renal function for contrast excretion. A plain abdominal radiograph may be useful, however, to identify evidence of urolithiasis or even to see surgical clips that could have inadvertently obstructed a ureter.

Sonography is the imaging modality of choice, because it does not rely on renal function. The kidney can be assessed for size, parenchymal thickness, and dilatation of the collecting system.

It may not be appropriate to perform ultrasound examination of all patients with acute renal failure (Ritchie et al., 1988). Patients more likely to have obstructive causes include those with histories of urolithiasis, bladder outlet obstruction, pelvic tumors, or recent pelvic surgery. Patients presenting with acute renal colic also deserve radiographic evaluation for possible ureteral obstruction.

Not all patients with ureteral obstruction have dilatation of the collecting system (Kamholtz et al., 1989). This nondilated form of obstructive uropathy

occurs most often in patients with retroperitoneal fibrosis or extensive retroperitoneal lymph node metastases that encase the ureters (Lalli, 1977). In these patients retrograde pyelography with ureteral stent placement or percutaneous nephrostomy is needed to reverse renal failure and preserve renal function (Naidich et al., 1986).

CT can also be helpful in this setting. Demonstration of para-aortic lymphadenopathy adjacent to or encasing the ureters suggests obstructive uropathy. Retroperitoneal fibrosis is readily detected by CT as a mantle of soft tissue surrounding the great vessels and encasing the adjacent ureters (Degesys et al.,

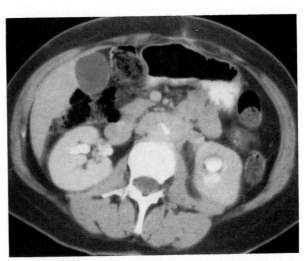

Figure 19–8. Retroperitoneal fibrosis. The mantle of soft tissue surrounding the great vessels is typical for retroperitoneal fibrosis.

1986) (Fig. 19–8). In retroperitoneal fibrosis the ureters are usually retracted medially. Involvement is typically most marked at the level of the lower lumbar spine, but it may occur anywhere from the pelvis to the renal hilum. The CT appearance of retroperitoneal fibrosis is not pathognomonic and may be mimicked by retroperitoneal lymph node metastases. Biopsy is need for confirmation.

Acute cortical necrosis may also be identified on CT. Renal failure is due to severe vasoconstriction of the renal cortical vessels. It is seen most often as part of a hemorrhagic shock syndrome. Only the renal cortex is involved and the medulla is spared. With intravenous contrast injection, there is preservation of the enhancement of the renal medulla but no enhancement of the renal cortex and no contrast excretion (Jordan et al., 1990).

ACUTE VASCULAR ABNORMALITIES

Renal Artery Infarction

Acute renal infarction may be due to either blunt or penetrating injury. The trauma might also occur as part of an iatrogenic injury including surgery, percutaneous biopsy, and arteriography. Patients with underlying heart disease may have an embolic cause. Renal infarction from vasculitis is usually segmental. The predominant clinical features of acute arterial infarction are flank pain, fever, and hematuria.

Acute occlusion of a segmental renal artery with infarction results in a wedge-shaped defect that extends from the medulla to the renal cortex (Fig. 19–9). Acutely there is swelling, but this subsides in 4 to 10 days and is followed by atrophy and scarring.

Acute infarction of the main renal artery results in global enlargement of the kidney due to edema. A thin peripheral rim may be preserved because of supply by unaffected capsular vessels.

The appearance of renal infarction on imaging studies depends on the amount of renal tissue affected. Excretory urography shows no function on the ipsilateral side if the main renal artery is occluded. Segmental infarction affects contrast excretion only in involved areas. The remainder of the kidney may appear normal. Edema from involved segments may cause swelling and reduce perfusion to the kidney.

An enlarged swollen kidney can be detected with sonography, and Doppler studies may be used to demonstrate the absence of normal blood flow.

The most useful imaging study is usually CT. An enhanced CT examination demonstrates which portions of the kidney are affected. The thin peripheral rim of renal parenchyma opacified by unaffected capsular vessels is also delineated (Hilton et al., 1984). This is occasionally helpful in distinguishing renal infarction from other possible causes of wedge-shaped hypoperfusion such as acute bacterial nephritis. If there is associated hemorrhage, this is also well defined with CT. However, this cortical rim sign may

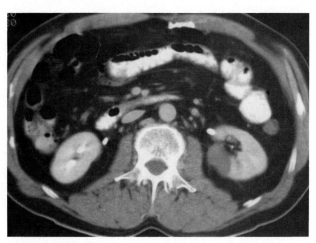

Figure 19–9. Renal infarction. A focal defect is present in the posteromedial aspect of the left kidney.

also be seen with renal vein thrombosis or in patients with acute tubular necrosis (Hann and Pfister, 1982).

Arteriography may be used to document this process but is usually not necessary. It is most helpful in patients with an underlying vasculitis or with segmental infarction, because it may occasionally identify the underlying cause. Vascular aneurysms and emboli are usually detected with arteriography.

Although magnetic resonance imaging (MRI) may also detect renal infarction, it does not provide information that cannot be gained with CT or arteriography. Because its availability is often limited, particularly in the acute setting, it is seldom used.

Renal Vein Thrombosis

Renal vein thrombosis may be due to trauma, but in adults it is often due to underlying renal disease such as membranous glomerulonephritis. Renal neoplasms, such as renal adenocarcinoma, may also cause renal vein thrombosis, but this is usually due to tumor extension into the renal vein. In children, renal vein thrombosis is most often due to dehydration.

The sequelae of renal vein thrombosis depend on the degree of collateral vascular supply. If the thrombosis develops slowly and adequate venous collaterals are recruited, there may be no adverse effect on the kidney. With acute occlusion and inadequate venous collaterals, however, a hemorrhagic infarction may ensue. These patients may present with acute flank pain, fever, and hematuria. Chronic renal vein thrombosis may cause the nephrotic syndrome because of excessive protein loss. It is not uncommon, however, for a patient with renal vein thrombosis to have insignificant proteinuria (Keating and Althausen, 1985).

The findings on excretory urography are nonspecific. The involved kidney is usually enlarged as a result of intrarenal edema, and function is poor. Increased pressure within the kidney reduces arterial inflow and results in delayed contrast excretion. When visualized, the underlying calyces are normal to attenuated. This helps to distinguish renal vein thrombosis from ureteral obstruction as both may demonstrate delayed contrast excretion and a persistent nephrogram.

Sonography may also demonstrate an enlarged kidney and can be helpful in excluding dilatation of the intrarenal collecting system. In some patients, clot may also be appreciated in the main renal vein (Gatewood et al., 1986). Doppler techniques can identify the absence of venous flow.

An enhanced CT scan may demonstrate both the venous thrombosis and its effect on the kidney. With a good bolus injection, clot is identified as a tubular filling defect within the main renal vein. Extension into the inferior vena cava can also be detected (Fig. 19–10). Venous collaterals, especially when the left kidney is involved, may be seen as enlargement of the gonadal, inferior phrenic, or other retroperitoneal veins. Because fewer veins enter the right renal vein, it is less likely that adequate collateralization will protect the right kidney (Keating and Althausen, 1985). Thus, the incidence of hemorrhagic infarction is higher on the right side than the left. The degree of opacification of the kidney and contrast excretion by the kidney depend on the adequacy of the capsular vessels.

MRI can also detect renal vein thrombosis. Limited flip-angle techniques, which can be acquired quickly, demonstrate absence of flow.

Spontaneous Renal Hemorrhage

Hemorrhage without an obvious cause such as trauma or anticoagulation is termed *spontaneous*. In the retroperitoneum, this includes both subcapsular and perinephric hematomas. The most common causes are neoplastic and vascular (Bosniak, 1989). Angiomyolipoma and renal adenocarcinoma are the most common tumors that present with a subcapsular or perinephric hemorrhage (Belville et al., 1989). Vascular causes include arterial venous malformations and vasculitides.

The usual clinical presentation is with the acute onset of flank pain. Hematuria may or may not be present.

Excretory urography may be obtained in this clinical setting, since the clinical symptoms may mimic acute renal colic. The urogram is often normal. If the hematoma is large enough, displacement of the kidney could be recognized. If the hematoma is subcapsular in location, pressure generated within the renal capsule may be sufficient to impede arterial inflow and cause delayed contrast excretion.

Sonography can detect the hematoma and often determine whether it is subcapsular or perinephric.

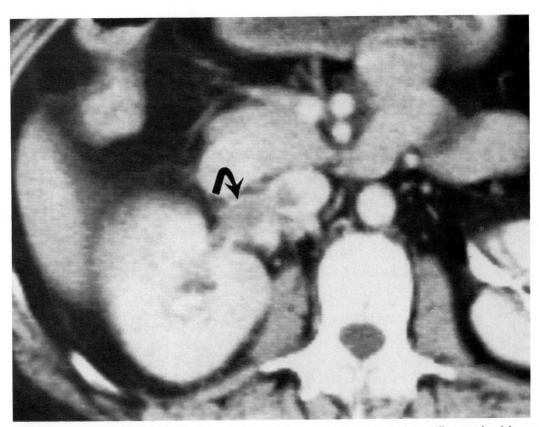

Figure 19–10. Renal vein thrombosis. Enhanced CT scan showing a tubular filling defect *(arrow)* extending out the right renal vein into the inferior vena cava.

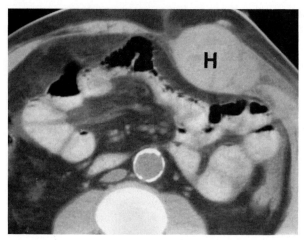

Figure 19–11. Rectus hematoma. After removal of a peritoneal dialysis catheter, an enlarged left rectus abdominis muscle (H) is most consistent with a hematoma.

CT is the most definitive examination for retroperitoneal hemorrhage (Fig. 19–11). An acute bleed often demonstrates the increased density associated with acute clot formation. As the hematoma matures, it may liquefy and gradually be reabsorbed. In some patients, however, a fibrous lining develops around the liquefied hematoma, creating a seroma. If this collection is subcapsular, the pressure generated may result in renin-mediated hypertension (Page kidney).

A subcapsular collection can often be distinguished from a perinephric collection by CT. If the hematoma is immediately adjacent to the renal parenchyma it is likely to be subcapsular. If the capsule remains intact, it is strong enough to deform the renal contour (Dunnick and Korobkin, 1984) (Fig. 19–12). This finding confirms its subcapsular location.

A perinephric hematoma extravasates through the renal capsule into the perinephric space. The blood

is contained by Gerota's fascia. In addition, multiple septations within the perinephric space keep the hematoma from diffusing throughout the entire perinephric fat (Kunin, 1986; McClennan et al., 1986) (see Fig. 19–12). These septations occasionally create confusion in the distinction between a subcapsular and perinephric hematoma. Thus, deformity of the renal contour is the most reliable sign.

Arteriography is no longer required to diagnose perinephric or subcapsular hematoma, because this can be done reliably with CT. Arteriography may be used, however, to identify the underlying cause. An avascular mass is appreciated by displacement of the capsular vessels away from the normal renal parenchyma. If the hematoma is largely perinephric, however, the arteriogram may be normal. Although MRI can also detect a retroperitoneal hematoma, it is not necessary and is rarely used for this purpose.

Identification of a subcapsular or perinephric hematoma as the cause for the patient's acute symptoms is only the first step. An effort should also be made to identify the underlying cause. An unenhanced CT scan is most useful for identifying the hematoma. If there are no contraindications, intravenous contrast material should also be given to examine the renal parenchyma. Even small (2-cm) renal adenocarcinomas are usually seen with an enhanced CT examination. Contiguous 1-cm sections should be used but some authors suggest even more finely collimated sections (5 mm) to minimize the partial volume artifact. This is most important in trying to make the diagnosis of an angiomyolipoma. These hamartomas are composed of several different tissues, and their radiographic appearance depends on the proportion of each tissue in them. The diagnosis rests on the demonstration of macroscopic fat (Bosniak et al. 1988). Thus, narrow collimated images, occasionally as small as 1.5 mm, may be needed.

If no mass can be detected on enhanced CT examination, a renal arteriogram could be obtained to detect vascular disease. The most common vascular cause is renal involvement by a vasculitis, such as polyarteritis nodosa. In these patients multiple small aneurysms are identified in intrarenal vessels.

TRAUMA

Kidney

The distinction of blunt from penetrating trauma is useful in understanding and investigating the effect of these injuries. Penetrating injury may be further categorized by the nature of the penetrating object and whether it occurred during a surgical or percutaneous interventional procedure.

Blunt Trauma

Most patients with significant nonpenetrating renal trauma also sustain injury to other abdominal organs,

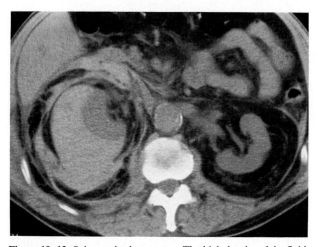

Figure 19–12. Subcapsular hematoma. The high density of the fluid collection in the perinephric space indicates a hematoma. Compression of the kidney is due to the subcapsular component, and additional blood is seen adjacent to septations in the perinephric fat.

such as the liver, spleen, or pancreas. For this reason, CT is the single most valuable modality since all of these organs can be evaluated with a single examination. Intravenous contrast, used to enhance the evaluation of the liver and spleen, is essential in evaluating possible renal injury (Lang et al., 1985). The major drawback in using CT to evaluate the acutely injured patient is the time required for oral contrast to opacify the bowel. In many patients it is not feasible to wait 2 hours to achieve bowel opacification, because examination of the solid viscera is needed more urgently.

Excretory urography can be used to evaluate patients with renal trauma. Unless an isolated renal injury is suspected, however, CT should be performed to examine the entire abdomen. Excretory urography has been advocated in stable patients with isolated flank trauma. Hematuria is frequently the compelling indication for evaluation of the kidneys. Any patient who has sustained significant trauma, however, is likely to have hematuria whether or not there is demonstrable renal injury. In the absence of shock, microhematuria is rarely associated with significant renal damage.

Although excretory urography tends to understage renal injury, it may be sufficient in the patient with a normal or near-normal urogram. In these patients, conservative therapy is indicated. Renal contusions and even mild parenchymal lacerations heal spontaneously, and surgery is not indicated. If there is more severe renal injury, however, CT must be performed for better evaluation.

Sonography has only a limited role in the patient with suspected acute renal injury. If there is no evidence of renal function on an excretory urogram, sonography may be used to confirm that a kidney is present and the patient does not have renal agenesis. However, this should not delay a more definitive examination, such as CT or arteriography.

Even minor renal injuries are well defined with CT (Sandler and Toombs, 1981). A renal contusion is seen as an unenhancing region within the kidney. An unenhanced scan may demonstrate the high density of acute clot, but there will be no contrast enhancement. Occasionally, extravasation of concentrated contrast material may occur, indicating a urinoma.

Renal laceration is an injury that reaches the renal cortex (Fig. 19–13). A subcapsular hematoma or urinoma may develop. If the renal capsule remains intact, the collection will not extend into the perinephric space.

The renal fracture is a severe form of renal laceration in which the kidney is completely separated into two or more fractions (Fig. 19–14). This is a severe form of renal injury in which surgical revascularization may be required. CT clearly defines those portions of kidney that are receiving blood supply, but fragments that have been totally avulsed may be indistinguishable from retroperitoneal hematoma.

Renal arteriography is superior to CT in demonstrating a vascular injury. It is useful in planning the

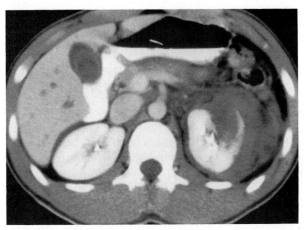

Figure 19–13. Renal laceration. The kidney is intact, but a deep laceration has resulted in a large perinephric hematoma.

surgical operation to repair a renal fracture (see Fig. 19–14). It may also be useful in defining intimal tears in which the renal artery is compromised but still patent. It is the only method of reliably diagnosing post-traumatic pseudoaneurysms or arteriovenous fistulae.

Most renal injuries are minor and may be treated conservatively. Major renal injuries, including severe lacerations or fracture, may require surgical intervention. Only a small minority of patients have vascular pedicle injuries that require emergent surgery (Bretan et al., 1986).

Penetrating Trauma

Although CT may not be able to define the tract of the penetrating injury, it is an excellent method of detecting its effects. Renal contusion, laceration, extravasation, and perinephric hematomas are all well defined by CT. If CT fails to demonstrate evidence

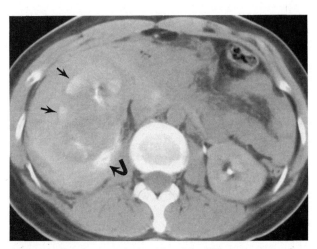

Figure 19–14. Renal fracture. The right kidney has been fragmented. Several portions are opacified by excreted contrast material *(arrows)*. Contrast extravasation can also be detected *(curved arrow)*.

of renal damage, surgical exploration is seldom indicated. Hematuria, especially if microscopic, is insufficient as an indication for exploration. Even among those patients in whom renal injury can be detected, only a few require surgical treatment.

Opacification of the renal parenchyma after intravenous contrast injection is evidence that the renal artery is patent. Absence of enhancement indicates that the renal artery is occluded, but it does not differentiate an acute injury from a chronic process. A perinephric hematoma, which is centered on the renal hilum, suggests injury to the vascular pedicle. Hematomas resulting from traumatic renal laceration are usually posterolateral to the kidney.

Significant renal injury can also be due to a number of iatrogenic causes. The most common is percutaneous renal biopsy, but similar injury may result from percutaneous nephrostomy or a surgical procedure. The acute onset of a perinephric hematoma after renal biopsy indicates damage to a major renal vessel. Emergency renal angiography may be required to identify the site of bleeding. If the catheter can be positioned close enough to the offending vessel, embolization can occlude the bleeding site and still preserve renal function.

Ureter

Ureteral injury from blunt trauma is unlikely. Avulsion of the renal pelvis from the ureter at the ureteropelvic junction has been reported and is more common in children than adults. This is presumably due to a higher incidence of injury to the vascular pedicle when the same mechanism of injury occurs in adults.

Most ureteral injuries are due to penetrating trauma. The ureter may be damaged by penetration from a stab wound or a missile or as a result of the blast effect of the missile.

With increasing use of ureteroscopy, cystoscopic ureteral catheterization, and percutaneous interventional procedures, iatrogenic ureteral injuries are becoming more common (Fig. 19–15). During pelvic surgery the ureter may be inadvertently ligated, clipped, or severed.

Excretory urography is the simplest method of assessing patients with suspected ureteral injury. Unless there is damage to the ipsilateral kidney, the ureter should be well opacified and sites of extravasation or obstruction easily detected. Antegrade pyelography after percutaneous nephrostomy may be useful to define more precisely the site of injury.

Percutaneous nephrostomy with urine diversion is often all that is needed to heal perforations in the ureter (see Fig. 19–15). Ureteral stenting may be performed in an effort to prevent subsequent ureteral stricture.

Bladder

The chance of bladder injury is roughly proportional to the degree of distention. An empty bladder

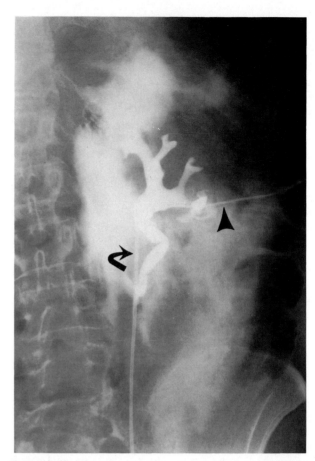

Figure 19–15. Ureteral perforation. A ureteral stent catheter has perforated the ureter *(curved arrow)*. A percutaneous nephrostomy was placed *(arrowhead)* to divert urine flow. Antegrade pyelography demonstrates extravasation.

is much less likely to be damaged than a distended bladder.

The bladder may be damaged as a result of blunt, penetrating, or iatrogenic injury. Most injuries are due to blunt pelvic trauma and accompany a pelvic fracture (Cass and Luxenberg, 1987).

Bladder contusion is an incomplete tear of the mucosa, which results in a localized hematoma in the bladder wall. The radiographic examination is usually normal.

Bladder rupture may result in intraperitoneal or extraperitoneal extravasation. With an acute rise in intravesicular pressure, bladder rupture may occur. If the bladder is distended, the rupture is likely to be in the dome where the bladder is in contact with the peritoneal surface. This results in intraperitoneal extravasation.

Extraperitoneal bladder rupture is more commonly associated with pelvic fracture in which one or more of the fracture fragments perforate the bladder. However, the bladder laceration is often found away from the site of the fracture (Corriere and Sandler, 1988). Both intraperitoneal and extraperitoneal bladder extravasation may occasionally occur with the same injury.

The bladder may be evaluated as part of the

excretory urogram. Delayed films that allow filling of the bladder are required. The post-voiding radiograph may be particularly helpful to demonstrate subtle bladder extravasations.

Cystography, performed on a fluoroscopic table, is the ideal method of detecting bladder injury (Fig. 19–16). A minimum of 300 ml of diluted (30%) contrast material must be used for adequate bladder distention. A radiograph including the entire abdomen should be obtained to detect intraperitoneal rupture that flows away from the bladder. Bladder injury is detected only on a post-draining film in as many as 10% of cases.

CT may also be used to detect bladder extravasation, particularly if the patient is undergoing CT to examine other abdominal organs. Extravasation can be detected as contrast material surrounding the bladder or in the peritoneal space.

Intraperitoneal bladder extravasation results in contrast material in the peritoneal cavity. On an abdominal radiograph, it may be seen medial to the properitoneal fat line and may outline loops of intestine. The contour is smooth, because it reflects the surface of the peritoneal cavity.

Extraperitoneal bladder extravasation results in contrast material in the immediate perivesical space. It has an irregular feathery appearance as it dissects into the adjacent tissue spaces (Fig. 19–17). Because it is usually associated with a pelvic fracture, the bony fragments can also be detected.

Urethra

Urethral injury may also result from either blunt or penetrating trauma. It often occurs in association with pelvic fracture but may be an isolated injury. Hematuria, blood at the urethral meatus, elevation

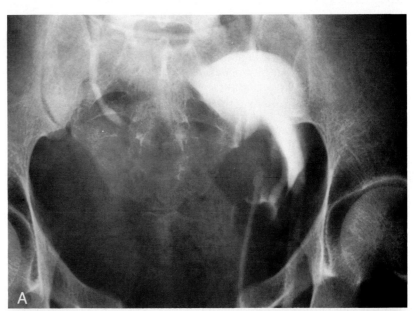

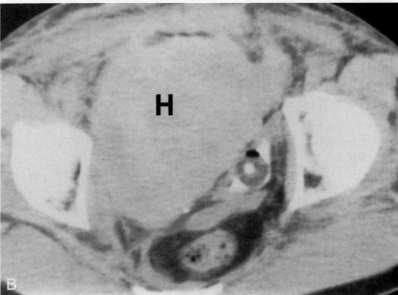

Figure 19–16. Pelvic hematoma. *A,* Cystogram demonstrates displacement of an intact bladder. *B,* CT scan reveals a huge pelvic hematoma *(H).*

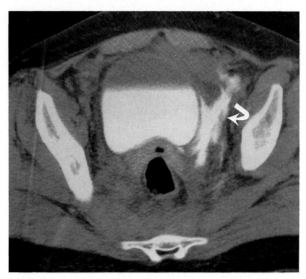

Figure 19–17. Extraperitoneal bladder extravasation. Contrast *(arrow)* is seen outside the bladder. The feathery appearance indicates an extraperitoneal location.

of the prostate gland on digital examination, or elevation of the bladder during excretory urography suggests the possibility of urethral injury. If urethral injury is suspected, a retrograde urethrogram should be performed before any attempt to pass a Foley catheter through the urethra into the bladder. If there is urgent need to catheterize the bladder, a suprapubic puncture should be performed.

The most common urethral injury (Type I) occurs at the proximal bulbous urethra, below the urogenital diaphragm (Sandler et al., 1981). During trauma the prostate gland is displaced in a cephalad direction and carries with it the fibrous connection to the external sphincter. The proximal bulbous urethra is supported only by fat and loose connective tissue, such that rupture usually occurs at this point.

Retrograde urethrography should be performed using a Foley catheter with the balloon distended by 1 to 2 ml of contrast material at the fossa navicularis. Contrast should be injected under fluoroscopic guidance, and spot films can be obtained for documentation.

In some patients the urethra remains intact but is compressed by a hematoma. There may be contusion in the wall of the urethra.

In Type II injury, the urethra is ruptured at the junction of the membranous and prostatic urethra, above the urogenital diaphragm. The retrograde urethrogram demonstrates extravasation of contrast material into the true pelvis rather than the perineum.

The most common injury is Type III, in which the tear in the urethra occurs below the urogenital diaphragm (Sandler et al., 1981). A retrograde injection of contrast material into the urethra demonstrates extravasation in the perineum (Fig. 19–18) and occasionally the scrotum.

The female urethra is rarely injured as a result of

trauma. Most cases of urethral injury occur during instrumentation or obstetric surgery.

Adrenal Gland

Acute traumatic injury to the adrenal glands is uncommon. Although retroperitoneal, they are located near the center of the upper abdomen, adjacent to the lumbar spine. They are surrounded by perinephric fat and located anteromedial to the upper poles of the kidneys.

Acute adrenal injury involves the right adrenal gland more frequently than the left. This may be due to direct transmission of acutely elevated caval pressures out the right adrenal vein to the adrenal gland. The left adrenal vein has a less direct route to the inferior vena cava, because it enters the inferior phrenic vein, which enters the left renal vein before joining the inferior vena cava.

Unless massive, adrenal hemorrhage cannot be seen on plain radiographs or excretory urography. Sonography can be used to identify adrenal hematomas, especially in children. With ultrasound, an echogenic mass is appreciated in the region of the adrenal gland.

In adults CT is most frequently used to detect adrenal injury. A high-density mass is appreciated on unenhanced scans (Fig. 19–19). Over weeks to months the adrenal hematoma slowly resolves. In some patients the hematoma is not resorbed but liquefies and forms a fibrous capsule. This is probably one of the more common causes of an adrenal pseudocyst.

Right adrenal hemorrhage is frequently seen in patients undergoing liver transplantation. In these patients, the right adrenal vein or even right adrenal gland may be oversewn during transplantation surgery

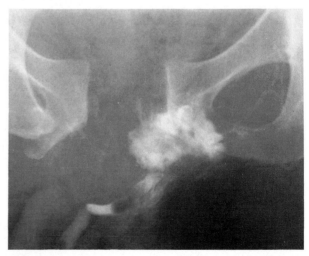

Figure 19–18. Urethral injury. A fracture of the right pubic ramus was seen on the preliminary radiograph. A retrograde urethrogram reveals Type III injury with extravasation of contrast into the perineum.

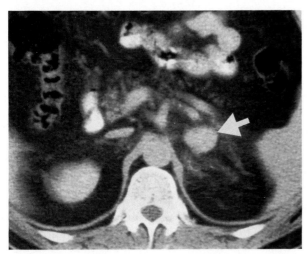

Figure 19–19. Adrenal hematoma. The high density indicates hematoma as the cause of the left adrenal mass *(arrow)*.

(Soloman and Sumkin, 1988). Because there is only one central right adrenal vein, its ligation results in vascular congestion and hemorrhage.

INTERVENTIONAL URORADIOLOGY

A myriad of percutaneous interventional techniques have been developed to accomplish therapeutic goals without surgery. A complete review of these procedures is beyond the scope of this text. However, percutaneous nephrostomy and percutaneous aspiration or abscess drainage are commonly used procedures for the care of patients with acute urinary tract disease. Other percutaneous procedures, such as stone removal, ureteral stent placement, and transcatheter embolization, are more specialized procedures performed by the vascular/interventional radiologist.

Percutaneous Nephrostomy

Percutaneous nephrostomy has been used for the relief of supravesicular obstruction for many years. With the introduction of percutaneous nephrostolithotomy techniques, many new procedures have been developed that use the percutaneous nephrostomy for access to the collecting system. The knowledge and skill used in these procedures have given radiologists confidence to apply them to additional problems, such as urinary diversion for urinary leak or fistula, infusion chemotherapy, ureteral stricture dilatation, or neoureterocystostomy.

Percutaneous nephrostomy may be indicated for patients presenting with acute ureteral obstruction. It may also be used as an emergent procedure in patients with chronic ureteral obstruction and a superimposed acute process such as infection or renal failure with electrolyte imbalance. The procedure may be performed under fluoroscopic, sonographic, or CT guidance. Fluoroscopy is the most efficient of these guidance systems but requires opacification of the collecting system to provide a target for needle placement. If the patient is in renal failure or is acutely obstructed, there may not be sufficient contrast excretion by the kidney to opacify the collecting system. In this setting, ultrasound may be used to guide needle placement initially (Matalon and Silver, 1990) with subsequent procedures performed under fluoroscopy. CT may be used in a similar capacity in specialized situations or may be used to mark the skin and provide assistance for blind needle placement in the fluoroscopy suite. If there is a question of unusual anatomy in which an intra-abdominal organ, such as the liver, spleen, or colon, may lie in the proposed route from the skin to the renal collecting system, CT may be used to define the optimal nephrostomy tract.

The precise method of performing the nephrostomy is a function of the desired goal of the procedure, as well as a personal preference (Pfister, 1986). Most interventional uroradiologists prefer the needle guide wire exchange system, because it usually provides more precise tract placement than the trocar system. The initial puncture of the collecting system is made with a 20- or 22-gauge fine needle. If a 22-gauge needle is chosen, direct puncture of the renal pelvis may be performed without passing through the renal parenchyma. This is then used to opacify the collecting system, either through the 22-gauge needle or through a no. 3 French catheter passed over an 0.018-inch guide wire. The needle hole in the renal pelvis is so small that it does not require the overlying renal parenchyma for tamponade after removal of the needle or catheter.

If there is good opacification of the collecting system, either by means of intravenously injected contrast material excreted by the kidney or retrograde injection of contrast material into the ureter, the initial puncture may be the definitive nephrostomy tract through the kidney. It is preferable to enter from a posterolateral position and pass along the avascular line of Brödel, which is the least vascular portion of the kidney (Dunnick et al., 1989). This line is usually 1 to 2 cm posterior to the lateral convex border of the kidney.

The needle should enter either a calyx or infundibulum (Fig. 19–20). Withdrawal of urine through the needle confirms its location in the collecting system. A 22-gauge needle accepts a 0.018-inch guide wire, which should be passed down the ureter if possible. A variety of systems can then be used to enlarge the tract to a size that can accommodate a 0.038-inch guide wire. This guide wire should be stiff enough to allow dilatation of the nephrostomy tract. The size and type of catheter placed for ultimate drainage depends on the goal of the procedure. Simple relief of urinary obstruction can be accomplished with a

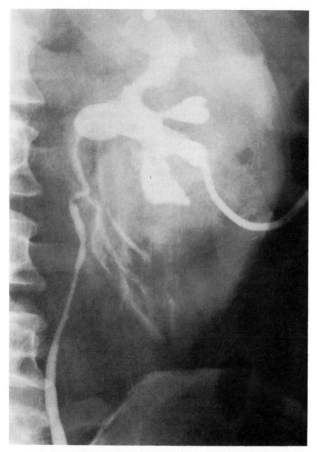

Figure 19–20. Percutaneous nephrostomy. The nephrostomy catheter enters the collecting system at a calyx. There is a small amount of extravasation into the perinephric space.

no. 5 French catheter. Most interventionalists, however, prefer to use a slightly larger (no. 8 French) self-retaining catheter for this purpose. If the contents of the collecting system are purulent, a slightly larger catheter (no. 10 French) may be used to prevent occlusion of the catheter by debris. If subsequent intrarenal manipulations are planned, a larger tract often is required. However, additional dilatation may be performed at a later date.

The results of percutaneous nephrostomy drainage for relief of supravesical obstruction are excellent. The adverse obstructive effects on the kidney are relieved, and renal function returns toward normal. Septic patients usually show prompt clinical improvement, and culture of the infected urine allows selection of the most appropriate antibiotic.

The complication rate for percutaneous nephrostomy is low. Major complications are seen in less than 2% of cases, and the mortality is less than 0.5%.

Contrast or urine extravasation is the most common complication but is self-limiting if adequate urine drainage is established. Vascular complications occur in about 1% of patients undergoing percutaneous nephrostomy. With additional dilatation and manipulation, the incidence of this complication increases. Septic complications also account for approximately

1% of cases. However, these usually occur in patients with underlying urinary tract infections or pyonephrosis, in which case relief of an obstructed infection is essential.

Abscess Drainage

Retroperitoneal abscesses, particularly in the kidney or perinephric space, are amenable to percutaneous drainage. The most common cause of such an abscess is a urinary tract infection, and the underlying cause of the abscess must be sought and treated.

A patient with suspected retroperitoneal abscess should be examined with CT. Although intravenous contrast injection is not essential, it is particularly helpful in evaluating the kidneys. In a septic patient, any abnormal fluid collection may be infected. If the fluid collection is confined to normal anatomic structures, it will not be walled off and may not be amenable to percutaneous drainage. Even in this setting, however, aspiration may be helpful because it provides fluid for culture.

A well-defined fluid collection with a thick wall and mass effect indicates abscess. Although the presence of gas suggests an infection by a gas-forming organism (Fig. 19–21), most intra-abdominal abscesses do not contain gas. Thus, aspiration of any abnormal fluid collection should be performed in a patient suspected of having an abdominal abscess.

Percutaneous aspiration of a suspected abscess should be performed with an 18-gauge needle. If a smaller needle is used, the abscess material may be too viscous to pass through it, and a false-negative aspiration could be obtained. If pus is withdrawn through a smaller needle, a larger needle will be needed to allow passage of an 0.038-inch guide wire for subsequent dilatation and drainage (see Fig. 19–21). Once pus is withdrawn from the abscess, the first sample should be sent for culture (before it becomes contaminated). Only a small amount of pus should be removed, and dilatation of the tract and placement of the drainage catheter should be performed before evacuating the cavity. A no. 8.3 French catheter is large enough to adequately drain most abscesses (Gobien et al., 1985). If the material is unusually viscous, larger catheters may be used. Although some authors advocate use of a sump catheter, most interventionalists find the self-retaining no. 10 French Cope catheter to be easy to use and adequate for abscess drainage.

The results of percutaneous abscess drainage have been excellent. Most patients can be cured with a combination of adequate drainage and appropriate antibiotic coverage (Lang, 1990). The underlying cause for the development of the abscess must also be treated. Unusually difficult, multiloculated, or poorly defined abscess cavities may also be drained, but the success rate may be lower. It still may be a useful procedure, however, because it can be used as

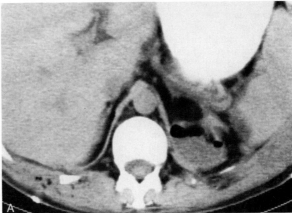

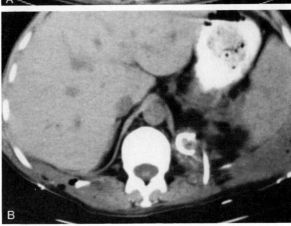

Figure 19–21. Abscess drainage. *A,* A retroperitoneal abscess is seen in the left renal fossa after nephrectomy. *B,* A percutaneous drainage catheter has been placed, and the cavity has been evacuated.

a temporizing measure to improve the patient's medical status and make subsequent surgery safer.

Complications are usually related to sepsis. Manipulation of the abscess cavity is likely to force bacteria into the bloodstream and to create a septicemia. For this reason, preparation of the patient with antibiotics before aspiration is indicated. The antibiotic does not reach the abscess cavity and does not interfere with growth of the bacteria on culture media. To minimize septicemia, the abscess cavity should be evacuated as gently as possible at the initial setting. Once control has been gained and appropriate antibiotic therapy has been instituted, more vigorous lavage can be performed to evacuate the abscess cavity completely.

Although each patient must be treated individually, the success of percutaneous abscess drainage has been excellent, and it has largely replaced surgical treatment. The radiologist must be prepared not only to diagnose the retroperitoneal abscess but also to institute prompt therapy in the form of percutaneous drainage.

ACKNOWLEDGMENT

The efforts of my diligent secretary, Mrs. Beverly R.J. Harris, greatly facilitated the production of this chapter. She cheerfully endured the numerous changes made during its writing and revision.

References

Belville, J.S., Morgentaler, A., Loughlin, K.R., and Tumeh, S.S.: Spontaneous perinephric and subcapsular renal hemorrhage: Evaluation with CT, US, and angiography. Radiology 172:733–738, 1989.

Bosniak, M.A.: Spontaneous subcapsular and perirenal hematomas. Radiology 172:601–602, 1989.

Bosniak, M.A., Megibow, A.J., Hulnick, D.H., et al.: CT diagnosis of renal angiomyolipoma: The importance of detecting small amounts of fat. AJR 151:497–501, 1988.

Bretan, P.N., Jr., McAninch, J.W., Federle, M.P., and Jeffrey, R.B., Jr.: Computerized tomographic staging of renal trauma: 85 consecutive cases. J. Urol. 136:561–565, 1986.

Cass, A.S., and Luxenberg, M.: Features of 164 bladder ruptures. J. Urol. 138:743–745, 1987.

Corriere, J.N., Jr., and Sandler, C.M.: Mechanisms of injury, patterns of extravasation and management of extraperitoneal bladder rupture due to blunt trauma. J. Urol. 139:43–44, 1988.

Degesys, D.E., Dunnick, N.R., Silverman, P.M., et al.: Retroperitoneal fibrosis: Use of CT in distinguishing among possible causes. AJR 146:57–60, 1986.

Dunnick, N.R., Illescas, F.F., Mitchell, S., et al.: Interventional uroradiology. Invest. Radiol. 24:831–841, 1989.

Dunnick, N.R., and Korobkin, M.: Computed tomography of the kidney. Radiol. Clin. North Am. 22:297–313, 1984.

Dunnick, N.R., McCallum, R.W., and Sandler, C.M.: Textbook of Uroradiology. Baltimore, Williams & Wilkins, 1991.

Edell, S.L., and Bonavita, J.A.: The sonographic appearance of acute pyelonephritis. Radiology 132:683–685, 1979.

Federle, M.P., McAninch, J.W., Kaiser, J.A., et al.: Computed tomography of urinary calculi. AJR 136:255–258, 1981.

Gatewood, O.M.B., Fishman, E.K., Burrow, C.R., et al.: Renal vein thrombosis in patients with nephrotic syndrome: CT diagnosis. Radiology 159:117–122, 1986.

Gobien, R.P., Stanley, J.H., Schabel, S.I., et al.: The effect of drainage tube size on adequacy of percutaneous abscess drainage. Cardiovasc. Interven. Radiol. 8:100–102, 1985.

Gold, P.M., McClennan, B.L., and Rottenberg, R.R.: CT appearance of acute inflammatory disease of renal interstitium. AJR 141:343–349, 1983.

Goldman, S.M., Hartman, D.S., Fishman, E.K., et al.: CT of xanthogranulomatous pyelonephritis: Radiologic–pathologic correlation. AJR 141:963–969, 1984.

Hann, L., and Pfister, R.C.: Renal subcapsular rim sign: New etiologies and pathogenesis. AJR 138:51–54, 1982.

Hill, M.C., Rich, J.I., Mardiat, J.G., and Finder, C.A.: Sonography vs. excretory urography in acute flank pain. AJR 144:1235–1238, 1985.

Hilton, S., Bosniak, M.A., Raghavendra, N., et al.: CT findings in acute renal infarction. Urol. Radiol. 6:158–163, 1984.

Hoddick, W., Jeffrey, R.B., Goldberg, H.I., et al.: CT and sonography of severe renal and perirenal infections. AJR 140:517–520, 1983.

Jordan, J., Low, R., and Jeffrey, R.B., Jr.: CT findings in acute renal cortical necrosis. J. Comput. Assist. Tomogr. 14:155–156, 1990.

Kamholtz, R.G., Cronan, J.J., and Dorfman, G.S.: Obstruction and the minimally dilated renal collecting system: US evaluation. Radiology 170:51–53, 1989.

Keating, M.A., and Althausen, A.F.: The clinical spectrum of renal vein thrombosis. J. Urol. 133:938–945, 1985.

Kunin, M.: Bridging septa of the perinephric space: Anatomic, pathologic, and diagnostic considerations. Radiology 158:361–365, 1986.

Lalli, A.F.: Retroperitoneal fibrosis and inapparent obstructive uropathy. Radiology 122:339–342, 1977.

Lang E.K.: Renal, perirenal, and pararenal abscesses: Percutaneous drainage. Radiology 174:109–113, 1990.

Lang, E.K., Sullivan, J., and Frentz, G.: Renal trauma: Radiological studies (Comparison of urography, computed tomography, angiography, and radionuclide studies). Radiology 154:1–6, 1985.

Matalon, T.A.S., and Silver, B.: US guidance of interventional procedures. Radiology 174:43–47, 1990.

McClennan, B.L., Lee, J.K.T., and Peterson, R.R.: Anatomy of the perirenal area. Radiology 158:555–557, 1986.

Morgan, W.R., and Nyberg, L.M., Jr.: Perinephric and intrarenal abscesses. Urology 26:529–536, 1985.

Naidich, J.B., Rackson, M.E., Mossey, R.T., and Stein, H.L.: Nondilated obstructive uropathy: Percutaneous nephrostomy performed to reverse renal failure. Radiology 160:653–657, 1986.

Pfister, R.C.: Percutaneous nephrostomy. In Lang, E.K. (ed.): Percutaneous and Interventional Urology and Radiology. Berlin, Springer-Verlag, 1986.

Ritchie, W.W., Vick, C.W., Glocheski, S.K., and Cooke, D.E.: Evaluation of azotemia patients: Diagnostic yield of initial US examination. Radiology 167:245–247, 1988.

Rosenfield, R.T., Glickman, M.G., Taylor, K.J.W., et al.: Acute focal bacterial nephritis (acute lumbar nephronia). Radiology 132:553–561, 1979.

Sandler, C.M., Harris, J.H., Jr., Corriere, J.N., Jr., and Toombs, B.D.: Posterior urethral injuries after pelvic fracture. AJR 137:1233–1237, 1981.

Sandler, C.M., and Toombs, B.D.: Computed tomographic evaluation of blunt renal injuries. Radiology 141:461–466, 1981.

Silver, T.M., Kass, E.J., Thornbury, J.R., et al.: The radiological spectrum of acute pyelonephritis in adults and adolescents. Radiology 118:65–71, 1976.

Soloman, N., and Sumkin, J.: Right adrenal gland hemorrhage as a complication of liver transplantation: CT appearance. J. Comput. Assist. Tomogr. 12:95–97, 1988.

Tolia, B.M., Iloreta, A., Freed, S.Z., et al.: Xanthogranulomatous pyelonephritis: Detailed analysis of 29 cases and a brief discussion of atypical presentations. J. Urol. 126:437–442, 1981.

ACUTE NEUROLOGIC DISEASE

PART VI

20

Imaging Evaluation of Acute Neurologic Disease

■

Virgil B. Graves
Curtis R. Partington

The initial assessment of the neurologic status of a patient is an essential component of the intensive care unit (ICU) admission. This is often difficult in the comatose or poorly responsive patient and requires close attention to detail. Any abnormal motor function, sensory deficit, cranial nerve dysfunction, or altered state of consciousness that has no known cause should be evaluated with imaging studies. Surprisingly large lesions can cause fairly subtle neurologic abnormalities in the already compromised patient. These lesions must be aggressively searched for, since many are surgically correctable, progressive, or both. Often in comatose patients or those with no localizing signs, the clinical history is the only tool available to guide the examination. The central nervous system (CNS) is unforgiving once it is damaged, so acting quickly to limit the extent of damage is essential. The added hospital cost of a computed tomographic (CT) scan or magnetic resonance imaging (MRI) examination is small when compared to an additional day in the ICU.

The neuroradiologic evaluation of the ICU patient is undergoing considerable change because of the development and greater availability of MRI and transcranial Doppler. MRI is insensitive to acute hemorrhage and fractures, but its superb soft-tissue depiction makes it the imaging modality of choice provided that acute hemorrhages or fractures are not items of concern. MRI requires either a mobile and stable patient or the availability of a mid- or low-field-strength resistive or permanent magnet system that is capable of imaging intubated patients with respirators, infusion pumps, and monitoring equipment present in the scanner room. MRI plays the major role in the evaluation of complications and progressive changes in ICU patients, and CT scanning plays the major role in their initial acute evaluation.

CT provides a much more rapid evaluation of the ICU patient than does MRI. Time outside the ICU for the critically ill patient is an important factor. Because specialized MRI capability for the ICU patient is not widely available, the CT findings are primarily described and MRI correlation is provided where appropriate.

We cannot overemphasize the necessity of clinical localization of the lesion and communication of this information to the radiologist so that the appropriate tailored examination can be performed. If localizing signs are present, detailed examination of the area in question (e.g., spinal cord, brachial plexus) has a much higher yield than global screening techniques. If, however, there are no localizing signs, evaluation of the brain has the highest yield. In the sections that follow we describe the initial radiologic findings in the more commonly encountered conditions and the radiologic findings associated with complications or new conditions likely to be encountered in the ICU setting.

STROKE

Infarction is the most common disease affecting the brain. It can be caused by any condition that compromises the continuous supply of blood to and from a region of the brain. This can be due to arterial thrombosis, embolic occlusion, hypotension, compression of arteries or veins, arterial spasm, or venous outlet obstruction. Stroke can usually be diagnosed accurately on the basis of clinical history and physical findings, but these are often lacking in the ICU patient. The major role of imaging studies in the evaluation of an acute stroke is to distinguish between a bland infarction and a hemorrhagic infarction and

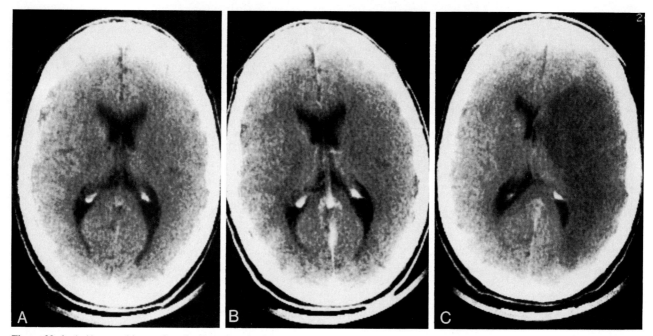

Figure 20–1. A 41-year-old man found unconscious by family members. Noncontrast (*A*) and contrast-enhanced (*B*) CT scans are normal. (*C*) Three days later, a noncontrast CT scan shows a low-density area in the left middle cerebral distribution with mass effect characteristic of a subacute ischemic infarction.

to detect intracerebral hemorrhage that may present clinically as a stroke (Larson et al., 1978).

Noncontrast CT scans are the method of choice for evaluating acute cerebral infarction (Figs. 20–1 and 20–2), because CT is sensitive to small amounts of hemorrhage. Contrast administration can mask areas of low density and may obscure subtle parenchymal hemorrhage. It may even worsen the prognosis of

patients with ischemic cerebral infarcts or intracerebral hemorrhage because of the incomplete blood-brain barrier in the ischemic area and the leakage of neurotoxic contrast into the brain parenchyma (Kendall and Pullicino, 1980). Contrast enhancement is therefore undesirable, although not absolutely contraindicated in the examination of a patient with a suspected stroke. The diagnosis of an acute cerebral

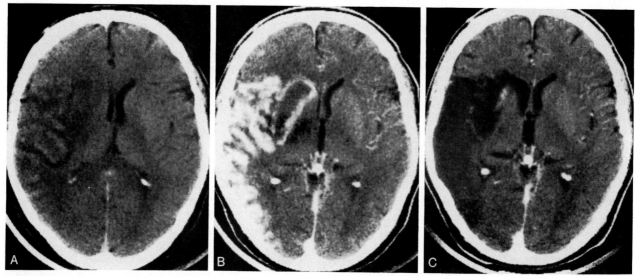

Figure 20–2. A 49-year-old woman with sudden onset of left hemiplegia. *A,* Noncontrast CT scan done 18 hours after the event shows irregular low-density area with mass effect (note loss of sulci and asymmetry of ventricles) involving the right hemisphere. *B,* Contrast-enhanced CT scan done the same time as *A* shows intense enhancement of the cortex and borders of the basal ganglia on the right, typical of a subacute infarct. *C,* Follow-up contrast-enhanced CT scan 4 months later shows the typical evolution of a right middle cerebral artery ischemic infarction, which now has sharply defined borders, negative mass effect, and no significant contrast enhancement.

infarct on CT is difficult during the first 24 hours. In as many as half of cases the initial CT scan is normal and follow-up CT scans are needed to document the location and extent of the ischemic injury (Drayer et al., 1977; Inoue et al., 1980). MRI shows promise in the early detection of stroke, but its sensitivity in detecting acute hemorrhage is limited, so that it has not found a role as a primary screening modality.

The extent of injury to the brain is determined by two main factors: the proximity of the obstruction and the presence of collateral pathways of circulation. The more proximal the arterial obstruction, the less likely that there will be infarction. Twenty-five percent of internal carotid artery occlusions show no clinical symptoms or evidence of infarction. The presence of diminished collateral circulation (hypotension, hypoxia, and incomplete circle of Willis) can result in larger areas of infarction in the arterial distribution of the affected artery, and the presence of collateral circulation (complete circle of Willis, leptomeningeal anastomosis, and external carotid–internal carotid anastomosis) may decrease the extent of infarction (Drayer et al., 1984).

Embolic strokes are generally caused by arterial occlusion from emboli arising from atherosclerotic plaques, the heart, or its valves. The emboli consist of fibrin, platelet aggregates, atheromatous material and, in rare cases, tissue fragments as from an atrial myxoma. The onset of clinical symptoms is usually rapid, and maximal deficit is reached within minutes. Hemorrhage may occur in embolic infarcts (Fig. 20–3) as a result of leptomeningeal collateral circulation or reperfusion as the embolus dissolves, fragments, or moves.

Thrombic stroke is the result of arterial thrombosis in a region of a vessel compromised by atherosclerosis or in a patient with a coagulation abnormality (such as protein C deficiency). Atherosclerotic thrombosis most commonly occurs in the middle cerebral artery (MCA) (50%), the internal carotid artery (ICA) (25%), and the vertebral basilar system (25%).

Thrombic occlusion of the anterior cerebral artery (ACA) is unusual. Thrombic stroke usually has a prolonged onset over hours or days so that aggressive measures to halt its progression (anticoagulation and thrombolysis) are frequently warranted.

Watershed infarcts occur in the border zones between the territories perfused by the ACA, the MCA, and the posterior cerebral artery (PCA) where there are insufficient collateral vessels to maintain perfusion. Infarcts also occur in the putamen, the head of the caudate nucleus, and occipital lobes, because these regions are supplied by distal penetrating arteries that do not form collateral pathways. The infarct generally is the result of some hemodynamic compromise (hypotension, hypoxia, arrhythmia) in conjunction with a compromised flow in the major parent vessel (generally atherosclerotic).

Lacunar infarctions are small (2- to 15-mm) cerebral infarcts usually seen in the basal ganglia, internal capsule, thalamus, and brain stem of older patients with hypertension. They occur most frequently in the distribution of the lenticulostriate, thalamoperforate, and paramedian penetrating arteries, which have a diameter of 50 to 200 μm and have nonbranching distal distributions with little if any collateral supply. The arterial abnormality consists of fibrinoid necrosis, lipohyalinosis, and microatheroma. These infarcts may be precipitated by systemic factors such as hypertension, hypotension, hypoxia, and anemia (Fisher, 1982).

Vasospasm associated with subarachnoid hemorrhage or migraines can produce infarction that is frequently in the distribution of a major arterial branch (Fig. 20–4). (See next section on subarachnoid hemorrhage.) Arterial compression leading to infarction most frequently occurs along the borders of the tentorium and the falx where the major arteries can be compressed and obstructed during times of brain swelling and herniation. This is most frequently seen along the anterior falx (ACA infarct) and the tentorial incisura (PCA infarct).

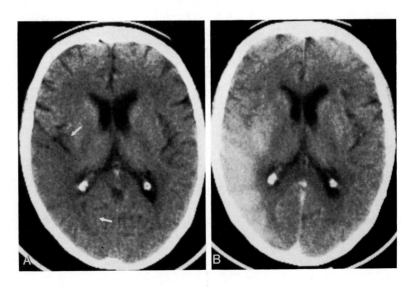

Figure 20–3. A 66-year-old man who presented with left hemiplegia. *A,* Noncontrast CT made at presentation shows a poorly defined lucency (*arrows*) in the posterior right middle cerebral artery distribution, typical of an acute infarct. *B,* Follow-up noncontrast CT scan done 5 days later shows increased density in the distribution of the infarct typical of hemorrhage into an ischemic infarct.

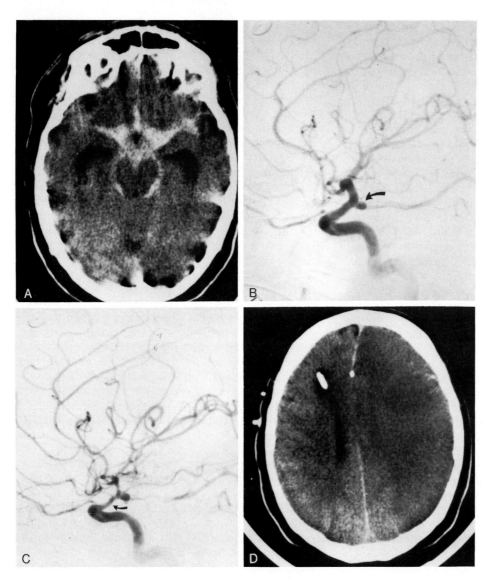

Figure 20–4. A 42-year-old man with sudden onset of severe headache. *A,* Noncontrast CT scan showing blood in the basal cisterns and sylvian fissures and hydrocephalus. *B,* Lateral subtraction film from a left internal carotid arteriogram shows a posterior communicating artery aneurysm (*arrow*) and no evidence of arterial spasm. *C,* Left internal carotid artery arteriogram done 8 days later when the patient's intracranial pressures were markedly elevated shows severe spasm (*arrow*) of the supraclinoid internal carotid artery, middle cerebral artery, and posterior cerebral artery. *D,* Noncontrast CT scan done 1 day after *C* shows a subacute infarct in the left carotid distribution (anterior and middle cerebral distribution) with mass effect. A ventriculoperitoneal shunt catheter is present in the right frontal region.

Venous thrombosis of the superficial cortical veins or the dural sinuses can cause cerebral infarction because of venous outlet obstruction. These infarcts are typically placed symmetrically about the obstructed vein or sinus and frequently have a hemorrhagic component. Predisposing factors include patients with coagulopathies, macroglobulinemia, tumors, sepsis, dehydration, and reatment with certain chemotherapeutic agents such as L-asparaginase.

The CT and MRI appearance of all bland infarcts is essentially the same (see Figs. 20–1 through 20–4 and 20–10), with the only differences being related to their location. The ischemic changes in neurons and glial elements are associated with cytotoxic edema initially and later with vasogenic edema. This condition causes an increase in the water content of the infarcted brain parenchyma and corresponding decreases in the density on CT scans and signal on T1-weighted MRI; signal intensity increases, however, on spin density and T2-weighted MRI. During the initial 6 to 12 hours after infarction, the increase in water content is sufficiently small that there may

be no detectable decrease in density on CT scanning (see Fig. 20–1), but there may be an obvious signal abnormality on MRI. In 1 to 7 days after infarction, tissue liquefaction and proliferation of the microglia begin to occur. Brain edema occurs secondary to blood-brain barrier disruption and leakage of water and large protein molecules into the interstitium of the brain and is maximal during this time. Herniation and compressive effects are most likely to occur during this time (1 to 7 days). Contrast used during this period may cause the low-density infarct to become isodense with brain parenchyma and therefore more difficult to detect. During the subacute period 7 to 21 days after the infarct, the brain edema begins to decrease and there is restoration of the blood-brain barrier in the infarcted zone. Administration of contrast material during this period shows a serpiginous, ribbon-like band of abnormal contrast enhancement following a gyral pattern in the vascular distribution of the infarct (see Fig. 20–2B). This is a result of arterial venous shunting, loss of autoregulation, and residual blood-brain barrier disruption at the border zones of the ischemia, as well as neovascularity in areas of active gliosis (Kawase et al., 1981). The infarct itself on noncontrast CT scans is a sharply defined area of decreased density in an arterial distribution.

Chronic infarcts show complete absence of mass effect and evidence of tissue atrophy with focal ventricular and sulcal enlargement (see Fig. 20–2C). Gliosis, cellular loss, microcystic changes, demyelination, increased extracellular space, and an increase in the local water content are the features of a chronic infarct. This usually produces the characteristic CT image of a low-density region of brain with negative mass effect, no edema, and no contrast enhancement. The characteristics of chronic infarcts on MRI scans are due to the increased water content. This produces low signal intensity regions on T1-weighted images and high signal intensity regions on spin density and T2-weighted images. Acute reinfarction superimposed on or adjacent to areas of chronic infarction is difficult to detect with either CT or MRI. This is because of the marked distortion of the normal anatomy and the extensive space to accommodate the swelling provided by the existing atrophic changes.

Hemorrhagic infarction (see Fig. 20–3) is a distinct entity from spontaneous intracerebral hemorrhage. These disorders have different causes, and they differ in the timing and amount of hemorrhage. Large secondary hemorrhage may complicate a primary ischemic insult in some instances. This is usually the result of the resumption of high-pressure flow into an ischemically damaged vascular bed after the break-up of a large embolus. Most instances of hemorrhage into an infarct are subclinical and petechial in nature. This usually occurs in the first or second week. Such petechial hemorrhages are frequent and may occur in as many as 40% of infarctions if serial CT scans are made. MRI suggests that this may be even more frequent than is suggested by CT images. The paramagnetic effects of blood breakdown products increase the sensitivity of MRI to detect these subclinical hemorrhagic changes (Hecht-Leavitt et al., 1986). The significance of detecting these subclinical hemorrhages is likely nil in terms of therapeutic management (Hornig et al., 1986; Weisberg, 1980).

The complications associated with infarcts are primarily related to their mass effect, either from edema or hemorrhage. This mass effect can lead to secondary infarcts from compression of major arteries and to herniation. The mass effect is often difficult to manage since the edema does not respond to osmotics, so that temporal or frontal lobectomy may be required. Non-CNS complications of infarcts include noncardiogenic pulmonary edema, cardiac arrhythmias, and gastric ulceration.

SUBARACHNOID HEMORRHAGE

The presence of blood in the subarachnoid space is a grave finding that requires a diligent search for its cause. Blood in the cerebrospinal fluid (CSF) is best seen with CT scanning, where acute and subacute bleeding is hyperdense relative to brain and CSF and hyperacute (active) bleeding is isodense with brain parenchyma. Both acute and subacute blood in the subarachnoid space is isointense with the brain parenchyma on MRI and thus difficult to detect. This is due to the high P_{O_2} of CSF, which keeps the hemoglobin in the oxyhemoglobin state for a prolonged period. Small amounts of blood tend to accumulate in dependent locations such as the basal cisterns (Fig. 20–5A; see Fig. 20–4A), the interpeduncular cistern

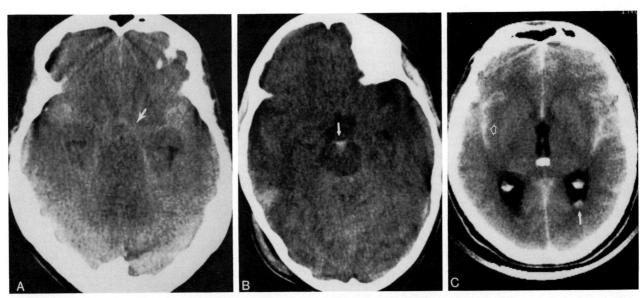

Figure 20–5. Noncontrast CT scans of three different patients who presented with severe headaches caused by subarachnoid hemorrhage. *A,* Obscuring of the basal cisterns (*arrow*) by isodense to slightly hyperdense blood. *B,* Blood in the interpeduncular cistern (*arrow*). *C,* Blood in the sylvian fissures (*open arrow*) and occipital horns (*arrow*) of the lateral ventricles bilaterally. Early hydrocephalus is present in *A* and *C.*

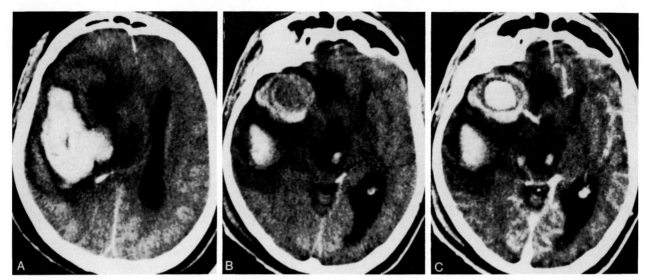

Figure 20–6. A 56-year-old unresponsive man involved in a motor vehicle accident. *A* and *B,* Noncontrast CT scans show a high-density mass with surrounding low-density areas in the right basal ganglia and hemisphere typical of a hematoma. *C,* Contrast-enhanced CT scan shows that the anterior component of this mass enhances intensely in the configuration of a giant aneurysm. The patient had an aneurysmal hemorrhage, which led to the motor vehicle accident.

(see Fig. 20–5*B*), and the occipital horns of the lateral ventricles (see Fig. 20–5*C*) in the supine patient. These areas should be examined for the presence of blood on each CT scan of the head.

There are three primary means for blood to escape the intradural vascular system and enter the subarachnoid space: (1) direct traumatic injury to the arteries or veins as they traverse the subarachnoid space, (2) arterial rupture (ruptured aneurysms), and (3) venous bleeding (bleeding from arteriovenous malformations [AVMs] and dural fistulas). In the case of trauma, the cause of the subarachnoid hemorrhage is often obvious (the presence of skull fractures, and so forth). Pre-existing conditions that have led to the trauma must be kept in mind, however. A patient who is driving an automobile when the aneurysm ruptures and has a subarachnoid hemorrhage will be brought to the emergency department labeled primarily as a motor vehicle accident (Fig. 20–6).

Subarachnoid blood accumulates in locations that reflect its cause (Table 20–1) so that analysis of the distribution of the subarachnoid blood can help to

guide further studies. Angiography is a definitive study for nontraumatic subarachnoid hemorrhage since it accurately defines aneurysms, AVMs, and dural fistulae and helps to guide further treatment planning. The timing for angiography (emergent versus delayed) varies with the local neurosurgical practice, the size of the intracranial hematoma, and the clinical condition of the patient. There is a general trend developing in which patients with subarachnoid hemorrhages are managed medically until routine working hours when first-case angiography can be done more safely and urgent surgery can be completed by the rested neurosurgical team.

A small percentage of patients with subarachnoid hemorrhage have normal arteriograms at the time of presentation. This is due to localized vasospasm, hematoma obscuring the aneurysm, or to other unsuspected sources of bleeding (e.g., spinal AVM or dural arteriovenous fistula when only internal carotid arteriograms were done as the initial angiography procedure). In this circumstance, repeat angiography in 10 to 14 days frequently shows the aneurysm. If

Table 20–1. SUBARACHNOID BLOOD ACCUMULATION LOCATIONS

Blood	Localization
Interhemispheric fissure, cistern of the lamina terminalis, lateral ventricle with little in the third or fourth ventricle, ± parenchymal hematoma in frontal lobe or septum pellucidum	Anterior communicating aneurysm
Basal cisterns, ± temporal horn of lateral ventricles ± parenchymal hematoma in basal ganglia and medial temporal lobe	Posterior communicating aneurysm
Sylvian fissure and basal cisterns, ± hematoma in temporal lobe	Middle cerebral aneurysm
Basal cisterns, interpeduncular cistern, third ventricle, parenchyma of the midbrain	Basilar tip aneurysm
Basal cisterns, fourth ventricle, ± cerebellar hemispheric hematoma	Posterior inferior cerebellar artery aneurysm
Overlying convexities, ± lobar hematoma	Mycotic aneurysm
	Amphetamine- or cocaine-related aneurysm
Basal cisterns, posterior fossa	Spinal arteriovenous malformation, dural fistula

repeated angiography is normal, a complete myelogram is warranted to search for abnormal vessels in the thecal sac. A normal MRI scan of the spine does not rule out a spinal AVM or arteriovenous fistula (AVF). If this is the case, a spinal arteriogram is necessary to define the abnormal spinal AVM or AVF. A small percentage of patients have subarachnoid hemorrhages with no known cause despite extensive and thorough evaluation. These patients appear to be at no increased risk for repeated hemorrhage and suffer only the ill effects of the initial event and its complications.

There are three major cerebral complications of subarachnoid hemorrhage: (1) herniation from the mass effect of the hematoma, (2) the development of hydrocephalus (see Figs. 20–4A and 20–5A and C), and (3) vasospasm leading to infarction (see Fig. 20–4). Hydrocephalus occurs because of obstruction of the arachnoid granulations, basilar cisterns, or the aqueduct of Sylvius by clot and red blood cells in the acute period and subsequently to adhesive arachnoiditis, which may occur weeks or even years after the subarachnoid hemorrhage. Shunting of the ventricular system with a ventricular peritoneal shunt is frequently required.

Vasospasm is a lethal complication of subarachnoid hemorrhage that is initiated by the presence of red blood cell breakdown products in the CSF surrounding the vessel. It may occur at any time from 6 hours to 3 weeks after subarachnoid hemorrhage and has a peak incidence between 7 and 10 days after the acute event. It frequently leads to large-vessel ischemic infarctions. Serial monitoring of the blood flow in the major intracranial vessels with transcranial Doppler examinations shows promise in evaluating the degree of spasm in guiding medical and interventional (balloon dilatation) therapy.

The non-CNS complications of subarachnoid hemorrhage are pulmonary edema, cardiac arrhythmias, and gastrointestinal bleeding. These three events occur independently in as many as 70% of patients with subarachnoid hemorrhages and contribute to the mortality and difficulty in management of these patients. The cause of each of these appears to be through centrally mediated independent mechanisms. Pulmonary edema is noncardiogenic in nature and is not associated with radiographic or cardiac indices of congestive heart failure.

PARENCHYMAL HEMORRHAGE

Bleeding into the brain substance is the third most frequent cause of stroke. Most of these are due to hypertensive rupture of Charcot-Bouchard false aneurysms in the perforating arteries of the basal ganglia (Fig. 20–7), thalamus, pons, and subcortical white matter. There are many other causes of parenchymal hemorrhage, however, including trauma, ruptured aneurysm, (see Fig. 20–6) or AVM, arterial amyloidosis, and hemorrhage into tumors or areas of ische-

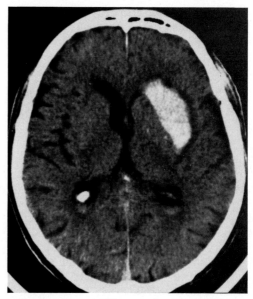

Figure 20–7. Noncontrast CT scan of a 77-year-old man found unresponsive with a blood pressure of 220/170. High-density mass in the left putamen with a surrounding low-density rim typical of a basal ganglia hematoma with surrounding edema.

mic infarction. Some parenchymal hemorrhages remain idiopathic despite exhaustive evaluation. Patients with bleeding diatheses, those taking anticoagulants, and those with markedly elevated blood pressures are at particular risk for bleeding from any of these causes (Dolinskas et al., 1977; Weisberg, 1979).

CT reliably demonstrates acute intracerebral hemorrhage as a sharply marginated area of increased density (35 to 80 HU) with a surrounding rim of low density that represents edema in the adjacent brain substance. One week after the bleed, the hematoma shows some decrease in mass effect and a decrease in its density. A thin rim of contrast enhancement may also be present. After 3 weeks the hematoma becomes isodense with adjacent brain substance, but it still has a prominent area of low density adjacent to it from edema and a contrast enhancing rim. With time the hematoma itself is resorbed, leaving only a low-density cavity in the brain substance that is considerably smaller than the original hematoma. There is no significant contrast enhancement of these chronic hematoma cavities. During the interval of 1 to 3 weeks after a hemorrhage, it may be difficult to distinguish a hematoma from a brain abscess because of the rim enhancement.

Because of the paramagnetic properties of the breakdown products of blood, MRI can accurately diagnose parenchymal hemorrhage. A hyperacute hematoma (oxyhemoglobin) has a nonspecific appearance (Cohen et al., 1986; Dooms et al., 1986) with a signal that is isointense to gray matter on T1-weighted images and hyperintense on T2-weighted images. With the conversion of oxyhemoglobin to intracellular deoxyhemoglobin and intracellular methemoglobin, the hematoma becomes low signal intensity on the T2-weighted images and remains isointense to slightly hyperintense on T1-weighted images. At the subacute stage (about 7 days after hemorrhage) hemolysis begins, and the extracellular methemoglobin released into the hematoma cavity results in a marked hyperintensity on both T1- and T2-weighted images. As the hematoma evolves, the hematoma cavity becomes encircled with hemosiderin-laden macrophages, which produces a striking rim of decreased signal intensity on both T1- and T2-weighted images that is directly proportional to the field strength of the instrument and the extent of T2 and T2* weighting. This hypointensity may remain for years after a hemorrhage (Gomori et al., 1986). The hypointense rim should be examined in each suspected hematoma, because a complete rim around a hematoma is a good indicator of its benign cause, and any disruption of this rim raises the possibility of an underlying neoplasm (Atlas et al., 1987).

The location of a hematoma frequently provides a clue to its cause. Most hemorrhages into the basal ganglia, thalamus, and brain stem have hypertensive causes. These frequently extend into the ventricles but only rarely into the subarachnoid space. Hematomas associated with an enhancing mass are generally secondary to bleeding from a ruptured AVM, aneurysm (including giant aneurysms), or tumor (most frequently glioblastoma or metastatic melanoma, renal cell carcinoma, choriocarcinoma, or bronchogenic carcinoma). Lobar hemorrhages are usually secondary to hypertension, amyloid angiopathy, mycotic aneurysms, or hemorrhage into an infarct.

Complications associated with parenchymal hemorrhage are primarily acute in nature and related to the mass effect of the hematoma and the surrounding edema. Hemorrhages that extend into the ventricles may cause hydrocephalus through the same mechanisms as subarachnoid hemorrhage. The scarring associated with the hematoma cavity may serve as a focus for seizures. Non-CNS complications associated with parenchymal hemorrhage are centrally mediated gastric ulceration and hemorrhage and noncardiogenic pulmonary edema.

The mortality associated with a parenchymal brain hemorrhage is 30% to 35%, but patients who survive often have surprisingly small neurologic deficits. The parenchymal hematoma appears to expand and displace the brain substance rather than destroying it. The management of the elevated intracranial pressure and mass effect is essential for preservation of brain substance and function.

INFECTION

Infectious processes that affect the CNS are a continuing problem in the ICU and are increasing in their frequency with the increasing population of immunocompromised patients. Bacteria and fungi gain entry to the nervous system and its coverings either by means of direct inoculation (e.g., trauma, surgery, lumbar puncture) spread from an adjacent site of infection (e.g., sinusitis, mastoiditis, osteomyelitis) or through hematogenous seeding to produce meningitis, ventriculitis, epidural abscess, subdural empyema, and brain abscess.

Epidural abscesses occur most frequently as a result of traumatic inoculation associated with a skull fracture, but they may occur through direct spread from an adjacent sinusitis or osteomyelitis. On CT and MRI they appear as biconvex lenticular extra-axial fluid collections with a limiting membrane toward the brain parenchyma, which enhances intensely with intravenous contrast material (Sharif and Ibrahim, 1982). In the spine they frequently extend over many segments as a result of the less tight application of the dura to the vertebral bodies. Subdural empyema and subdural abscess are localized infectious collections in the subdural extra-arachnoid space. They occur most frequently after surgery or trauma. Their spontaneous origin is almost exclusively secondary to spread from frontal sinusitis in adults or from bacterial seeding of subdural effusions associated with *Haemophilus influenzae* meningitis in children. On CT and MRI they appear as fluid collections that follow the contours of the brain and skull with adjacent parenchymal low densities from adjacent brain edema (high signal intensity on T2-weighted MRI) with intensely enhancing overlying membranes (Davidson and Steiner, 1985; Moseley and Kendall, 1984). The complications and morbidity associated with epidural abscess, subdural empyema, and subdural abscess are related to the mass effect of the abscess itself and to the mass effect induced by adjacent edema causing herniation and cord compression as well as to their contributing to the continuing episodes of sepsis. They may spread to the adjacent venous structures to produce septic phlebitis and venous infarctions.

Meningitis and ventriculitis are infections of the meninges and ventricular linings. Imaging generally plays only a secondary role in the presence of meningitis in that it allows the clinician to rule out intracranial mass lesions or signs of elevated intracranial pressure that may prohibit performing a lumbar puncture, the diagnostic test of choice. The contrast-enhanced CT scan may show marked contrast enhancement of the meninges that are affected by meningitis, but the absence of this enhancement does not rule out meningitis. Diagnostic imaging is important in the evaluation of complications from meningitis, however (Fig. 20–8). The primary complications of meningitis are (1) arterial spasm leading to focal areas of ischemia and infarction, (2) development of septic phlebitis leading to venous infarctions, (3) hydrocephalus from adhesive arachnoiditis, and (4) abscess formation.

Brain abscess may arise from direct spread from an adjacent area of infection or through hematogenous seeding. Patients with right to left vascular

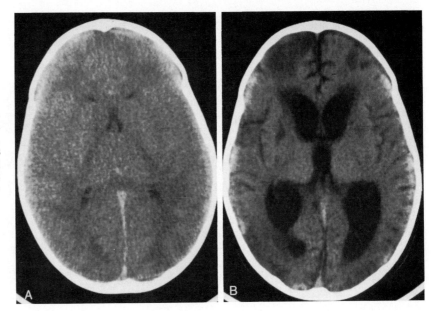

Figure 20–8. A 2-year-old boy with *Haemophilus influenzae* meningitis. *A,* Contrast-enhanced CT scan at presentation is normal. *B,* Four weeks later a noncontrast CT scan shows marked enlargement of the ventricles and sulci as well as wedge-shaped low-density regions typical of cortical infarction secondary to vasospasm.

shunts from congenital heart disease or pulmonary AVMs are at increased risk for formation of brain abscesses as a result of the lack of the normal filtering function of the lungs. Patients who are immunosuppressed or who have decreased immune function are also at increased risk. Brain abscesses that are hematogenous in origin have their epicenter at the gray-white junction. They occur in a distribution directly related to the blood volume (increased incidence in the middle cerebral artery distribution and decreased incidence in the brain stem and spinal cord). The formation and development of brain abscesses have been elucidated by Britt and Enzmann (1983), who found four stages in their development: (1) early cerebritis occurring 1 to 3 days after inoculation characterized by a poorly defined focus of contrast enhancement with surrounding low-density brain edema; (2) late cerebritis occurring 4 to 6 days after inoculation characterized by intense homogeneous contrast enhancement surrounded by low density from brain edema; (3) early abscess formation occurring 10 to 13 days after inoculation characterized by a poorly defined rim of contrast enhancement with a low-density, nonenhancing center representing early abscess cavity and surrounding low density from edema; and (4) mature abscess formation occurring more than 14 days after inoculation characterized by a well-defined rim of contrast enhancement with a low-density center representing the true abscess cavity and a surrounding low-density area representing edema in the brain parenchyma (Figs. 20–9 and 20–10).

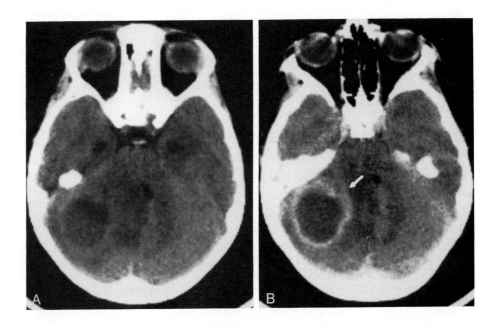

Figure 20–9. A 4-year-old girl with a history of urinary tract infection presented with headaches and a staggering gait. *A,* Noncontrast CT scan shows a round low-density mass in the right cerebellar hemisphere with displacement of the fourth ventricle. *B,* Contrast-enhanced CT scan shows ring enhancement of this mass with a thicker rim of enhancement (*arrow*) toward the ventricle typical of a mature brain abscess.

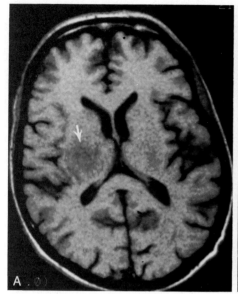
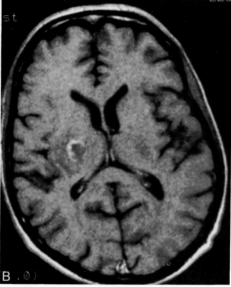

Figure 20–10. A 32-year-old HIV-positive man with headaches. *A,* Axial T1-weighted (TR = 600, TE = 20) MRI scan shows a poorly defined low-signal-intensity mass (*arrow*) in the right basal ganglia. *B,* An identical image done after intravenous contrast shows ring enhancement of the center of this mass typical of CNS toxoplasmosis.

TRAUMA

Head trauma is the most common cause of death in people less than 45 years of age and is the third leading cause of death in the general population. Patients with severe head injury frequently have additional injuries to the face, chest, abdomen, pelvis, and extremities (Baker et al., 1980; Barkay and Glasauer, 1980). The recent advances in emergency medicine and acute resuscitation have allowed many of these patients to survive the initial insult. Their subsequent management in the ICU requires recognition of the extent of the initial injuries, prognosis, and the potential for delayed complications.

In patients with acute head injuries, the abnormalities can be divided into the following categories:

Extra-axial injury
  1. Subdural hematoma
  2. Epidural hematoma
  3. Subarachnoid hemorrhage
Intra-axial injury
  1. Diffuse axonal injury (sheer injury)
  2. Cortical contusion
  3. Intracerebral hematoma
  4. Subcortical gray matter injuries
  5. Primary brain stem injuries
Secondary injuries
  1. Herniation syndromes
  2. Hydrocephalus
  3. Duret's midbrain hemorrhage
  4. Vascular injuries and CSF leaks

In patients with acute head trauma (less than 72 hours since injury), CT is the imaging study of choice, even though MRI has been shown to be more sensitive in the detection of intracranial injuries. CT is more widely available, can be easily performed with unstable patients on multiple monitors, and has a high sensitivity for acute hemorrhage, fractures, and blood collections, which may be less well visualized on MRI (French and Dublin, 1977; Kelly et al., 1988).

MRI should be the primary imaging technique used in evaluating head injury patients in the subacute (3 to 10 days), chronic (11 to 30 days), and remote (more than 30 days) stages after head injury. At these periods, MRI is more sensitive and demonstrates the extent and complexity of the injury better than CT. Secondary injuries, complications of the initial event, and superimposed nonrelated events are also better depicted with MRI (Gentry et al., 1988a, 1988b; Zimmerman et al., 1986).

EXTRA-AXIAL HEMORRHAGE

Subdural hematomas occur most commonly as a result of movement of the brain within the cranial vault with tearing of the subdural veins that pass between the cerebral cortex and the dural sinuses (Strich, 1976). Subdural hematoma may occur after the relief of the tamponading effect after surgical evacuation of an intracerebral hematoma, or an intracerebral hematoma may develop after the evacuation of a subdural hematoma (Davis et al., 1976). This results in bleeding into the subdural extra-arachnoid space so that the inner border of a subdural hematoma is defined by the arachnoid membrane and the outer border by the dura, which is closely applied to the inner skull table. Subdural hematomas are crescentic; have smooth, well-defined margins; and conform to the inner table of the skull. They may extend along the falx and tentorium to produce interhemispheric and tentorial subdural hematomas. The density of subdural hematomas on CT scanning is related to the hemoglobin concentration, clot retraction, and their age (Bergstrom et al., 1977). Clot retraction removes the lower-density serum and concentrates the higher-density proteins and red blood cells, resulting in a high-density (40- to 90-HU) lesion. Acute (0 to 3 days) subdural hematomas are hyperdense on CT (Fig. 20–11A), but patients with coagulopathies, those taking anticoagulants, and those with hemoglobin levels of less than 10 g/dl may develop isodense or even hypodense acute subdural hematomas. Hyperacute blood (active bleeding) is isodense with brain parenchyma so that the area of mixed density within a hyperdense subdural hematoma suggests active bleeding.

The subdural hematoma begins to decrease in density from day 3 to 13 as the blood elements in the clot are broken down. At some point (usually 7 to 13 days, depending on the size of the subdural hematoma), the subdural hematoma becomes isointense with normal brain matter (25 to 40 HU) and may be difficult to detect (see Fig. 11B). This is particularly true when the subdural hematoma is bilateral so that the asymmetries of mass effect become balanced.

Chronic (14 to 30 days) and remote (more than 30 days) subdural hematomas have completed the degradation of blood products and have low density (15 to 30 HU) on CT (Fig. 20–12; see Fig. 20–11C). At this time differentiation from a hygroma (CSF leak through a ball valve tear in the arachnoid membrane into the subdural extra-arachnoid space) may be impossible without MRI or the administration of intravenous contrast material. The membrane surrounding a subdural hematoma is vascular and shows intense contrast enhancement on both CT (see Fig. 20–11D) and MRI, whereas hygromas have no enhancing membrane. The paramagnetic characteristics of subdural hematoma follow closely those previously described for parenchymal hematomas so that their characterization on MRI is relatively straightforward (Fig. 20–13).

The secondary effects and complications of subdural hematomas are primarily related to their mass effect on the adjacent brain. These effects are a

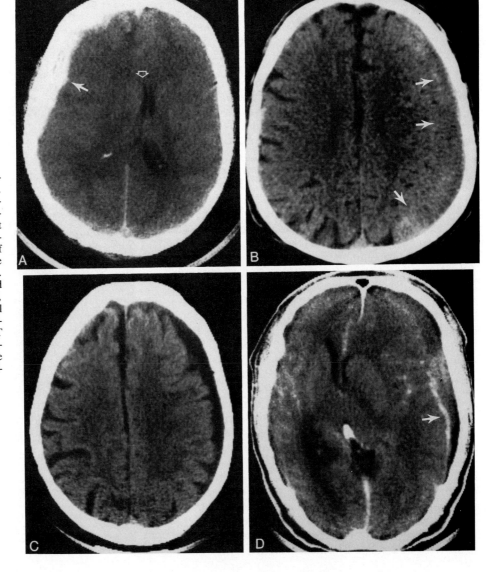

Figure 20–11. Four different patients with subdural hematomas. *A,* Acute, hyperdense mass overlying the right frontal region (*arrow*) with considerable mass effect displacing the right lateral ventricle (*open arrow*) to the left of midline. *B,* Subacute, isodense left subdural hematoma (*arrows*). Note loss of cortical markings and sulci over left convexity. *C,* Chronic, low-density left subdural hematoma, with a mild mass effect. *D,* Contrast-enhanced CT scan of a chronic subdural hematoma showing enhancement of the membranes (*arrow*) and mass effect.

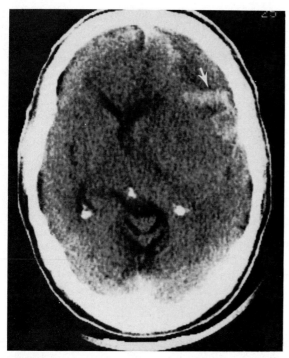

Figure 20–12. Axial noncontrast CT scan showing a low-density extra-axial collection over the left hemisphere with patches of high density within it (*arrow*) indicating rebleeding into a chronic subdural hematoma.

function of the amount of space available for the hematoma, its size, and its location. When located in the posterior fossa or over the convexities in a young person, a relatively small subdural hematoma may have considerable deleterious effect, whereas a large subdural hematoma may be well tolerated in a patient with underlying atrophy and enlarged CSF spaces.

Epidural hematomas occur as a result of bleeding into the potential space between the inner table of the skull and the dura. They are usually the result of a skull fracture that tears a branch of the middle meningeal artery, but they may occur as a result of venous bleeding from the diploic space or a lacerated dural sinus. Skull fractures are present in 80% of adults and 40% of children with epidural hematomas. An arterial epidural hematoma develops rapidly as the high-pressure arterial bleeding strips the dura from the inner skull table, but a venous epidural hematoma may be insidious in onset, increasing in size over hours or days. Epidural hematomas have a characteristic biconvex/lenticular shape (Fig. 20–14) and abut the inner skull table. Their density on CT scanning and appearance on MRI are identical to those described for subdural hematomas, but chronic epidural hematomas are rarely encountered since most are immediately surgically evacuated. MRI has limited usefulness in evaluating epidural hematomas except in cases that involve the dural sinuses and skull base, in which the sagittal and coronal capabilities of MRI have considerable advantage over CT.

The secondary effects and complications of epidural hematomas are related to their mass effect and loca-tion (identical to those described for subdural hema-tomas), associated injuries (fractures, subdural he-matoma, contusions), and their propensity for rapid expansion. Epidural hematomas nearly always re-quire immediate surgical evacuation.

Post-traumatic subarachnoid hemorrhage results from tearing of the veins or arteries as they traverse the subarachnoid space. It is frequently associated with subdural hematoma, epidural hematoma, and brain contusions. Post-traumatic subarachnoid hem-orrhage is rarely of as large a volume as subarachnoid hemorrhage from other causes, but the delayed com-plications of blood in the subarachnoid space (hydro-cephalus, vasospasm) are the same, regardless of the source.

INTRA-AXIAL INJURY

Shear injuries (diffuse axonal injuries) are the most frequent traumatic injury to the brain (Gentry et al., 1988; Kelly et al, 1988). The brain lacks rigidity, and there is a differential in the density of gray matter relative to white matter. Axonal stretching, separa-tion, and disruption of nerve and vascular tracks may occur secondary to the differential movements of the

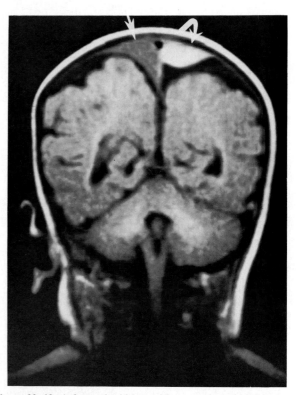

Figure 20–13. A 3-month-old boy with a question of birth trauma and developmental delay. Coronal T1-weighted (TR = 600, TE = 20) MRI scan shows bilateral extra-axial fluid collections. The collection on the right has low signal intensity (*arrow*) of an acute subdural hematoma, whereas the left collection (*curved arrow*) has high signal intensity of a more remote subdural hematoma. There is enlargement of the cortical sulci and ventricles indicating a chronic change. This constellation raises the possibility of child abuse with multiple episodes of injury.

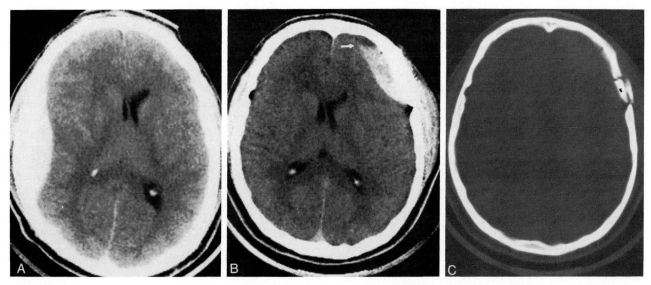

Figure 20–14. An 18-year-old man who lost consciousness after being struck by a baseball. *A,* Noncontrast CT scan shows a high-density extra-axial mass with a biconvex shape typical of an epidural hematoma. Note the mass effect with shift of the right lateral ventricle to the left of midline. *B* and *C,* A 27-year-old man was unconscious after a motor vehicle accident. Noncontrast CT scan shows a biconvex high-density extra-axial mass with a sedimentation level (*arrow*) ("hematocrit level") within it typical of an epidural hematoma. *C,* Bone windows demonstrate the comminuted skull fracture crossing the course of the middle meningeal artery.

hemispheres relative to one another and the gray matter relative to the white matter when the brain is subjected to rotation and acceleration-deceleration forces (Holbourn, 1943, 1945). These lesions are rarely seen on CT unless hemorrhagic, but on MRI they appear as multiple 5- to 15-mm diameter areas of increased signal intensity on T2-weighted images. They are found most frequently at the gray-white junction, the corpus callosum, and the corona radiata.

They may be hemorrhagic, in which case they are visible on CT as areas of high density located at the gray-white junction (Fig. 20–15*A*), and on MRI they have the characteristics of small parenchymal hematomas. Their distribution is 50% at the gray-white junction (most frequently frontal and temporal lobe), 30% at the corona radiata and internal capsule, and 20% in the corpus callosum.

Shear injuries are an indicator of severe brain

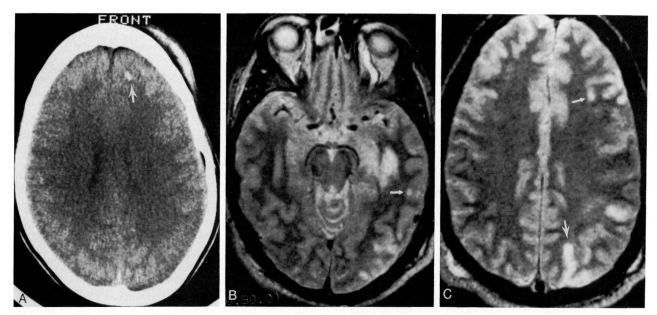

Figure 20–15. An 18-year-old man unresponsive after a motor vehicle accident. Noncontrast CT scan (*A*) shows focal tiny hemorrhages at the gray-white junction (*arrow*) and diffuse loss of cortical sulci associated with diffuse brain swelling. (*B* and *C*), T2-weighted (TR = 2000, TE = 80) MRI scan in a different patient shows multiple areas of increased signal in the cortex and at the gray-white junction (*arrows*) characteristic of cortical contusions and shear injuries.

injury and a relatively poor prognosis. They are acutely and subacutely associated with diffuse or focal brain swelling (see Fig. 20–15B and C), mass effect, and herniation, and they evolve into focal or generalized regions of brain atrophy.

Cortical contusions are the second most frequent brain injury. They are the result of direct impact forces causing deformation of the skull and brain at the impact site and are frequently found contralateral to the impact site (coup-contrecoup injuries). Cortical contusions are multiple, often hemorrhagic, and involve the cortical gray matter with relatively less involvement of the underlying white matter. Those that arise remote from the site of impact are generally located along the surfaces of the frontal and temporal lobes where the brain is damaged as it slides along the bony surfaces of the anterior and middle cranial fossa. As many as half of cortical contusions are not detected by CT; when seen, they appear as ill-defined areas of mixed high and low signal intensity located in the cerebral cortex. This mixed density reflects the varying amounts of edema and hemorrhage as well as the stage of breakdown of hemoglobin at the injury site. On MRI (see Fig. 20–15B and C) these injuries have the mixed signal intensity of brain edema (high signal intensity on T2-weighted images) and parenchymal hemorrhage.

Cortical contusions are frequently associated with subarachnoid hemorrhage. They are acutely and subacutely associated with focal and diffuse brain swelling and herniation and may evolve into areas of brain atrophy. Delayed or acute hydrocephalus may occur because of the subarachnoid blood.

Intracerebral hematomas in head trauma may be thought of as cortical contusions in which a large blood vessel has been damaged and results in a significant accumulation of blood within the brain substance. They are usually more irregular in shape than spontaneous parenchymal hematomas (as described earlier), but they have the same imaging characteristics, evolution, and complications.

Subcortical gray matter injuries and primary brain stem injuries are best detected by MRI. They are rarely seen with CT scanning. They represent a variety of shear injury located in the subcortical gray matter and the dorsal lateral pons, respectively. They have the imaging characteristics of shear injuries and are indicators of serious brain injury and a poor prognosis for recovery. Secondary injuries of the brain occur and can be difficult to differentiate from primary traumatic brain injury. Several rather characteristic secondary injuries are frequently detected.

SECONDARY INJURIES

The skull is a rigid structure that contains two relatively immobile septations (the falx and the tentorium) and a single outlet (the foramen magnum). The brain is soft and is susceptible to compressive injury when either symmetric (as in hydrocephalus or diffuse brain edema) or asymmetric (edema and swelling associated with infarcts, contusions, focal masses, or hematomas) shifts in the mass of the intracranial contents occur. These injuries occur at characteristic locations where the brain and its vessels are easily compressed. The cingulate and parahippocampal gyri are susceptible to pressure necrosis from compression against the tentorium and free edge of the falx. The anterior cerebral arteries may be obstructed by herniation of the frontal lobes across midline below the falx, and the posterior cerebral artery may be obstructed by herniation of the medial temporal lobe through the tentorial incisura. Herniation of the medulla and cerebellar tonsils through the foramen magnum may compromise blood supply to the brain stem and the posterior fossa. Each of these events begins a vicious cycle in which the mass effect causes infarction, which causes more severe mass effect, worsening the herniation and extending the infarction.

The signs of increased intracranial pressure must be searched for on each CT and MRI scan of the brain so that aggressive measures may be taken to avoid herniation and the associated damage to the brain. The primary signs of increased intracranial pressure are (1) effacement of the cortical sulci, (2) small slit-like ventricles in cerebral swelling, (3) large ventricles in hydrocephalus, (4) shift of intracranial structures from their normal location, and (5) abnormally small suprasellar, prepontine, and basal cisterns. These signs are indicators of increased intracranial pressure and impending herniation, but their absence does not indicate a normal pressure. A patient with a normal CT scan may have a markedly elevated pressure so that other clinical findings (e.g., papilledema) must be taken into account. Based only on imaging studies, it is not possible to conclusively state that intracranial pressure is not elevated.

In each case in which there is radiographic or clinical evidence of elevated intracranial pressure, a detailed examination of the scan is required to attempt to identify a cause. In cases of hydrocephalus the lateral third and fourth ventricles must be examined for any asymmetries that may suggest a cause. The fourth ventricle is in a confined space so that it shows smaller changes than the other components of the ventricular system, but these changes may give an important clue to the cause of the hydrocephalus (i.e., posterior fossa mass or cerebellar infarct causing compression of the fourth ventricle). A single lateral ventricle may become trapped if its outlet (foramen of Monroe) is obstructed by unilateral mass effect in herniation while its choroid plexus continues to produce CSF. This produces worsening mass effect, herniation, and pressure necrosis.

The imaging signs of herniation are (1) obliteration of the basal cisterns, (2) obliteration of the suprasellar cistern, (3) distortion of the uncus and brain stem, and (4) extension of the cerebellum and midbrain into the foramen magnum. These ominous signs indicate compression of the vessels at the base of the brain that will lead to irreversible damage and death if not corrected immediately. Aggressive treatment with osmotics, emergent shunting, and hyperventilation is essential. Associated injuries include ventral midline and pons hemorrhages (Duret's hemorrhages), which occur secondary to anoxia and compression of the paramedian arteries and veins. These hemorrhages are frequently too small to be detected on CT but may be detected on MRI. They are associated with a high mortality.

VASCULAR INJURIES AND CSF LEAKS

The major vessels are relatively immobile at their entrance into the skull base and are thus more susceptible to injury at these points. Fractures through the skull base frequently cross the carotid canals and lacerate the petrous and cavernous carotid arteries. This may lead to carotid occlusion, massive hemorrhage, pseudoaneurysm formation, or development of a carotid cavernous fistula.

Massive hemorrhage is frequently fatal, but in some instances the blood may be contained within the cranial vault. If the rent in the carotid artery remains patent, a pseudoaneurysm may form. Pseudoaneurysms such as this consist of a contained collection of blood in communication with the carotid artery. They frequently have multiple areas of laminated thrombus lining their walls but not true arterial wall elements. They cause symptoms by repeated bleeding and mass effect. They may expand slowly over many years, producing bony remodeling at the skull base. The imaging signs of a post-traumatic pseudoaneurysm are those of a mass in the paracavernous region that has a central enhancing component that shows contrast enhancement identical to that of the carotid artery. On MRI, the patent lumen may be identified, and the multiple layers of laminated thrombus in the walls have a characteristic alternating bright and dark appearance. These are usually discovered only later in the patient's course. The initial signs are those of a soft-tissue mass in the skull base and an associated fracture lying crossing the carotid canal.

Carotid occlusions may be asymptomatic in patients with good collateral circulation, but they may cause massive infarction, particularly if associated with significant hypotension. On CT, the only hint of a carotid occlusion is frequently a fracture line crossing the carotid canal, although the occluded carotid artery will not enhance with intravenous contrast material. On MRI, there is an absence of the characteristic flow void in the occluded carotid whose lumen is filled with clot.

Carotid cavernous fistulae frequently are discovered some days after the trauma when the patient has progressive proptosis, vascular congestion of the eyes (one or both), bruits, and headache. They result from laceration of the carotid artery in its intracavernous segment, where brisk arterial bleeding occurs into the confines of the cavernous sinus. Venous outlets of the cavernous sinus (superior ophthalmic vein, petrosal sinuses, intracavernous sinuses) become engorged by the excessive arterial flow and distend as a result of venous hypertension. Carotid cavernous fistulas cause glaucoma and blindness, compression of the chiasm and optic nerves by the massively dilated venous sinuses, and venous hypertension of the brain parenchyma, which may lead to seizures or venous infarction. The imaging signs of carotid cavernous fistulae on both CT and MRI rely on visualization of the dilated cavernous sinus, superior ophthalmic vein, and petrosal sinuses. Proptosis of the affected eye may be identified, but there is rarely an associated abnormality of the brain itself.

Chronic CSF leaks occur after laceration of the dura by a fracture fragment. These occur most frequently in the temporal bone (producing CSF otorrhea) and in the cribriform plate (producing CSF rhinorrhea). Clinically, patients have a clear drainage from the nose or ears that is frequently position-dependent. Imaging shows only the fracture and an adjacent fluid-filled middle ear and mastoid air cells or paranasal sinus. Contrast installation in the subarachnoid space followed by CT scanning in the position of most active drainage is necessary to identify absolutely the site of leakage and to aid in surgical repair. The primary complications of CSF leaks are caused by repeated bacterial seeding and meningitis.

SPINE

Traumatic injury to spinal axis is often associated with head trauma. Most traumatic injuries to the spinal axis are the result of fractures and subluxations of the vertebral bodies that cause compromise of the spinal canal and compression of the spinal cord and nerve roots. Plain radiographs should be used to initially evaluate the patient with spine trauma since they accurately depict bony alignment and fractures that will direct a more specific CT or MRI examination. In unusual cases (e.g., obese patients, presence of metallic fixation devices), CT may be required to accurately depict the bony spinal axis. Both CT and MRI provide excellent ways to evaluate the spine. CT offers the advantage of accurately depicting the bony anatomy (e.g., fractures, bony alignment, displaced fragments), but it has the disadvantage of being unable to evaluate the spinal cord. MRI has the advantage of evaluating injury to the cord itself (Figs. 20–16 and 20–17), although small bone fragments may not be detected on MRI evaluation. MRI does have the advantage of determining the cause of the injury to the cord in that it can differentiate between hematoma, edema in the spinal cord, traumatic disc herniation, and canal compromise by subluxations and bone fragments. The use of MRI, however, requires the use of non-ferromagnetic traction and immobilization devices.

Patients often present to the acute care unit with nontraumatic spine and spinal cord symptoms. These are due most often to osseous lesions and to acute

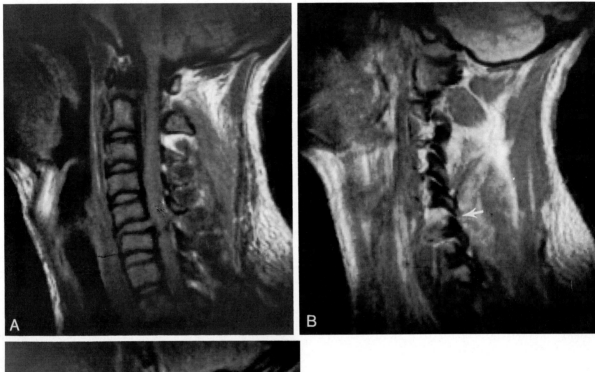

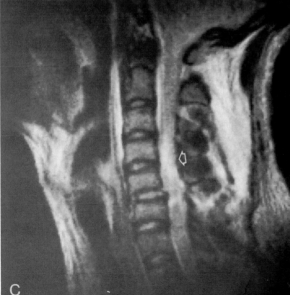

Figure 20–16. A 24-year-old woman quadriplegic after a motor vehicle accident. *A* and *B,* Sagittal T1-weighted (TR = 600, TE = 20) MRI scan shows the malalignment of C5 on C6, (*arrow in B*) and shows the disrupted C5, C6 facets. *C,* T2-weighted (TR = 2000, TE = 80 msec) MRI scan shows extensive signal abnormality (*arrow*) in the cervical spinal cord extending from C4 to C6 characteristic of edema and acute hemorrhage in the cord substance.

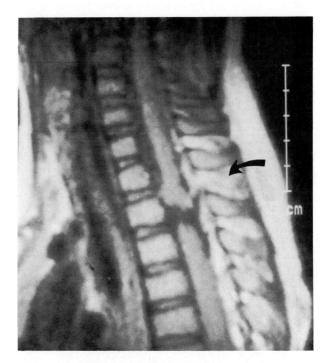

Figure 20–17. An 8-year-old girl with complete cord dysfunction below T2 after a motor vehicle accident. Sagittal T1-weighted (TR = 600, TE = 20) MRI scan shows transection of the cord at the T1-T2 level. Plain radiographs and CT were normal in this patient, but the ligamentous injury to the spine is shown by the abnormal increased signal (blood) in the dorsal ligaments (*arrow*).

cord compression from extradural or intradural metastatic disease. MRI is the imaging technique of choice for evaluation of these patients because it allows a timely evaluation of the entire spinal axis and demonstrates the osseous, soft-tissue, paraspinal, and cord involvement in a single examination. Myelography and CT provide a rapid evaluation of small areas of interest and can be useful techniques when there is a contraindication to MRI.

Osseous metastases are clearly delineated as areas of alteration of normal MRI signal from the marrow space of the vertebrae. In general, osseous metastases appear as discrete areas of low signal intensity on T1-weighted images that contrast markedly with the normal bright signal from fatty marrow. These lesions contain more water than does normal marrow; as a result they show increased signal intensity on spin density and T2-weighted images (Fig. 20–18). Con-

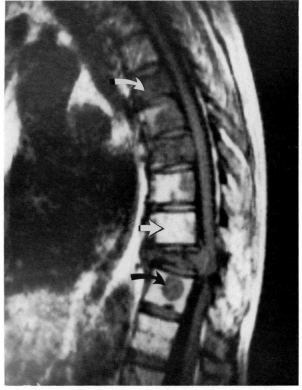

Figure 20–18. A 50-year-old woman with breast carcinoma, leg weakness, and urinary incontinence. Sagittal T1-weighted (TR = 600, TE = 20) MRI scan of the thoracic spine shows multiple bone metastases as areas of low signal (*curved arrows*) compared with the normal marrow signal (*straight arrow*). There is a compression fracture of one of the lower thoracic vertebral bodies with cord compression by a retropulsed fragment and epidural metastatic tumor.

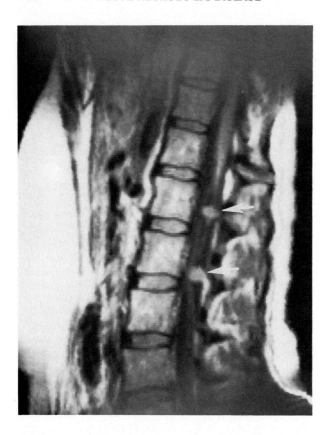

Figure 20–19. A 42-year-old woman with breast carcinoma and bilateral leg weakness. Sagittal T1-weighted (TR = 600, TE = 20) MRI scan of the upper lumbar spine shows intradural metastatic tumor (*arrows*) displacing the nerve roots.

trast enhancement is not routinely used in the initial MRI evaluation of patients with metastatic disease because of the high sensitivity of noncontrast MRI. Contrast enhancement in bony metastases may increase its signal intensity to such an extent that it becomes isointense with the fatty marrow and thus not detectable. Contrast enhancement can be helpful in selected cases in which the noncontrast scan does not fully explain the patient's symptoms. This usually occurs in patients that have small or plaque-like lesions in the epidural or intradural spaces.

Epidural masses that may be compressing the subarachnoid space, nerve roots, and spinal cord may be evaluated with either myelography and CT scanning

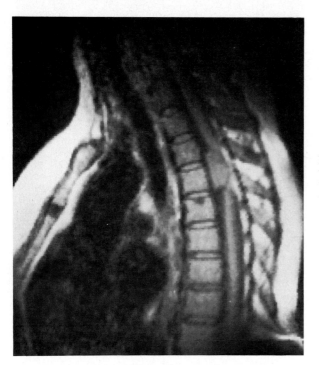

Figure 20–20. A 58-year-old woman with bilateral progressive leg weakness. Sagittal T1-weighted (TR = 600, TE = 20) MRI scan of the upper thoracic spine shows an isointense soft tissue mass in the spinal canal that is compressing the thoracic spinal cord. This was found to be an intraspinal meningioma.

or MRI. Again, MRI has the advantage of being able to visualize a large segment of the spinal axis on a single examination and to characterize more accurately the extradural compressive lesion as well as to demonstrate additional lesions not previously suspected (Fig. 20–19).

Primary tumors of the spinal axis are less frequent causes of compressive spinal cord symptoms. MRI also demonstrates these lesions with high sensitivity (Fig. 20–20).

References

Atlas, S.W., Grossman, R.I., Gomori, J.M., et al.: Hemorrhagic intracranial malignant neoplasms: Spin echo MR imaging. Radiology 164:71, 1987.

Baker, C.C., Oppenheimer, L., and Stevens, B.: Epidemiology of trauma deaths. Am. J. Surg. 140:144–150, 1980.

Barkay, L., and Glasauer, F.E.: Head Injury. Boston, Little, Brown & Co., 1980.

Bergstrom, M., Ericson, K., Levander, B., et al.: Computed tomography of cranial subdural and epidural hematomas: Variation of attenuation related to time and clinical events such as rebleeding. J. Comput. Assist. Tomogr. 1:449–455, 1977.

Britt, R.H., and Enzmann, D.R.: Clinical stages of human brain abscesses on serial CT scans after contrast infusion: Computerized tomographic, neuropathological, and clinical correlations. J. Neurosurg. 59:972–989, 1983.

Cohen, M.D., McGuire, W., Cory, D.A., and Smith, J.A.: MR appearance of blood and blood products: An in vitro study. AJR 146:1293, 1986.

Davidson, H.D., and Steiner, R.E.: Magnetic resonance imaging in infection of the central nervous system. AJNR 6:499–504, 1985.

Davis, K.R., Taveras, J.M., Robertson, G.H., et al.: Some limitations of computerized tomography in the diagnosis of neurological disease. AJR 127:111–123, 1976.

Dolinskas, C.A., Bilaniuk, L.T., Zimmerman, R.A., et al.: Computed tomography of intracerebral hematomas. I. Transmission CT observations on hematoma resolution. AJR 129:681–688, 1977.

Dooms, G.C., Uske, A., Brant-Zawadzki, M., et al.: Spin-echo MR imaging of intracranial hemorrhage. Neuroradiology 28:132, 1986.

Drayer, B.P. Diseases of the cerebral vascular system. In Rosenberg R.N. (ed.): The Clinical Neurosciences, vol. 4. New York, Churchill Livingstone, 1984, pp. 247–360.

Drayer, B., Dujovny, M., Boehnke, M., et al.: The capacity for computer tomography diagnosis of cerebral infarction. Radiology 125:393–402, 1977.

Fisher, C.M.: Lacunar strokes and infarcts: A review. Neurology 32:871–876, 1982.

French, B.N., and Dublin, A.B.: The value of computerized tomography in the management of 1000 consecutive head injuries. Surg. Neurol. 7:171–183, 1977.

Gentry, L.R., Godersky, J.D., and Thompson, B.: MR imaging of head trauma: Review of the distribution and radiologic features of traumatic lesions. AJNR 9:101–110, 1988a.

Gentry, L.R., Godersky, J.D., and Thompson, B.: Prospective comparative study of intermediate-field MR and CT in the evaluation of closed head trauma. AJNR 9:91–100, 1988b.

Gomori, J.M., Grossman, R.I., Goldberg, H.I., et al.: Intracranial hematomas: Imaging by high-field MR. Radiology 157:443, 1986.

Hecht-Leavitt, C., Grossman, R.I., et al.: High field MRI of hemorrhagic cortical infarction. AJNR 7:581–585, 1986.

Holbourn, A.H.S.: Mechanics of head injury. Lancet 2:438–441, 1943.

Holbourn, A.H.S.: The mechanics of brain injury. Br. Med. Bull. 3:147–149, 1945.

Hornig, C.R., Dorndorf, W., and Agnoli, A.: Hemorrhagic cerebral infarction: A prospective study. Stroke 17:179–186, 1986.

Inoue, Y., Takemoto, K., and Miyamoto, T.: Sequential computed tomography scans in acute cerebral infarction. Radiology 135:655–662, 1980.

Kawase, T., Mizukami, M., Maki, G., et al.: Mechanisms of contrast enhancement in cerebral infarctions: Computerized tomography, regional cerebral blood flow, fluoroscein angiography, and pathological study. Adv. Neurol. 30:149–158, 1981.

Kelly, A.B., Zimmerman, R.D., Snow, R.B., et al.: Head trauma: Comparison of MR and CT in 100 patients. AJNR 9:699–708, 1988.

Kendall, B.E., and Pullicino, P.: Intravascular contrast injection in ischaemic lesions. I. Relationship to prognosis. II. Effect on prognosis. Neuroradiology 19:235–243, 1980.

Larson, E.B., Omenns, G.S., and Loop, J.W.: Computerized tomography in patients with cerebrovascular disease: Impact of a new technology on patient care. AJR 131:35–40, 1978.

Moseley, I.F., and Kendall, B.E.: Radiology of intracranial empyema. Neuroradiology 26:333–345, 1984.

Sharif, H.S., and Ibrahim, A.: Intracranial epidural abscess. Br. J. Radiol. 55:81–84, 1982.

Strich, S.J.: Cerebral Trauma, Greenfield's Neuropathology. London, Edward Arnold, 1976.

Weisberg, L.A.: Computerized tomographic enhancement patterns in cerebral infarction. Arch. Neurol. 37:21–24, 1980.

Weisberg, L.A.: Computerized tomography in intracranial hemorrhage. Arch. Neurol. 36:630–634, 1979.

Zimmerman, R.A., Bilaniuk, L.T., Hackney, D.B., et al.: Head injury: Early results comparing CT and high-field MR. AJNR 7:757–764, 1986.

THE NEONATE

PART
VII

21

Imaging Evaluation of the Neonate

∎

Gerald A. Mandell

Pulmonary disease is a major cause of life-threatening illness in both preterm and full-term neonates. The differentiation of the medical and surgical causes of respiratory distress and the possible iatrogenic complications of treatment are discussed. Because aberrations of the cardiovascular, gastrointestinal (GI), genitourinary, central nervous system (CNS), and musculoskeletal system can also affect the ultimate course of the neonate, the imaging descriptions of the more commonly occurring pathologic entities are also briefly addressed. Conventional radiography as well as ultrasound, computed tomography (CT), and even magnetic resonance imaging (MRI) are helpful in the management of the neonate.

MEDICAL AND SURGICAL CAUSES OF RESPIRATORY DISTRESS

Respiratory Distress Syndrome

Respiratory distress syndrome (RDS) is the preferred term for hyaline membrane disease because the hyaline membrane formation is a nonspecific response of the lung to varied insults. Prematurity, cesarean section delivery, and diabetic mothers are predisposing factors. Common to all infants with RDS are decreased number of terminal air spaces, lack of the tension-reducing substance surfactant, and a highly compliant chest wall (Stark and Frantz, 1986). Surfactant reduces the surface tension within the air sacs, allowing the air spaces to stay open during exhalation and producing a more uniform expansion of these air spaces. Without surfactant the air spaces collapse on exhalation, creating uneven ventilation and resulting in hypoxia and acidosis. Complications of severe hypoxia include intracranial hemorrhage, disseminated intravascular coagulation (DIC), pul-

monary hemorrhage, and congestive heart failure (CHF) due to a patent ductus arteriosus (PDA). Continuous positive airway pressure and positive end-expiratory pressure (PEEP) not only open up the alveoli but lead to other complications such as pneumothorax, pneumomediastinum, pulmonary interstitial emphysema (PIE), pneumoperitoneum, massive gas embolism, and bronchopulmonary dysplasia (BPD).

Clinically, infants with RDS show signs of respiratory distress in the first few hours of life. The disease runs a spectrum from very mild to very severe. The symptoms consist of progressively increasing dyspnea, tachypnea, grunting, nasal flaring, and retractions (intercostal, suprasternal, and substernal). Radiographic changes are usually minimal in the mild forms of the disease. The classic roentgenographic findings in moderate to severe RDS consist of underaeration, finely granular appearance of pulmonary parenchyma (collapsed alveoli and alveolar ducts), and bilateral symmetric branching air bronchograms (Ellis and Nadelhaft, 1957; Peterson and Pendleton, 1955). Air bronchograms beyond the main stem right bronchus and the first bifurcation of the left bronchus are abnormal. Secondary air hunger signs include pneumoesophagus and sternal retractions (Fig. 21–1). The pneumoesophagus can also be seen in H-type tracheoesophageal fistula and gastroesophageal reflux. With mild to moderate RDS, emphysema of the distal airways may cause overaeration rather than the expected under-ventilation. Sometimes the roentgenographic picture is altered by therapy. Sometimes in moderate to severe disease, the lung may be overaerated as a result of mechanical ventilation. The lung density decreases markedly when mechanical ventilation is instituted (Giedion et al., 1973). The pressure necessary to keep terminal air spaces open is provided by mechanical ventilation.

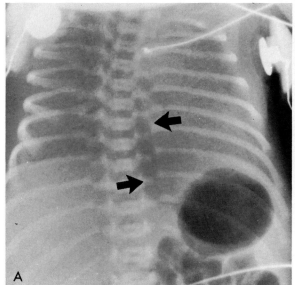
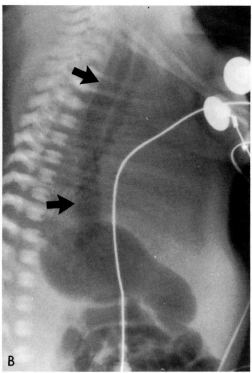

Figure 21–1. *A,* Anteroposterior (AP) view of the chest with air-filled esophagus *(arrows),* bilateral fine granularity, and peripherally extending air bronchograms in the lungs. *B,* Lateral view showing aeroesophagus *(arrows)* and sternal retraction indicative of air hunger in a patient with the respiratory distress syndrome.

The application of exogenous surfactant either preventilatory (shortly after birth) or post-ventilatory (after development of RDS) has also altered roentgenographic patterns in RDS. Early installation of surfactant can result in four distinct patterns of radiographic abnormality—diffuse granularity and air bronchograms (30%), central clearing (14%) (Fig. 21–2), disproportionate clearing in the right lung (8%), and complete clearing (49%). Clarke et al. (1989) found that 66% of infants with severe RDS achieve a lasting response to surfactant, 11% a transient response, and 22% no response. Poor or transient responses were associated with early PDA and air leaks (pneumothorax and PIE) (Charon et al., 1989). Early reports of multiple doses of pre- and post-ventilatory surfactant claim a reduction in the incidence of BPD (Kendig and Shapiro, 1988).

High-frequency jet ventilation can be used in neonates with respiratory failure. It can deliver adequate oxygenation at lower peak airway pressures. The intent is to prevent the development of BPD (Wetzell and Gioia, 1987). In one series high-frequency jet ventilation reduced airway pressure and partial pressure of arterial carbon dioxide but did not improve outcome or affect the incidence of BPD when compared with conventional ventilation (Carlo et al., 1989). The incidence of intraventricular cerebral hemorrhage (grades III and IV) was increased. Controversy exists about whether high-frequency jet ventilation can cause necrotizing tracheobronchitis in the mucosa near the distal end of the endotracheal tube (Kercsmar et al., 1988). Laryngotracheomalacia and nodular vocal cords are the most common abnormalities in both groups.

Muscle relaxation with pancuronium is controversial but is generally used in infants who are fighting the ventilator and who require high ventilatory pressures for RDS (Stark and Frantz, 1986). The benefits include improved gas exchange and reduction of the complications of barotrauma, BPD (oxygen toxicity), and severe intraventricular hemorrhage. Radiographically, pancuronium therapy is recognized by airless abdomen (lack of swallowing), edema of chest wall (fluid retention) (Fig. 21–3), and tower-shaped chest (lack of intercostal muscle movement). Skeletal muscle atrophy can occur as a consequence of the therapy (Rutledge et al., 1986).

Extracorporeal membrane oxygenation (ECMO) is a technique of supporting patients with a high likelihood of death (less than 20% chance of survival) but with potentially reversible respiratory failure by using a partial venoatrial (cardiopulmonary) bypass. ECMO can be applied to neonates with meconium aspiration syndrome, persistent fetal circulation, congenital diaphragmatic hernia, sepsis, and RDS. ECMO allows the diseased lungs to rest without the iatrogenic effects of high oxygen and ventilator therapy. Chest radiographs can be used to determine the placement of the arterial catheter in the aorta through the right carotid artery and the venous catheter in the right atrium through the right jugular vein (Hall et al., 1985) (Fig. 21–4). Pulmonary opacification on chest radiographs occurs and probably correlates with decreased ventilator settings (Schlesinger et al., 1986) rather than clinical status. Interstitial air collections usually disappear on the lowered settings. Improved lung function is evidenced by improved blood gases or a trailing off of ECMO. Continuous heparinization

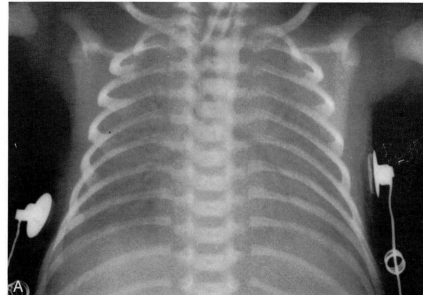
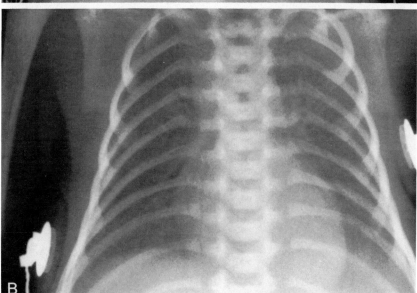

Figure 21–2. *A,* Anteroposterior radiograph of chest during first few hours of life demonstrating bilateral air bronchograms and a granular appearance to the lungs suggestive of respiratory distress syndrome. *B,* Anteroposterior radiograph of chest after administration of surfactant with some central clearing of lungs resulting in more distinct margins of mediastinum.

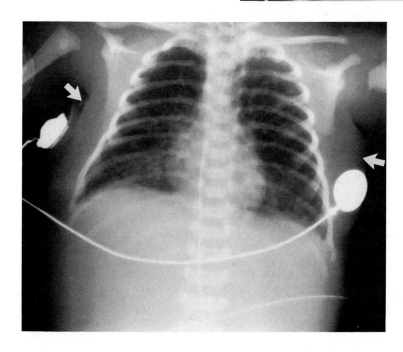

Figure 21–3. Anteroposterior view of chest and upper abdomen exhibiting an airless abdomen and swollen soft tissues *(arrows)* about the chest secondary to iatrogenic paralysis (pancuronium therapy) in a newborn with respiratory distress.

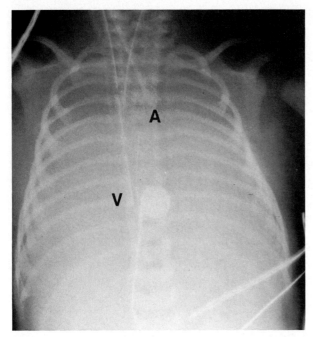

Figure 21–4. Anteroposterior radiograph showing dense unaerated lungs in patient on extracorporeal membrane oxygenator. Note the jugular line extending down to the right atrium (V) and the arterial line from the carotid to the aorta (A) (Courtesy of George Gross, M.D., Thomas Jefferson University Hospital, Philadelphia, PA.)

and thrombocytopenia as well as unilateral carotid artery and jugular vein catheterization during ECMO impose an increased risk of intracranial hemorrhage (Ortiz et al., 1987; Taylor et al., 1987).

Transient Respiratory Distress of the Newborn (Transient Tachypnea, Wet Lung Disease)

Transient respiratory distress of the newborn (TRDN) is probably more common than RDS. As the name *wet lung syndrome* implies, there is delayed clearance of physiologic fluid from the newborn infant's lungs (Swischuk, 1970). During vaginal delivery, part of the lung fluid is expressed into the airways and cleared. After birth, most fluid is cleared by lymphatics and veins. Infants delivered by cesarean section commonly have TRDN because a substantial volume of fluid is not eliminated from their lungs by the usual uterine squeeze. Extra fluid can also be seen in vaginally delivered infants, especially those newborns who are relatively small in comparison with the uterine confines or who are delivered rapidly. Polycythemia from intrauterine placental transfusion or excessive milking of the cord, hypervolemia in infants of diabetic mothers, and hypoproteinemia (Steele and Copeland, 1972) with reduced oncotic pressure have been proposed as other predisposing factors. Aspiration of clear amniotic fluid secondary to fetal distress or breech delivery can cause clinical

and radiographic conditions indistinguishable from wet lung.

TRDN is present by 2 to 4 hours of age. Symptoms include tachypnea, nasal flaring, grunting, retractions, and in some cases, cyanosis. Resolution of TRDN usually occurs between 24 and 72 hours after birth, and these infants need minimal supportive oxygen therapy. An association has been reported between TRDN and later development of childhood asthma (Shohat et al., 1989).

The roentgenographic findings consist of symmetric parahilar patches or streaks, mild to moderate over-aeration, and, occasionally, mild cardiomegaly or pleural effusions (Steele and Copeland, 1972) (Fig. 21–5). Diagnosis is more difficult when the parahilar pattern is predominantly in the right lung or when there is a localized air-space disease (Wesenberg et al., 1971). The radiograph is almost always clear by 48 to 72 hours. If the wet lung pattern and cardiomegaly persist beyond 72 hours, hypoplastic left-sided heart syndrome, cor triatriatum, and myocardial dysfunction must be considered. The initial radiographic appearances of sepsis and TRDN are similar.

Pulmonary Hemorrhage

Pulmonary hemorrhage is usually due to capillary damage in response to severe hypoxia. Factors that contribute to pulmonary hemorrhage include DIC (hypoxia, acidosis, hypotension, and sepsis), thrombocytopenia (sepsis, DIC, and exchange transfusion), decreased hepatic function, and decreased vitamin K levels. Pulmonary hemorrhage may accompany RDS, neonatal pneumonia, congenital heart disease, and hypoxia after a difficult or prolonged delivery. Massive pulmonary hemorrhage in the newborn may result in death.

Pulmonary hemorrhage is heralded by sudden deterioration with shock, cyanosis, bradycardia, and apnea. Pink or red fluid is found in the mouth or in the tracheal aspirate.

Small areas of hemorrhage are difficult to identify when superimposed on pre-existing pulmonary disease. Massive pulmonary hemorrhage is characteristically homogeneous, opaque, and airless on the chest radiograph (Fig. 21–6). Differentiation from pneumonia is made by the more rapid clearance of hemorrhage, often within 12 to 24 hours. Massive pulmonary hemorrhage in the newborn may be indistinguishable from pulmonary edema (Bomsel et al., 1975).

Neonatal Pneumonia

Neonatal pneumonia is predominantly bacterial in origin, Group B *Streptococcus* being the major pathogen. These bacteria colonize about 25% of pregnant women at the time of labor. Prolonged labor, premature rupture of the membranes, vaginal infection,

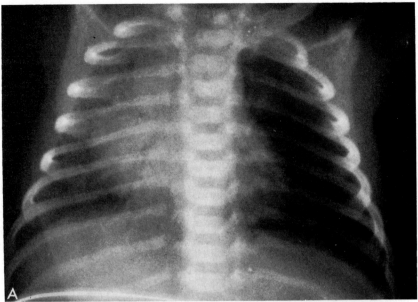

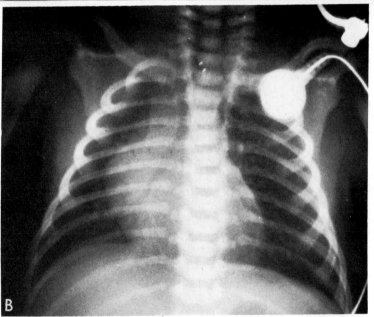

Figure 21–5. *A,* Anteroposterior view of the chest of a 4-hour-old infant with increased markings in the right lung. *B,* A radiograph made 2 days later with remarkable clearing of wet lung.

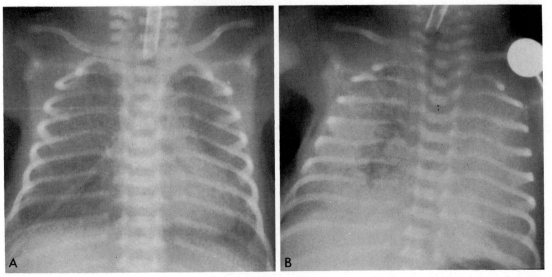

Figure 21–6. *A,* Initial AP radiograph of respiratory distress syndrome. *B,* One day later the increased opacity is due to pulmonary hemorrhage.

417

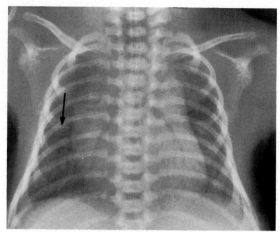

Figure 21–7. Anteroposterior radiograph showing bilateral lower lobe air bronchograms, some fluid in minor fissure *(arrow)*, and overaeration in a neonate with streptococcal pneumonia.

placental infection, and contamination with maternal fecal material or bacteria from improper cleaning of the perineum are the predisposing factors. Other pathogens usually superimpose themselves on acquired lung disease. *Escherichia coli, Candida albicans* (Kassner et al., 1981), and *Pneumocystis carinii*, as well as respiratory viruses, are included in this group. Infants who are intubated have a high incidence of bacterial colonization in their airways. Premature infants are affected more than full-term neonates.

Diagnosis of sepsis depends greatly on radiographic demonstration of infiltrates together with a clinical suspicion. The infants are often afebrile and occasionally are hypothermic. Shortly after birth, tachypnea, retractions, and cyanosis may be evident. Neutropenia sometimes accompanies Group B streptococcal infections.

In Group B streptococcal infections the chest radiograph may show initially clear lungs, a diffusely granular pattern with air bronchograms mimicking RDS (Fig. 21–7), or parahilar haziness and streakiness mimicking TRDN or heart failure (Ablow et al., 1976). Radiologically, differentiation of the air bronchograms of Group B streptococcal pneumonia from RDS depends on the presence of hyperaeration in the former as opposed to hypoaeration in the latter. The aeration criteria depend largely on ventilation unaltered by mechanical means (Ablow et al., 1976). Coarse, patchy, or diffusely nodular lesions may also be seen (Fig. 21–8). Lobar consolidation is an infrequent radiographic manifestation. Small pleural effusions and worsening consolidations support the diagnosis of Group B streptococcal pneumonia and differentiate it from TRDN or transient tachypnea of the newborn. Pleural effusions are present 10% of the time (Haney et al., 1984). Infants with gradually elevating right diaphragms should be suspected of having acquired diaphragmatic hernias (McCarten et al., 1981) (Fig. 21–9). Premature infants with diffuse disease have the worst prognosis. *E. coli* pneumonia may present with pneumatocele formation. Staphylococcal pneumonia can exhibit a miliary pattern in the lungs (Flores, 1988). Fungal pneumonia causes a sudden worsening of already abnormal lungs.

Meconium Aspiration and Hypoxia

Intrauterine fetal distress (e.g., hypoxemia, bradycardia, unusual traumatic delivery) induces rapid respirations and defecation. Meconium in the amniotic fluid is inhaled, leading to respiratory distress. These neonates are usually postmature and have CNS damage. A chemical pneumonitis prevails, and superimposed infection can occur if early antibiotic coverage is not instituted.

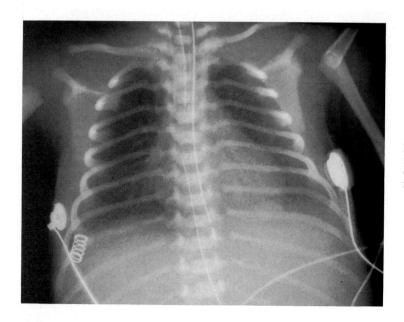

Figure 21–8. Anteroposterior radiograph of chest of neonate with interstitial bilateral diffuse micronodular disease consistent with miliary pattern that can be seen in streptococcal pneumonia.

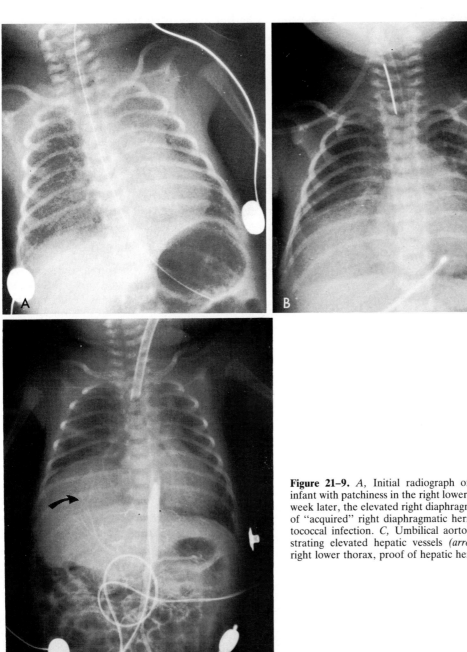

Figure 21–9. *A,* Initial radiograph of a 1-day-old infant with patchiness in the right lower lung. *B,* One week later, the elevated right diaphragm is indicative of "acquired" right diaphragmatic hernia poststreptococcal infection. *C,* Umbilical aortogram demonstrating elevated hepatic vessels *(arrow)* over the right lower thorax, proof of hepatic herniation.

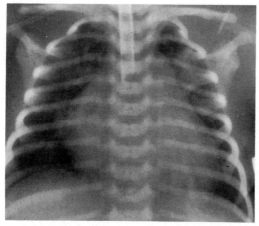

Figure 21–10. Anteroposterior radiograph showing patchy consolidation and an enlarged heart in a patient with anoxia and meconium aspiration syndrome.

Depending on the severity of the aspiration, the symptoms are variable and may include tachypnea, grunting, retractions, and even cyanosis. Suction of the tracheobronchial passages is necessary to remove as much debris as possible.

Roentgenographically, hyperaeration is an expression of air trapping secondary to obstruction of the smaller bronchi by particles of meconium. Coarse nodular or streaky atelectasis is most common. Occasionally, "cystic" changes representing streaky disease interspersed with areas of compensatory overaeration can be seen (Gooding et al., 1971; Hoffman et al., 1974) (Fig. 21–10). Mild cases may simply manifest overaeration with small streaks or patches. Pleural effusions are sometimes evident. Pneumothorax and pneumomediastinum may result from sudden attempts to clear bronchi of meconium. The roentgenographic presence of the proximal humeral ossification centers (38 weeks of gestation) identifies the possibility of post-maturity. The lungs take weeks to clear, and a "dirty" chest radiograph persists long after clinical recovery from meconium aspiration.

Right to left shunting from increased pulmonary vascular resistance (persistent fetal circulation [PFC]) may occur (see section on PFC). Hypoxia can lead to cardiomegaly because of myocardial ischemia, actual infarction, and transient myocardial dysfunction. For the most part, with conservative therapy the changes are reversible. Hypoxic sequelae include bell-shaped chest configurations secondary to poor intercostal muscle movement (Fig. 21–11A), hydrocephalus secondary to intracranial bleeding and tissue damage, and even pylorospasm mimicking pyloric stenosis (see Fig. 21–11B and C).

Patent Ductus Arteriosus

See section on left to right shunts.

Bronchopulmonary Dysplasia (Oxygen Toxicity, Ventilator Lung)

BPD is usually the end result of therapy of patients with RDS who have elevated concentrations of oxygen, mechanical ventilation, and endotracheal intubation. These patients required the additional therapy because their pulmonary disease (RDS) failed to resolve. Clinically, cyanosis, oxygen dependency, and respiratory distress are present. Most authors indicate that less than 20% of premature infants who weigh less than 1,500 g at birth develop the disease (O'Brodovich and Mellins, 1985). There is a difference of opinion regarding the relative contributions of high oxygen exposure and mechanical ventilator injury to the development of BPD (Edwards et al., 1977; Stocks et al., 1978). In these studies the neonates with RDS who developed BPD tended to be more premature than the group without evidence of BPD, and those succumbing to BPD were the most premature. Stiffening of the lungs by the increased perfusion through a PDA or by diffuse interstitial emphysema (see section on PIE) necessitates increased ventilatory pressures and increased oxygen concentrations, which predispose the patient to BPD. Gastroesophageal reflux may contribute to the severity of the disease (Sindel et al., 1989).

Eighty percent of infants that progress to BPD do not experience all four of the stages described by Northway and Rosan (1968; Heneghan et al., 1986). Stage I consists radiologically of classic RDS with bilateral fine granular changes, air bronchograms, and small lungs (Fig. 21–12A). Pathologically, hyaline membranes, hyperemia, atelectasis, and lymphatic dilatation are present. Stage II (the exudative phase) develops 4 to 10 days after birth. The chest radiograph (see Fig. 21–12B) becomes more diffusely opaque until it reaches a complete whiteout with obscuring of the cardiomediastinal silhouette. Interstitial edema, intraluminal eosinophilic exudate, some hyaline membranes, and patchy bronchiolar necrosis are noted pathologically. There is pulmonary edema probably secondary to vascular damage, with seepage of fluid into the interstitium and alveoli. Between the 10th and 20th day of life, Stage III appears with cyst-like changes and a sponge-like appearance (Williams and Cumming, 1986) (see Fig. 21–12C). It lasts 10 to 30 days. Pathologically, bronchial and bronchiolar mucosal metaplasia and hyperplasia with macrophagic and histiocytic exudate are seen. Bronchiolitis and bronchiectasis produce the small emphysematous radiolucent air spaces. These air bubbles collapse with exhalation, differentiating them from relatively fixed PIE. Occasionally, persistent foci of tension PIE can be seen in BPD. Schwartz and Graham (1986) reported improvement in the emphysema with lateral decubitus positioning of the neonate with the emphysematous side down. In Stage IV disease, dense areas of fibrosis and atelectasis radiate from hila intermixed with diffuse hyperaeration. This stage lasts months or

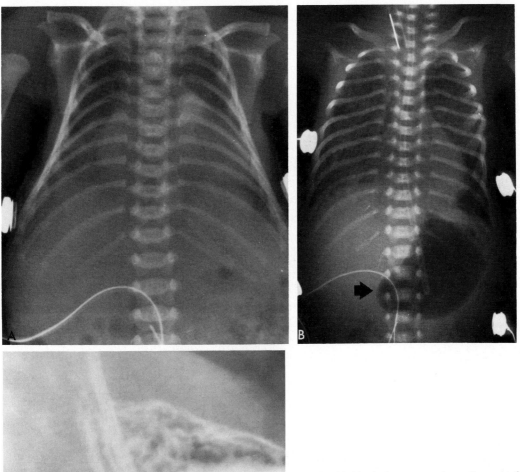

Figure 21–11. *A,* Anteroposterior radiograph of a chest with bell-shaped configuration in an anoxic neonate. *B,* In another neonate the stomach is distended by air *(arrow)* secondary to pylorospasm. *C,* Barium-filled stomach confirming the pylorospasm, narrowed pyloric channel.

years and may gradually clear or may progress to pulmonary hypertension or to cor pulmonale and death. Chronic alveolar hypoxia leads to an alteration in the structure of the pulmonary vascular bed with abnormal muscularization of small pulmonary arteries and intimal proliferation (Goodman et al., 1988).

The radiographic features and evolution of clinical BPD often vary from Northway's original description. Most patients do not show evolution through four discrete radiographic stages. Most patients never manifest radiologic Stage II but immediately develop lungs with large areas of atelectasis alternating with areas of emphysema (Heneghan et al., 1986). Varia-

tion in the radiologic appearance of BPD relates to the amount of pre-existing disease in the lungs and to the severity of iatrogenic damage. When atelectasis protects a portion of the lung, the disease may be asymmetric (Sickler and Gooding, 1976). Follow-up of patients with BPD reveals increased incidence of reactive airway disease and lower respiratory tract infections (Bader et al., 1987). Long-term diuretic therapy seems to improve the outcome in infants with BPD (Albersheim et al., 1989). A narrow anteroposterior diameter of the chest of children with chronic BPD has been reported (Edwards and Hilton, 1987) and is thought to be attributable to demineralized

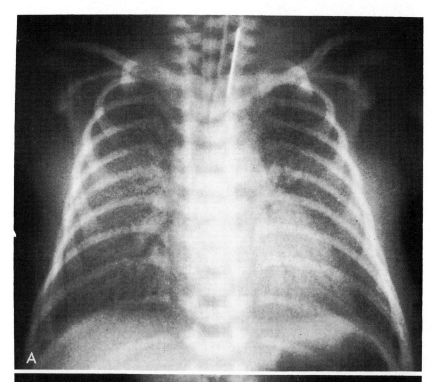

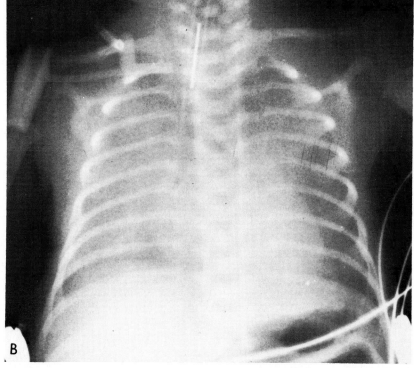

Figure 21–12. *A*, Initial AP radiograph demonstrating typical granularity and air bronchograms of respiratory distress syndrome. *B*, Seven days later, increasing density of lungs indicates the second stage of bronchopulmonary dysplasia.

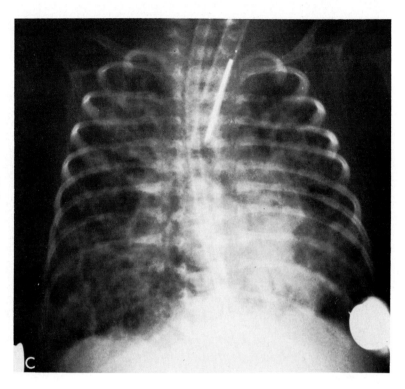

Figure 21–12 *(Continued) C,* The advanced third stage disease of bronchopulmonary dysplasia with a diffuse cystic pattern.

thoracic cage, prolonged recumbency, and chronic sternal retraction. This abnormal chest shape may be deleterious because of its interference in normal chest dynamics.

COMPLICATIONS OF MECHANICAL VENTILATION

After mechanical ventilation and PEEP a dramatic diminution usually occurs in the degree of respiratory distress. The effects of PEEP are to increase arterial oxygenation and lower the requirements for supplemental oxygen (McCloud and Ravin, 1977). The lung volume is increased to functional residual capacity. The elevated pressure is transmitted to the small airways and alveoli to prevent atelectasis, to reduce shunting during the expiratory phase, and to press alveolar fluid against the alveolar walls. In theory the elevation of the pressure gradient between the alveolus and pulmonary capillary results in water entering the capillaries from the alveoli and interstitial spaces.

Alveolar hyperinflation may rupture the alveoli, resulting in interstitial emphysema, pneumomediastinum, pneumothorax, pneumopericardium, pneumoperitoneum, and even intravascular air embolism (Giedion et al., 1973). Extra-alveolar collections of air may occur singly or in combination. RDS is the most common underlying condition associated with extra-alveolar dissection of air. Meconium aspiration, neonatal pneumonia, and BPD also predispose the patient to develop extra-alveolar air collections.

Pulmonary Interstitial Emphysema

With alveolar rupture, air travels initially along the perivascular sheaths toward the pleura, mediastinum, or pericardium. When the air is trapped in the interstitium of the lung, the radiograph may show bubbles of air in the lung that may be unilateral or bilateral, localized or diffuse. The lenticular chaotic pattern of interstitial air helps to differentiate PIE from the air bronchograms characteristic of RDS and pneumonia. The diffuse air bubbles in the interstitium (Swischuk, 1977) (Fig. 21–13), some localized in dilated lymphatics, stiffen the lungs and make ventilation more difficult. Pneumomediastinum or pneumothorax usually follows. Localized air collections can be small, ovoid, or round and are sometimes referred to as pseudocysts (Clark and Edwards, 1979). These may decompress with pneumothorax or pneumomediastinum or may just spontaneously disappear, usually in 3 to 18 days (Fig. 21–14). These lesions vary from 0.5 to 3 cm and are predominantly right parahilar (Williams et al., 1988). Areas of PIE can coalesce or, because of a check valve mechanism secondary to the damaged lung tissue, can develop into larger extra-alveolar interstitial collections (Fig. 21–15). Sometimes the abnormal emphysematous region is of such magnitude that it compresses ipsilateral and contralateral normal portions of the lungs and leads to worsening respiratory distress (Magilner et al., 1974). After conservative therapy, perhaps with selective bronchial intubation, emphysematous areas may have to be decompressed by a chest tube (Brooks et al., 1977) or removed by surgical means (Bauer et al.,

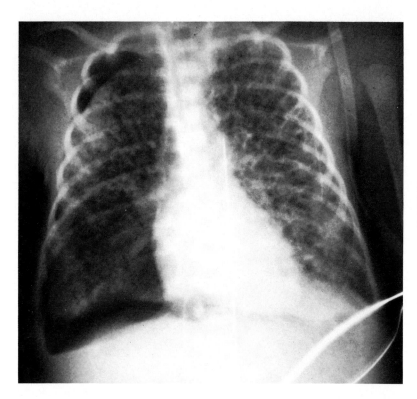

Figure 21–13. Diffuse lenticular air collections of pulmonary interstitial emphysema throughout both lungs. An associated right pneumothorax and pneumoperitoneum are also present.

1978). Lung perfusion scanning has been reported to aid in the selection of patients for surgical intervention (Leonidas et al., 1978). A large perfusion defect in areas of emphysema is suggestive of a lung with permanent dysfunction.

Pneumomediastinum

The pneumomediastinum, usually of no clinical significance per se, may be the first indicator of barotrauma. It is characteristically recognized in the superior mediastinum by its uplifting of the lobes of the thymus gland, producing the "spinnaker sail sign" (Fig. 21–16). Mediastinal air can dissect under tension to deep cervical regions, subcutaneous tissues, and extraperitoneal spaces. A crescentic epiphrenic collection of air that outlines the muscle bundles of the diaphragm is either extrapleural or extraperitoneal (Christensen and Landay, 1980). It is important to distinguish between subpulmonic pneumothorax needing pleural drainage and pneumoperitoneum probably secondary to a ruptured viscus. Extraperitoneal air remains fixed on decubitus films, whereas intraperitoneal or intrapleural air moves. Mediastinal

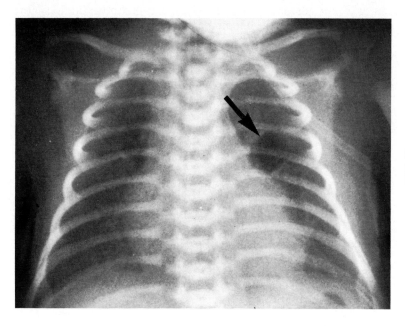

Figure 21–14. In the left upper lung is a small pseudocyst, a localized interstitial extra-alveolar collection *(arrow)*.

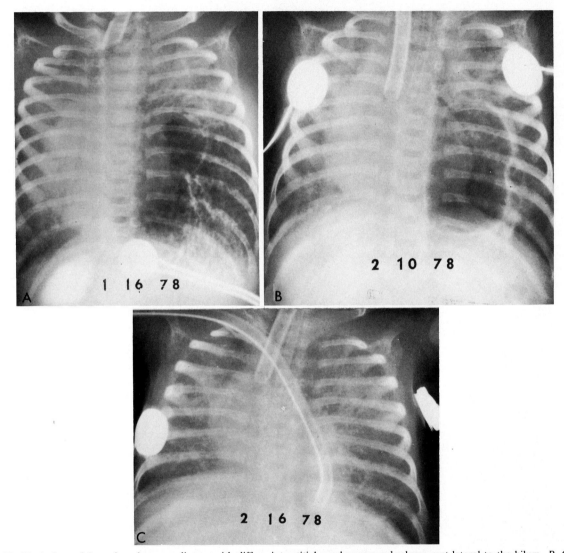

Figure 21–15. *A*, Stage 3 bronchopulmonary disease with diffuse interstitial emphysema and a large cyst lateral to the hilum. *B*, Over the next 3 weeks the cyst enlarged. *C*, Subsequently, a chest tube was inserted to drain the cyst. (Courtesy of A. E. O'Hara, M.D., Philadelphia, PA.)

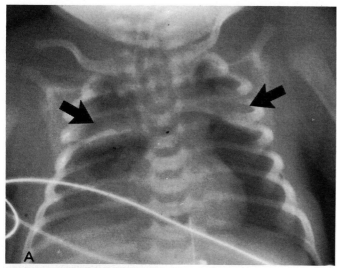

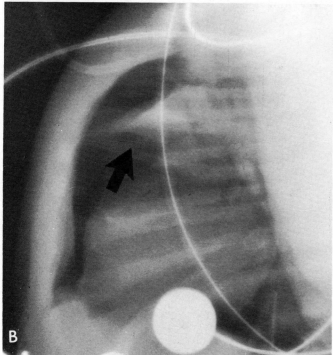

Figure 21–16. Thymic lobes uplifted by anterior pneumome-diastinum on AP *(A)* and lateral *(B)* views, so-called spinnaker sails *(arrows)*.

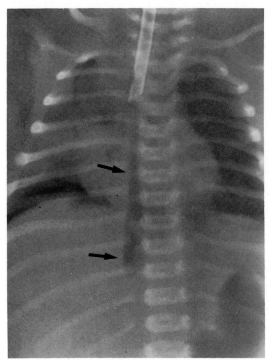

Figure 21–17. A linear streak of air dissecting from the mediastinum toward the peritoneum *(arrows).*

air may dissect in linear streaks along the descending aorta to the retroperitoneum and peritoneum (Fig. 21–17). The inferior pulmonary ligament, a double layer of visceral pleural extending from the hilum to diaphragm and anchoring the lung, is a potential space for air dissecting from the mediastinum. An alternative explanation for this paramediastinal pneumatocele was offered by CT. The air collection was suggested to be a medial pneumothorax behind the pulmonary ligament or a posterior pneumomediastinum (Goodwin et al., 1985) (Fig. 21–18).

Pneumothorax

The incidence of pneumothorax may be as high as 33% in low-birth-weight infants receiving mechanical ventilatory assistance and PEEP for treatment of RDS (Ogata et al., 1976). Half of these infants had prior evidence of PIE. An infant with contralateral PIE at the time of a unilateral pneumothorax is at risk for developing a contralateral pneumothorax (Ryan et al., 1987). The commonly recognized pneumothorax in the supine neonate is lateral. In about 75% of cases, however, air may be seen anteromedial to the lung (Mandell and Chawla, 1981). The appearance of the medial pneumothorax is well described by Moskowitz and Griscom (1976). In the supine neonate it rises anterior to the stationary lung, which is anchored by pulmonary vessels and the pulmonary ligament. The pleural air causes a hyperlucent hemithorax (Fig. 21–19). With further accumulation, the air in the pleural space may cross the

midline in the upper or lower portions of the mediastinum (Fletcher, 1978) (Fig. 21–20). Anterior pneumothoraces may be under tension and require immediate insertion of a pleural chest tube to relieve dyspnea. A posterolaterally positioned chest tube may not relieve the pneumothorax. Anterior placement of chest tubes in the herniated pleural space (Fig. 21–21) has been demonstrated by Mandell and Chawla (1981) to clear the pneumothorax rapidly, usually within 30 minutes of insertion. The chest tube can subsequently be withdrawn more proximally.

Pneumopericardium

The pneumopericardium usually occurs in preterm infants with RDS. The collection of air in the pericardial cavity can be sufficient to compromise the pulmonary venous return to the heart and cause cardiac tamponade. With tension pneumopericardium there is abrupt onset of bradycardia, hypotension, and cyanosis. Radiographically, a lucent halo surrounds the heart (Fig. 21–22). Differentiation from pneumomediastinum is usually made by visualization of the halo continuous below the inferior cardiac surface. If the location of the extra-alveolar air is in question, a lateral decubitus projection moves the air to the nondependent side in the freely communicating pericardial cavity. Mediastinal air does not mobilize readily. In cardiac tamponade the heart size becomes markedly reduced secondary to the diminished blood return (Higgins et al., 1979). Mortality from untreated neonatal pneumopericardium is 86% (Lawson et al., 1980), and rapid needle aspiration of the pericardium is necessary to prevent sudden death. Smaller collections of pericardial air may be treated conservatively. If symptoms recur after pericardiocentesis, a catheter may be required to drain the pericardial cavity. As reported by Brans et al. (1976), patients with pneumopericardium treated by pericardiocentesis had a 79% survival; those treated conservatively had a 32% survival.

Pneumoperitoneum

Mechanical ventilators may drive mediastinal air along vascular sheaths across the diaphragm, with a resultant pneumoperitoneum (Campbell et al., 1975). The classic pneumoperitoneum consists of a "football sign" (Fig. 21–23), distended flanks, and the ligamentum teres outlined by the free peritoneal air. It is of utmost importance to differentiate between ventilator-induced pneumoperitoneum and enteric perforation. Cross-table supine lateral views are sometimes helpful. If a large air–fluid level is seen, it implies peritonitis secondary to intestinal perforation. Pneumoperitoneum secondary to mediastinal dissection, however, lacks a fluid component. Nonetheless, the absence of a fluid level does not exclude the possibility of a perforated viscus: Kaufman et al. (1976) found

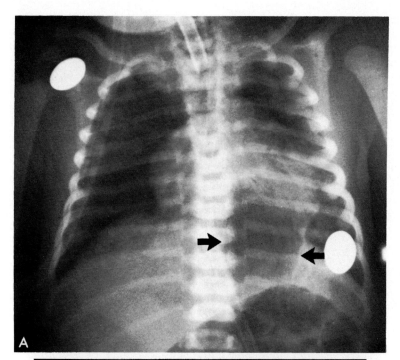

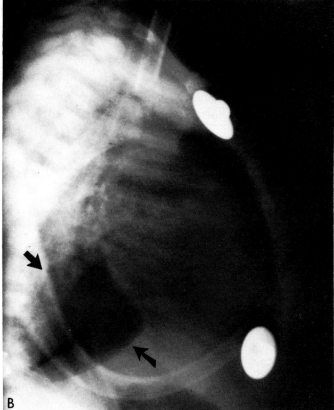

Figure 21–18. A large medial inferior collection of air in the left pulmonary ligament on the AP view *(A)* *(arrows)* and posteriorly placed on the lateral view *(B)* *(arrows)*.

Figure 21–20. *A,* On the AP view the pleural space, which is distended with air, has herniated from right to left, in a retrosternal potential location *(arrows)*. *B,* The lateral view shows the hyperlucent retrosternal space. *C,* The left lateral decubitus view demonstrates that the air in the freely communicating pleural space moves from medial to lateral *(arrows)*.

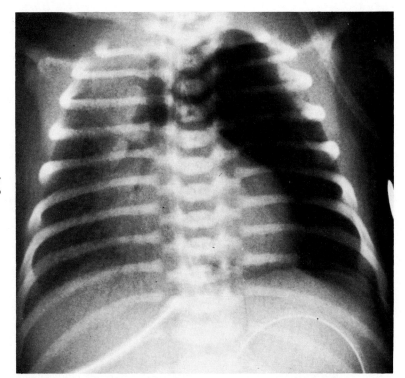

Figure 21–19. Hyperlucent left hemithorax secondary to air accumulating in the pleural space anterior to the lung.

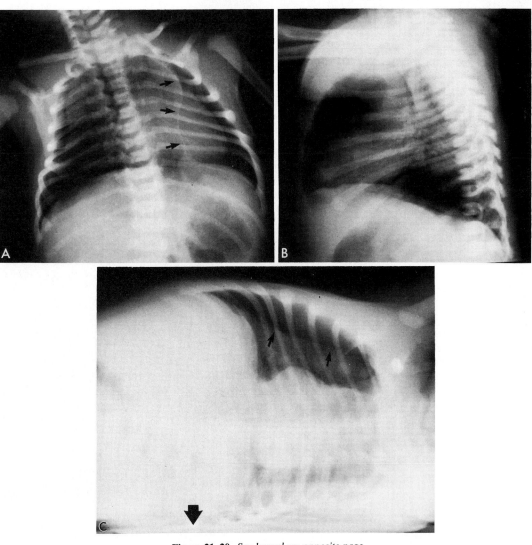

Figure 21–20. *See legend on opposite page*

429

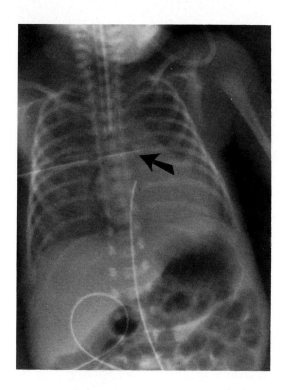

Figure 21–21. The chest tube has crossed the midline, in the medial right pleural space. The retrosternal location was confirmed on a lateral radiograph.

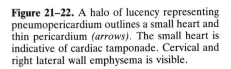

Figure 21–22. A halo of lucency representing pneumopericardium outlines a small heart and thin pericardium *(arrows)*. The small heart is indicative of cardiac tamponade. Cervical and right lateral wall emphysema is visible.

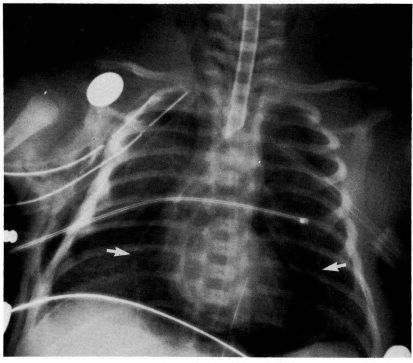

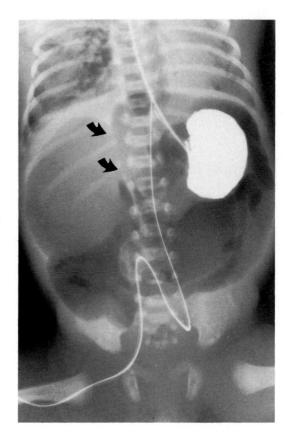

Figure 21–23. "Football sign" with large pneumoperitoneum. The ligamentum teres *(arrows)* is outlined by air. Water-soluble contrast material in the stomach shows no evidence of gastric perforation.

that only 43% of neonatal GI perforations had a demonstrable air–fluid level. If the amount of intraperitoneal air is small, even a large amount of peritoneal fluid will not be easily detected (see section on gastric perforation).

When there is a large pneumoperitoneum and a pneumomediastinum in an infant with ventilator-assisted peak inspiration of over 30 cm H_2O, the lung is usually the source of the abdominal air (Knight and Abdenour, 1981). If a ventilated infant has less

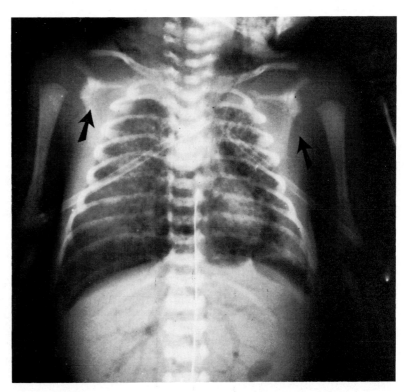

Figure 21–24. Evidence of systemic air embolism with air in the hepatic, splenic, and brachial vessels *(arrows)* and in the heart.

than 28 cm H_2O peak inspiratory pressure, gastric perforation should be excluded with an aqueous contrast agent instilled through the feeding tube (see Fig. 21–22). Usually there is no time to study the entire GI tract, and laparotomy is performed. Paracentesis can be done to measure the oxygen concentration in the peritoneal gas and to sample any intra-abdominal fluid.

Systemic Air Embolism

Systemic intravascular air embolism secondary to respirator therapy, a rare occurrence, is incompatible with life. Air in the vascular system most likely results from formation of either alveolar-capillary or bronchovenous fistulae after alveolar rupture. When the intra-alveolar pressure exceeds the left atrial pressure, air enters the pulmonary veins and travels to the heart and then into the systemic circulation. The radiologic diagnosis is made by visualization of air within the systemic vascular circulation (Fig. 21–24). Air is simultaneously present in both arterial and venous circulations. Intracardiac air is a consistent finding. The air can also be seen in the cerebral ventricles, apparently having crossed the blood-brain barrier. Only one infant has been reported to have survived this insult (Oppermann et al., 1979).

COMPLICATIONS OF TUBES AND CATHETERS

Life support in intensive care units (ICUs) frequently involves the use of endotracheal tubes, intravascular catheters, pleural drainage tubes, and feeding tubes. Malposition of these tubes can be readily detected by radiography. Improper placement of these conduits can lead to rapid deterioration of the neonate.

Endotracheal Tube Position

The polyvinylchloride orotracheal tube is usually identified by a radiopaque lead line at its tip. The tip should be located between the first thoracic vertebra and the carina. Adequate securing of the tube at the mouth with adhesive tape prevents proximal movement. A cadaver study (Donn and Kuhns, 1980) noted movement of the tube on flexion, extension, and rotation of the head. Most of the head and neck motion occurs primarily at the level of the first four cervical vertebrae. The tube tip moves caudad with flexion and cephalad with extension on the radiographs for endotracheal tube placement (Fig. 21–25). Therefore, when assessing tube position on the radiograph, the position of the head and neck should also be evaluated (Todres et al., 1976).

Most endotracheal tube mishaps are due to placement in the larynx or right bronchus (Fig. 21–26A

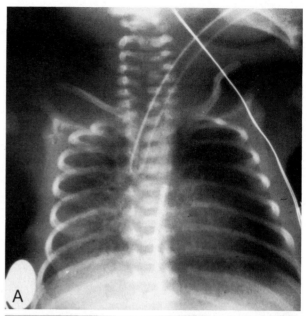

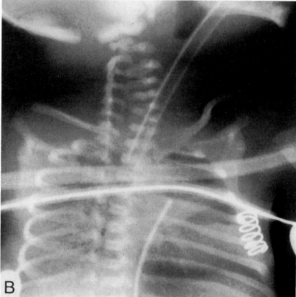

Figure 21–25. *A,* Anteroposterior view of neck and chest with neck in flexion, the tip of the ET tube enters right bronchus. *B,* With extension the ET tube is positioned at T3 in the same infant.

and *B*). Occasionally, the esophagus or stomach is intubated, reducing the aeration of the lungs (see Fig. 21–26C).

Endotracheal Tube Complications

Complications of intubation include perforation of the pharynx, usually the posterior pharyngeal wall or piriform sinuses (Clark et al., 1980) (Fig. 21–27). Immediate problems include cervical emphysema, pneumomediastinum, and pneumothorax. These usually heal spontaneously after 7 to 10 days. Rarely, vigorous intubations can result in tracheal perfora-

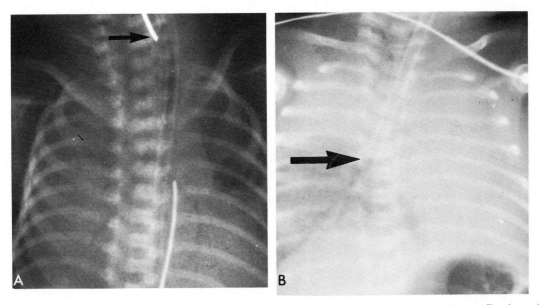

Figure 21–26. Endotracheal tube malposition (two patients). *A,* In the larynx *(arrow).* *B,* In the bronchus intermedius *(arrow).* Note the airless left lung and right upper lobe.

tion, an often lethal occurrence (Serlin and Daily, 1975). Suctioning catheters introduced through the endotracheal tube can be threaded too far, rupturing a bronchus and causing a pneumothorax. This usually occurs on the right, because the right bronchus is in more direct continuity with the trachea (Fig. 21–28). Perforation will often heal with conservative treatment with a pleural drainage tube. In other cases,

surgery is required to close the bronchopleural fistula (Anderson and Chandra, 1976).

Complications of traumatic or prolonged intubation in the neonate can result in subglottic granulomas and membranes or cartilaginous stenoses. Some stenoses have been reported after as little as 72 hours of intubation (Holinger et al., 1976). Other factors influencing formation of a postintubation tracheal

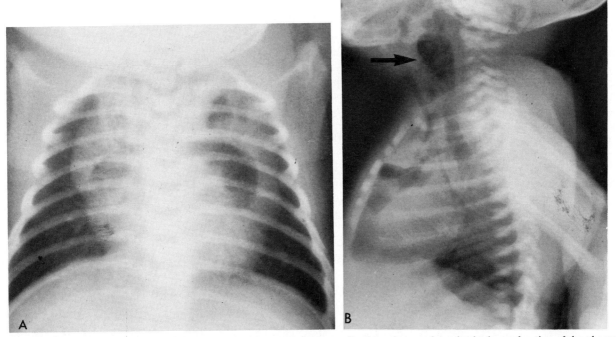

Figure 21–27. *A,* Anteroposterior view of the chest demonstrates pneumomediastinum from endotracheal tube perforation of the pharynx. *B,* On the lateral view, air is visible in the retropharyngeal and mediastinal spaces, and a large air collection is seen in the neck *(arrow).*

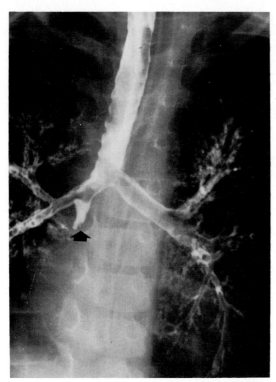

Figure 21–28. Bronchogram showing a ruptured bronchus from excessive suctioning through an endotracheal tube *(arrow)*. (Courtesy of Marie Capitanio, M.D., St. Christopher's Hospital for Children, Philadelphia, PA.)

narrowing are the size of the tube in relation to the size of the lumen of the airway, the number of tube changes, the tube material (rubber or plastic), and the type of sterilization (gas or chemical). Acquired subglottic stenoses are becoming more common with the aggressive use of PEEP and endotracheal intubation in the neonate. In Holinger's series of subglottic stenoses, approximately one third were acquired, and 86% of these were from endotracheal intubations. The acquired lesions were usually more severe than their congenital counterparts. Circumferential subglottic stenosis with a concomitant glottic web or stenosis was the most common endoscopic finding (see section on tracheal stenosis) (Holinger et al., 1976). Tracheotomies have been used in a large percentage of acquired subglottic stenoses as a temporizing procedure pending adequate growth of the airway.

Endobronchial granulation tissue formation can obstruct a bronchus and lead to acquired lobar emphysema (Miller et al., 1981) Tracheobronchomalacia can develop as a sequela to the mechanical injury incurred after intubation and ventilation in BPD (McCubbin et al., 1989). Mechanical injury has been implicated in the production of tracheobronchomegaly (Bhutani et al., 1986) (Fig. 21–29).

Feeding Catheters

Feeding catheters in neonates are usually threaded through the mouth and ultimately land in either the

stomach, duodenum, or jejunum, depending on their proposed functions. These polyvinyl tubes are frequently malpositioned in the pharynx or esophagus and can result in traumatic perforation of either, with concurrent pneumomediastinum, cervical emphysema, and pneumothorax. The perforation is usually on the right because the esophagus in the posterior mediastinum contacts the right parietal pleura just below the bifurcation of the trachea (Kassner et al., 1977). Clark et al. (1980) proposed that the rightward deviation and inadequate extramural support of the esophagus on the right predisposed the infant to perforation of the right wall of the esophagus. Most pharyngeal perforations occur on the posterior wall or piriform sinus. Traumatic pharyngeal and cervical esophageal pseudodiverticulum can mimic esophageal atresia and fistula (Lynch et al., 1974). Differentiation can sometimes be made by the associated extra-alveolar collection of air, the absence of a posterior impression on the trachea, and an increased distance between the trachea and esophagus (Lucaya et al., 1979).

The most common indication of perforation is difficulty in passing a feeding tube. The most common symptoms are respiratory distress, excessive salivation, choking, coughing, stridor, and increased oral

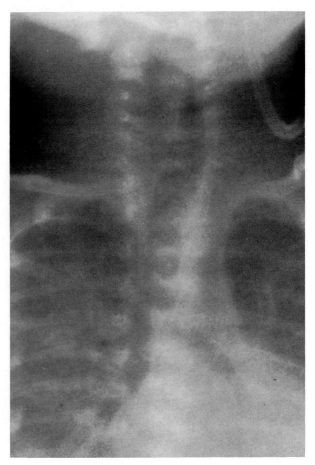

Figure 21–29. Anteroposterior view of the trachea and bronchi with tracheobronchomegaly secondary to chronic ventilatory therapy and bronchopulmonary disease.

secretions. There is usually a delay in diagnosis because the radiographic signs and clinical symptoms are not recognized. The false passage sometimes may be submucosal or retroesophageal. It can be localized to the neck or occasionally may extend below the diaphragm into the retroperitoneal space (Fig. 21–30). A small amount of water-soluble contrast material injected through the tube can identify the location of the perforation. Surgery is not usually required once the tube has been repositioned in the esophagus and the patient has been placed on antibiotic therapy and maintained on intravenous hyperalimentation for 10 days. A repeat contrast material examination should be performed after 10 to 14 days. Occasionally, the patient may develop a post-traumatic abscess that has to be surgically drained. Included in the differential diagnosis are spontaneous esophageal rupture, esophageal tracheal fistula with or without atresia, and congenital diverticula. Gastric pneumatosis has been reported as a complication of submucosal placement of the catheter (Mandell and Finkelstein, 1988).

Transpyloric polyvinyl tubes are used for feeding low-birth-weight infants in the intensive care nursery, to prevent aspiration pneumonitis and avoid the need for parenteral alimentation (Pereira and Lemons, 1981). Merten et al. (1980) reported on five infants with perforation of the duodenum from this procedure. Altered radiographic configuration of the tube

in the region of the superior or inferior flexure, associated with clinical deterioration, pneumoperitoneum, peritonitis, or a retroperitoneal fistula is diagnostic of duodenal perforation. Tubes should be positioned beyond the inferior flexure in the distal duodenum, avoiding the fixed portions of duodenum and consequent possible perforation (Siegle et al., 1976).

Pleural Drainage Tubes

Pleural drainage tubes are usually placed to relieve a respirator-induced tension pneumothorax. The most frequent complication is lung perforation. A review of autopsies of newborn infants (Moessinger et al., 1978) showed that 25% of percutaneous pleural drainages for relief of a pneumothorax perforate the lung. The clinical diagnosis of lung perforation is extremely difficult. Recovery of blood from the tracheostomy tube or the persistence of a large air leak suggests the diagnosis.

It is important to recognize lung perforation because it is potentially correctable. Increased density representing atelectasis or hemorrhage can be sometimes found around the tip of the tube on the radiograph (Strife et al., 1983). Radiographic determination of the penetrated lung position is difficult in the neonate. Two views of the chest (anteroposterior and

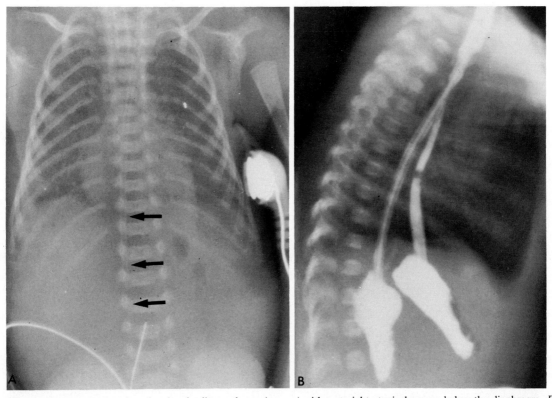

Figure 21–30. *A,* Anteroposterior view showing feeding catheter *(arrows)* with a straight atypical course below the diaphragm. *B,* Lateral view with aqueous contrast material placed through the feeding tube shows the retroperitoneal catheter. Contrast material is also seen anteriorly in the stomach and esophagus.

lateral) are sometimes helpful in the differentiation if the drainage tube seems not to have the ordinary peripheral course (Bowen and Zarabi, 1985).

Umbilical Catheters

Umbilical intravascular catheters are routinely used for exchange transfusions, monitoring of blood gases, hyperalimentation, and pressure estimation, and as a source of blood samples. No. 3.5 to 5 French radio-opaque polyvinyl catheters with end-holes to prevent clot formation are used for umbilical catheterization. The vessels usually remain patent for the first 4 days of life, but in hypoxic infants they may remain patent for longer. Fluoroscopy or anteroposterior and lateral radiographs should be used to verify proper catheter position (Baker et al., 1969).

The umbilical venous line is seldom used because of the risk of hepatic fibrosis, portal hypertension, and portal vein thromboembolism. The tip of the umbilical venous line should be positioned in the inferior vena cava near the right atrium after traversing a mild reverse "S" through the ductus venosus (Fig. 21–31). Liver necrosis and clot formation can result from improper positioning and infusion of hypertonic solutions and bicarbonate into the hepatic bed. Ultimately, hepatic calcifications (portal vein thromboemboli, ischemic infarcts, or ductus venosus) may form (Ablow and Effman, 1972; Rizzo et al., 1989). Perforation and hemorrhage can also occur with umbilical vein catheterization (Kanto and Parrish, 1977) (Fig. 21–32). Intracardiac catheters may produce cardiac arrhythmias, damage the cardiac valves, cause endocarditis, and perforate the myocardium (Symchych et al., 1977) (Fig. 21–33). Other less frequent complications include pulmonary emboli, infection, and colonic perforation after exchange transfusions (Sommerschild, 1971). Scott (1965) reported a 20% overall incidence of complications with the use of venous catheterization.

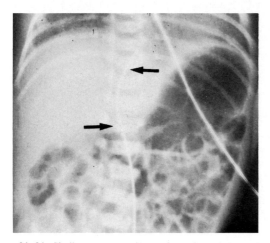

Figure 21–31. Shallow reverse "S" configuration of the umbilical venous line through the ductus venosus to the inferior vena cava (*arrows*).

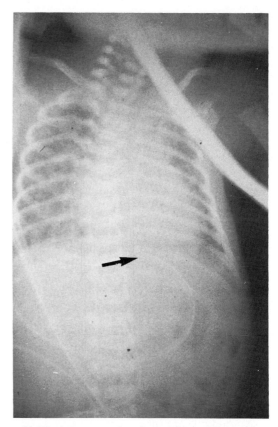

Figure 21–32. Anteroposterior view of the umbilical venous line in abnormal course, probably in the peritoneal cavity (*arrow*).

Umbilical arterial catheters ideally should be positioned between the upper vertebral plate of L3 and the lower plate of L4, avoiding the origins of the major abdominal arteries and the bifurcation of the aorta (Fig. 21–34). The catheter loops through the hypogastric–internal iliac arteries to reach the abdominal aorta. The alternative position is the sixth and seventh thoracic vertebral level in the descending aorta (Weber et al., 1974). The longer tubing probably increases the propensity toward thromboembolism. One should carefully avoid placing arterial lines in the left common carotid artery, innominate artery, external iliac artery, femoral artery, or pulmonary artery by means of the ductus arteriosus (Fig. 21–35). Thrombotic complications after umbilical artery catheterization ranged from 3.5% (Gupta et al., 1968) and 16% (Cochran et al., 1968) in clinical series. In an autopsy series Goetzman et al. (1975) found thrombotic complications in 24% of their patients. Although angiography shows an even higher incidence (Williams et al., 1972), most of the arteriographically demonstrated lesions are without clinical manifestations. Thromboses of the aorta and iliac, renal, celiac, splenic, and pulmonary arteries have been reported. Other complications of umbilical arterial catheterization include perforation of vessels with or without massive bleeding, peritoneal cavity perforation (Miller et al., 1979), umbilical arteriovenous fistulae, false aneurysms of the aorta (Spangler

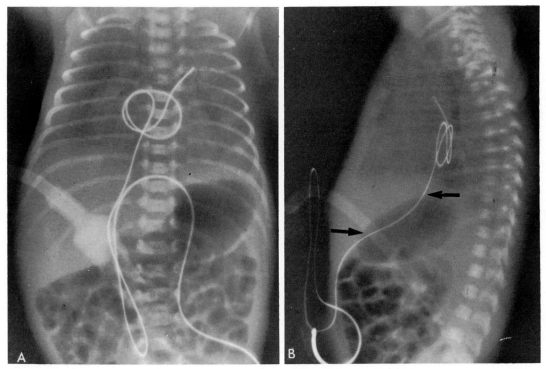

Figure 21–33. A coiled umbilical venous line in the left atrium, ending in the left superior pulmonary vein on AP *(A)* and lateral *(B)* views. A shallow "S" configuration coursing through the liver is seen on the lateral view *(arrows)*. The venous line traveled through the right atrium and foramen ovale to get to the left atrium and left pulmonary vein.

Figure 21–34. Lateral view depicting the umbilical artery catheter going from anterior (umbilicus) *(white arrow)* through the umbilical artery through the hypogastric-iliac artery complex to the aorta *(black arrow)*. The tip of the catheter is placed too high.

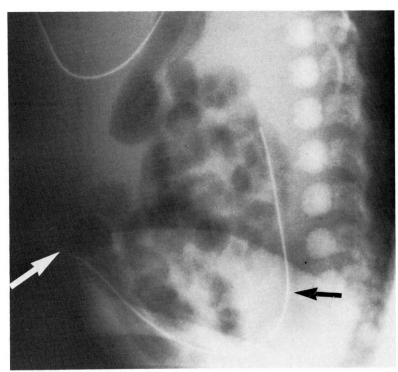

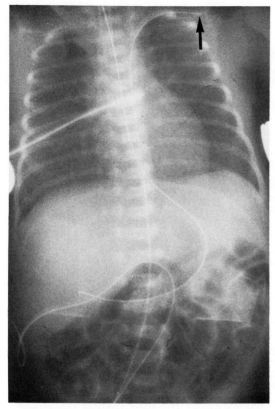

Figure 21–35. An umbilical artery line malpositioned in the left subclavian artery *(arrow).*

et al., 1977), infection and thromboembolic disease such as renal artery thrombosis with hypertension (Merten et al., 1978), gangrene of the buttock, spinal cord damage with paraplegia (Aziz and Robertson, 1973), and complete obstruction of the aorta.

Neonatal bladder rupture is a rare complication of umbilical artery catheterization (Diamond and Ford, 1989). The urachus arising from the dome of the neonatal bladder is in proximity to the umbilical arteries. The arteries and the urachus share the umbilical vesical fascia. The mortality is 18%. Surgical repair is necessary.

LUNG UNDERDEVELOPMENT

Bilateral Pulmonary Hypoplasia

Bilateral pulmonary hypoplasia commonly occurs secondary to some form of uterine compression of the fetal thorax that inhibits lung development. The causes include extrathoracic fetal compression, thoracic cage compression of the fetal lung, intrathoracic fetal compression of the lungs, and primary pulmonary hypoplasia with no obvious cause of compression.

Potter syndrome (Potter, 1946) is the best known cause of secondary pulmonary hypoplasia. Bilateral renal agenesis, severe polycystic kidney disease or

obstructive uropathy, and prune-belly syndrome can result in anuria or oliguria, oligohydramnios and compression of the fetal thorax and lungs by the uterus (Perlman and Levin, 1974). The cramped, compressed intrauterine environment also leads to abnormal facies, rib and spinal deformities, and abnormal foot configurations. Hypoplastic lungs can result in pneumomediastinum or pneumothorax on initiating respiration. Other causes of oligohydramnios such as amniotic fluid leakage and enlarged abdomen (ascites, mass) can lead to bilateral pulmonary hypoplasia (Perlman et al., 1976).

Bony dysplasias such as asphyxiating thoracic dystrophy, achondrogenesis, thanatophoric dwarfism, severe achondroplasia, hair-cartilage syndrome, and severe osteogenesis imperfecta can lead to pulmonary hypoplasia secondary to intrauterine compression of the lungs by the fetal thorax (Swischuk et al., 1979). Intrathoracic compression occurs with congenital diaphragmatic hernia or bilateral eventrations (see Figs. 21–41 and 21–42). Space occupying lesions such as bilateral fetal hydro-chylothorax, tumor or gigantic heart can result in pulmonary hypoplasia.

In primary or idiopathic pulmonary hypoplasia of the lungs, the neonates have respiratory distress, tachypnea, mild to moderate cyanosis, and abnormal blood gasses (Swischuk et al., 1979). The lungs are clear but small on radiographic examination. When several examinations show persistence of small lungs, the diagnosis of primary pulmonary hypoplasia is justified (Fig. 21–36).

Unilateral Pulmonary Agenesis and Hypoplasia

Some infants with unilateral pulmonary agenesis can have respiratory distress from the beginning (see Fig. 21–36). Pulmonary agenesis can occur on either side. Sometimes the chest cage development and configuration can be symmetric. In utero compensation for the expansion of one lung apparently has occurred. Right-sided agenesis with ipsilateral pulmonary artery agenesis is usually a greater problem than left-sided agenesis. The pronounced mediastinal shift to the right side causes more kinking of the great arteries, veins, and major bronchi (Fig. 21–37). Tracheal compression by the displaced aorta can occur. Severe complex cardiac and venous anomalies are more prevalent with right-sided agenesis. However, tetralogy of Fallot is frequently associated with left-sided involvement and ipsilateral pulmonary artery hypoplasia or agenesis. In addition to cardiac and vascular anomalies it is not unusual to find spinal, renal, genitourinary, and GI aberrations.

When there is unilateral agenesis the trachea continues directly into the opposite bronchus, and the ipsilateral pulmonary artery and veins are absent. No aeration of the agenetic lung is seen roentgenographically. The contralateral lung overdistends and usually herniates across the midline. Unilateral pulmonary

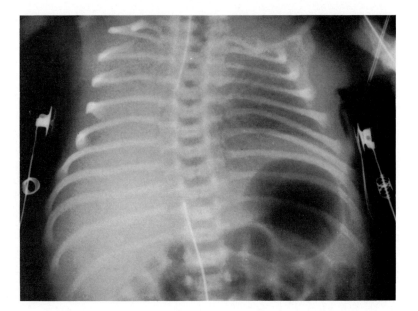

Figure 21–36. Anteroposterior radiograph with opacity of right lung due to lung fluid and shallow inspiration of left lung in 3-hour-old infant with primary pulmonary hypoplasia.

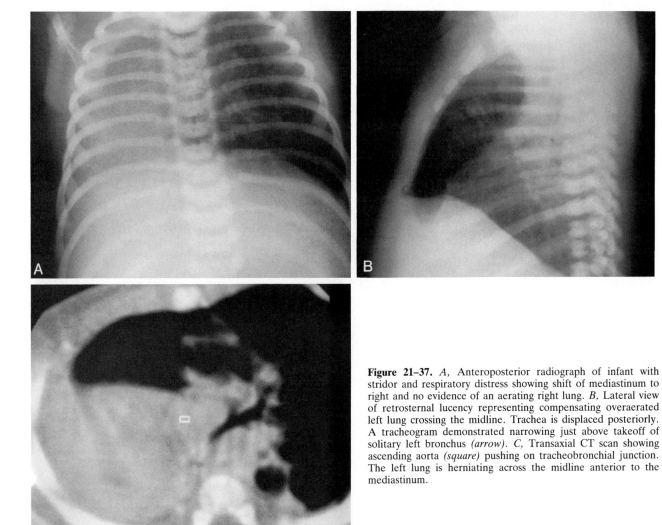

Figure 21–37. *A,* Anteroposterior radiograph of infant with stridor and respiratory distress showing shift of mediastinum to right and no evidence of an aerating right lung. *B,* Lateral view of retrosternal lucency representing compensating overaerated left lung crossing the midline. Trachea is displaced posteriorly. A tracheogram demonstrated narrowing just above takeoff of solitary left bronchus *(arrow). C,* Transaxial CT scan showing ascending aorta *(square)* pushing on tracheobronchial junction. The left lung is herniating across the midline anterior to the mediastinum.

hypoplasia can involve a lobe or an entire lung. Some of the pulmonary veins on the hypoplastic side may enter the vena cava. The "scimitar syndrome" consists predominantly of the anomalous pulmonary vein, the "scimitar shadow," or "Turkish sword," on the same side as the hypoplastic lung (usually on the right side) (Bourassa, 1963) (Fig. 21–38). The right bronchial tree may mimic the left. The upper or middle lobe bronchus may be hypoplastic or absent, and the right pulmonary artery is hypoplastic, stenosed, or absent. In some patients the abdominal aorta supplies the right lower lobe, simulating a sequestration. The degree of dextraposition of the heart depends on the severity of the right pulmonary hypoplasia. Associated anomalies include cardiac lesions, arteriovenous malformation, bronchiectasis, and duplication of the diaphragm (Bessolo and Maddison, 1969). The compartment formed between the two diaphragms contains the lower lobe or middle and lower lobes (Davis and Allen, 1968) (Fig. 21–39). An opening medially allows for passage of bronchi and vessels. On the anteroposterior radiograph of the chest, the right mediastinal-cardiac border may be indistinct as a result of the associated accessory diaphragm. On the lateral roentgenogram a retrosternal soft-tissue density parallels the sternum (Cremin and Bass, 1975). This represents extrapleural fibroalveolar tissue that adds to the right thorax because the accessory diaphragm prevented normal anterior development of the lung bud in utero.

With unilateral pulmonary hypoplasia, clinical findings can range from mild to moderate respiratory distress to no symptoms at all. The lungs are aerated but smaller than normal. Sometimes the lung appears radiographically hyperlucent because of pulmonary artery hypoplasia and decreased perfusion.

Diaphragmatic Hernia

A foramen of Bochdalek hernia of the diaphragm results from an incomplete closure of the pleuroperitoneal communication and accounts for 86% of congenital diaphragmatic hernias (Simpson and Eckstein, 1985). This failure of proper development of the posterolateral aspect of the diaphragm with abdominal contents in the chest usually results in cyanosis and tachypnea soon after birth. Death may occur suddenly as a result of cardiac and respiratory compression. Immediate radiologic recognition is imperative. An anteromedial retrosternal herniation via the foramen of Morgagni is rarer but can cause the same symptoms as the more common Bochdalek hernia.

The radiologic appearance of the chest and abdomen in anteroposterior and lateral projections is usually diagnostic in herniations of the diaphragm in the newborn. In most cases multiple gas-filled segments of intestine produce a cystic bubbly appearance in the left hemithorax (Fig. 21–40). The herniated contents may include stomach, small intestine, colon,

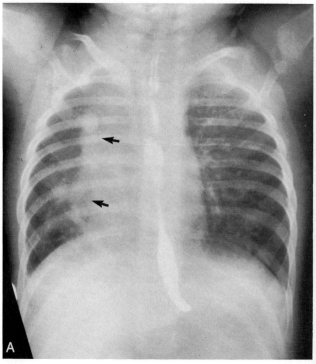
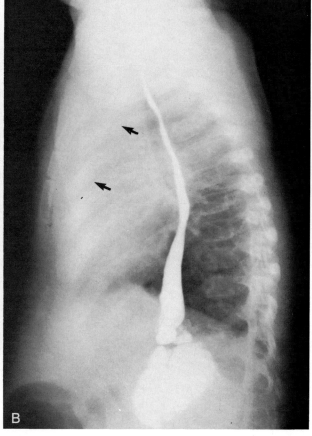

Figure 21–38. *A,* Anteroposterior radiograph showing "scimitar" sign (anomalous pulmonary vein draining below the diaphragm [*arrows*]). Mediastinal shift to right secondary to hypoplastic right lung. *B,* Lateral view with increased soft-tissue density *(arrows)* retrosternally representing extrapleural fibroalveolar tissue.

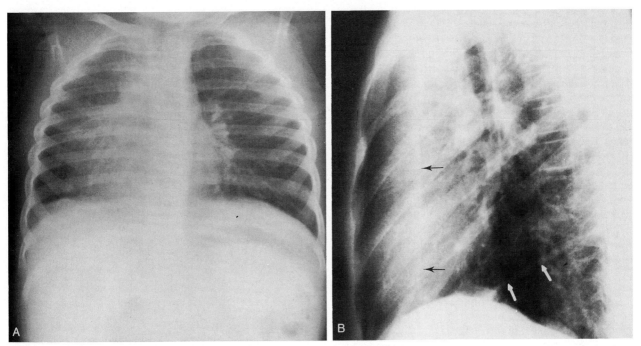

Figure 21–39. *A,* Anteroposterior radiograph with indistinct right mediastinal cardiac border secondary to anterior fibroalveolar tissue. Hypoplastic right lung allows shift of mediastinum to the right. *B,* Retrosternal parallel soft-tissue density on lateral view *(black arrows)* represents extrapleural fibroalveolar tissue. An accessory diaphragm is present *(white arrows).*

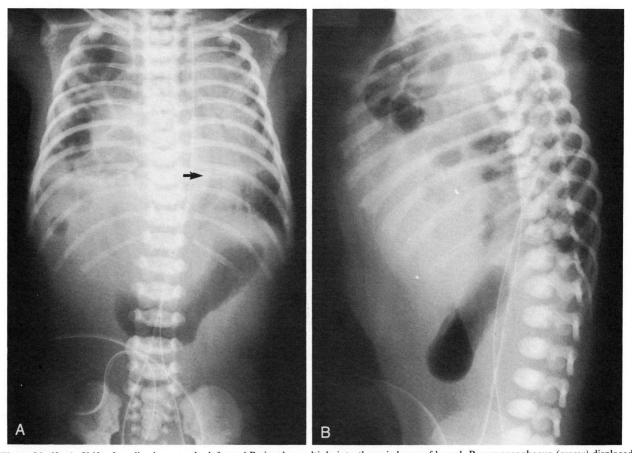

Figure 21–40. *A,* Shift of mediastinum to the left on AP view by multiple intrathoracic loops of bowel. Pneumoesophagus *(arrow)* displaced to the left. *B,* Scaphoid abdomen on lateral view.

liver, and spleen. An erect radiograph may depict multiple air–fluid levels in the chest. The mediastinum is displaced to the opposite hemithorax by the mass of herniated abdominal contents. The abdomen is usually scaphoid, lacking most of the customary viscera. Eighty-three to 96% of Bochdalek hernias occur on the left side. Acquired hernias (presenting after the newborn period) occur more commonly on the right, the large neonatal liver probably intervening as a protective organ (Wiseman and MacPherson, 1977). Morgagni hernias occur mostly on the right and can also have delayed presentation (Mandell and Finkelstein, 1989).

Herniated abdominal contents in the chest may prevent the normal formation of bronchi and alveoli, resulting in pulmonary hypoplasia. Herniation before the 16th week of gestation results in the greatest interference in the bronchial divisions. Infants with Type I hypoplasia have little, if any, hypoplasia and have the best prognosis (Berdon et al., 1965). Type II is severe bilateral pulmonary hypoplasia with resultant acidosis, hypoxia and death. The majority of patients have Type III with unilateral hypoplasia and survival depends on the degree of pulmonary underdevelopment.

There is a 30% to 40% survival rate of infants who undergo surgery in the first 24 hours. Immediate postoperative use of chest tube prevents significant pneumothorax and maintains stability until the hypoplastic lung expands to fill the hemithorax. The abdomen at surgery may be too small to accommodate the repositioned viscera, and a ventral abdominal wall defect is created with a temporary Silastic or skin covering, allowing the gradual enlargement of the abdomen (approximately 7 to 10 days).

Some patients may be initially asymptomatic with the appearance of the chest relatively normal for a few days up to several months after birth. In infants, acquired diaphragmatic hernias with delayed presentation can follow streptococcal infection (McCarten et al., 1981).

Congenital Eventration of the Diaphragm

Eventration of the diaphragm is an abnormal elevation of all or part of the intact diaphragm. The diaphragm is usually deficient in muscle fibers, giving it a membranous appearance. Eventration can be unilateral or bilateral (Garbaccio et al., 1972). Partial eventrations are usually right-sided and total eventrations are predominantly left-sided. Most eventrations are asymptomatic, but very large or bilateral deficiencies occasionally cause respiratory distress (Avnet, 1962; Lundstrom and Allen, 1966).

Radiologically, eventrations present as localized bulges of the diaphragm, either anteriorly with obliteration of the cardiac silhouette, or posteriorly as a diaphragmatic bulge. Total eventration elevates the whole diaphragm. The eventration may include stom-

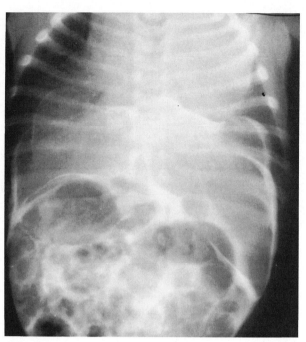

Figure 21–41. Anteroposterior radiograph shows bilaterally elevated diaphragms and small lung volumes due to eventration.

ach, colon, kidney, small intestine, spleen, liver, and adrenal gland (Wayne et al., 1974). Under fluoroscopy, the localized bulge usually enlarges with deeper inspiration (more abdominal contents protruding through the area of weakness). Total eventration displays paradoxical motion of the involved diaphragm. Peritoneography with water-soluble iodine contrast medium (Otherson and Lorenzo, 1977) can differentiate a hernia from an eventration. In some Bochdalek hernias the contrast medium penetrates the pleural space. Ultrasound can also detect an eventration, especially on the right side (Moccia et al., 1981).

Surgical intervention is necessary if medical management fails to impede the progression of the respiratory insufficiency. Some total eventrations, similar to Bochdalek hernias, result in pulmonary hypoplasia (Fig. 21–41).

Phrenic Nerve Paralysis (Acquired Eventration)

Cervical nerve root trauma at birth and phrenic nerve injury during thoracic surgery are the most common causes of diaphragmatic paralysis (Fig. 21–42). The right diaphragm is affected more commonly than the left and can be associated with Erb palsy (Adams and Gyepes, 1971). Diaphragmatic paralysis has also been reported after chest tube placement (Phillips et al., 1981). Paralysis is usually mild, and symptoms are virtually absent. Paradoxical cephalad motion of the diaphragm on inspiration prevents normal air entry into the lung on the affected side

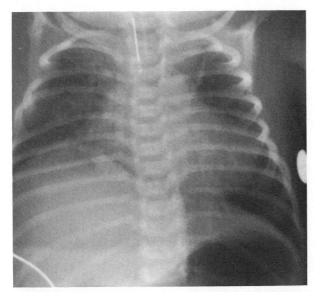

Figure 21–42. Postoperative AP view after repair of tetralogy of Fallot. Note elevation of the right diaphragm representing acquired traumatic phrenic palsy. Surgical plication was required.

and produces a marked shift of the mediastinum to the opposite side with impairment of the contralateral lung. In the very young patient, weak intercostal musculature and the recumbent position contribute to the respiratory distress.

Diagnosis of diaphragmatic paralysis can be made by routine chest radiographs, perhaps aided by fluoroscopy. The marked elevation of the affected diaphragm is apparent when the right diaphragm is two interspaces above the left or when the left hemidiaphragm is one interspace above the right. Fluoroscopy shows paradoxical motion of the affected side. Ultrasonography can be used to demonstrate diaphragmatic paralysis and monitor diaphragmatic activity (Ambler et al., 1985).

Paralysis of the diaphragm requires intervention with plication if the infant requires prolonged mechanical ventilation (usually about 2 weeks) (Schwartz and Fille, 1978). Many paralyzed diaphragms return to normal function after 6 to 12 months. Some diaphragms resume normal physiology even after surgical trauma to the phrenic nerve.

Cystic Adenomatoid Malformation

Cystic adenomatoid malformation is a cystic dysplastic process with abnormal proliferation of the bronchioli that fail to join alveolar mesenchyma, causing cysts of varying size, absence of normal bronchial cartilage, absence of bronchial tubular glands, abundance of terminal bronchiolar structures, and tremendous enlargement of the affected lobe (Hueck-Parodi et al., 1969). No inflammation is present (Heij et al., 1990). The lesion is usually unilateral, involving all or part of a lung. In the early neonatal period the involved lung can be opaque because it is filled by physiologic fluid. The cysts gradually fill with

air from direct bronchial connections or collateral aeration (Fig. 21–43).

Bubbles or cysts become large and radiographically mimic pneumatoceles of staphylococcal pneumonia or the air-filled loops of congenital diaphragmatic hernia. There is shift of the mediastinum (indicated by the position of the nasogastric tube) to the contralateral side. The abdominal gas pattern in cystic adenomatoid malformation is normal as opposed to the scaphoid abdomen in diaphragmatic hernia. The differentiation sometimes is difficult and requires placement of contrast media in the GI tract. Staphylococcal pneumatoceles are uncommon in the neonatal period.

Most commonly the child presents with respiratory distress at birth and the enlarging cystic structures gradually compress the contralateral lung with a shift of the mediastinum. As many as two thirds of patients with cystic adenomatoid malformation can present later in life (Hulnick et al., 1984).

Therapy is the immediate extirpation of the involved segment, because displacement of the heart may interfere with normal venous return and cardiac function. No long-term impairment of pulmonary function occurs in these patients.

Congenital Lobar Emphysema

Some infants are asymptomatic, but others present with severe respiratory distress. Breath sounds are

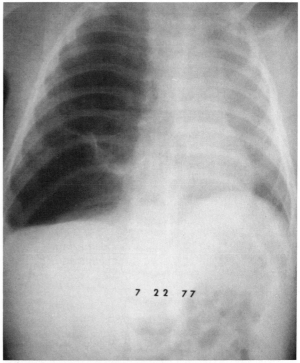

Figure 21–43. Anteroposterior radiograph of chest with hyperlucent right lung containing septa indicative of multiple cysts of cystic adenomatoid malformation. The mediastinum is displaced to left with some compression of the left lung.

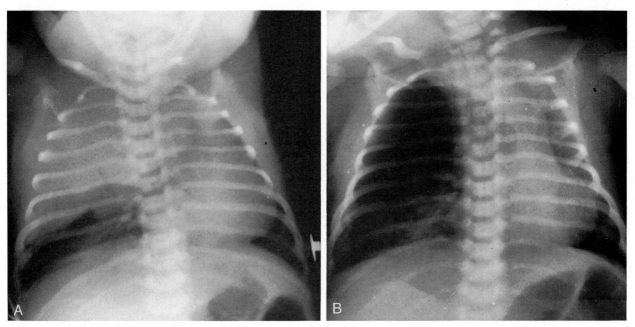

Figure 21–44. *A,* Anteroposterior chest radiograph with fluid in the upper two thirds of the right hemithorax producing mass effect with displacement of mediastinum to the left in first day of life. *B,* The next day, the fluid resorbed. There is right upper lobe hyperaeration due to congenital lobar emphysema.

usually diminished over the hyperexpanded, hyperresonant hemithorax. The upper lobes, especially the left, are more frequently involved, but middle lobe involvement is not uncommon. There is a high association of lobar emphysema with congenital heart disease, with involvement of the middle lobe and lingula. The emphysema could be secondary to the large right pulmonary artery or left atrium pressing on the bronchial tree (Jones et al., 1965).

Most cases result from collapse of the bronchus secondary to segmental bronchial cartilage underdevelopment. This leads to bronchial wall collapse and a ball valve obstruction and air trapping. Other causes of bronchial obstruction include stenosis, mucus plugs, and extrinsic masses. The polyalveolar form exhibits excessive alveolar multiplication. In the usual case of congenital lobar emphysema the affected hyperlucent, overdistended lobe with widely dispersed pulmonary vasculature usually shifts the mediastinum to the contralateral side. Secondary compression of the ipsilateral lower lobe is seen with upper lobe emphysema. In some cases the involved overdistended lungs are opaque rather than hyperlucent (Fig. 21–44). Fluid accumulates proximal to the obstruction, but later on the fluid clears and the lung configuration is transformed to the classic chest appearance.

Conservative therapy without surgical intervention results in a mortality of 50%. Most often treatment consists of an emergency lobectomy. Some cases of congenital emphysema, however, can remain static and asymptomatic for years (Leape and Longino, 1964).

AIRWAY OBSTRUCTION

Choanal Obstruction

Choanal atresia is the most common congenital anomaly of the nose. It is usually bilateral, the obstruction being osseous 90% of the time. Bilateral choanal atresia is commonly associated with other congenital anomalies such as craniofacial anomalies, congenital heart disease, and tracheoesophageal fistula. Severe respiratory distress with asphyxia can result. The diagnosis is strongly suggested by the inability to pass a firm catheter through each nostril. Diagnosis by plain radiography with oily contrast material has been virtually replaced by CT (Fig. 21–45). In a plane 10 to 15 degrees to the hard palate, the diagnosis can be made (Chinwuba et al., 1986; Slovis et al., 1985). There is medial bowing and thickening of the lateral wall of the nasal cavity on CT. In membranous atresia the air passage between the lateral wall of the nasal cavity and the vomer is reduced. Secretions in the nose can accumulate and result in a falsely thickened appearance of the narrowed segment.

Congenital Masses Associated With Stridor

A normal and frequently observed mass of soft tissue in the anterior mediastinum on the chest radiograph in the neonate is the thymus. The thymus

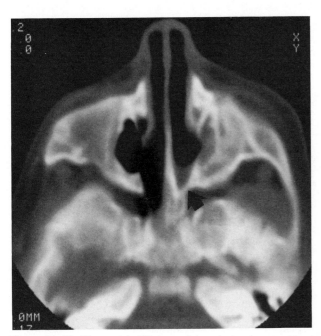

Figure 21–45. Transaxial CT scan demonstrates bony septum *(arrow)* with associated secretions on left side.

increases in size in the first few months. The cardinal difference between thymus and other mediastinal masses is its soft texture. The classic appearance of thymus on the posteroanterior chest radiograph is one of bilateral, smoothly outlined superior mediastinal fullnesses blending in with the cardiac silhouette. Occasional unilateral prominence produces the classic "sail sign" on radiograph. On the lateral projection, the thymus fills the anterosuperior mediastinal space. The sail configuration is sometimes seen radiographically when one lobe predominates. The undulating

pattern produced by the anterior ribs pressing on the thymus is evidence of its soft character. Thymic tissue is flexible, changing dramatically in size under fluoroscopy or on inspiration–expiration chest radiographs (Fig. 21–46). Firmer masses are fairly static in size and produce impressions or compressions of the tracheobronchial tree. The pliable thymus does not interfere with the airway. When the thymus starts to compress or narrow the trachea or bronchus with resultant atelectasis, thymic infiltration with lymphosarcoma, leukemia, and histiocytosis should be suspected.

A prominent right thymic lobe may be confused with upper lobe consolidation. Rarely, an aberrant thymus can extend posteriorly or into the cervical region and mimic a superior mediastinal or neck mass (Malone and Fitzgerald, 1987; Shackelford and McAlister, 1974) or upper lobe atelectasis (Lanning and Heikkinen, 1980) (Fig. 21–47). The posterior mediastinal thymus can deviate the esophagus and trachea while the cervical thymus sharply displaces the cervical trachea to the right (left thymic lobe usually dominant) and posteriorly at the thoracic inlet. The posterior mediastinal thymus can be differentiated from other masses by CT or MRI (Cohen et al., 1983; Rollins and Currarino, 1988). Cervical thymus lends itself to real-time ultrasonography (Mandell et al., 1991).

Posterior pharyngeal soft-tissue masses can impinge on the airway and displace it anteriorly. The most common tumor, cystic hygroma, is a congenital malformation of the cervical lymph sac (Fig. 21–48A). Sonographically, these tumors are sonolucent and multicystic or multiseptated. Echogenicity can occur from bleeding into the cysts. MRI defines the boundaries of the cystic hygroma well for the surgeon (Fig. 21–48B). Some hygromas extend from the neck down

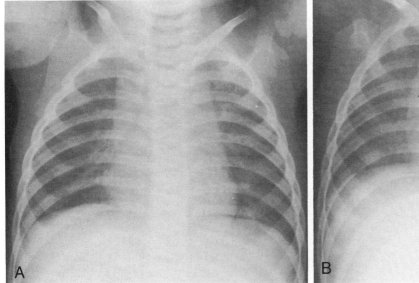 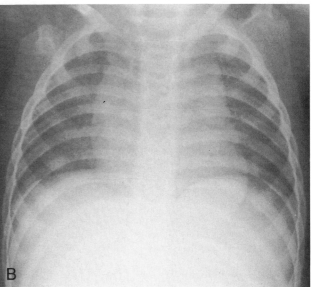

Figure 21–46. Normal change of neonatal thymus on inspiration *(A)* with decrease in dimension and on exhalation *(B)* with increased size.

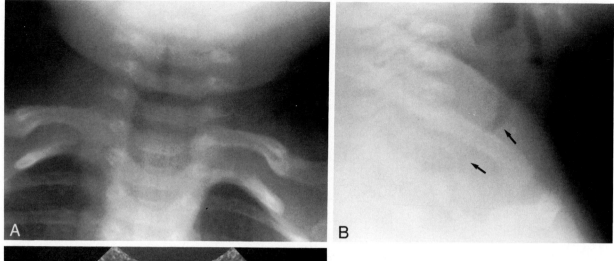

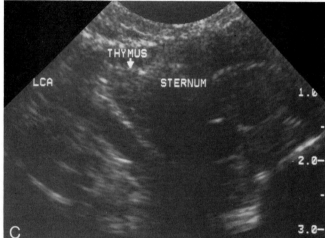

Figure 21–47. *A,* Anteroposterior view of neck and upper chest with 90-degree bend of trachea due to right cervical thymus. *B,* Lateral view of neck showing posterior displacement and impression on trachea at thoracic inlet *(arrows).* *C,* Real-time sagittal ultrasound confirmation of homogeneous textured mass of cervical thymus *(arrow)* projecting cephalad to the sternum.

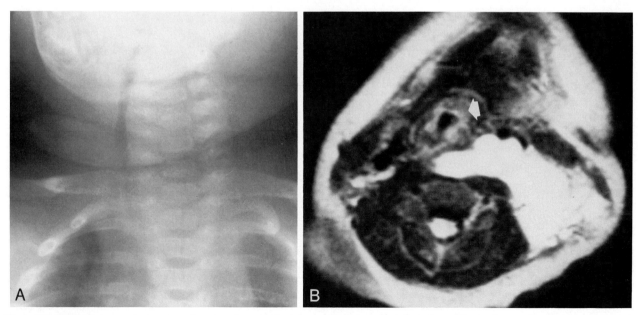

Figure 21–48. *A,* Anteroposterior view of neck and upper chest demonstrating marked deviation of the trachea to the right by a large soft-tissue mass occupying the left side of the neck. *B,* T2-weighted, MRI scan with high-signal multiseptated mass (compatible with cystic hygroma) emanating from left side and pushing larynx *(arrow)* to the right.

to the mediastinum. Hemangiomas of the neck are less common. Ultrasound usually shows homogeneous echogenicity of these tumors. Hemangiomas can be treated with steroids but naturally regress in some instances. Other congenital neck masses include teratoma and goiter.

Hemangiomas can also occur in the subglottic portion of the airway. The subglottic hemangioma is the most common soft-tissue mass causing airway obstruction in infancy. Half have associated cutaneous lesions (Benjamin and Carter, 1983). Dyspnea, croupy cough, and inspiratory stridor are the earliest and most common symptoms. The lesion characteristically is a smooth nodule a few millimeters below the cords that projects anteriorly off the posterolateral wall of the trachea.

Other Mediastinal Masses

This group includes bronchopulmonary and foregut malformations as well as neurogenic tumors. These are beyond the scope of this chapter.

Laryngomalacia

Laryngomalacia, a soft, flaccid larynx, produces inspiratory stridor from birth. Laryngomalacia is the most common abnormality of the larynx in infancy. The stridor usually improves with crying and activity. An infolding of the soft, redundant aryepiglottic folds leads to collapse of the airway and minor obstruction. With maturation the folds become firmer and more resistant to the inspiratory forces. By 2 years of age, 90% of infant stridor resolves (Lane et al., 1984). Persistence of laryngomalacia in older children can be associated with underlying neuromuscular disease (i.e., cerebral palsy) (Smith and Cooper, 1981). Anteromedial bending of the bellies of the aryepiglottic folds with ballooning of the pyriform sinuses on lateral airway examination is suggestive of laryngomalacia (Fig. 21–49).

Congenital Tracheal Stenosis

Congenital tracheal stenosis involves intrinsic narrowing of the lumen of the trachea due to small and inflexible cartilaginous rings. The patient may have wheezing or inspiratory stridor. There is an association with H-type tracheoesophageal fistulae and pulmonary slings (Berdon et al., 1984). High-kilovoltage magnification imaging and MRI can show the length of the stenosis (Hernandez and Tucker, 1987). Fluoroscopy of the airway can demonstrate dynamics. Tracheal size can be assessed with MRI or CT (Effman et al., 1983). Most stenoses are acquired secondary to intubation.

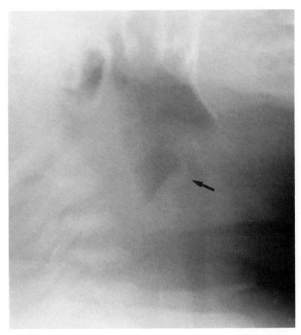

Figure 21–49. Lateral view of airway showing redundant aryepiglottic folds bowed forward *(arrow)*.

Tracheomalacia

Tracheomalacia is thought to be a weakness in the trachea caused by a softening of the supporting cartilage (Baxter and Dunbar, 1963; Benjamin, 1984) from intrinsic or extrinsic causes. Tracheomalacia is usually due to extrinsic compression from vascular anomalies (double aortic arch, anomalous innominate artery, and pulmonary sling) or mass effect (esophageal atresia, cystic hygroma, bronchogenic cyst, duplication cyst, and cervical thymus). In children with esophageal atresia and tracheoesophageal fistulae, the tracheomalacia is produced by the dilated proximal esophagus, which pushes the trachea into the crossing innominate artery. The tracheomalacia can persist for many months after the corrective surgery. The vascular causes usually result in stridor, wheezing, or respiratory distress; feeding difficulties may also accompany tracheomalacia. Radiographically, the segment of malacia collapses on exhalation and distends on inhalation (Fig. 21–50).

Double Aortic Arch

The double aortic arch is the most common vascular ring. It represents a persistence of both a right and a left aortic arch and is a true vascular ring because it encircles the trachea and the esophagus. The ascending aorta arises anterior to the trachea, divides into an anterior and posterior branch and joins posteriorly to form a common descending aorta. The descending aorta may be on the left or the right. Variables include the size of the arches, the patency, and

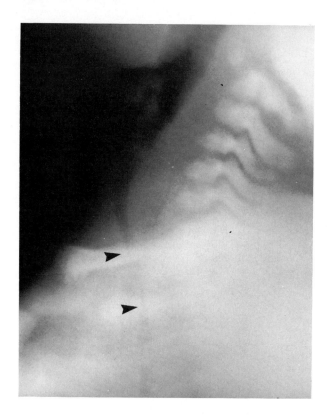

Figure 21–50. Lateral radiograph of airway demonstrating collapse of trachea at thoracic inlet on exhalation indicative of tracheomalacia. The trachea was normal, and no vascular ring was present on barium swallow.

position of the upper descending aorta, and the sight of the ductus arteriosus. The right arch is usually the largest and passes posterior to the trachea and esophagus. Radiographically, the trachea can be indented on its right side and malpositioned in the middle of the mediastinum or slightly displaced to the left. An anterior bowing can be seen by the retrotracheal aorta (Fig. 21–51). The esophagram shows bilateral indentations on the anteroposterior view. The right indentation is usually higher and larger because of the larger right aortic arch. A variation of the double aortic arch is a right aortic arch with an aberrant left subclavian with or without a diverticulum and a left ductus arteriosus. MRI can define the anomaly well enough for a surgical approach (Coscina et al., 1986; Gomes et al., 1987).

Anomalous Innominate

In young children the right innominate artery normally arises to the left of the trachea and crosses the trachea anteriorly and to the right as it ascends into the mediastinum and neck. Less commonly the left carotid arises at a point more proximal than normal and the vessel courses from right to left anterior to the trachea. In a small percentage of children the airway is narrowed by tracheomalacia and extrinsic compression secondary to this crossing vessel. Radiographically, there is an anterior tracheal indentation (Fig. 21–52). Persistent anterior tracheal collapse and indentation can be seen on fluoroscopy. MRI can also demonstrate extent of trachea narrowing and its

relationship to the innominate vessel (Fletcher et al., 1986). A few patients require surgery because of persistent respiratory distress (Strife et al., 1981).

Right Aortic Arch

The right aortic arch basically consists of two types. In the first type the right arch arises anterior and to the right of the trachea and esophagus. It is associated with cyanotic heart disease. There is no large posterior indentation. A small posterior indentation can occur with an anomalous left subclavian vessel crossing obliquely from right to left. The second type of right aortic arch exhibits a large posterior indentation and may be associated with a ring depending on the presence of an anomalous left subclavian artery or a diverticulum and the position of the ductus arteriosus. The position of the right aortic arch is inferred from the location of the trachea toward the left. However, half of all right aortic arches have normal position of the trachea (Strife et al., 1989). High-kilovoltage roentgenograms (Wolfe et al., 1978) and the unilateral dense thoracic spine pedicles (indicating side of descent) are sometimes helpful in locating the elusive aorta.

Pulmonary Sling

The pulmonary sling consists of the left pulmonary artery arising from the right pulmonary artery and crossing between the trachea and the esophagus

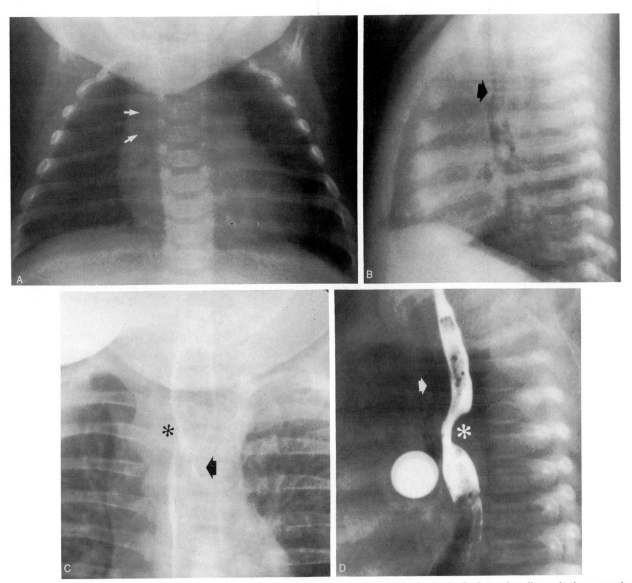

Figure 21–51. *A,* Anteroposterior view of patient with stridor and right aortic arch *(arrows). B,* Lateral radiograph demonstrating constriction of trachea *(arrow)* at the aortic arch level. *C,* Esophagogram in AP view with large, more superior impression on the right side *(asterisk)* and smaller, inferior impression on the left side *(arrow)* of the double aortic arches. *D,* Lateral view of esophagogram with large posterior vascular impression *(asterisk)* and indentation of anterior tracheal wall by the vascular ring *(arrow).*

slightly above the carina (Capitanio et al., 1971). The distal trachea and carina are usually displaced to the left. The anomalous vessel can indent the right bronchus or distal trachea posteriorly. Barium-filled esophagus shows posterior indentation of the trachea and anterior impression (Fig. 21–53). Bronchogenic cysts can occasionally produce a similar appearance when wedged between the trachea and esophagus. CT, MRI, and angiography can be performed to demonstrate the anomaly (Malmgren et al., 1988).

Vocal Cord Palsy

In vocal cord palsy, there are often associated anomalies of the CNS (usually myelomeningocele and

hydrocephalus) or cardiovascular anomalies predisposing to vagus or recurrent laryngeal nerve injury. Birth injury with stretching of the neck has also been associated with vocal cord palsy, as have surgical trauma and infection. Rare causes of congenital laryngeal abductor paralysis due to brain stem dysgenesis have been reported. Unilateral vocal cord palsy occurs in 38% to 47% of all cases. Left-sided palsy (79% to 91%) occurs much more often than right-sided palsy. The difference has been attributed to the longer, more vulnerable pathway of the left recurrent laryngeal nerve. Vocal cord dysfunction can occur secondary to the cannulation procedures for ECMO. The incidence of spontaneous recovery from palsy is 40% to 48%. Rounding of the laryngeal ventricle may be visible on the lateral neck radiograph (Cohen et al., 1982; Dedo, 1979) (Fig. 21–54).

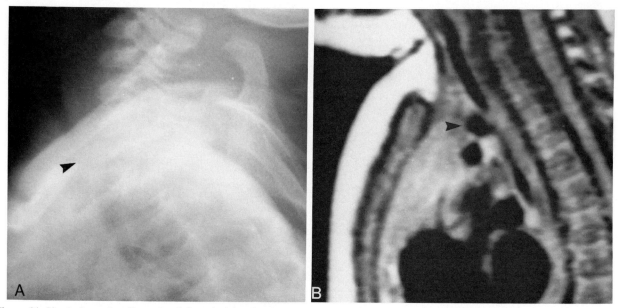

Figure 21–52. *A,* Lateral radiograph of thoracic inlet showing collapse of trachea *(arrow)* at point of impression of crossing vessel on exhalation. *B,* Sagittal T1-weighted MRI scan with anomalous innominate artery *(arrow)* pressing on anterior trachea at thoracic inlet.

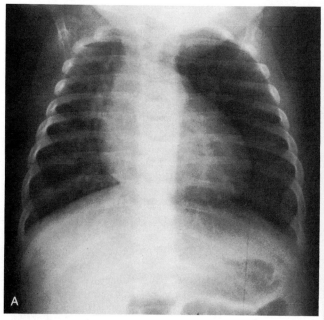

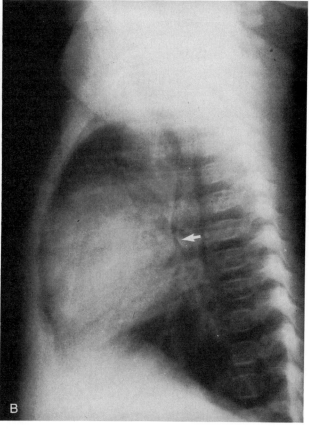

Figure 21–53. *A,* Anteroposterior radiograph showing a hyperlucent left lung in patient with stridor. *B,* Lateral view of chest showing both carina *(arrow)* and right bronchus being bowed forward by anomalous pulmonary artery.

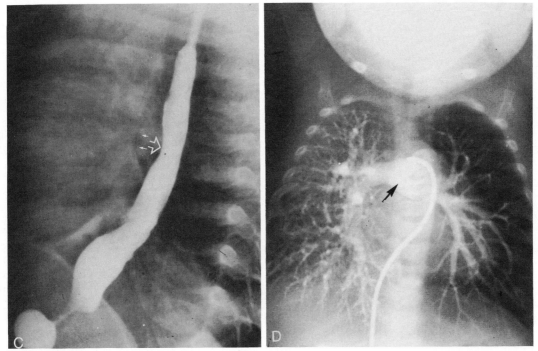

Figure 21–53. *Continued C,* Esophagogram in lateral view showing anterior impression on upper esophagus *(open arrow)* and again anterior bowing of the carina *(small arrows). D,* Arteriogram demonstrating left pulmonary artery originating from the right side *(arrow).*

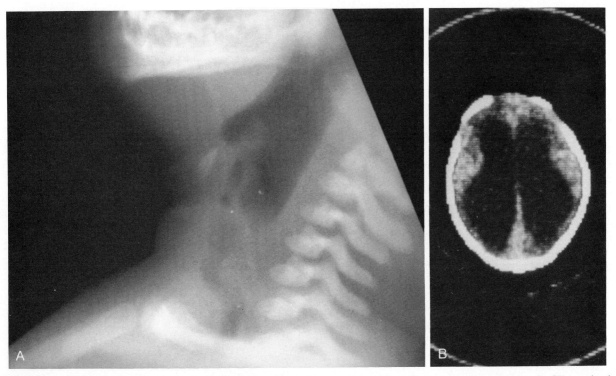

Figure 21–54. *A,* Lateral radiograph of upper airway showing rounded laryngeal ventricle indicative of vocal cord palsy. *B,* CT examination of brain demonstrates marked associated hydrocephalus.

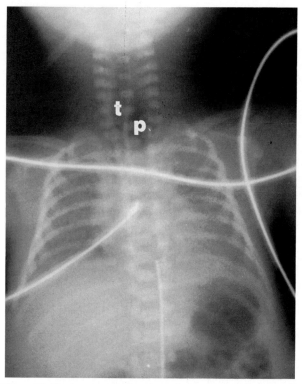

Figure 21–55. Anteroposterior view of chest showing trachea (t) deviated to right by air-filled pouch (p) of the esophageal atresia. Gas in the abdomen indicates an associated fistula.

GASTROINTESTINAL PROBLEMS

Tracheoesophageal Fistula

Tracheoesophageal fistula is part of the esophageal atresia complex. About 90% of lesions consist of a proximal esophageal atresia with a distal fistula from the distal esophageal segment to the tracheobronchial tree. Esophageal atresia is suspected on the basis of polyhydramnios, inability to swallow saliva or formula, aspiration during early feedings, or inability to pass a catheter successfully into the stomach. Naturally occurring air can be used to demonstrate the atresia (Fig. 21–55). Contrast material should seldom be used because of probability of aspiration. Radiographically, the trachea can be deviated by the proximal esophageal pouch. A distal fistula may be evidenced by an overaerated GI tract. Determination of aortic arch placement is helpful in deciding the approach for anastomosis of the proximal and distal esophageal segments as well as ligation of the fistula.

Chalasia

Lack of closure of the distal esophageal sphincter at rest produces gastroesophageal reflux. Clinical features include vomiting, aspiration pneumonia, apneic spells, chronic pulmonary disease, failure to thrive, rumination, and Sandifer's syndrome (torsions of head and neck mimicking torticollis or seizure activity). A barium swallow can demonstrate gastroesophageal reflux. Minor reflux occurs in the distal esophagus. Major reflux into the upper esophagus is responsible for chronic aspiration and refractory pulmonary disease (Fig. 21–56). Either type can result in esophagitis and stricture. An aeroesophagus on chest radiograph usually is indicative of esophageal sphincter dysfunction. Achalasia, H-type tracheoesophageal fistula, and air hunger in the premature infant with hyaline membrane disease (see Fig. 21–1) are other causes of aeroesophagus.

Congenital Gastric Anomalies

Antral duplication, antral diaphragm or web, and microgastria can cause vomiting. Antral duplications are usually located in the antropyloric region. The mass of the cyst can encroach on the barium-filled stomach and cause a thin barium track (Pruksapong et al., 1979). Gastric atresia is rare. Most diaphragms are considered forms of atresia but are usually non-obstructing. Data suggest that the membrane is secondary to intrauterine stress, vascular insult, or anoxia (Cremin, 1969; Santulli and Blanc, 1961). Radiographically, the double-bulb appearance is sometimes seen (Fig. 21–57). Microgastria is a rare

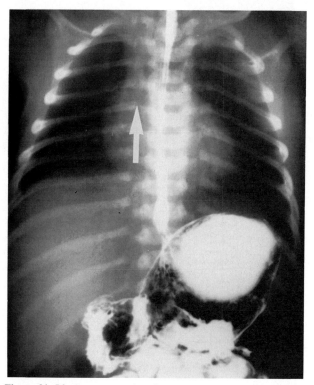

Figure 21–56. Anteroposterior view of chest and upper abdomen demonstrating a barium-filled esophagus secondary to significant reflux from stomach to above the thoracic inlet.

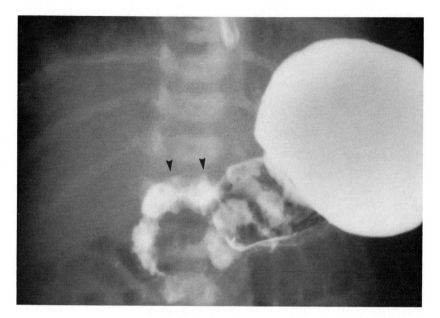

Figure 21–57. Anteroposterior view of the stomach and duodenum showing a double-bulb configuration *(arrows)* indicative of an antral web.

condition in which the stomach is midline in position and rudimentary in size. Gastroesophageal reflux is common because food collects in the esophagus as a result of the low storage capacity of the stomach. Microgastria is associated with asplenia-polysplenia syndrome (Kessler and Smulewicz, 1973).

Pylorospasm

Pylorospasm is radiographically similar to pyloric stenosis. It has a propensity to occur in the adreno-genital syndrome and in infants with severe neurologic damage usually secondary to cerebral hemorrhage. The caliber of the pyloric channel in pylorospasm in some cases is changeable (see Fig. 21–11*C*). In tight cases ultrasound is useful in showing normal thickness of the muscle of the antrum. (See section on meconium aspiration.)

Gastric Volvulus

Gastric volvulus can occur in early infancy and produces acute gastric obstruction. Most cases are of the mesenteroaxial type, wherein the stomach twists and flips into an inverted position. Radiographically, the distended stomach is inverted (Ziprkowski and Teele, 1978). Gastric volvulus is associated with asplenia and diaphragmatic hernia.

Gastric Perforation

Neonatal gastric ulcerations and perforations, usually secondary to anoxia or stress, result in the largest intraperitoneal air collections from enteric sources

(see also section on pneumoperitoneum) (James et al., 1976). Perforations of the ileum are next in frequency. Indomethacin therapy for ductus closure has also been implicated to cause focal ischemia and perforation (Gray, 1980). A large pneumoperitoneum, absence of gastric air, and (usually) absence of ventilator support help to confirm the diagnosis of gastric perforation. A nasogastric tube that extends beyond the contour of the stomach is definite evidence of perforation (Coopersmith and Rabinowitz, 1973).

The radiographic detection of pneumoperitoneum and the differentiation of enteric and mediastinal causes is discussed in the section on pneumoperitoneum.

Duodenal Obstructions

Duodenal atresia and stenosis are relatively common causes of congenital GI tract obstruction. Children with these aberrations usually present with bilious vomiting in the first few hours of life. Many affected children have Down syndrome. A double-bubble sign on radiography signifies atresia or stenosis of the duodenum (Fig. 21–58), annular pancreas, and malrotation secondary to crossing Ladd bands. Barium enema can be helpful in defining the location of the cecum if malrotation is contemplated.

Rotational Anomalies

Some rotational anomalies are asymptomatic, but others can result in ischemia and necrosis of the bowel. The GI tract is located outside the abdomen during fetal development. As the bowel gradually

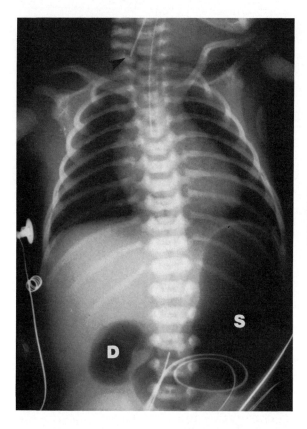

Figure 21–58. Anteroposterior radiograph of chest and upper abdomen showing the presence of a double bubble (stomach [S] and duodenum [D]) indicative of duodenal atresia. In neck, feeding tube *(arrow)* in proximal esophageal pouch is indicative of concurrent tracheoesophageal atresia and fistula.

enters the abdomen the duodenum is fixed retroperitoneally on the right. The small intestine extends along a mesentery from the left upper quadrant to the right lower quadrant of the abdomen. The transverse colon lies most anteriorly, and the cecum becomes retroperitonealized last in the right lower quadrant. Rotational anomalies consist of nonrotation and reversed rotation. In nonrotation the small intestine lies entirely on the right and the large intestine on the left. This condition often is asymptomatic. In malrotation the cecum and terminal ileum are generally misplaced upwardly and medially. The small intestine is abnormally fixed and mainly right-sided. The duodenum is often fixed by bands, and the abnormally fixed small intestine is predisposed to midgut volvulus. When this occurs the entire gut twists around the superior mesenteric artery and vascular compromise occurs.

Infants with duodenal bands, with or without volvulus, usually present with bilious vomiting. Barium study of the proximal bowel demonstrates linear indentation of the third portion of the duodenum and a beaked, tapered appearance if volvulus is also present (Simpson et al., 1972). In volvulus, plain radiographic findings vary from normal-appearing abdomen to a gastric outlet obstruction to a small intestinal obstruction. The appearance depends on number of twists of intestine and its viability. The barium enema can be performed to demonstrate the cecum malpositioned high under the transverse colon. Ultrasonic examination can show the midgut volvulus (Hayden et al., 1984).

Necrotizing Enterocolitis

Necrotizing enterocolitis (NEC) is a disease of unknown origin usually affecting premature infants (90% born at less than 36 weeks of gestation) (Kliegman and Fanaroff, 1984). Epidemiologic observations emphasize the potential roles of infection, enteric feeding, and local vascular compromise of the GI tract in the pathogenesis of this disease. For the most part, NEC is sporadic, but it can be epidemic.

The neonate presents with systemic signs and symptoms suggestive of sepsis and shock. The GI manifestations include abdominal tenderness and distention, GI hemorrhage, emesis, gastric residuals, intestinal perforation, and peritonitis (Kliegman, 1990).

Acute ischemia of the intestine can result from arterial occlusion secondary to volvulus or intussusception, or thromboembolic disease associated with sepsis, DIC, emboli from a closing ductus or umbilical vessel catheterization, and dehydration. Chronic hypoperfusion is more common and results from hypoxia-induced vasospasm of the splanchnic arteries (dive reflex). During hypoxia, blood is shunted away from the splanchnic circulation to the CNS and cardiac muscle. The intestine, especially the terminal small intestine and ascending colon, becomes ischemic. Other causes of hypoperfusion include stress, hypothermia, hyperviscosity, hypovolemia, shunting of blood from the systemic circulation by large left to right shunts through a PDA, decreased left ventricular output as in hypoplastic left-sided heart syndrome, sepsis, dehydration, and shock (Swischuk, 1989).

Over 90% of infants with NEC develop the disease after enteric feeding begins. Oral administration of IgA has reduced the incidence of NEC (Eibl et al., 1988). The NEC can occur in epidemics. Epidemics have been associated with single pathogens such as *E. coli*, *Klebsiella pneumoniae*, *Salmonella* species, *Staphylococcus epidermidis*, *Clostridium butyricum*, coronavirus, enterovirus, and rotavirus. Blood cultures are positive in about one third of patients with NEC (Kliegman, 1990).

The first radiographic finding of NEC is general intestinal distention consistent with a paralytic ileus. The bowel loop distention sometimes originates in the right lower quadrant (Fig. 21–59). The loops become more tubular and may exhibit bowel wall thickening. Pneumatosis cystoides intestinalis may appear at any time in several different configurations including bubbly, linear, curvilinear, or foamy collections of gas (see Fig. 21–59). The intestinal wall, having lost the integrity of its mucosa, allows entry of gas-forming bacteria. Pneumatosis cystoides intestinalis is best seen in the colon but can occur anywhere from the stomach to the rectum. Portal vein gas (see Fig. 21–59) is not as ominous as thought previously. Ultrasound can also demonstrate portal venous gas (Lindley et al., 1986). A pneumoperitoneum indicates intestinal perforation and the necessity for surgical intervention (see Fig. 21–59). Sometimes free air in the abdomen is small and decubitus views are needed in addition to cross-table lateral supine examination. In some infants with perforation, free intraperitoneal air is not recognized, but the presence of increased density of the abdomen usually indicates development of peritonitis and peritoneal fluid. If focal loops of dilated bowel persist, necrotic bowel must be inferred and surgery is necessary (Wexler, 1978).

Atresias and Stenoses of Small and Large Intestine

A local vascular accident in utero is the probable cause of small intestinal atresias and stenoses, since they are associated with wedge-shaped mesenteric defects (Santulli and Blanc, 1961). Duodenal atresia, however, may be a failure of recanalization. Atresia is more common than stenosis, and the ileum is involved more frequently than the jejunum. A rare form of small bowel atresia is "apple peel" bowel, in which a long segment of atresia and a large mesenteric defect coexist. The distal end of the small bowel is spiraled (Dickson, 1970) and is supplied by the ileocolic artery. Colonic atresias and stenoses are rarer than their small intestinal counterparts. Plain radiographs demonstrate multiple dilated loops of bowel. More loops are involved in an ileal obstruction than in a jejunal obstruction (Fig. 21–60). An enema examination can be performed to better define the site of obstruction. The colon is usually unused (microcolon) when the obstruction is distal to the mid-jejunum, preventing the progression of succus enter-

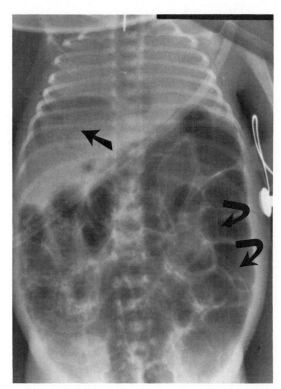

Figure 21–59. Anteroposterior abdominal radiograph with branching lucent shadows in the hepatic region *(arrow);* distended loops of bowel with a bubbly, streaky pattern of pneumatosis intestinalis on the right side of the abdomen; and evidence of free air, sharply defined serosal surface of loops of bowel *(curved arrows).*

icus in utero. Meconium ileus can produce a similar unused appearance in the large intestine because of the inspissation of meconium in the distal small intestine.

Meconium Ileus

Meconium ileus denotes intraluminal obstruction by the colon and lower small intestine by hard meconium pellets. The term implies the presence of cystic fibrosis in which a deficiency of pancreatic enzymes allows the meconium to become abnormal. Vomiting and abdominal distention are the presenting complaints. The plain radiographs show dilated small bowel loops and sometimes bubbly meconium (Leonidas et al., 1970). Lack of air–fluid levels in the cross-table projections may also suggest the diagnosis. Repeated enema examinations with high-osmolar water-soluble contrast material may alleviate the obstruction and obviate the necessity for a laparotomy (Frech et al., 1970). Complicated meconium ileus can include volvulus and atresia with cyst formation and meconium peritonitis (Fig. 21–61). Meconium peritonitis occurs when the fetal gut ruptures and the contents evoke peritonitis and calcification (Fig. 21–62). The perforation sometimes heals spontaneously with preservation of intestinal continuity. Meconium peritonitis can occur in normal neonates as well as those with cystic fibrosis.

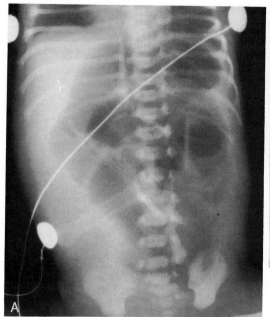

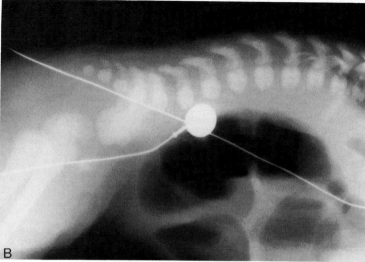

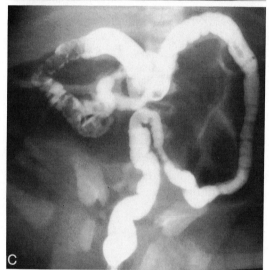

Figure 21–60. *A*, Anteroposterior view of abdomen with multiple distended bowel loops. *B*, Prone cross-table lateral view with obstruction indicated by no gas in rectum. *C*, Retrograde contrast study shows small colon and distal ileum indicative of more proximal ileal atresia.

Hirschsprung's Disease (Aganglionosis)

The intestine may be aganglionic in the lowest portion of the rectum, or there may be involvement of the entire colon and some of the intestine. The sigmoid colon is the most common site for transition to normal intestine. Initially, the neonate may fail to pass meconium or may have diarrhea (Swenson et al., 1973). Because Hirschsprung's disease causes only partial obstruction, the problem may not come to medical attention until after the first month of life. Plain radiographs may show dilated intestinal loops or an unusual variation in intestinal caliber (Fig. 21–63*A*). A prone cross-table lateral radiograph of the abdomen may show a rectum void of feces and air. The morbidity and mortality of neonatal Hirschsprung's disease are high. Therefore, barium enema examinations should be performed readily when the

diagnosis is suspected. Radiographic signs of Hirschsprung's disease include irregular contractions in the aganglionic segment, transition zone between dilated and normal bowel, transverse contractions in the proximal part of the colon, irregularities of mucosa, and failure of prompt evacuation of contrast material and even marked retrograde movement (see Fig. 21–63*B*). The demonstration of a rectosigmoidal transition zone is the most reliable sign.

URINARY PROBLEMS

Ureteropelvic Junction Obstruction

The most common location of obstruction in the upper urinary tract is the ureteropelvic junction. The obstruction may result from abnormal ureteral insertion, intrinsic narrowing, and extrinsic compression

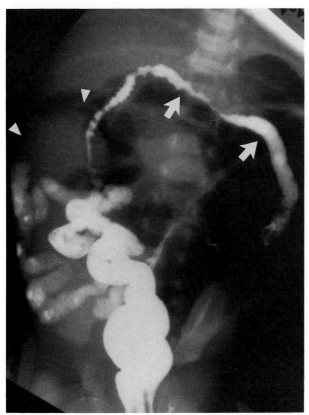

Figure 21–61. Anteroposterior view of abdomen demonstrating a retrograde water-soluble contrast study of a microcolon *(arrows)*. Several loops of ileum are opacified in right lower quadrant ending in a cystic structure *(arrowheads)* representing an atretic portion of ileum complicating a meconium ileus.

by a vessel. Boys are more commonly affected, and obstruction is bilateral in 18% of children (Bernstein et al., 1988). In the immediate postnatal period, ureteropelvic junction obstruction is noticed on clinical examination by detection of a palpable mass on

the affected side. Urinary infection may occur. Obstructions detected at this time tend to be moderate to severe.

Ultrasound examination can reveal the cystic or solid nature of the renal or extrarenal mass. In ureteropelvic junction obstruction, the renal pelvis should be centrally positioned and contain the largest of the fluid collections. In the other fluid collections, the calyces are approximately the same size and communicate with the renal pelvis. If there is enlargement of the ipsilateral ureter, other diagnoses such as megaureter, simple ureterocele, and vesicoureteral reflux should be included. Ureteropelvic junction obstruction can coexist with vesicoureteral reflux or distal ureteral obstruction (Lebowitz and Blickman, 1983). Additional diagnostic studies include ultrasound of bladder (looking for ureterocele), voiding cystourethrogram (diagnosing vesicoureteral reflux or bladder outlet obstruction), and renal scintigraphy (assessing function and level of obstruction).

Multicystic Dysplastic Kidney

This noninheritable cystic renal disease can present as a palpable irregular flank mass. When hydronephrosis is excluded the most common cause of abdominal mass in the newborn is the multicystic kidney. The affected kidney does not function and is composed of cysts of varying size and number, connective tissue, cartilage, and primitive tubules. The ipsilateral ureter or renal pelvis is atretic. The contralateral kidney is frequently abnormal, commonly a mild ureteropelvic junction obstruction. Bilateral multicystic kidneys are incompatible with life.

Ultrasound is usually sufficient to make the diagnosis of multicystic kidney. On longitudinal and transverse scans, the cysts of varying size are arranged in no specific configuration (Fig. 21–64). This helps differentiate a multicystic dysplastic kidney from an

Figure 21–62. Anteroposterior view of abdomen showing multiple calcifications *(arrows)* within the abdomen characteristic of meconium peritonitis. There is also free air with the ligamentum teres outlined *(arrowheads)*.

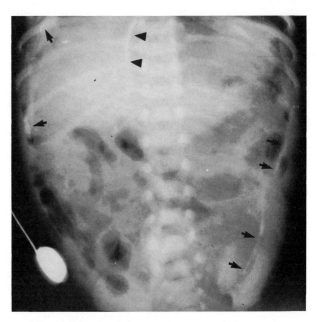

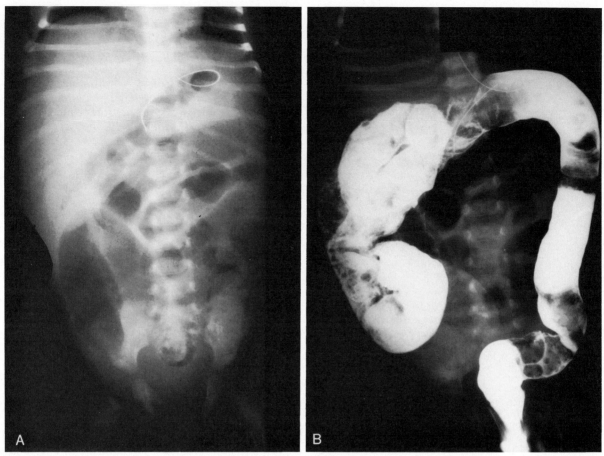

Figure 21–63. *A,* Anteroposterior radiograph of abdomen with multiple distended loops and no air in the rectum. *B,* Retrograde barium water examination of the colon showing some foreshortening of the sigmoid and similar caliber to the entire colon in patient with total colonic aganglionosis. A 24-hour radiograph showing characteristic retrograde propulsion of the barium water mixture into the proximal small bowel.

obstructed kidney (Sanders and Hartman, 1984). When the cysts are small or few in number and there is a question of a parenchymal rim, the sonographic diagnosis is more difficult. Other imaging modalities such as renal scintigraphy may be contributory.

There has been increasing willingness not to extirpate the kidney when the diagnosis is clear. In one series of 21 patients there was no increased morbidity in 2 to 101 months of follow-up examination (Vinocur et al., 1988).

Infantile Polycystic Disease

Infantile polycystic disease is inherited as an autosomal recessive trait. Infants presenting in the immediate neonatal period have a poor prognosis with large kidneys and poor renal function. Hypoplasia of the lungs results from the so-called fetal compression syndrome of Potter. Oligohydramnios results in hypoplasia of lungs, abnormal facies, and abnormal feet. Ultrasonography has replaced intravenous urography (Hayden et al., 1986) for the diagnosis of infantile polycystic disease (Fig. 21–65). The kidneys are enlarged and highly echogenic. Calyces are sel-

dom seen, and the corticomedullary differentiation is obscured. Increased echogenicity is due to numerous dilated radiating tubules (Melson et al., 1985). The bladder is often hypoplastic. Infants who have the juvenile form with less tubular involvement with cysts live longer but have hepatic fibrosis and the complications of cirrhosis.

Absent Abdominal Musculature (Prune-Belly Syndrome, Eagle Barrett Syndrome)

The prune-belly syndrome occurs almost exclusively in males. The lack of development of the abdominal musculature has been attributed to the chronic intrauterine massive distention of the abdomen caused by ascites or dilatation of the urinary tract. There appears to be two groups of patients. The first group has an obstructing lesion of the urethra and generally do poorly; the second group has a functional abnormality of bladder but no urethral obstruction and survives the neonatal period (Berdon et al., 1977). In the former group the problem is usually posterior urethral valve atresia or urethral

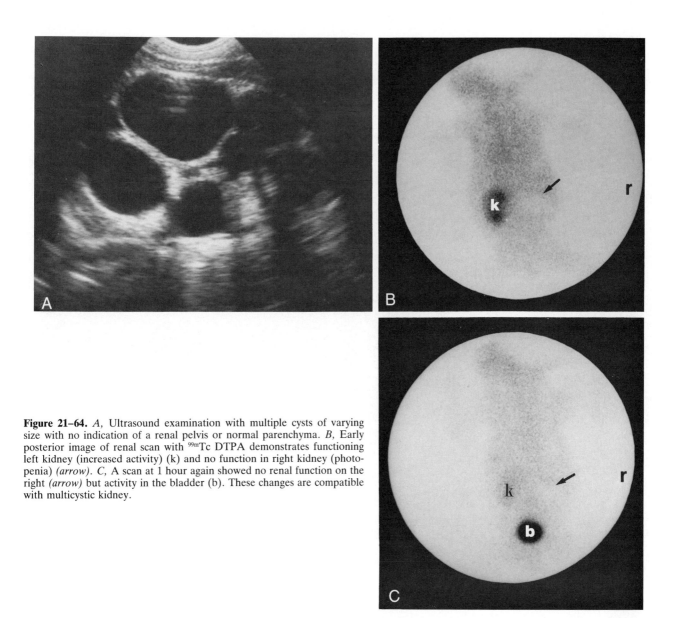

Figure 21–64. *A,* Ultrasound examination with multiple cysts of varying size with no indication of a renal pelvis or normal parenchyma. *B,* Early posterior image of renal scan with ^{99m}Tc DTPA demonstrates functioning left kidney (increased activity) (k) and no function in right kidney (photopenia) *(arrow). C,* A scan at 1 hour again showed no renal function on the right *(arrow)* but activity in the bladder (b). These changes are compatible with multicystic kidney.

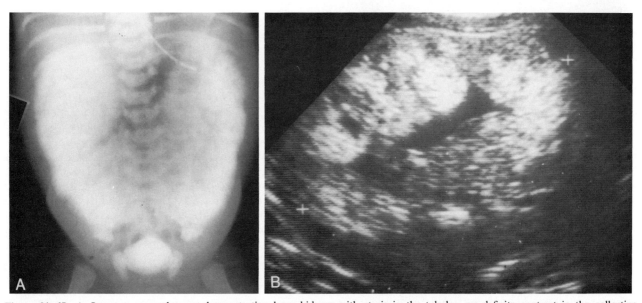

Figure 21–65. *A,* Intravenous pyelogram demonstrating huge kidneys with stasis in the tubules, no definite contrast in the collecting systems, and a small bladder indicative of infantile polycystic kidney disease. *B,* Increased echogenicity of parenchyma of enlarged kidney on ultrasound examination.

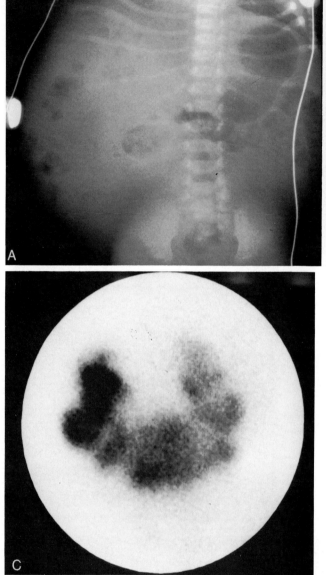

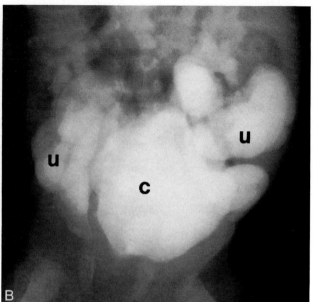

Figure 21–66. *A,* Anteroposterior radiograph of abdomen exhibiting broadened flanks secondary to deficient abdominal musculature and paucity of gas in lower abdomen. *B,* Intravenous pyelogram showing megaureters (u) and megacystis (c). *C,* Posterior image of a nuclear renogram with activity in redundant ureters and bladder. More activity in left proximal ureter related to stasis. A urethrogram demonstrated the distended prostatic urethra.

atresia. The kidneys are severely hydronephrotic and may become dysplastic and multicystic. The Potter syndrome, as described with infantile polycystic kidney disease, can develop with fetal compression and hypoplastic lungs secondary to renal nonfunction (Pramanik et al., 1977). The second group of infants, who have no obstructing lesion of the urethra, have abnormal bladder emptying. The posterior urethra is enlarged and bulbous, probably secondary to hypoplasia of the prostate gland. Associated findings include undescended testicles, club-foot deformity, and dislocated hips.

Radiographically, the abnormally broadened belly is identified as well as a large distended urinary bladder, bilateral hydroureters and hydronephrosis, and sometimes persistence of the urachal remnant (Fig. 21–66). Cystography identifies the associated vesicoureteral reflux in as many as 60% of cases (Nunn and Stephens, 1961). The ureters tend to be tortuous and poorly peristaltic. Eighty percent of ureters would be classified as megaureters. Diverticula of the urethra can also occur (Cremin, 1971), as can occasional calcifications in the bladder and urachal remnant (Kirks and Taybi, 1975). Renal scintigraphy determines accurately the function of the kidneys and the necessity of surgical drainage. Ultrasonography demonstrates a large bladder, megaureters, and urinary ascites (Garris et al., 1980).

Posterior Urethral Valves

Posterior urethral valves occur mainly in males. A poor urinary stream is a clue to their presence. Some infants are born with poor renal function secondary to the obstruction of the valves. The classification divides posterior urethral valves into three types. Type I is most common and occurs below the verumontanum; Type II occurs above the verumontanum; and Type III consists of a diaphragm below the verumontanum. Type II has been questioned as being a real cause of obstruction (Williams et al., 1973).

The bladder is markedly thickened and grossly trabeculated. The posterior urethra is markedly dilated on cystourethrography (Fig. 21–67), and reflux of contrast material into the seminal vesicles and prostatic ducts is sometimes seen. Ultrasonography can demonstrate all the abnormalities of the posterior urethral valve complex (Cremin, 1986). Gross hydronephrosis is frequently present, and vesicoureteral reflux can occur into massively dilated ureters. Poorly functioning hypoplastic or dysplastic kidneys are not unusual, and Potter syndrome can occur (see section on infantile polycystic kidneys) (Henneberry and Stephens, 1980).

Urine Ascites

Most infants with urine ascites are male and have some form of bladder outlet or urethral obstruction (Cremin, 1975). The most common problem is posterior urethral valves. Urine ascites can result from either spontaneous or iatrogenic perforation of the bladder (McDonald and Murphy, 1975). The perforation most often occurs in the upper tracts secondary to a distal obstruction. The urine escapes around the kidney defined by perirenal fascia and then through a peritoneal defect or tear into the free peritoneal space. Intravenous urography in association with cystourethrography usually demonstrates the extravasation.

CONGENITAL HEART DISEASE

Persistent Fetal Circulation Syndrome

Sometimes an abnormal persistent elevation of the pulmonary vascular resistance results in right to left shunting through the patent foramen ovale or the PDA (persistence of the fetal circulatory pathway) in full-term infants. The primary form has elevated pulmonary pressures with no underlying pulmonary problem. These infants experience respiratory distress and cyanosis in the first 24 hours of life. In most cases (Silverstein et al., 1981), perinatal hypoxia is the stimulus for the pulmonary vasoconstriction. Other factors that influence the development of persistent fetal circulation (PFC) syndrome are hypoglycemia, acidemia, and hyperviscosity. Radiographically, the lungs are usually clear, which helps to differentiate PFC syndrome from pulmonary disease. Venous congestion, patchy infiltrates, pleural effusions, hepatomegaly, or even mild hyaline membrane disease may be present, however (Nielson et al., 1976). Mild to moderate cardiomegaly is usually seen (Bauer et al., 1974), and differentiation of PFC syndrome from cyanotic heart disease may be difficult. Angiography can exclude transposition of the great vessels, hypoplastic left-sided heart syndrome, and right ventricular outflow tract obstruction as the causes of cyanosis. Treatment usually consists of oxygen therapy, correction of acidosis, and vasodilators such as tolazoline. The patient generally improves in 2 to 6 days, with lung clearance and disappearance of the cardiomegaly. Conditions leading to secondary persistence of the fetal circulation include aspiration syndromes, congenital diaphragmatic her-

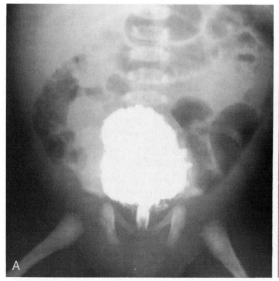
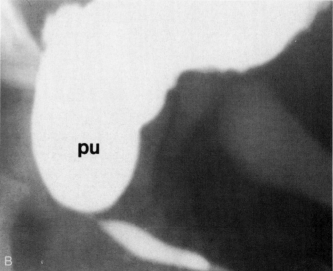

Figure 21–67. *A,* Cystogram demonstrating markedly trabeculated bladder with mural thickening. *B,* Urethrogram showing marked discrepancy between enlarged posterior urethra *(pu)* and distal urethra indicative of a posterior urethral valve. A renal scan with ^{99m}Tc DTPA shows dilated collecting systems and ureters due to obstruction distally.

nia, hypoplastic lung, and ischemic myocardial dysfunction.

Hypoplastic Left-Sided Heart Syndrome and Coarctation of the Aorta

Underdevelopment of the left side of the heart may range from the severe combined aortic and mitral valve atresia to relatively mild stenosis of both valves. Other variations include aortic atresia, mitral atresia with normal aortic valve, and hypoplasias of the ascending and transverse portions of the aorta. Hypoplastic left-sided heart syndrome is the most common cause of congestive heart failure in the first few days of life (Fig. 21–68). Wet lungs that do not clear but become progressively worse with enlargement of the heart in the first 24 hours suggest a left-sided cardiac obstruction. Angiography and ultrasonography are used to make the diagnosis.

Coarctation is the most common cause of congestive heart failure after the first week of life. Many coarctations of the aorta are associated with either a ventricular septal defect or PDA, producing an extra burden and therefore congestive failure. The rarer infantile (preductal) type of coarctation is the coarctation proximal to the ductus arteriosus and may be of considerable length. The adult (postductal) type is a short segment just distal to the ductus arteriosus. Plain radiographic changes consist of congestion and cardiomegaly. Rib notching is usually not present. The diagnosis depends heavily on angiocardiography and MRI.

Total anomalous pulmonary venous return below the diaphragm as well as bilateral pulmonary venous

atresia can produce clinical and radiographic findings such as pulmonary congestion that are similar to those of the lesions described earlier. Cardiomegaly is usually not present.

Cardiomyopathies

Neonatal hypoxia can in association with acidosis lead to pulmonary arteriolar vasoconstriction and pulmonary hypertension. Hypoxia can also lead directly to myocardial ischemia and transient myocardial dysfunction. Another myocardial abnormality is transient hypertrophic (septal) subaortic stenosis in infants of diabetic mothers. Radiographically, these infants exhibit a nonspecific cardiomegaly. Primary endocardial fibroelastosis presents with marked endocardial thickening and myocardial fibroelastosis, predisposing to failure of the left side of the heart. When the left ventricular dilatation is aneurysmal, the cardiomegaly can be massive at birth. Most children are diagnosed in the first few days of life and die before age 1 (Johnstrude and Carey, 1965).

Aberrant left coronary artery with its origin from the pulmonary artery presents with congestive heart failure and cardiomegaly secondary to damage of the anterolateral myocardium. Angiography can demonstrate a large dilated right coronary artery and retrograde filling of the aberrant coronary artery (Hawker et al., 1976).

Left-to-Right Shunts Including PDA

This group of lesions includes mainly atrial septal defect, ventricular septal defect, endocardial cushion defect, and PDA. These lesions, except for PDA, do not present a problem in the immediate neonatal period. In most full-term infants, unless the lesions are extremely large, the pulmonary vascular resistance remains high enough to prevent significant left-to-right shunting in the first few weeks. The premature infant does not possess the same degree of hypertrophy of the media of the pulmonary arteries as does the full-term infant. The ventricular septal defect and PDA in the premature infant can be significant. Children with large left-to-right shunts are often hyperaerated with flattened hemidiaphragms, a bowed sternum, and increased retrosternal air space (Markowitz et al., 1988).

The complete endocardial cushion defect consists of a single confluent atrioventricular orifice, a continuous cleft between the anterior leaflet of the mitral valve and the septal leaflet of the tricuspid valve, and fusion of the valve segments into a common atrioventricular valve. The partial endocardial cushion defect consists of portions of this complex. These lesions usually occur in Down syndrome. Skeletal configurations of 11 ribs and hypersegmented manubrial ossification centers are frequent. Radiographically,

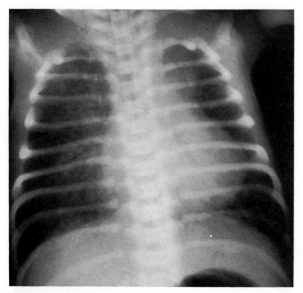

Figure 21–68. Anteroposterior view of chest with persistent congestive heart failure (wet lungs) in patient with left heart obstruction (aortic atresia).

cardiomegaly is present. Pulmonary vascularity is increased, and the left atrium is not usually enlarged. The right atrial appendage enlargement may contribute to a characteristic shelved appearance to the right upper margin of the cardiac silhouette. Endocardial cushion defects can be evaluated by echocardiographic and angiographic techniques.

The ductus remains open longer in all premature infants and infants with pulmonary disease such as hyaline membrane disease (19%) (Thieboult et al., 1975), BPD, meconium aspiration, and so forth. Sequential radiographs of infants with hyaline membrane disease are often helpful in early diagnosis of PDA (Slovis and Shankaran, 1980). The increased perfusion causes an engorgement of the pulmonary vascular bed, which diminishes compliance and ventilation; ventilatory pressures then usually have to be elevated. Indomethacin therapy or surgical intervention may be necessary to prevent the progression of lung disease to BPD.

Radiographically, cardiomegaly is not usually striking. Instead, increased pulmonary vascularity, pulmonary edema, and congestion are evident. With a PDA, preferential shunting sometimes occurs to the right lung with unilateral edema, perihilar haze, and overaeration (Fig. 21–69). Elevation of the left bronchus signifies left atrial enlargement. Chest radiographs may detect the PDA 24 to 48 hours before its clinical presentation in more than half of the patients with PDA. Ultrasonography with demonstration of the ductus, or umbilical arteriography with 1 to 2 ml of contrast medium, can substantiate the diagnosis (Edwards et al., 1978; Silverman et al., 1974).

Lesions With Decreased Vascularity

Lesions with decreased vascularity are caused by some form of right outflow tract obstruction, anywhere from the tricuspid valve to the pulmonary artery. The right side pressures are usually high with resultant right to left shunting. Perfusion of the pulmonary vessels depends on the patency of the ductus arteriosus. Even though tetralogy of Fallot is the most common cause of cyanotic heart disease, it is not commonly seen in neonates. The main problem of outflow tract obstruction is infundibular or mixed infundibular and valvular stenosis. A few cases with atresia of the pulmonary valve may present early. All patients have ventricular septal defects. The overriding aorta is more a function of aortic size than abnormal aorta position. The aorta is right-sided in 25% of cases (Daves, 1968).

There are two types of pulmonary atresia, that with a small right ventricle and that with a normal or enlarged right ventricle. Patients with normal or enlarged right ventricles usually show dilatation of the tricuspid annulus and gross tricuspid insufficiency. Right atrial enlargement depends on the size of the tricuspid insufficiency and the size of the atrial defect.

The largest right atrium results from a small atrial septal defect and a large amount of tricuspid insufficiency. Radiographically, there usually is cardiomegaly and small concave main pulmonary artery as well as decreased pulmonary vasculature (Fig. 21–70). The aorta is usually on the left (Davignon et al., 1961).

In tricuspid atresia there is complete atresia of the tricuspid valve and usually underdevelopment of the right ventricle and right outflow tract. Blood is usually shunted across an atrial septal defect and out the left ventricle. Sometimes an associated small ventricular defect is present, but the outflow tract and pulmonary artery are underdeveloped. Tricuspid atresia is divided into two groups, that associated with transposition of the great vessels and that which has no transposition. The larger group of patients has no transposition and pulmonary stenosis, whereas the smaller group have transposition and no pulmonary stenosis. Cardiac enlargement, concave main pulmonary artery segment and decreased pulmonary vasculature are similar in the larger group of patients (no transposition, pulmonary stenosis) to pulmonary atresia (Elliott et al., 1968). Left atrial enlargement depends on the size of the associated atrial defect.

Congenital (In Utero) Infections

Generalized in utero infection with rubella, syphilis, and cytomegalovirus (CMV) can cause osseous manifestations that are recognized after birth. Longitudinal radiolucent streaks with occasional interposed trabeculae, an appearance characterized as "celery stalking," can be seen with congenital rubella (Singleton et al., 1966). The osseous appearance of CMV may be similar to rubella with poorly mineralized, irregularly, striated metaphyses (Merten and Gooding, 1970). When CMV infection is suspected, CT of the brain may reveal periventricular calcifications. In congenital syphilis, symmetric polyostotic periostitis of the long bones is a common radiographic finding (Solomon and Rosen, 1978). In the metaphyses there are dystrophic bands, erosions, and serrations at the ends of the bones (Fig. 21–71). With metaphyseal granulation tissue disrupting the periosteum, corner fractures can also be present. Bilateral erosions in the medial metaphyses of the proximal tibiae (Wimberger sign) have been noted. The bony changes of CMV and syphilis can be delayed in appearance for several weeks to months after birth.

Neonatal Osteomyelitis

Neonatal osteomyelitis has an indolent presentation with no systemic signs or symptoms. Osteomyelitis that occurs during the neonatal period is an especially serious condition that can leave a child with permanent musculoskeletal deformity (Fox and Sprunt, 1978). Multiple sites of involvement are present in half of infants and occur simultaneously half of the

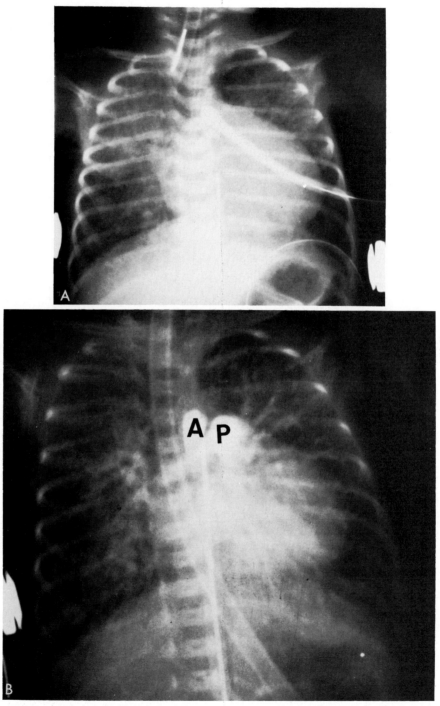

Figure 21–69. *A*, Preferential perfusion of patent ductus arteriosus demonstrated by increased markings in the right lung. *B*, Umbilical aortogram confirming the left-to-right shunt at the ductus level. P, Pulmonary artery; A, Aorta.

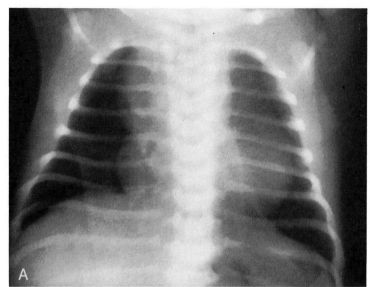

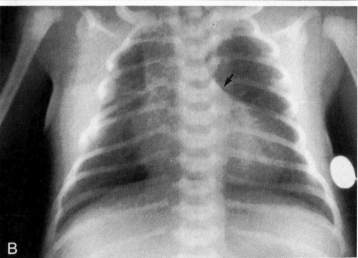

Figure 21–70. *A,* Anteroposterior radiograph of chest showing lung fields with decreased vascularity in a cyanotic newborn with pulmonary atresia. The aorta is left-sided. *B,* Postoperative AP view of chest with rib changes secondary to right thoracotomy, concave pulmonary outflow tract related to infundibular stenosis *(arrow),* and increased perfusion from a right Waterston shunt (ascending aorta to right pulmonary artery). Note the shrinkage of thymus gland from stress.

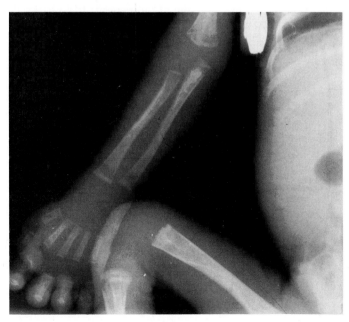

Figure 21–71. Anteroposterior view of right wrist and knee with irregular metaphyses and regional deossification indicative of the metaphysitis of congenital syphilis.

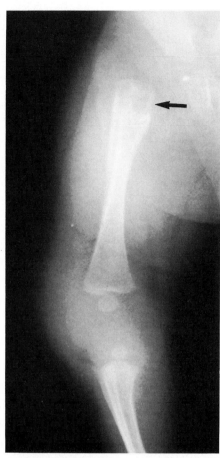

Figure 21–72. Anteroposterior view of legs showing lytic lesion *(arrow)* in proximal right femur and subluxation secondary to neonatal osteomyelitis and septic arthritis. Concurrently there is a septic arthritis of the right knee with appreciable soft-tissue swelling.

time. *Staphylococcus aureus* is the most frequent organism, with Group B beta-hemolytic streptococcal infections on the increase. Metaphyseal involvement with crossing of the growth plate by the vascular route or direct destruction of the growth plate with entrance into the epiphysis can occur. Soft-tissue swelling occasionally accompanied by pseudoparesis when an arm or leg is affected is the most common radiographic finding. A full skeletal survey or bone scintigraphy looking for unsuspected sites of bone destruction in the metaphyses and epiphyses should be performed (Mok et al., 1982) (Fig. 21–72).

CENTRAL NERVOUS SYSTEM PROBLEMS

Brain Injury in Premature Infants

Being born prematurely is the greatest risk factor for intracranial hemorrhage. In infants born at less than 32 weeks of gestation, the incidence of hemorrhage is 35% to 55%. Being male increases the risk.

Ischemia is postulated to be the cause of most types of hemorrhage. Positron emission tomography shows a large area of poorly perfused brain in the presence of a small germinal matrix hemorrhage (Volpe et al., 1983). Sudden reperfusion of an ischemic area may result in hemorrhagic infarction. Screening of all infants of less than 32 weeks' gestation should be performed with ultrasound, because most hemorrhage occurs centrally and can be diagnosed easily. The screening can occur at the end of the first week of life unless clinical reasons require earlier evaluation. Most hemorrhage episodes occur in the first 3 days of life (Rumack et al., 1985).

Subependymal germinal matrix hemorrhage (Grade I) is the most common type of hemorrhage in the premature infant (Fig. 21–73). The germinal matrix, a loosely organized tissue with thin-walled vessels, develops into neurons and glia of the cerebral cortex. On sonograms the subependymal hemorrhage is a highly echogenic focal lesion (Fig. 21–74), usually in the caudothalamic groove. Intraventricular hemorrhage often results from the rupture of subependymal hemorrhage or, less commonly, from choroid plexus hemorrhage into the ventricular system (Grade II with no ventricular dilatation, Grade III with ventricular dilatation) (Rumack et al., 1985). The diagnosis of intraventricular hemorrhage can be made if there is echogenic material in the occipital or frontal horns where there is normally no choroid plexus (see Fig. 21–74). As the intraventricular hemorrhage resolves, the clot disintegrates, resulting in debris in the ventricular system than may settle into the occipital horn as a fluid level or may be seen as low-level intraventricular echoes. An echogenic rim that forms around the ventricle 1 or 2 weeks after the hemorrhage represents a chemical ventriculitis in response to the blood. Secondary hydrocephalus occurs in 70% of patients with intraventricular hemorrhage. The hydrocephalus may be due to a clot within the ventricular system, obstruction of the outlets, or failure of resorption due to blood's coming over the surface of the brain from the circulation of the intraventricular blood (Rumack et al., 1985). One third of cases of hydrocephalus return to normal, and ventriculoperitoneal shunting is necessary in another third. Porencephalic cyst formation can occur from bleeding into periventricular parenchyma (Grade IV). Grades III and IV have the worst prognoses, including atrophy, hydrocephalus, gliosis, and porencephaly.

Periventricular leukomalacia is necrosis of cerebral white matter adjacent to the lateral edges of the lateral ventricles, particularly the frontal (near the foramen of Monro) and peritrigonal (optic radiations) regions (Volpe et al., 1983). With major degrees of periventricular leukomalacia, cystic cavities may develop; with less severe degrees, only diminished cerebral myelin with dilated ventricles is seen. The two principle diagnostic procedures used to identify periventricular leukomalacia are cranial sonography and CT. In the coronal projection on sonograms the areas of leukomalacia appear as echoic densities adjacent

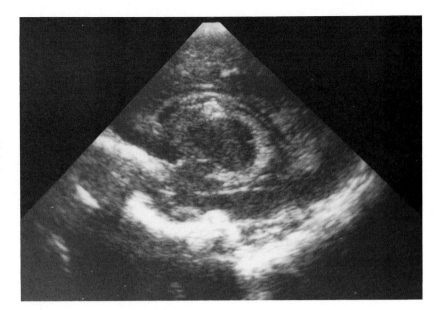

Figure 21–73. Sagittal ultrasound examination of side of lateral ventricular system with hyperechogenic area of germinal matrix hemorrhage *(arrow).*

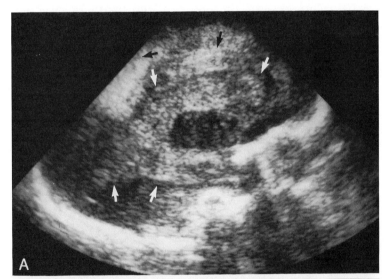

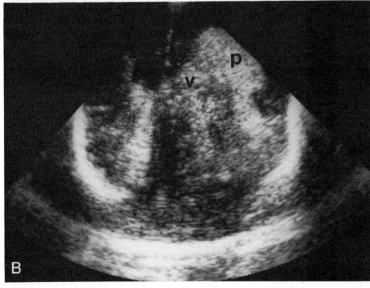

Figure 21–74. *A,* Sagittal ultrasound image demonstrating dilated lateral ventricle containing echogenic material *(white arrows).* Increase echogenicity is in brain parenchyma above the frontal horn and trigone (Grade IV) regions of left lateral ventricle *(black arrows). B,* Coronal image showing left lateral ventricle *(v)* with echogenicity and extension into adjacent brain parenchyma *(p).*

to the external angles of the lateral ventricles or adjacent to the ventricles near the level of the foramina of Monro. Cyst formation occurs 2 or 3 weeks after the appearance of the echoic densities. It is common for relatively small, circumscribed cysts, to disappear after 1 to 3 months. CT and MRI may not show early periventricular leukomalacia because of the large amount of brain water present. After several weeks or more have passed, the extent of major lesions can be determined when the degree of white matter atrophy can be assessed. It is difficult to differentiate lucencies caused by periventricular leukomalacia from those normally seen on CT scans of neonates. The major long-term clinical correlates of periventricular leukomalacia are spastic diplegia and, to a lesser extent, intellectual deficits.

Congenital Brain Anomalies

In the newborn the classic Arnold-Chiari Type II malformation (downward displacement of the cerebellum, medulla oblongata, lower pons, and fourth ventricle into the spinal canal) is almost always associated with spinal or cranial meningocele or meningomyelocele. Hydrocephalus is frequently associated but can be mild until about a week after the repair of the spinal defect because of a change in CSF dynamics. Secondary obstruction probably results from narrowing and downward stretching of the aqueduct.

Plain radiographs demonstrate a large head but small posterior fossa. Lacunar skull and an enlarged foramen magnum are common features. Posterior scalloping of the petrous pyramids can be seen. Hydrocephalus can be more definitively examined with ultrasound, MRI, and CT. The third ventricle, the fourth ventricle, and the aqueduct of Sylvius are usually elongated and stretched downward. The lateral ventricles characteristically are larger posteriorly and pointed anteriorly and inferiorly. The choroid plexus is usually prominent, and a large massa intermedia may reside in an enlarged third ventricle. Aqueductal stenosis can present with severe obstructive hydrocephalus. Agenesis of the corpus callosum is a common anomaly associated with other major malformations. The classic findings are separation of the lateral ventricles and superior displacement of the third ventricle in the midline. Complete agenesis can be diagnosed with ultrasound but partial agenesis probably requires MRI for definitive diagnosis. Many other rare anomalies can occur and be diagnosed with appropriate imaging techniques.

Congenital Central Nervous System Infection

Cytomegalic inclusion disease is a viral infection transmitted from the mother to an infant in utero.

Usually infants are delivered prematurely and are quite ill. Hepatosplenomegaly, ecchymoses, and petechiae, as well as jaundice, can be present. Definitive diagnosis depends on demonstration of large inclusion bodies within desquamated renal epithelial cells and elevated antibody titers in the infant. CMV causes diffuse brain damage, which usually results in calcification in the periventricular regions of varying involvement (Sackett and Ford, 1956) (Fig. 21–75). All patients with cytomegalic inclusion virus infection do not demonstrate calcification, however. Microcephaly usually occurs secondary to poor brain development.

Toxoplasmosis is a protozoal infection caused by the organism *Toxoplasma gondii*. The infection is transmitted to the fetus by the maternal circulation. Skin hemorrhages, hepatosplenomegaly, and chorioretinitis may be present. The skull may be large or small. Radiographically, the calcifications can be anywhere, including the basal ganglia, choroid plexus, subependyma, and meninges. The calcifications tend to be irregular and flaky (Mussbichler, 1968). Periventricular distribution is unusual.

In herpesvirus infection there is diffuse echogenicity of brain on sonogram with poorly defined sulci and necrosis. The lateral ventricles can enlarge secondary to the brain destruction. Massive calcifications of the brain have been described in herpes simplex encephalitis (South et al., 1969).

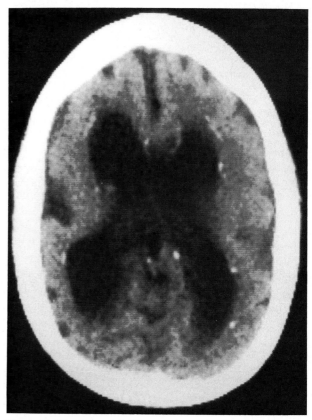

Figure 21–75. Transaxial CT scan demonstrating periventricular calcifications of cytomegalic inclusion disease.

References

Ablow, R.C., Driscoll, S.G., Effman, E.L., et al.: Comparison of early onset group-B streptococcal neonatal infection and the respiratory distress syndrome of the newborn. N. Engl. J. Med. 294:65, 1976.

Ablow, R.C., and Effman, E.L.: Hepatic calcifications associated with umbilical vein catheterization in the newborn infant. AJR 114:380, 1972.

Adams, F.H., and Gyepes, M.J.: Diaphragmatic paralysis in the newborn infant simulating cyanotic heart disease. J. Pediatr. 78:119, 1971.

Albersheim, S.G., Solimano, A.J., Sharma, A.K., et al.: Randomized, double-blind, controlled trial of long-term diuretic therapy for bronchopulmonary dysplasia. J. Pediatr. 115:615, 1989.

Ambler, R., Gruenewald, S., and John, E.: Ultrasound monitoring of diaphragm activity in bilateral diaphragmatic paralysis. Arch. Dis. Child. 60:170, 1985.

Anderson, K.D., and Chandra, R.: Pneumothorax secondary to perforation of sequential bronchi by suction catheters. J. Pediatr. Surg. 11:687, 1976.

Avnet, N.L.: Roentgenologic features of congenital bilateral anterior diaphragmatic eventration. AJR 88:743, 1962.

Aziz, E.M., and Robertson, A.F.: Paraplegia: A complication of umbilical arterial catheterization. J. Pediatr. 82:1051, 1973.

Bader, D., Ramos, A.D., Lew, C.D., et al.: Childhood sequelae of infant lung disease: Exercise and pulmonary function abnormalities after bronchopulmonary dysplasia. J. Pediatr. 110:693, 1987.

Baker, D.H., Berdon, W.E., and James, L.S.: Proper localization of umbilical arterial and venous catheters by lateral roentgenograms. Pediatrics 43:34, 1969.

Bauer, C.R., Brennan, M.J., Doyle, C., and Poole, C.A.: Surgical resection for pulmonary interstitial emphysema in the newborn infant. J. Pediatr. 93:656, 1978.

Bauer, C.R., Tsipuras, D., and Fletcher, B.D.: Syndrome of persistent pulmonary vascular obstruction of the newborn: Roentgen findings. AJR 120:285, 1974.

Baxter, J.D., and Dunbar, J.S.: Tracheomalacia. Ann. Otol. Rhinol. Laryngol. 72:1013, 1963.

Benjamin, B.: Tracheomalacia in infants and children. Ann. Otol. Rhinol. Laryngol. 93:438, 1984.

Benjamin, B., and Carter, P.L.: Congenital laryngeal hemangioma. Ann. Otol. Rhinol. Laryngol. 92:448, 1983.

Berdon, W.E., Baker, D.H., and Amoury, R.: The role of pulmonary hypoplasia in the prognosis of newborn infants with diaphragmatic hernia and eventration. AJR 103:413, 1965.

Berdon, W.E., Baker, D.H., Jen-Tien, W., et al.: Complete cartilage ring trachea stenosis associated with anomalous pulmonary artery: The ring-sling complex. Radiology 152:57, 1984.

Berdon, W.E., Baker, D.H., Wigger, H.J., et al.: The radiologic and pathologic spectrum of the prune belly syndrome: The importance of the obstruction in prognosis. Radiol. Clin. North Am. 1:83, 1977.

Bernstein, G.T., Mandell, J., Lebowitz, R.L., et al.: Ureteropelvic junction obstruction in the neonate. J. Urol. 140(Part 2):1216, 1988.

Bessolo, R.J., and Maddison, F.E.: Scimitar syndrome. AJR 103:572, 1969.

Bhutani, V.K., Richie, W.G., and Shaffer, T.H.: Acquired tracheobronchomegaly in very premature neonates. Am. J. Dis. Child. 140:449, 1986.

Bomsel, F., Gouchard, M., Larroche, J.C., and Magder, L.: Radiologic diagnosis of massive pulmonary hemorrhage of the newborn. Ann. Radiol. 18:419, 1975.

Bourassa, M.G.: The scimitar syndrome: Report of two cases of anomalous venous return from a hypoplastic right lung to the inferior vena cava. Can. Med. Assoc. J. 88:115, 1963.

Bowen, A., and Zarabi, M.: Radiographic clues to chest tube perforation of the neonatal lung. Am. J. Perinatol. 2:43, 1985.

Brans, Y.W., Pitts, M., and Cassady, G.: Neonatal pneumopericardium. Am. J. Dis. Child. 130:393, 1976.

Brooks, J.G., Bustamante, S.A., Koops, B.L., et al.: Selective bronchial intubation for the treatment of severe localized pulmonary interstitial emphysema in newborn infants. J. Pediatr. 91:648, 1977.

Campbell, R.E., Boggs, T.R., Jr., and Kirkpatrick, J.A., Jr.: Early neonatal pneumoperitoneum from progressive massive pneumomediastinum. Radiology 114:121, 1975.

Capitanio, M.A., Ramos, R., and Kirkpatrick, J.A.: Pulmonary sling: Roentgen observations. AJR 112:28, 1971.

Carlo, W.A., Beoglos, A., Chatburn, R.L., et al.: High-frequency jet ventilation in neonatal pulmonary hypertension. 143:233, 1989.

Charon, A., Taeusch, H.W., Fitzgibbon, C., et al.: Factors associated with surfactant treatment response in infants with severe respiratory distress syndrome. Pediatrics 83:348, 1989.

Chinwuba, C., Wallman, J., and Strand, R.: Nasal airway obstruction: CT assessment. Radiology 159:503, 1986.

Christensen, E.E., and Landay, M.J.: Visible muscle of the diaphragm: Sign of extraperitoneal air. AJR 135:121, 1980.

Clark, T.A., Coen, R.W., Feldman, B., and Papile, L.: Esophageal perforations in premature infants and comments on the diagnosis. Am. J. Dis. Child. 134:367, 1980.

Clark, T.A., and Edwards, D.R.: Pulmonary pseudocysts in newborn infants with respiratory distress syndrome. AJR 133:417, 1979.

Clarke, E.A., Siegle, R.L., and Gong, A.K.: Findings on chest radiographs after prophylactic pulmonary surfactant treatment of premature infants. AJR 153:799, 1989.

Cochran, W.D., Davis, H.T., and Smith, C.A.: Advantages and complications of umbilical artery catheterization in the newborn. Pediatrics 42:769, 1968.

Cohen, M.D., Weber, T.R., Sequeira, F.W., et al.: Diagnostic dilemma of the posterior thymus: CT manifestations. Radiology 146:691, 1983.

Cohen, S.R., Geller, K.A., Birns, J.W., et al.: Laryngeal paralysis in children: A long term retrospective study. Ann. Otol. Rhinol. Laryngol. 91:417, 1982.

Coopersmith, H., and Rabinowitz, J.G.: A specific sign for neonatal gastric perforation. J. Can. Assoc. Radiol. 24:141, 1973.

Coscina, W.F., Kressel, H.Y., Gefter, W.B., et al.: MR imaging of the double aortic arch. J. Comput. Assist. Tomogr. 10:673, 1986.

Cremin, B.J.: Congenital pyloric membranes in infancy. Radiology 92:509, 1969.

Cremin, B.J.: The urinary tract anomalies associated with agenesis of the abdominal walls. Br. J. Radiol. 44:767, 1971.

Cremin, B.J.: Urinary ascites and obstructive uropathy. Br. J. Radiol. 48:113, 1975.

Cremin, B.J.: A review of the ultrasonographic appearances of posterior urethral valve and ureteroceles. Pediatr. Radiol. 16:357, 1986.

Cremin, B.J., and Bass, E.M.: Retrosternal density: A sign of pulmonary hypoplasia. Pediatr. Radiol. 3:145, 1975.

Daves, M.L.: Roentgenology of tetralogy of Fallot. Semin. Roentgenol. 3:377, 1968.

Davignon, A.L., Greenwold, W.E., Du Shane, J.W., et al.: Congenital pulmonary atresia with intact ventricular septum: Clinicopathologic correlation of two anatomic types. Am. Heart. J. 62:591, 1961.

Davis, W.S., and Allen, R.P.: Accessory diaphragm. Radiol. Clin. North Am. 6:253, 1968.

Dedo, D.D.: Pediatric vocal cord paralysis. Laryngoscope 89:1378, 1979.

Diamond, D.A., and Ford, C.: Neonatal bladder rupture: A complication of umbilical artery catheterization. J. Urol. 142:1543, 1989.

Dickson, J.A.S.: Apple-peel small bowel: An uncommon variant of duodenal and jejunal atresia. J. Pediatr. Surg. 5:595, 1970.

Donn, S.M., and Kuhns, L.R.: Mechanism of endotracheal tube movement with change of head position in the neonate. Pediatr. Radiol. 9:37, 1980.

Edwards, D.K., Dyer, W.M., and Northway, W.H., Jr.: Twelve years' experience with bronchopulmonary dysplasia. Pediatrics 59:839, 1977.

Edwards, D.K., Higgins, C.B., and Gilpin, E.A.: The cardiothoracic ratio in newborn infants. (Abstract.) Radiology 137:16, 1980.

Edwards, D.K., Higgins, C.B., Meritt, A., et al.: Radiographic and echocardiographic evaluation of newborns treated with indomethacin for patent ductus arteriosus. AJR 131:1009, 1978.

Edwards, D.K., III, and Hilton, S.W.: Flat chest in chronic bronchopulmonary dysplasia. AJR 149:1213, 1987.

Effmann, E.L., Fram, E.K., Vock, P., et al.: Tracheal cross-sectional area in children: CT determination. Radiology 149:137, 1983.

Eibl, M., Wolf, H., Furnkranz, H., et al.: Prevention of necrotizing enterocotis in low birth weight infants by IgA-IgG feeding. N. Engl. J. Med. 319:1, 1988.

Elliott, L.P., Van Mierop, L.H.S., Gleason, D.C., et al.: The roentgenology of tricuspid atresia. Semin. Roentgenol. 3:399, 1968.

Ellis, K., and Nadelhaft, J.: Roentgenographic findings in hyaline membrane disease in infants weighing 2000 grams and over. AJR 78:444, 1957.

Fletcher, B.D.: Medial herniation of the parietal pleura: Useful sign of pneumothorax in supine neonates. AJR 130:469, 1978.

Fletcher, B.D., Earborn, D.G., and Mulopulos, G.P.: MR imaging in infants with airway obstruction: Preliminary observations. Radiology 160:245, 1986.

Flores, J.A.M.: Miliary pattern in neonatal pneumonia. Pediatr. Radiol. 18:355, 1988.

Fox, L., and Sprunt, K.: Neonatal osteomyelitis. Pediatrics 62:535, 1978.

Frech, R.S., McAllister, W.H., Ternberg, J., et al.: Meconium ileus relieved by 49% water soluble contrast enemas. Radiology 94:341, 1970.

Garbaccio, C., Gyepes, M.T., and Fonkalsrud, E.W.: Malfunction of the intact diaphragm in infants and children. Arch. Surg. 105:57, 1972.

Garris, J., Kangarloo, H., Sarti, D., et al.: The ultrasound spectrum of prune-belly syndrome. J. Clin. Ultrasound 8:117, 1980.

Giedion, A., Hoefliger, H., and Dangel, P.: Acute pulmonary x-ray changes in hyaline membrane disease treated with artificial ventilation and positive end-expiratory pressure (PEEP). Pediatr. Radiol. 1:145, 1973.

Goetzman, B.W., Stadalnik, R.C., Bogren, H.G., et al.: Thrombotic complications of umbilical artery catheters: A clinical and radiographic study. Pediatrics 56:374, 1975.

Gomes, A.S., Lois, J.F., George, B., et al.: Congenital abnormalities of the aortic arch. MR imaging. Radiology 165:691, 1987.

Gooding, C.A., Gregory, G.A., Tabor, P., et al.: Clinical and experimental studies of meconium aspiration of the newborn. Ann. Radiol. 14:162, 1971.

Goodman, G., Perkin, R.M., Anas, N.G., et al.: Pulmonary hypertension in infants with bronchopulmonary dysplasia. J. Pediatr. 112:67, 1988.

Goodwin, J.D., Merten, D.F., and Baker, M.E.: Paramediastinal pneumatocele: Alternative explanations to gas in the pulmonary ligament. AJR 145:525, 1985.

Gray, P.H.: Gastric perforation associated with indomethacin therapy in pre-term infants. Aust. Paediatr. J. 16:65, 1980.

Gupta, J.M., Robertson, N.R., and Wigglesworth, J.S.: Umbilical artery catheterization in the newborn. Arch. Dis. Child. 43:382, 1968.

Hall, J.A., Hartenberg, M.A., and Kodroff, M.B.: Chest radiographic findings in neonates on extracorporeal membrane oxygenation. Radiology 157:75, 1985.

Haney, P.J., Bohlman, M., and Chjen-Chih, J.S.: Radiographic findings in neonatal pneumonia. AJR 143:23, 1984.

Hawker, R.E., Bowdler, J.D., Celermajer, J.M., et al.: Angiographic assessment of anomalous origin of the left coronary from the pulmonary artery in infancy and childhood. Pediatr. Radiol. 5:69, 1976.

Hayden, C.K., Jr., Boulden, T.F., Swischuk, L.E., et al.: Sonographic demonstration of duodenal obstruction with midgut volvulus. AJR 142:9, 1984.

Hayden, C.K., Jr., Swischuk, L.E., Smith, T.H., et al.: Renal cystic disease in childhood. Radiographics 6:97, 1986.

Heij, H.A., Ekkelkamp, S., and Vos, A.: Diagnosis of congenital cystic adenomatoid malformation of the lung in newborn infants and children. Thorax 45:122, 1990.

Heneghan, M.A., Sosulski, R., and Baquero, J.M.: Persistent pulmonary abnormalities in newborns: The changing picture of bronchopulmonary dysplasia. Pediatr. Radiol. 16:180, 1986.

Henneberry, M.O., and Stephens, F.D.: Renal hypoplasia and dysplasia in infant with posterior urethral valves. J. Urol. 123:912, 1980.

Hernandez, R.J., and Tucker, G.F.: Congenital tracheal stenosis: Role of CT and high KV films. Pediatr. Radiol. 17:192–196, 1987.

Higgins, C.B., Broderick, T.W., Edwards, D.K., and Shumaker, A.: The hemodynamic significance of massive pneumopericardium in pre-term infants with respiratory distress syndrome. Radiology 133:363, 1979.

Hoffman, R.R., Jr., Campbell, R.E., and Decker, J.P.: Fetal aspiration syndrome: Clinical roentgenologic and pathologic features. AJR 122:90, 1974.

Holinger, P.H., Kutnick, S.L., Schild, J.A., and Holinger, L.D.: Subglottic stenosis in infants and children. Ann. Otol. 85:591, 1976.

Hueck-Parodi, L., Densler, J.F., Reed, R.C., et al.: Congenital cystic adenomatoid malformation of the lung. Clin. Pediatr. 8:327, 1969.

Hulnick, D.H., Naidich, D.P., McCauley, D.I., et al.: Late presentation of congenital cystic adenomatoid malformation of the lung. Radiology 151:569, 1984.

James, A.E., Heller, R.M., White, J.J., et al.: Spontaneous rupture of the stomach in the newborn: Clinical and experimental evaluation. Pediatr. Res. 19:79, 1976.

Johnstrude, I.S., and Carey, L.S.: Roentgenographic manifestations of endocardial fibroelastosis. AJR 94:109, 1965.

Jones, J.C., Almond, C.H., Snyder, H.M., et al.: Lobar emphysema and congenital heart disease in infancy. J. Thorac. Surg. 49:1, 1965.

Kanto, W.P., Jr., and Parrish, R.A., Jr.: Perforation of the peritoneum and intra-abdominal hemorrhage: A complication of umbilical vein catheterizations. Am. J. Dis. Child. 131:1102, 1977.

Kassner, E.G., Baumstark, A.E., Balsam, D., and Haller, J.O.: Passage of feeding catheters into the pleural space: Radiographic sign of trauma to the pharynx and esophagus in the newborn. AJR 128:19, 1977.

Kassner, E.G., Kauffman, S.L., Yoon, J.J., et al.: Pulmonary candidiasis in infants: Clinical, radiologic and pathologic features. AJR 137:707, 1981.

Kaufman, R.A., Kuhns, L.R., Poznanski, A.K., and Holt, J.F.: Gastrointestinal perforation without intraperitoneal air-fluid level in neonatal pneumoperitoneum. AJR 127:915, 1976.

Kendig, J.W., and Shapiro, D.L.: Surfactant therapy in the newborn. Pediatr. Ann. 17:504, 1988.

Kercsmar, C.M., Martin, R.J., Chatburn, R.L., et al.: Bronchoscopic findings in infants treated with high-frequency jet ventilation versus conventional ventilation. Pediatrics 82:884, 1988.

Kessler, H., and Smulewicz, J.J.: Microgastria associated with agenesis of the spleen. Radiology 107:393, 1973.

Kirks, D.R., and Taybi, H.: Prune belly syndrome: An unusual case of neonatal abdominal calcification. AJR 123:778, 1975.

Kliegman, R.M.: Models of the pathogenesis of necrotizing enterocolitis. J. Pediatr. 116:S2, 1990.

Kliegman, R.M., and Fanaroff, A.A.: Necrotizing enterocolitis. N. Engl. J. Med. 310:1093, 1984.

Knight, P.J., and Abdenour, G.: Pneumoperitoneum in the ventilated neonate: Respiratory or gastrointestinal origin? J. Pediatr. 98:972, 1981.

Lane, R.W., Weider, D.J., Steinem, C., et al.: Laryngomalacia: A review and case report of surgical treatment with resolution of pectus excavatum. Arch. Orolaryngol. 110:546, 1984.

Lanning, P., and Heikkinen, E.: Thymus simulating left upper lobe atelectasis. Pediatr. Radiol. 9:177, 1980.

Lawson, E.E., Gould, J.B., and Taeusch, H.W., Jr.: Neonatal pneumopericardium: Current management. J. Pediatr. Surg. 15:181, 1980.

Leape, L.L., and Longino, L.A.: Infantile lobar emphysema. Pediatrics 34:246, 1964.

Lebowitz, R.L., and Blickman, J.G.: The coexistence of uretero-pelvic junction obstruction and reflux. AJR 140:231, 1983.

Leonidas, J.C., Berdon, W.E., Baker, D.H., et al.: Meconium ileus and its complications: A reappraisal of plain film roentgen diagnostic criteria. AJR 108:598, 1970.

Leonidas, J.C., Fergus, M.B., Moylan, B., et al.: Ventilation-perfusion scans in neonatal regional pulmonary emphysema complicating ventilatory assistance. AJR 131:243, 1978.

Lindley, S., Mollitt, D.K., Seiber, J.J., et al.: Portal vein ultrasonography in the early diagnosis of necrotizing enterocolitis. J. Pediatr. Surg. 21:530, 1986.

Lucaya, J., Herrera, M., and Salcedo, S.: Traumatic pharyngeal pseudodiverticulum in neonates and infants: Two case reports and review of the literature. Pediatr. Radiol. 8:65, 1979.

Lundstrom, C.H., and Allen, R.P.P.: Bilateral congenital eventration of the diaphragm. AJR 97:216, 1966.

Lynch, E.P., Coran, A.G., Cohen, S.R., and Lee, F.A.: Traumatic esophageal pseudodiverticula in the newborn. J. Pediatr. Surg. 9:675, 1974.

Magilner, A.D., Capitanio, M.A., Wertheimer, I., et al.: Persistent localized intrapulmonary interstitial emphysema: An observation in three infants. Radiology 111:379, 1974.

Malmgren, M., Lavrin, S., and Lundstrom, N.R.: Pulmonary artery sling: Diagnosis by magnetic resonance imaging. Acta Radiol. 29:7, 1988.

Malone, P.S., and Fitzgerald, R.J.: Aberrant thymus: A misleading mediastinal mass. J. Pediatr. Surg. 22:130, 1987.

Mandell, G.A., and Chawla, M.S.: Chest tube positioning in neonatal pleural herniation. AJR 137:1029, 1981.

Mandell, G.A., and Finkelstein, M.S.: Gastric pneumatosis secondary to an intramural feeding catheter. Pediatr. Radiol. 18:418, 1988.

Mandell, G.A., Boulden, M.E., and Hercke, H.T.: Intermittent cervical thymus: Radiographic/sonographic correlation. (Abstract.) J. Ultrasound Med. 10:521, 1991.

Markowitz, R.I., Johnson, K.M., and Weinstein, E.M.: Hyperinflation of the lungs in infants with large left-to-right shunts. Invest. Radiol. 23:354, 1988.

McCarten, K.M., Rosenberg, H.K., Borden, S., IV, and Mandell, G.A.: Delayed appearance of right diaphragmatic hernia associated with group-B streptococcal infection in newborns. Radiology 139:385, 1981.

McCloud, T.C., and Ravin, C.E.: PEEP: Radiographic features and associated complications. AJR 129:209, 1977.

McCormick, T.L., and Kuhns, L.R.: Tracheal compression by a normal aorta associated with right lung agenesis. Radiology 130:659, 1970.

McCubbin, M., Frey, E.E., Wagener, J.S., et al.: Large airway collapse in bronchopulmonary dysplasia. J. Pediatr. 114:304, 1989.

McDonald, J., and Murphy, A.V.: Neonatal ascites from spontaneous rupture of the bladder. Arch. Dis. Child. 50:956, 1975.

Melson, G.L., Shackelford, G.D., Cole, B.R., et al.: The spectrum of sonographic findings in infantile polycystic kidney disease with urographic and clinical correlation. J. Clin. Ultrasound 13:113, 1985.

Merten, D.F., Goetzman, B.W., and Wennberg, R.P.: Persistent fetal circulation: An evolving clinical and radiographic concept of pulmonary hypertension of the newborn. Pediatr. Radiol. 6:74, 1977.

Merten, D.F., and Gooding, C.A.: Skeletal manifestations of congenital cytomegalic inclusion disease. Radiology 95:333, 1970.

Merten, D.F., Mumford, L., Filston, H.C., et al.: Radiological observations during transpyloric tube feeding in infants of low birth weight. Radiology 136:67, 1980.

Merten, D.F., Vogel, M.M., Adelman, R.D., et al.: Renovascular hypertension as a complication of umbilical arterial catheterization. Radiology 126:751, 1978.

Miller, D., Kirkpatrick, B.U., Kodroff, M., et al.: Pelvic exsanguination following umbilical artery catheterization in neonates. J. Pediatr. Surg. 14:264, 1979.

Miller, K.E., Edwards, D.K., Hilton, S., et al.: Acquired lobar emphysema in premature infants with bronchopulmonary dysplasia: An iatrogenic disease? Radiology 138:589, 1981.

Moccia, W.A., Kaude, J.V., and Felman, A.H.: Congenital eventration of the diaphragm: Diagnosis by ultrasound. Pediatr. Radiol. 10:197, 1981.

Moessinger, A.C., Driscoll, J.M., Jr., and Wigger, H.J.: High incidence of lung perforation by chest tube in neonatal pneumothorax. J. Pediatr. 92:635, 1978.

Mok, P.M., Reilly, B.J., and Ash, J.M.: Osteomyelitis in the neonate: Clinical aspects and the role of radiography and scintigraphy in the diagnosis and management. Radiology 145:677, 1982.

Moskowitz, P.S., and Griscom, N.T.: The medial pneumothorax. Radiology 120:143, 1976.

Mussbichler, H.: Radiologic study of intracranial calcifications in congenital toxoplasmosis. Acta. Radiol. Diagn. 7:369, 1968.

Nielson, H.C., Riemenschneider, T.A., and Jaffe, R.B.: Persistent transitional circulation. Radiology 120:649, 1976.

Northway, W.H., Jr., and Rosan, R.C.: Radiographic features of pulmonary oxygen toxicity in the newborn: Bronchopulmonary dysplasia. Radiology 91:49, 1968.

Nunn, I.N., and Stephens, F.D.: The triad syndrome: Composite anomaly of the abdominal wall, urinary system and testes. J. Urol. 86:782, 1961.

O'Brodovich, H.M., and Mellins, R.B.: Bronchopulmonary dysplasia: Unresolved neonatal acute lung injury. Am. Rev. Respir. Dis. 132:694, 1985.

Ogata, E.S., Gregory, G.A., Kitterman, J.A., et al.: Pneumothorax in respiratory distress syndrome: Incidence and effect on vital signs, blood gases and pH. Pediatrics 58:177, 1976.

Oppermann, H.C., Wille, L., Obladen, M., and Richter, E.: Systemic air embolism in respiratory distress syndrome of the newborn. Pediatr. Radiol. 8:139, 1979.

Ortiz, R.M., Cilley, R.E., and Bartlett, R.H.: Extracorporeal membrane oxygenation in pediatric respiratory failure. Pediatr. Clin. North Am. 34:39, 1987.

Otherson, H.B., Jr., and Lorenzo, R.L.: Diaphragmatic paralysis and eventration: New approaches to diagnosis and operative correction. J. Pediatr. Surg. 12:309, 1977.

Pereira, G.R., and Lemons, J.A.: Controlled study of transpyloric and intermittent gavage feeding in small preterm infants. Pediatrics 67:68, 1981.

Perlman, M., and Levin, M.: Fetal pulmonary hypoplasia, anuria, and oligohydramnios: Clinicopathologic observations and review of literature. Am. J. Obstet. Gynecol. 118:1119, 1974.

Perlman, M., Williams, J., and Hirsch, M.: Neonatal pulmonary hypoplasia after prolonged leakage of amniotic fluid. Arch. Dis. Child. 51:349, 1976.

Peterson, H.G., Jr., and Pendleton, M.E.: Contrasting roentgenographic pulmonary pattern of hyaline membrane and fetal aspiration syndromes. AJR 74:800, 1955.

Phillips, A.F., Rowe, J.C., and Raye, J.R.: Acute diaphragmatic paralysis after chest tube placement in a neonate. AJR 136:824, 1981.

Potter, E.L.: Facial characteristics of infants with bilateral renal agenesis. Am. J. Obstet. Gynecol. 51:885, 1946.

Pramanik, A.K., Alshuler, G., Light, I.J., et al.: Prune belly associated with Potter (renal nonfunction) syndrome. Am. J. Dis. Child. 131:672, 1977.

Pruksapong, C., Donovan, R.J., Pinit, A., et al.: Gastric duplication. J. Pediatr. Surg. 14:83, 1979.

Rizzo, A.J., Haller, J.O., Mulvihill, D.M., et al.: Calcification of the ductus venosus: A cause of right upper quadrant calcification in the newborn. Radiology 173:89, 1989.

Rollins, N.K., and Currarino, G.: MR imaging of the posterior mediastinal thymus. J. Comput. Assist. Tomogr. 12:518, 1988.

Rumack, C.M., Manco-Johnson, M.L., Manco-Johnson, M.J., et al.: Timing and course of neonatal intracranial hemorrhage using real-time ultrasound. Radiology 154:101, 1985.

Rutledge, M.L., Hawkins, E.P., and Langston, C.: Skeletal muscle growth failure induced in premature newborn infants by prolonged pancuronium treatment. J. Pediatr. 109:883, 1986.

Ryan, C.A., Barrington, K.J., Phillips, H.J., et al.: Contralateral pneumothoraces in the newborn: Incidence and predisposing factors. Pediatrics 79:417, 1987.

Sackett, G.L., and Ford, M.M.: Cytomegalic inclusion disease with calcification outlining the cerebral ventricles. AJR 76:512, 1956.

Sanders, R.C., and Hartman, D.S.: The sonographic distinction between neonatal multicystic kidney and hydronephrosis. Radiology 151:621, 1984.

Santulli, T.V., and Blanc, W.A.: Congenital atresia of intestine: Pathogenesis and treatment. Ann. Surg. 154:939, 1961.

Schlesinger, A.E., Cornish, J.D., and Null, D.M.: Dense pulmonary opacification in neonates treated with extracorporeal membrane oxygenation. Pediatr. Radiol. 16:448, 1986.

Schwartz, A.N., and Graham, C.B.: Neonatal tension pulmonary interstitial emphysema in bronchopulmonary dysplasia treatment with lateral decubitus positioning. Radiology 161:351, 1986.

Schwartz, M.Z., and Fille, R.M.: Plication of the diaphragm for symptomatic phrenic nerve paralysis. J. Pediatr. Surg. 13:259, 1978.

Scott, J.M.: Iatrogenic lesions in babies following umbilical vein catheterization. Arch. Dis. Child. 40:426, 1965.

Serlin, S.P., and Daily, W.J.R.: Tracheal perforation in the neonate: Complication of endotracheal intubation. J. Pediatr. 86:596, 1975.

Shackelford, G.D., and McAlister, W.H.: The aberrantly positioned thymus: A cause of mediastinal or neck masses in children. AJR 120:291, 1974.

Shohat, M., Levy, G., Schonfeld, T.D., et al.: Transient tachypnea of the newborn and asthma. Arch. Dis. Child. 64:277, 1989.

Sickler, E.A., and Gooding, C.A.: Asymmetric lung involvement in bronchopulmonary dysplasia. Radiology 118:379, 1976.

Siegle, R.L., Rabinowitz, J.G., and Sarasohn, C.: Intestinal perforation secondary to nasojejunal feeding tubes. AJR 126:1229, 1976.

Silverman, N.H., Lewis, A.B., Heymann, M.A., et al.: Echocardiographic assessment of ductus arteriosus in premature infants. Circulation 50:821, 1974.

Silverstein, E.F., Ellis, K., Casarella, W.J., et al.: Persistence of the fetal circulation: Radiologic considerations. AJR 137:497, 1981.

Simpson, A.J., Leonidas, J.C., Krasna, I.H., et al.: Roentgen diagnosis of midgut malrotation: Value of upper gastrointestinal radiographic study. J. Pediatr. Surg. 7:243, 1972.

Simpson, J.N.L., and Eckstein, H.B.: Congenital diaphragmatic hernia: A 20 year experience. Br. J. Surg. 72:735, 1985.

Sindel, B.D., Maisels, M.J., and Ballantine, V.N.: Gastroesophageal reflux to the proximal esophagus in infants with bronchopulmonary dysplasia. Am. J. Dis. Child. 143:1103, 1989.

Singleton, E.B., Rudolph, A.J., Rosenberg, H.S., et al.: The roentgenographic manifestations of the rubella syndrome in newborn infants. AJR 97:82, 1966.

Slovis, T.L., Renfro, B., Wats, F.B., et al.: Choanal atresia: Precise CT evaluation. Radiology 155:345, 1985.

Slovis, T.L., and Shankaran, S.: Patent ductus arteriosus in hyaline membrane disease: Chest radiography. AJR 135:307, 1980.

Smith, G.L., and Cooper, D.M.: Laryngomalacia and inspiratory obstruction in later childhood. Arch. Dis. Child. 56:345, 1981.

Solomon, A., and Rosen, E.: Focal osseous lesions in congenital lues. Pediatr. Radiol. 7:36, 1978.

Sommerschild, H.C.: Intestinal perforation in the newborn infant as a complication in umbilical vein infusion or exchange transfusion. Surgery 70:609, 1971.

South, M.A., Tompkins, W., Morris, R., et al.: Congenital malformation of the central nervous system associated with genital type (type II) herpes virus. J. Pediatr. 75:13, 1969.

Spangler, J.G., Kleinberg, F., Fulton, R.E., et al.: False aneurysm of the descending aorta: Complication of umbilical artery catheterization. Am. J. Dis. Child. 131:1258, 1977.

Stark, A.R., and Frantz, I.D., III: Respiratory distress syndrome. Pediatr. Clin. North Am. 33:533, 1986.

Steele, R.W., and Copeland, G.A.: Delayed resorption of pulmonary alveolar fluid in the neonate. Radiology 103:637, 1972.

Stocks, J., Godfrey, S., and Reynolds, E.O.R.: Airway resistance in infants after various treatment for hyaline membrane disease: Special emphasis on prolonged high levels of inspired oxygen. Pediatrics 61:178, 1978.

Strife, J.L., Baumel, A.S., and Dunbar, J.S.: Tracheal compression by the innominate artery in infancy and childhood. Radiology 139:73, 1981.

Strife, J.L., Matsumoto, J., Bisset, G.S., et al.: The position of the trachea in infants and children with right aortic arch. Pediatr. Radiol. 19:226, 1989.

Strife, J.L., Smith, P., Dunbar, J.S., et al.: Chest tube perforation of the lung in premature infants: Radiographic recognition. AJR 141:73, 1983.

Swenson, O., Sherman, J.O., Fisher, J.H.: Diagnosis of congenital megacolon: An analysis of 501 patients. J. Pediatr. Surg. 8:587, 1973.

Swischuk, L.E.: Transient respiratory distress of the newborn—TRDN: A temporary disturbance of a normal phenomenon. AJR 108:557, 1970.

Swischuk, L.E.: Bubbles in hyaline membrane disease: Differentiation of three types. Radiology 122:417, 1977.

Swischuk, L.E.: Imaging of the Newborn, Infant, and Young Child, 3rd ed. Baltimore, Williams & Wilkins, 1989, p. 496.

Swischuk, L.E., Richardson, C.J., Nichols, N.M., et al.: Primary pulmonary hypoplasia in the neonate. J. Pediatr. 95:573, 1979.

Swischuk, L.E., Richardson, C.J., Nichols, M.M., et al.: Bilateral pulmonary hypoplasia in the neonate (a classification). AJR 133:1057, 1979.

Symchych, P.S., Krauss, A.N., and Winchester, P.: Endocarditis following intracardiac placement of umbilical venous catheters in neonates. J. Pediatr. 90:287, 1977.

Taylor, G.A., Glass, P., Fitz, C.R., et al.: Neurologic status in infants treated with extracorporeal membrane oxygenation: Correlation of imaging findings with developmental outcome. Radiology 165:679, 1987.

Thieboult, D.W., Emmanouilides, G.C., Nelson, R.T., et al.: Patent ductus arteriosus complicating the respiratory distress syndrome in preterm infants. J. Pediatr. 86:120, 1975.

Todres, I.D., deBros, F., Kramer, S.S., et al.: Endotracheal tube placement in the newborn infant. J. Pediatr. 89:126, 1976.

Vinocur, L., Slovis, T.L., Perlmutter, A.D., et al.: Follow-up studies of multicystic dysplastic kidney. Radiology 167:391, 1988.

Volpe, J.J., Herscovitch, P., Perlman, J.M., et al.: Positron emission tomography in the newborn: Extensive impairment of regional cerebral blood flow with intraventricular hemorrhage and hemorrhagic intracerebral involvement. Pediatrics 72:589, 1983.

Wayne, E.R., Campbell, J.B., Burrington, J.D., et al.: Eventration of the diaphragm. J. Pediatr. Surg. 9:643, 1974.

Weber, A.L., DeLuca, S., and Shannon, D.C.: Normal and abnormal position of the umbilical artery and venous catheter on roentgenogram and review of complications. AJR 120:361, 1974.

Wesenberg, R.L., Graven, S.N., and McCabe, E.B.: Radiological findings in wet lung disease. Radiology 98:69, 1971.

Wetzell, R., and Gioia, F.R.: High frequency ventilation. Pediatr. Clin. North Am. 34:15, 1987.

Wexler, H.A.: The persistent loop sign in neonatal necrotizing enterocolitis: A new indication for surgical intervention? Radiology 126:201, 1978.

Williams, D.O., Whitaker, R.H., Barratt, T.M., et al.: Urethral valves. Br. J. Urol. 45:200, 1973.

Williams, D.W., Merten, D.F., Effman, E.L., et al.: Ventilator induced pulmonary pseudocysts in preterm infants. AJR 150:885, 1988.

Williams, H.J., Jarvis, C.W., Neal, W.A., and Reynolds, J.W.: Vascular thromboembolism complicating umbilical artery catheterization. AJR 116:475, 1972.

Williams, J.L., and Cumming, W.A.: Bronchopulmonary dysplasia. J. Thorac. Imag. 1:16, 1986.

Wiseman, W.E., and MacPherson, R.I.: "Acquired" congenital diaphragmatic hernia. J. Pediatr. Surg. 12:657, 1977.

Wolfe, E.L., Berdon, W.E., and Baker, D.H.: Improved plain film diagnosis of right aortic arch anomalies and high kilovoltage-selective filtration technique. Pediatr. Radiol. 7:141, 1978.

Ziprkowski, M.N., and Teele, R.L.: Gastric volvulus in childhood. AJR 132:921, 1979.

RADIOLOGIC PROCEDURES

PART
VIII

22

Systemic Effects of Radiologic Procedures

■

Michael A. Bettmann

The effects of radiologic procedures can be classified into three categories: those related to equipment, those related to diagnostic agents, and those related to therapeutic pharmaceuticals employed in conjunction with the procedures.

EQUIPMENT

The effects related to equipment are primarily those of radiation, and a detailed discussion is beyond the scope of this chapter. Currently available evidence suggests that doses of radiation from diagnostic procedures have no significant effect in regard to teratogenesis, induction of malignancies, or other distinct abnormalities. Whether cataract formation increases or longevity decreases is not clear, but no recent evidence has been found to support the occurrence of such adverse effects (Baverstock et al., 1981; Land et al., 1980; Miller et al., 1989; NRCP Report No. 100, 1989; Upton, 1977; Wagner, 1991). The information concerning the exposure received by interventionalists involved in large numbers of prolonged procedures is, however, scant. Similarly, there is relatively little information regarding the effect of radiation exposure on radiologists in the era of modern image intensifiers.

Catheter-related effects are generally local (e.g., vessel wall damage resulting in distal embolization or pseudoaneurysm formation). Systemic effects may be encountered in a few specific situations. Arterial procedures in which a catheter is advanced into the aortic root or advanced selectively into the innominate or carotid artery involve the potential risk of a cerebrovascular accident. Overall, this risk is low (Mani et al., 1978), but it may be increased in patients with extensive atherosclerosis of the aorta or great vessels. In patients with extensive atherosclerosis or

aneurysms of the abdominal aorta, catheter and wire manipulation may on rare occasion dislodge material into the mesenteric circulation. If thrombi are dislodged into the renal or lower extremity arteries, symptoms are usually local, and effective treatment can be symptomatic or may involve thrombolytic agents or surgical embolectomy, as indicated clinically. In the mesenteric circulation, however, there may be a relatively insidious onset of bowel ischemia, which can be extensive and sometimes fatal.

Catheter-induced cardiac arrhythmias are generally related to the direct contact between the catheter and the endocardium. They resolve when the catheter is moved. This phenomenon is seen most often during pulmonary angiography. As the right ventricle is traversed for selective catheterization of the pulmonary arteries, ectopy is very frequent but usually transient and unimportant. Particular care must be exercised, however, in patients with poorly controlled arrhythmias or left bundle branch block. In such patients, a temporary pacing wire may be advisable. Most other catheter- or wire-induced complications, including thrombosis, embolization, dissection, and vessel perforation, result in local effects that are usually self-limited (Bettmann, 1983; Fellmeth et al., 1991; Hessel et al., 1981; Leach et al., 1990).

CONTRAST AGENTS

Contrast agents are the most widely used medications in radiologic procedures. In addition, they are among the most widely used of all medications in terms of total volume. All contrast agents administered intravascularly produce systemic effects, although these are usually minor. The systemic effects of contrast media may be substantial, however, in certain situations (Bettmann, 1989; Katayama et al.,

1990). These situations include administration in particular parts of the body, such as the heart, or in particular patients, such as those in an unstable hemodynamic state. One must consider the potentially important systemic effects of contrast agents in a systematic fashion, and this task is perhaps best accomplished by considering four distinct categories of these effects: cardiac, vascular/hematologic, renal, and general.

The cardiac effects of contrast agents are most marked with intracardiac administration, as during cardiac catheterization or pulmonary angiography. Cardiac effects occur, however, whenever contrast agents are administered. Certain factors inherent to contrast agents lead to more marked effects. Additives to contrast media, such as sodium citrate, which avidly binds ionized calcium, lead to increased hemodynamic effects of contrast agents whenever they are administered (Bourdillon et al., 1985; Caulfield et al., 1975). It is also clear that in general, the higher the osmolality of contrast media, the greater are the hemodynamic effects, although the specific importance of this phenomenon is unclear.

The specific effects of contrast agents on the heart vary with the site of administration. Intracoronary injection invariably involves a decrease in blood pressure accompanied by a decrease in heart rate (Bettmann et al., 1984; Reagan et al., 1988). These are direct cardiac effects. Conversely, with pulmonary artery injection, with left ventricular injection, or with most other systemic injections, the decrease in blood pressure that generally occurs is accompanied by an increased heart rate, which suggests a reflex process. Knowledge of these effects allows predictions regarding which patients are most likely to suffer direct adverse effects of contrast injection. Such patients are those who have limited myocardial function or in whom cardiac compensation is borderline—for example, those with severe congestive heart failure, those with a recent large myocardial infarction, those with severe coronary artery disease or tight aortic stenosis (even with normal myocardial function), and those with pulmonary hypertension. In such patients, a decrease in blood pressure may result in significant hemodynamic compromise with resultant morbidity.

As in many other cases, the extent to which the specific use of a low-osmolality contrast agent reduces morbidity or mortality in such patients is unclear (Hlatky et al., 1990). Some sparse evidence indicates that high-risk cardiac patients, at least during cardiac catheterization, have a lower incidence of significant complications when a low-osmolality agent is used (Feldman et al., 1988). Although this small study must be looked at in light of larger studies that are less convincing (Hlatky et al., 1990; Katayama et al., 1990), it seems reasonable to suggest that the significant cardiac effects of contrast agents are lessened in high-risk cardiac patients through the use of a low-osmolality agent.

An additional systemic manifestation that deserves consideration is that of cardiopulmonary arrest. As is discussed subsequently, the most feared reaction to contrast agents is the "anaphylactoid" response, which involves cardiac arrest that is subsequent to contrast administration and independent of dose or site of administration. The cause of such reactions is not clear, in part because evidence indicates several possible etiologic factors. One pathophysiologic process alone is unlikely to explain all cases. Among the clear causes of cardiac arrest following contrast administration is electromechanical dissociation, which can be caused by sudden alteration in ionized calcium (Caulfield et al., 1975). This effect in turn may be related to calcium binding by the contrast agent, or, more specifically, by the additives noted previously, such as sodium citrate and sodium ethylenediaminetetra-acetic acid (EDTA). Most contrast agents no longer contain these additives, but instead contain calcium disodium EDTA, which does not bind calcium.

In general, other cardiac effects are more obviously related to underlying cardiac disease. Examples include patients with pulmonary hypertension who develop severe right heart failure following pulmonary angiography and patients with cardiomyopathies and marked compromise of left ventricular function who develop severe systemic hypotension. Other than calcium binding, cardiac effects remain incompletely explained. In most cases, they can be simply and effectively treated symptomatically as needed, as with hypotension and bradycardia following coronary angiography (treated with leg elevation, fluids, and, if necessary, intravenous atropine) and as with generally mild hypotension and tachycardia following carotid or peripheral angiography.

The renal effects of contrast agents are also feared. Despite extensive experimental and clinical attention to contrast-related renal failure, many questions remain. Although it is clear that pre-existing renal failure can be worsened following the administration of contrast, and that on rare occasions, renal failure may occur in patients with evidently normal renal function prior to contrast administration, the etiologic factors, frequency, and associated risk factors for these occurrences are not well understood. Patients with pre-existing renal failure are apparently more likely to develop worsening of renal function after contrast administration, and patients with normal renal function rarely develop renal failure (Miller et al., 1988; Parfrey et al., 1989). Many risk factors have been considered in the past, but the only one that is supported by reliable data is pre-existing renal failure. Such risk factors as hepatic dysfunction, congestive heart failure, and diabetes mellitus with normal renal function are not consistently associated (Brezis and Epstein, 1989; Gomes et al., 1989). Similarly, no clear dose–effect relationship has been found (Miller et al., 1988). Perhaps most surprisingly, and in contradistinction to the results of experimental studies, the use of low-osmolality contrast agents does not appear to produce a lower likelihood of contrast-induced renal dysfunction than does the use of conventional high-osmolality agents (Brezis and Epstein, 1989; Parfrey et al., 1989; Schwab et al., 1989). Studies are currently under way to determine whether these results are applicable to patients with severe renal failure, but currently available data suggest with reasonable certainty the accuracy of these results in patients with normal renal function, and even in those with mild renal failure.

The effects of contrast media on renal function are difficult to delineate accurately, either experimentally or clinically, for two primary reasons. First, neither the specific site nor the exact nature of the effect of contrast agents on the kidney is known. Second, clinical renal disease, and therefore the additive effects of contrast agents, vary widely in etiologic factors and location of damage. The osmotic effect of contrast agents may be important in regard to renal function, but it is more likely important in regard to cardiac function, as studies fail to demonstrate a substantial difference between high- and low-osmolality contrast agents or between patients receiving high and low doses of contrast material (Gomes et al., 1989; Miller et al., 1988; Schwab et al., 1989).

Vascular and hemotologic effects also occur with any injection of contrast agent. They occur because contrast comes in contact with both the blood and the blood vessel wall with all injections, whether the injection is central or peripheral, arterial or venous. The concern in reference to hematologic effects centers on the difference between ionic and nonionic contrast agents. Both high- and low-osmolality ionic contrast media substantially retard clotting in high concentrations. That is, during arteriography or when small amounts of blood are in contact with a large amount of contrast material, as in a catheter, ionic contrast agents prevent the blood from clotting for several minutes or longer (Stormorken, 1988). The effect of nonionic agents is somewhat different and is still poorly understood (Grollman et al., 1988; Kopko et al., 1990). The retardation of clotting is clearly not as great with nonionic agents. What remains to be determined is whether this difference is clinically significant. To date, large studies have shown no difference in the incidence of embolic or thrombotic phenomena in comparing ionic and nonionic agents, but such occurrences are often hard to detect. At this point, one must be aware that differences might exist and must ensure that optimal technique is used, particularly with nonionic agents used in angiography.

Vascular effects assume potential importance with the realization that has emerged over the past few years that the blood vessel wall is an extremely active organ. It produces many substances that are known to have systemic effects, including prostaglandins, heparin and heparin-like substances, urokinase, and various mitogens. Direct interaction of the vessel wall with markedly hyperosmolar contrast agents, which include both high- and low-osmolality agents, can potentially release vasoactive substances that might cause such relatively minor symptoms as flushing or pain or, conceivably, such serious effects as marked hypotension or bronchoconstriction. The causes of specific systemic effects are difficult to determine. At present, contrast agents are known to lead to relatively minor acute alterations in vascular wall function (Morgan et al., 1989), but such alterations are not likely to lead to significant systemic effects. Because of the known but incompletely defined metabolic activity of the vessel wall, further investigation of the role of the normal and abnormal vessel wall in systemic reactions is warranted.

As noted previously, many of the systemic effects of contrast injection, particularly intravenous injection, are widely considered to be anaphylactoid in origin, but direct cardiac and vascular effects are also known to cause important systemic effects. A true allergy to contrast agents is rare. Symptoms of such allergic reactions are probably primarily cutaneous or hematologic rather than classically anaphylactoid (Kendel et al., 1984). Life-threatening systemic reactions to contrast media may be caused by a poorly understood mechanism that involves the immune system (Lasser et al., 1987), may be related to anxiety and a neurocardiac interaction (Podrid, 1985; Samuels, 1987), or may be related to stimulation of the parasympathetic nervous system, with resultant hypotension and bradycardia.

Attempts to define the specific etiologic factors of symptomatic systemic reactions are important, so that appropriate prophylaxis can be used and appropriate therapy can be given when needed. Anxiety clearly has a significant role in radiologic procedures, as in other procedures. This must be recognized so that preventive measures can be taken (Podrid, 1985). The importance of anxiety cannot be overemphasized, although it is obviously difficult to quantitate. Similarly, a vagal response is relatively common and is usually easily treated, if recognized. Difficulty arises when hypotension is thought to be the result of an anaphylactoid reaction and is treated solely with measures such as epinephrine and bronchodilators. If a patient is hypotensive with normal cardiac rate or bradycardia, fluids and atropine must be administered instead (vanSonnenberg et al., 1987). If a severe systemic reaction is related to cardiac depression, appropriate systemic resuscitation in addition to appropriate cardiac medications must be considered. Such interventions may include antiarrhythmic agents such as lidocaine or quinidine.

The difference in incidence of systemic effects between high- and low-osmolality contrast agents is difficult to assess. There is clearly a higher incidence of nausea and vomiting with agents of higher osmolality (Bettmann, 1990), as well as an increase in other minor side effects such as urticaria. This difference may be sixfold to tenfold, but such reactions are almost invariably self-limited, require no or minimal treatment, and do not progress to severe reactions. Whether they can be used to predict severe reactions with subsequent contrast injections is not clear, but evidence suggests that in general they cannot. Also, a lower incidence of more serious systemic reactions is thought to occur with low- as compared with high-osmolality agents (Katayama et al., 1990). This difference appears to be approximately threefold to sixfold, depending on study design and definition of what constitutes a severe or very severe reaction. Most severe reactions, however, are not life-threatening and do not even require institution or prolongation of hospitalization (Powe et al., 1988). It is surprising, but reassuring, that there is no evidence of a difference in mortality rates between the two classes of contrast media (Bettmann, 1990). This lack of a difference in mortality reflects the high degree of safety of both low- and high-osmolality contrast media.

The use of contrast media for magnetic resonance imaging (MRI) is increasing. To date, almost all the intravascular agents are chelates of gadolinium, most often gadolinium diethylenetriaminepenta-acetic acid (Gd-DTPA). This compound is as high in osmolality as conventional contrast agents, but is usually administered in very small doses. Systemic reactions to this agent have been reported (Gibby, 1988), but the experience to date suggests that severe reactions are probably rare. Further experience with this class of agents must be gained before conclusions can be made.

One additional area of particular interest involves the use of barium (Gelfand, 1991). Reactions to oral barium, either local or systemic, are extremely rare. Between December 1988 and September 1990, however, nine fatal reactions related to barium enemas were reported. Five of these cases were thought to be related, at least in part, to the latex formulation used for the barium enema tips. Subsequently, this type of inflatable tip has been recalled and replaced. As with all diagnostic procedures, it is extremely disquieting to encounter a severe or fatal reaction. This incidence of fatality, however, is less than 1 in 2,000,000 procedures. By way of comparison, the major complication rate of colonoscopy, a frequently advocated alternative to barium enemas, is 0.2%, with a fatality rate of 0.02%, or 1 in 5000 (Habr-Gama and Waye, 1989).

Although minor systemic effects are common, the systemic effects of contrast agents, both intravascular and gastrointestinal, are thankfully rare, with very rare fatalities. Regarding intravascular use, the newer low-osmolality contrast agents have a lower incidence of minor side effects and probably a lower incidence of moderate to severe side effects, but no difference in mortality rate. Given the marked increase in their cost, they are most useful in patients with particular risks. Patients in this category include those with severe cardiac disease, those with a history of *significant* prior reaction to contrast agents (this excludes nausea and vomiting), those with a history of significant and active allergies, or those in a clinical situation in which discomfort or movement would pose a substantial risk. Indications are likely to change with the accrual of further data and with the development of newer, less expensive, and safer low-osmolality contrast media.

THERAPEUTIC AGENTS

Systemic effects of therapeutic agents are related to several specific categories. Many medications are encountered coincidentally during radiologic procedures, including antibiotics, various cardiac drugs, and antineoplastic agents. The most important medications, however, are those regularly employed during radiologic procedures. These include thrombolytic agents, anticoagulants, antiplatelet agents, vasodilators, vasoconstrictors, agents used directly for embolization procedures, sedatives, and analgesics. Most embolic agents, including absolute ethanol, surgical gelatin sponge (Gelfoam), microfibrillar collagen (Avitene), rapidly polymerizing plastics (e.g., cyanoacrylate) and stainless steel coils containing wool (Gianturco-Anderson-Wallace coils) have purely local effects when properly used. Secondary systemic effects occur when, for example, arteriovenous malformations are embolized from the arterial side and iatrogenic pulmonary embolization occurs (Chuang et al., 1981).

The various devices used for intravascular stenting or for inferior vena cava (IVC) filtration fall into a related category. Although adverse effects are well described, they are for the most part local. The most common complication of the various intravascular stents is occlusion. As pre-existent arterial occlusion or severe stenosis is usually the reason such stents are initially employed, sequelae tend to be minimal and nonsystemic. In the case of IVC filters, occlusion with consequent leg swelling is thought to occur in 5% to 12% of cases (Dorfman et al., 1989; Mewissen et al., 1989). This complication generally results in discomfort, which responds to the use of an elastic stocking. This complication may eventually lead to chronic venous stasis disease, but filters are used most often in patients with limited mobility (e.g., quadriplegics) or with limited life expectancy, so that this possibility is usually not a major consideration. Rarely, acute occlusion may lead to phlegmasia cerulea dolens (Aruny and Kandarpa, 1990). This condition causes venous gangrene due to occlusion of both iliac systems and is almost invariably fatal unless promptly treated with heparin anticoagulation.

Thrombolytic Agents

Thrombolytic agents are increasingly used in radiologic procedures (McNamara and Fischer, 1985; van Breda et al., 1987). Various types are available, and several methods of administration have been advocated. All types and methods, regardless of selectivity of administration, result in systemic effects. The agents currently available are streptokinase, urokinase, recombinant tissue plasminogen activator (r-tPA), and anisoylated plasminogen–streptokinase activator complex (APSAC, Eminase). Several other agents, including recombinant urokinase, pro-urokinase, and antibody-directed plasminogen activators, are being investigated. All of these agents have the primary function of catalyzing the conversion of plasminogen to plasmin. Plasmin in turn breaks down fibrin, which results in lysis of thrombi, which are formed on fibrin strands. Two problems are encountered with all of these agents. First, not all fibrin-based thrombi are pathologic. Those that result in pulmonary embolism or pulmonary artery occlusion clearly are pathologic, but those that form in response to normal daily activity represent a normal physiologic response. Even when administered locally, in all but very low doses, all available agents lyse both physiologic and pathologic thrombi. For this reason, thrombolytic agents are contraindicated in patients with recent surgery, cerebrovascular accident, or active bleeding. Similarly, arterial and venous punctures must be limited as much as possible in patients undergoing thrombolytic therapy.

Second, thrombolytic agents vary in their specificity. Streptokinase is a relatively nonspecific enzyme. It functions by combining with free plasminogen. The resulting streptokinase–plasminogen complex activates additional plasminogen molecules. This activation occurs not only with plasminogen, which is bound to thrombus, but also with circulating plasminogen. Furthermore, streptokinase catalyzes the breakdown of various other proteins, including fibrinogen. Reactive thrombosis may therefore occur, most often with the use of catheters for streptokinase infusion. Urokinase acts by direct plasminogen cleavage and is somewhat more specific as an enzyme, but not entirely so. The agent r-tPA acts by combining with fibrin-bound plasminogen in thrombi, rather than by directly activating plasminogen in circulation. It, too, has nonspecific effects, however, as well as effects on physiologic thrombi. The agent APSAC is also more specific than streptokinase, but additional enzymatic as well as systemic effects occur (Bassand et al., 1989).

Even when thrombolytic agents are directly infused into a peripheral arterial occlusion via catheter, a systemic lytic state is almost invariably achieved. This state may lead to various bleeding complications, ranging from oozing at venipuncture sites to major retroperitoneal or intracerebral bleeding. Also, as previously noted, reactive thrombi may form. In patients receiving prolonged thrombolytic therapy (i.e., for a period of more than 4 hours) concomitant heparinization has been empirically found to reduce this type of complication, which is generally catheter- or guidewire-related (McNamara and Fischer, 1985). Satisfactory methods of preventing systemic effects of prolonged infusion have yet to be developed. Measurement of levels of fibrinogen and of fibrin split products (the latter are themselves lytic) have not been found to have a predictive value for incipient bleeding (Bonnier et al., 1988). Similarly, monitoring of hematocrit may help to indicate the onset of major bleeding but does not prevent it. The most effective approach probably consists of limiting the dose and duration of infusion, but this measure may limit the efficacy of thrombolytic therapy, as higher doses have been found to lead to more rapid resolution of thrombotic occlusions (McNamara and Fischer, 1985). In addition, longer infusion times are related to higher complication rates (van Breda et al., 1987), but this finding may be related in part to the specific agent.

Much of the available literature comparing various agents in large numbers of patients concerns intravenous administration for acute myocardial infarction. The results of these studies differ from what is expected in radiologic use, both because of intravenous rather than intra-arterial infusion, and because thrombi treated angiographically are usually subacute or chronic. That is, patients with acute symptoms are usually treated surgically. Only those patients who do not have acutely threatened limbs (e.g., an acutely cold leg with loss of function or sensation) are treated angiographically. Such individuals usually have symptoms and thrombotic occlusions that have been present for 1 day to 3 months. Conversely, in the treatment of myocardial infarctions, thrombolysis is employed for acute thrombi and is effective only if begun within 4 to 6 hours of the onset of symptoms.

The specific thrombolytic agents differ quantitatively rather than qualitatively in systemic effects, despite the theoretic improvement in fibrin specificity of r-tPA and APSAC. Streptokinase, however, has the additional problem of being a foreign protein. Its currently used, purified form rarely, if ever, causes anaphylactic reactions. Most people, however, have antibodies due to prior streptococcal infections. The dose necessary to overcome antibodies and achieve a lytic effect, therefore, varies widely. This problem is partially obviated by selective infusion into thrombi, but in general, streptokinase has been found to have a lower success rate than urokinase in treating peripheral arterial occlusion (McNamara and Fischer, 1985; van Breda et al., 1987). Also, retreatment with streptokinase in less than 6 to 12 months is usually inadvisable because of the production of new antibodies. In addition, systemic effects have been found to vary with specific formulations, as reflected in the lower incidence of intracerebral bleeding with the currently used, single-chain r-tPA as compared with the double-chain form that was initially available. This finding is thought to be related to greater fibrin specificity with the single-chain form (Gurevich, 1989).

Anticoagulants

Heparin is another agent widely used in radiologic procedures, and it affects the hemostatic mechanism. The primary effect of this large, complex molecule is induction of a change in shape in antithrombin III (AT-III), which causes it to bind more readily to thrombin (Rosenberg and Lam, 1979). This change inactivates thrombin and thus blocks enzymatic conversion of fibrinogen into fibrin. Heparin–AT-III binding is reversible and noncatalytic, and the effect is not the conversion of AT-III to a different form, but rather an increase of its activity through alteration of the accessibility of its active site. Heparin, however, has a number of additional actions. It inactivates other components of the coagulation cascade, notably Factor Xa, and also affects smooth muscle cell proliferation (Clowes and Clowes, 1986). Like urokinase and r-tPA, heparin is a normal component of the endothelial cells that line the blood vessel wall, and it is thought to be one of the factors responsible for the nonthrombogenic character of normal endothelium (Vane et al., 1990).

The different functions of heparin are thought to involve different portions of the molecule. In theory, then, fractionation would allow production of smaller molecules with specific, limited activities. Fractionation has been attempted, both by molecular weight and by function. Although the former method is difficult at this time, the latter has been performed with some clinical success. In particular, a fraction with markedly decreased AT-III activity but preserved anti–Factor Xa action has been successfully used to achieve prophylaxis for patients at risk of developing deep vein thrombosis, without exposure to the risks of full heparin anticoagulation (Turpie et al., 1986). This fragment is also being investigated for use in the prevention of restenosis following angioplasty. The rationale for such use is that restenosis is primarily due to smooth muscle cell proliferation. In vitro, restenosis can be markedly lessened with either heparin or heparin fragments (Clowes and Clowes, 1986; Vane et al., 1990), but the effects in vivo remain to be proved.

Clinically, heparin is used during radiologic procedures both to prevent thrombosis during or immediately following angioplasty or stent placement and to prevent thrombosis induced by a combination of slow flow and the use of thrombogenic catheters during thrombolysis. It is effective in both of these situations. The dose used varies but is generally 5000 to 10,000 IU as a bolus, and if necessary, a constant infusion of about 1000 IU/hr, to achieve an activated partial thromboplastin time (aPTT) of 40 to 60 seconds (normal aPTT is 20 to 35 seconds). The biologic half-life of heparin is about 90 minutes (Hirsh et al., 1976); the dose necessary to achieve and maintain a therapeutic level of anticoagulation varies widely among individual patients. All patients receiving heparin, therefore, must be carefully monitored. If the aPTT is too low, no effective anticoagulation occurs. If the level is too high, the risk of bleeding substantially increases. As with thrombolytic agents, one must keep in mind that heparin is both an effective and a dangerous drug. The risk-benefit ratio for heparin use must be continually re-assessed.

Warfarin is increasingly used in radiologic procedures. It prevents conversion of prothrombin to thrombin, which is one step prior to the primary level of action of heparin. Recently, warfarin has been accepted as effective in preventing deep vein thrombosis in patients at risk when it is administered in doses that are usually considered subtherapeutic. This approach lessens the risk of full anticoagulation but provides adequate protection. Monitoring is more intense and difficult, and the onset of action is slower. Warfarin has been used in attempts to lessen the restenosis rate following angioplasty, primarily in the coronary arteries. Like heparin, it has not proved effective to date. Warfarin is most often encountered in radiologic procedures as a concurrently used medication having an effect that must be taken into consideration in the timing of interventional procedures. No clear guidelines exist for acceptable prothrombin times during angiography. A normal value is desirable, but elevations of 35% are generally considered safe. Rather than reversing the prothrombin time (PT) with parenteral vitamin K, most physicians prefer to allow the PT to decline gradually, and, if necessary, to cover patients temporarily with heparin if anticoagulation is necessary before and after the procedure. In contrast to warfarin, heparin is easily reversed with protamine and has a relatively short biologic half-life (Hirsh et al., 1976).

Antiplatelet Agents

Antiplatelet agents are increasingly used in patients with cardiovascular disease. Specific formulations are under investigation, but aspirin remains a mainstay that appears to be at least as effective as other, more expensive preparations (AIMS Trial Study Group, 1990). Among its many properties, aspirin irreversibly blocks platelet thromboxane synthesis, by acetylating the enzyme cyclo-oxygenase. Thus, a single oral aspirin effectively, albeit incompletely, blocks platelet aggregation and release. This action has been shown to lead to an overall decrease in cardiac morbidity (AIMS Trial Study Group, 1990). Because of its antiplatelet effects, aspirin at low to moderate doses (65 to 325 mg daily) has been used extensively in patients with prior cardiovascular events and in those undergoing angioplasty (Fuster et al., 1989; Relman, 1988). Aspirin apparently does not prevent restenosis, but it does lower the incidence of acute occlusion following coronary angioplasty (Ellis et al., 1987; Schwarz et al., 1988). It is inexpensive, generally safe in all patients except those with an aspirin allergy, and possibly helpful. It is, therefore, widely used at an empiric dose of 325 mg daily in patients with known cardiovascular disease, or following a vascular intervention. Dipyridamole, another widely used antiplatelet agent, does not seem to improve the efficacy of aspirin, either when used alone or when the two are used concurrently.

Other Vasoactive Agents

Various other vasoactive medications are used in vascular procedures, usually orally and with minimal systemic effects. These include nitroglycerin (NTG) and various calcium channel blockers, as well as other direct vasodilators such as papaverine, tolazoline (Priscoline), and nitroprusside. In patients with angina, NTG is an important agent. It should, therefore, be readily available in all radiology departments. Its action is thought to inhibit guanosine triphosphate (GTP) breakdown in smooth muscle cells in both coronary and peripheral arteries. It is most commonly administered sublingually at a dose of 1/150 or 1/300 g. If it is fresh, NTG acts within seconds to increase coronary flow and relieve angina in patients with coronary artery disease. In noncardiac patients, it usually leads to mild hypotension and headache. It is a useful adjunct to intravascular interventions in small vessels. At a dose of 100 μg, repeated at intervals of 1 to 5 minutes, it treats or prevents spasm in arteries below the knee or in distal upper extremity arteries, without systemic symptoms. Nifedipine is the calcium channel blocking agent most often used in radiology. Its mechanism of action is different from that of NTG, in that it partially blocks smooth muscle cell contraction by blocking one of the channels of influx of ionized calcium. It is most often administered orally at a dose of 10 mg. It is also a useful adjunct in vascular spasm and at this dose is rarely associated with systemic symptoms. Nitroprusside is particularly useful when administered parenterally for the short-term control of hypertension. It must be carefully monitored and adjusted. For a more thorough discussion of these medications, a textbook of pharmacology or clinical cardiology should be consulted.

Other vasoactive medications, such as vasopressin or papaverine, are particularly useful in diagnostic or therapeutic angiography but have a minimal role in daily practice. Vasopressin (Pitressin) has been widely used to control gastrointestinal bleeding. It is a posterior pituitary extract whose primary action is mesenteric vasoconstriction. Intra-arterially, it is used at a dose of 0.2 to 0.4 unit/min, as tolerated. In variceal bleeding, it is thought to be as effective when administered in a higher dose (0.4 to 0.6 unit/min) intravenously as when it is administered directly into the superior mesenteric artery. The major systemic concern is acute coronary vasoconstriction in patients with coronary artery disease; patients must be carefully monitored for electrocardiogram (ECG) changes or chest pain, so that the dose can be promptly reduced. If prolonged use is necessary, patients may develop a syndrome identical to inappropriate antidiuretic hormone secretion. Again, the dose must be reduced or treatment stopped, and fluid restriction must be instituted.

Sedatives, Analgesics, and Anesthetics

In all procedures, ranging from intravenous urography to interventional vascular radiology, sedation, analgesia, and anesthesia are major concerns. Patient preparation for the particular procedure is the primary consideration in this regard. Appropriate discussion and interaction with patients not only lessens discomfort, but also lessens both anxiety and complications (Egbert et al., 1963; Podrid, 1985; Samuels, 1987). Nonetheless, medications often prove to be an indispensable adjunct to explanation and reassurance.

Antihistamines with a primary histamine$_1$ (H$_1$)-receptor blocking effect, such as diphenhydramine or hydroxyzine, are frequently used to help achieve sedation (Forrest et al., 1977). They have relatively minor but prolonged sedative effects, so that they must be used with care in outpatients. They also have no analgesic effects, although they potentiate the analgesia produced by narcotics, which can therefore be used at lower dosage levels. They also have minor antiemetic effects. They have relatively little effect on blocking symptomatic histamine release unless they are administered at least several hours prior to contrast agent administration. If such an effect is the aim of using these antihistamines, histamine$_2$ (H$_2$)-receptor blockers, such as cimetidine or ranitidine, should also be used. No evidence has been found, however, that antihistamines of either category, used alone or in combination, decrease the incidence of severe or recurrent contrast agent reactions.

Benzodiazepines, such as diazepam or midazolam, are useful for producing both sedation and decreased anxiety. In contrast, barbiturates are relatively safe and effective sedatives but do not reduce anxiety as reliably (Forrest et al., 1977). Diazepam is widely used, either orally at a dose of 5 to 10 mg, 60 to 90 minutes prior to procedures, or intravenously at a dose of 5 to 10 mg via slow infusion. It is effective, but can lead to local pain and thrombophlebitis when administered intravenously. It also may cause respiratory depression, particularly in the elderly, or prolonged sedation in patients with hepatic dysfunction. Midazolam, a newer benzodiazepine, does not cause vascular damage when administered intravenously (Reves et al., 1985). It can be reliably administered intravenously or intramuscularly with rapid and usually short-lived (60- to 90-minute) effects. At a dose that produces sedative and anxiolytic effects comparable with those of diazepam (1 to 5 mg, administered in 1-mg increments), midazolam has the advantage, particularly in painful procedures, of producing a brief (20- to 90-minute) amnestic effect. Midazolam is usually preferred by patients as compared with diazepam, but it must be used with great care because it is thought to lead to hypoxia, which may be delayed in onset. When it is administered, then, the use of a pulse oximeter is advisable, particularly in older patients or in those with lung disease.

Droperidol is a useful adjunctive drug in radiologic procedures, partly for sedation but more for its antiemetic effects (Lind and Mushlin, 1987). The antiemetic effects can be achieved with intravenous doses of 0.625 to 1.25 mg. Narcotics are also useful for sedation but are more useful for pain control. Those commonly used are morphine, meperidine, and fentanyl. Morphine and meperidine have the selective advantage of longer duration of action, but they may cause profound sedation and respiratory depression, particularly after the sudden removal of the painful stimulus. Fentanyl is a potent, short-acting synthetic opioid that has proved useful in painful procedures. It is usually administered intravenously at doses of 25 to 50 μg, usually in conjunction with a benzodiazepine such as midazolam. In general, the use of narcotics is limited to painful procedures in inpatients. Monitoring and resuscitation equipment should always be available. A narcotic antagonist, such as naloxone, should also be on hand. If needed, it should be titrated 0.04 to 0.12 mg over 1 to 3 minutes to achieve the desired effect (Lind and Mushlin, 1987). Also, it has a 30- to 45-minute duration of action, so that patients who have received longer-acting narcotics such as morphine or meperidine must be carefully monitored for recurrence of symptoms.

Anesthetics have an important role in the preparation of pediatric patients, severely retarded patients, or others unable to cooperate fully, and occasionally in patients undergoing painful interventional procedures. In all of these situations, a trained anesthesiologist should administer the necessary medications. As a general guideline, all radiologists involved in procedures should be trained in life-support techniques, should ensure that equipment is readily available and functional for emergency treatment, and should carefully weigh the risk–benefit ratio for each procedure in each patient.

References

AIMS Trial Study Group: Long-term effects of intravenous anistreplase in acute myocardial infarction: Final report of the AIMS study. Lancet 335:427, 1990.

Aruny, J.E., and Kandarpa, K.: Phlegmasia cerulea dolens, a complication after placement of a bird's nest vena cava filter. AJR 154:1105, 1990.

Bassand, J.P., Machecourt, J., Cassgnes, J., et al.: Multicenter trial of intravenous anisoylated plasminogen streptokinase activator complex (APSAC) in acute myocardial infarction: Effects on infarct size and left ventricular function. J. Am. Coll. Cardiol. 13:988, 1989.

Baverstock, K.F., Papworth, D., and Vennart, F.: Risks of radiation at low dose rates. Lancet 1:430, 1981.

Bettmann, M.A. Complications of angiography in the thorax. In Herman, P.G. (ed.): Iatrogenic Thoracic Complications. New York, Springer-Verlag, 1983, p. 175.

Bettmann, M.A.: Adverse events and contrast media: Scope of the problem. In Enge, I., and Edgren, J. (eds.): Patient Safety and Adverse Events in Contrast Medium Examinations. Amsterdam, Excerpta Medica, 1989, p. 1.

Bettmann, M.A.: Ionic versus nonionic contrast agents for intravenous use: Are all the answers in? Radiology 175:616, 1990.

Bettmann, M.A., Bourdillon, P.D., Barry, W.H., et al.: The effects of a standard vs. a new nonionic contrast agent for cardiac angiography in man. Radiology 153:583, 1984.

Bonnier, H.J., Visser, R.F., Klomps, H.C., et al.: Comparison of intravenous anisoylated plasminogen streptokinase activator complex and intracoronary streptokinase in acute myocardial infarction. Am. J. Cardiol. 62:25, 1988.

Bourdillon, P.D., Bettmann, M.A., McCracken, S., et al.: Effects of a new nonionic and a conventional contrast agent on coronary sinus ionized calcium and left ventricular hemodynamics in dogs. J. Am. Coll. Cardiol. 6:845, 1985.

Brezis, M., and Epstein, F.H.: A closer look at radiocontrast-induced nephropathy. N. Engl. J. Med. 320:179, 1989.

Caulfield, J.B., Zir, L., and Harthorne, J.W.: Blood calcium levels in the presence of arteriographic contrast material. Circulation 52:119, 1975.

Chuang, V.P., Wallace, S., Gianturco, C., and Soo, C.S.: Complications of coil embolization: Prevention and management. AJR 137:809, 1981.

Clowes, A.W., and Clowes, M.M.: Kinetics of cellular proliferation after arterial injury. IV. Heparin inhibits rat smooth muscle cell mitogenesis and migration. Circ. Res. 58:839, 1986.

Dorfman, G.S., Cronan, J.J., Paolella, L.P., et al.: Iatrogenic changes at the venotomy site after percutaneous placement of the Greenfield filter. Radiology 173:159, 1989.

Egbert, L.D., Battit, G.E., Turudorf, H., and Beecher, H.K.: The value of the pre-operative visit by an anesthetist. JAMA 185:553, 1963.

Ellis, S.G., Roubin, G.S., Wilentz, J., et al.: Results of a randomized trial of heparin versus aspirin for prevention of acute closure and restenosis after PTCA. (Abstract.) Circulation 76:IV-213, 1987.

Feldman, R.L., Jalowiec, D.A., Hill, J.A., and Lambert, C.R.: Contrast media-related complications during cardiac catheterization using Hexabrix or Renografin in high-risk patients. Am. J. Cardiol. 61:1334, 1988.

Fellmeth, B.D., Roberts, A.C., Bookstein, J.J., et al.: Postangiographic femoral artery injuries: Nonsurgical repair with US-guided compression. Radiology 178:677, 1991.

Forrest, W.H., Brown, C.R., and Brown, B.W.: Subjective responses to six common pre-operative medications. Anesthesiology 47:241, 1977.

Fuster, V., Stein, B., Cohen, M., and Chesebro, J.: Post-angioplasty occlusion and restenosis: Mechanism and prevention by pharmacological therapy. Highlights 4:1, 1989.

Gelfand, D.W.: Barium enemas, latex balloons and anaphylactic reactions. AJR 156:1, 1991.

Gibby, W.A.: MR Contrast agents: An overview. Radiol. Clin. North Am. 26:1047, 1988.

Gomes, A.S., Lois, J.F., Baker, J.D., et al.: Acute renal dysfunction in high-risk patients after angiography: Comparison of ionic and nonionic contrast media. Radiology 170:65, 1989.

Grollman, J.H., Jr., Liu, C.K., Astone, R.A., and Lurie, M.D.: Thromboembolic complications in coronary angiography associated with the use of nonionic contrast medium. Cathet. Cardiovasc. Diagn. 14:159, 1988.

Gurevich, V.: Importance of fibrin specificity in therapeutic thrombolysis and the rational of using sequential and synergistic combinations of tissue plasminogen activator and pro-urokinase. Semin. Thromb. Hemost. 15:123, 1989.

Habr-Gama, A., and Waye, J.D.: Complications and hazards of gastrointestinal endoscopy. World J. Surg. 13:193, 1989.

Hessel, S.J., Adams, D.F., and Abrams, H.L.: Complications of angiography. Radiology 138:273, 1981.

Hirsh, J., van Aken, W.G., Gallus, A.S., et al.: Heparin kinetics in venous thrombosis and pulmonary embolism. Circulation 315:957, 1976.

Hlatky, M.A., Morris, K.G., Peiper, K.S., et al.: Randomized comparison of the cost and effectiveness of iopamidol and diatrizoate as contrast agents for cardiac angiography. J. Am. Coll. Cardiol. 16:871, 1990.

Katayama, H., Yamaguchi, K., Kozuka, T., et al.: Adverse reactions to ionic and nonionic contrast media: A report from the Japanese Committee on the Safety of Contrast Media. Radiology 175:621, 1990.

Kendel, F.A., Fraker, D.L., and Haynes, H.A.: Necrotizing vasculitis from radiographic contrast media. J. Am. Acad. Dermatol. 10:25, 1984.

Kopko, P.M., Smith, D.C., and Bull, B.S.: Thrombin generation in nonclottable mixtures of blood and nonionic contrast agents. Radiology 174:459, 1990.

Land, C.E., Boire, J.D., Jr., Shore, R.E., et al.: Breast cancer risk from low dose exposures to ionizing radiation: results of parallel analysis of three exposed populations of women. J. Natl. Cancer Inst. 65:353, 1980.

Lasser, E.C., Berry, C.C., Talner, L.B., et al.: Pretreatment with corticosteroids to alleviate reactions to intravenous contrast material. N. Engl. J. Med. 317:845, 1987.

Leach, K.R., Kurism, Y., Carlson, J.E., et al.: Thrombogenicity of hydrophilically coated guide wires and catheters. Radiology 175:675, 1990.

Lind, L.J., and Mushlin, P.S.: Sedation, analgesia, and anesthesia for radiologic procedures. Cardiovasc. Intervent. Radiol. 10:247, 1987.

Mani, R.L., Eisenberg, R.L., McDonald, E.J., Jr., et al.: Complications of catheter cerebral arteriography: Analysis of 5000 procedures. I. Criteria and incidence. AJR 131:861, 1978.

McNamara, T.O., and Fischer, J.R.: Thrombolysis of peripheral arterial and graft occlusions: Improved results using high-dose urokinase. AJR 144:769, 1985.

Mewissen, M.W., Erickson, S.J., Foley, W.D., et al.: Thrombosis at venous insertion sites after inferior vena caval filter placement. Radiology 173:155, 1989.

Miller, A.B., Howe, G.R., Sherman, G.J., et al.: Mortality from breast cancer after irradiation during fluoroscopic examinations in patients being treated for tuberculosis. N. Engl. J. Med. 321:1285, 1989.

Miller, D.L., Chang, R., Wells, W.T., et al.: Intravenous contrast media: Effect of dose on renal function. Radiology 167:607, 1988.

Morgan, D.M.L., Bettmann, M.A., and Gordon, J.L.: Effects of x-ray contrast media and radiation on human vascular endothelial cells in vitro. Cardiovasc. Intervent. Radiol. 12:154, 1989.

NCRP Report No. 100.: Exposure of the U.S. Population From Diagnostic Medical Radiation. National Council on Radiation Protection and Measurement, Bethesda, MD, 1989.

Parfrey, P.S., Griffiths, S.M., Barrett, B.J., et al.: Contrast material–induced renal failure in patients with diabetes mellitus, renal insufficiency or both: A prospective controlled study. N. Engl. J. Med. 320:143, 1989.

Podrid, P.J.: Role of higher nervous activity in ventricular arrhythmia and sudden cardiac death: Implications for alternative antiarrhythmic therapy. Ann. NY Acad. Sci. 432:296, 1985.

Powe, N.R., Steinberg, E.P., Erickson, J.E., et al.: Contrast-medium induced adverse reactions: Economic outcome. Radiology 169:163, 1988.

Reagan, K., Bettmann, M.A., Finkelstein, J., et al.: Double-blind study of a new nonionic contrast agent for cardiac angiography. Radiology 167:409, 1988.

Relman, A.S.: Aspirin for the primary prevention of myocardial infarction. N. Engl. J. Med. 318:245, 1988.

Reves, J.G., Fragen, R.J., Vinik, H.R., and Greenblatt, D.J.: Midazolam: Pharmacology and uses. Anesthesiology 62:310, 1985.

Rosenberg, R.D., and Lam, L.: Correlation between structure and function of heparin. Proc. Natl. Acad. Sci. USA 76:1218, 1979.

Samuels, M.A.: Neurogenic heart disease: A unifying hypothesis. Am. J. Cardiol. 60:15J, 1987.

Schwab, S.J., Hlatky, M.A., Pieper, K.S., et al.: Contrast nephrotoxicity: A randomized controlled trial of a nonionic and an ionic radiographic contrast agent. N. Engl. J. Med. 320:149, 1989.

Schwarz, L., Bourassa, M.A., Lesperance, J., et al.: Aspirin and dipyridamole in the prevention of restenosis after PTCA. N. Engl. J. Med. 318:1714, 1988.

Stormorken, H.: Effects of contrast media on the hemostatic and thrombotic mechanisms. Invest. Radiol. 23(Suppl. 2):S318, 1988.

Turpie, A.G., Levine, M.N., Hirsh, J., et al.: A randomized controlled trial of a low-molecular-weight heparin (enoxaparin) to prevent deep-vein thrombosis in patients undergoing elective hip surgery. N. Engl. J. Med. 315:925, 1986.

Upton, A.C.: Radiological effects of low doses: Implications for radiological protection. Radiat. Res. 71:51, 1977.

van Breda, A., Katzen, B.T., and Deutsch, A.S.: Urokinase versus streptokinase in local thrombolysis. Radiology 165:109, 1987.

vanSonnenberg, E., Neff, C.C., and Pfister, R.C.: Life-threatening hypotensive reactions to contrast media administration: Comparison of pharmacologic and fluid therapy. Radiology 162:15, 1987.

Vane, J., Jr., Angard, E.E., and Botting, R.M.: Regulatory functions of the vascular endothelium. N. Engl. J. Med. 323:27, 1990.

Wagner, L.K.: Absorbed dose in imaging: Why measure it? Radiology 178:622, 1991.

INDEX

Note: Page numbers in *italics* refer to illustrations;
page numbers followed by t refer to tables.

485